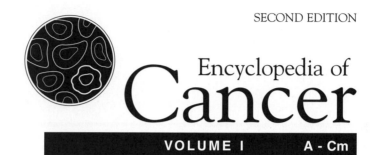

SECOND EDITION

Encyclopedia of
Cancer

VOLUME I   **A - Cm**

SECOND EDITION

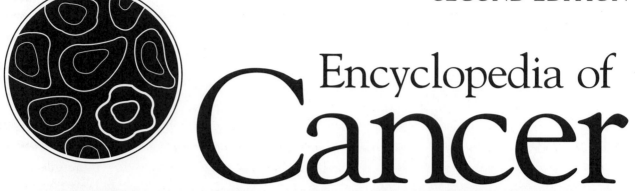

Encyclopedia of
Cancer

VOLUME I **A - Cm**

Editor-in-Chief

Joseph R. Bertino

The Cancer Institute of New Jersey
Robert Wood Johnson Medical School
New Brunswick, New Jersey

ACADEMIC PRESS

An imprint of Elsevier Science

Amsterdam   Boston   London   New York   Oxford   Paris   San Diego   San Francisco   Singapore   Sydney   Tokyo

Copyright © 2002, 1997, Elsevier Science (USA).

Academic Press
An imprint of Elsevier Science
525 B Street, Suite 1900, San Diego, California 92101-4495, USA
http://www.academicpress.com

Academic Press
84 Theobalds Road, London WC1X 8RR, UK
http://www.academicpress.com

Library of Congress Catalog Card Number: 2002102352

International Standard Book Number: 0-12-227555-1 (set)
International Standard Book Number: 0-12-227556-X (Volume 1)
International Standard Book Number: 0-12-227557-8 (Volume 2)
International Standard Book Number: 0-12-227558-6 (Volume 3)
International Standard Book Number: 0-12-227559-4 (Volume 4)

PRINTED IN THE UNITED STATES OF AMERICA
02   03   04   05   06   07   MM   9   8   7   6   5   4   3   2   1

Contents

B

C

VOLUME II

D

I

J

K

VOLUME III

L

M

VOLUME IV

R

Contents by Subject Area

VIRAL CARCINOGENESIS

Contributors

Sanjiv S. Agarwala
University of Pittsburgh Cancer Institute
Melanoma: Epidemiology

Siamak Agha-Mohammadi
University of Pittsburgh
Cytokine Gene Therapy

Jaffer A. Ajani
University of Texas M. D. Anderson Cancer
Center
Gastric Cancer: Epidemiology and Therapy

Anthony P. Albino
The American Health Foundation
Multistage Carcinogenesis

Jeffry R. Alger
University of California, Los Angeles Medical
Center
Brain Cancer and Magnetic Resonance Spectroscopy

Robert Amato
Baylor College of Medicine
Testicular Cancer

Howard Amols
Memorial Sloan-Kettering Cancer Center
*Dosimetry and Treatment Planning for
Three-Dimensional Radiation Therapy*

Darrell E. Anderson
Scientific Consulting Group, Inc., Gaithersburg,
Maryland
*Cancer Risk Reduction (Diet/Smoking
Cessation/Lifestyle Changes)*

Cristina R. Antonescu
Memorial Sloan-Kettering Cancer Center
TLS-CHOP in Myxoid Liposarcoma

Wadih Arap
University of Texas M. D. Anderson Cancer Center
Vascular Targeting

Ralph B. Arlinghaus
University of Texas M. D. Anderson Cancer
Center
BCR/ABL

Georg Aue
University of Pennsylvania School of Medicine
Antisense Nucleic Acids: Clinical Applications

Nicholas R. Bachur
University of Maryland Cancer Center
Anthracyclines

Richard Barakat
Memorial Sloan-Kettering Cancer Center
Endometrial Cancer

Fred G. Barker II
Massachusetts General Hospital
*Brain Tumors: Epidemiology and Molecular and
    Cellular Abnormalities*

Frederic G. Barr
University of Pennsylvania School of Medicine
*PAX3–FKHR and PAX7–FKHR Gene Fusions in
    Alveolar Rhabdomyosarcoma*

Michael T. Barrett
Fred Hutchinson Cancer Research Center
*Esophageal Cancer: Risk Factors and
    Somatic Genetics*

P. Leif Bergsagel
Weill Medical College of Cornell University
Multiple Myeloma

Leslie Bernstein
University of Southern California Keck School of
    Medicine
*Non-Hodgkin's Lymphoma and Multiple Myeloma:
    Incidence and Risk Factors*

Sandra H. Bigner
Duke University Medical Center
Genetic Alterations in Brain Tumors

R. Michael Blaese
ValiGen, Inc., Newtown, Pennsylvania
Suicide Genes

Eda T. Bloom
U.S. Food and Drug Administration
Gene Therapy Vectors, Safety Considerations

Clara D. Bloomfield
Roswell Park Cancer Institute
Chromosome Aberrations

Peter Blume-Jensen
Serono Reproductive Biology Institute
Kinase-Regulated Signal Transduction Pathways
*Signal Transduction Mechanisms Initiated by Receptor
    Tyrosine Kinases*

Paolo Boffetta
International Agency for Research on Cancer,
    Lyon, France
Lung, Larynx, Oral Cavity, and Pharynx

Melissa Bondy
University of Texas M. D. Anderson Cancer
    Center
Brain and Central Nervous System Cancer

David Boothman
University of Wisconsin–Madison
Radiation Resistance

Ernest C. Borden
Taussig Cancer Center
*Interferons: Cellular and Molecular Biology of
    Their Actions*

George J. Bosl
Memorial Sloan-Kettering Cancer Center
Germ Cell Tumors

Marc E. Bracke
Ghent University Hospital
Molecular Mechanisms of Cancer Invasion

Patrick J. Brennan
University of Pennsylvania School of Medicine
Her2/neu

Ricardo R. Brentani
Ludwig Institute for Cancer Research,
    Sao Paulo
Cell–Matrix Interactions

Norman E. Breslow
University of Washington, Seattle
Wilms Tumor: Epidemiology

Ronald Breslow
Columbia University
*Differentiation and the Role of Differentiation
    Inducers in Cancer Treatment*

Jacqueline F. Bromberg
Memorial Sloan-Kettering Cancer Center
STAT Proteins in Growth Control

Steven J. Burakoff
Dana-Farber Cancer Institute
T Cells and Their Effector Functions

Barbara Burtness
Yale Univesity School of Medicine
Head and Neck Cancer

Anna Butturini
Children's Hospital of Los Angeles
BCR/ABL

Blake Cady
Brown University School of Medicine
Endocrine Tumors

José Campione-Piccardo
National Laboratory for Viral Oncology, Canada
Viral Agents

Judith Campisi
Lawrence Berkeley National Laboratory
Senescence, Cellular

Eli Canaani
Kimmel Cancer Center
ALL-1

France Carrier
University of Maryland
Ataxia Telangiectasia Syndrome

JoAnn C. Castelli
University of California, San Francisco
HIV (Human Immunodeficiency Virus)

Webster K. Cavenee
University of California, San Diego
PTEN

R. S. K. Chaganti
Memorial Sloan-Kettering Cancer Center
Germ Cell Tumors

Roger Chammas
Ludwig Institute for Cancer Research,
Sao Paulo
Cell–Matrix Interactions

Paul B. Chapman
Memorial Sloan-Kettering Cancer Center
Anti-idiotypic Antibody Vaccines

Irvin S. Y. Chen
University of California, Los Angeles School of
Medicine
Human T-Cell Leukemia/Lymphotropic Virus

Seng H. Cheng
Genzyme Corporation, Framingham,
Massachusetts
Cationic Lipid-Mediated Gene Therapy

David A. Cheresh
The Scripps Research Institute
Integrin-Targeted Angiostatics

Rajas Chodankar
University of Southern California Keck School
of Medicine
Ovarian Cancer: Molecular and Cellular Abnormalities

Ting-Chao Chou
Memorial Sloan-Kettering Cancer Center
Chemotherapy: Synergism and Antagonism

Edward Chu
Yale University School of Medicine
*Resistance to Inhibitor Compounds of
Thymidylate Synthase*

John A. Cidlowski
National Institute of Environmental Health Sciences
Corticosteroids

Lena Claesson-Welsh
Uppsala University
*Anti-Vascular Endothelial Growth
Factor-Based Angiostatics*

Bayard Clarkson
Memorial Sloan-Kettering Cancer Center
*Chronic Myelogenous Leukemia: Etiology, Incidence,
and Clincal Features*
*Chronic Myelogenous Leukemia: Prognosis and
Current Status of Treatment*

Jack S. Cohen
The Hebrew University
*Magnetic Resonance Spectroscopy and Magnetic
Resonance Imaging, Introduction*

Peter Cole
Cancer Institute of New Jersey
Folate Antagonists

Susan P. C. Cole
Queen's University, Canada
Multidrug Resistance II: MRP and Related Proteins

Jerry M. Collins
U.S. Food and Drug Administration
PET Imaging and Cancer

O. Michael Colvin
Duke University
Akylating Agents

Raymond L. Comenzo
Memorial Sloan-Kettering Cancer Center
Stem Cell Transplantation

Abigail A. Conley
The Mayo Clinic
*Pancreatic Cancer: Cellular and
Molecular Mechanisms*

Louis Constine
University of Rochester Medical Center
Late Effects of Radiation Therapy

Leslie C. Costello
University of Maryland, Baltimore
*Metabolic Diagnosis of Prostate Cancer by Magnetic
Resonance Spectroscopy*

Wendy Cozen
University of Southern California Keck School of
Medicine
*Non-Hodgkin's Lymphoma and Multiple Myeloma:
Incidence and Risk Factors*

Carlo M. Croce
Kimmel Cancer Center
ALL-1

Stanley T. Crooke
Isis Pharmaceuticals, Inc.
*Antisense: Progress toward Gene-Directed
Cancer Therapy*

Lloyd A. Culp
Case Western Reserve University School
    of Medicine
Extracellular Matrix and Matrix Receptors:
    Alterations during Tumor Progression

Thomas J. Cummings
Duke University Medical Center
Genetic Alterations in Brain Tumors

David T. Curiel
University of Alabama at Birmingham
Targeted Vectors for Cancer Gene Therapy

Tom Curran
St. Jude Children's Research Hospital
fos Oncogene

George Q. Daley
Whitehead Institute
Cytokines: Hematopoietic Growth Factors

Chi V. Dang
The Johns Hopkins University School of
    Medicine
c-myc Protooncogene

James E. Darnell, Jr.
Rockefeller University
STAT Proteins in Growth Control

Michael David
University of California, San Diego
Jak/STAT Pathway

Roger G. Deeley
Queen's University, Canada
Multidrug Resistance II: MRP and
    Related Proteins

Samuel R. Denmeade
Johns Hopkins University School of Medicine
Hormone Resistance in Prostate Cancer

Christopher T. Denny
University of California, Los Angeles School
    of Medicine
EWS/ETS Fusion Genes

Channing J. Der
University of North Carolina at Chapel Hill
Ras Proteins

Mark W. Dewhirst
Duke University Medical Center
Hyperthermia

Frederick A. Dick
Massachusetts General Hospital Cancer Center
Retinoblastoma Tumor Suppressor Gene

John P. Dileo
University of Pittsburgh
Liposome-Mediated Gene Therapy

Eugene P. DiMagno
The Mayo Clinic
Pancreatic Cancer: Cellular and Molecular Mechanisms

Clark W. Distelhorst
Case Western Reserve University
Steroid Hormones and Hormone Receptors

Ethan Dmitrovsky
Dartmouth Medical School
Chemoprevention, Pharmacology of

M. Eileen Dolan
University of Chicago
Resistance to DNA-Damaging Agents

Alessia Donadio
Memorial Sloan-Kettering Cancer Center
Germ Cell Tumors

Zhongyun Dong
University of Texas M. D. Anderson Cancer
    Center
Macrophages

Harold O. Douglass, Jr.
Roswell Park Cancer Institute
Pancreas and Periampullary Tumors

Louis Dubeau
University of Southern California Keck School
    of Medicine
Ovarian Cancer: Molecular and
    Cellular Abnormalities

Anita K. Dunbier
University of Otago
Gastric Cancer: Inherited Predisposition

Nicholas J. Dyson
Massachusetts General Hospital Cancer Center
Retinoblastoma Tumor Suppressor Gene

Timothy J. Eberlein
Washington University School of Medicine,
    St. Louis
T Cells against Tumors

Randa El-Zein
University of Texas M. D. Anderson Cancer
    Center
Brain and Central Nervous System Cancer

Elaine A. Elion
Harvard Medical School
MAP Kinase Modules in Signaling

Volker Ellenreider
The Mayo Clinic
Pancreatic Cancer: Cellular and Molecular Mechanisms

Paul F. Engstrom
Fox Chase Cancer Center
Hepatocellular Carcinoma (HCC)

Zelig Eshhar
Weizmann Institute of Science
Antibodies in the Gene Therapy of Cancer

Conrad B. Falkson
McMaster University
Malignant Mesothelioma

Geoffrey Falkson
University of Pretoria
Malignant Mesothelioma

Gerold Feuer
State University of New York Upstate
Medical University
Human T-Cell Leukemia/Lymphotropic Virus

Isaiah J. Fidler
University of Texas M. D. Anderson Cancer
Center
Macrophages

Mary E. Fidler
The Mayo Foundation
Renal Cell Cancer

Richard Fishel
Thomas Jefferson University
Hereditary Colon Cancer and DNA Mismatch Repair

David FitzGerald
National Cancer Institute
Antibody–Toxin and Growth Factor–Toxin Fusion Proteins

Albert J. Fornace Jr.
National Cancer Institute
Ataxia Telangiectasia Syndrome

Ruben C. Fragoso
Dana-Farber Cancer Institute
T Cells and Their Effector Functions

Thomas S. Frank
Myriad Genetic Laboratories, Salt Lake City
Hereditary Risk of Breast and Ovarian Cancer: BRCA1 and BRCA2

R. B. Franklin
University of Maryland, Baltimore
Metabolic Diagnosis of Prostate Cancer by Magnetic Resonance Spectroscopy

Eric O. Freed
National Institute of Allergy and Infectious Diseases
Retroviruses

Michael L. Freeman
Vanderbilt University School of Medicine
Hyperthermia

Krystyna Frenkel
New York University School of Medicine
Carcinogenesis: Role of Active Oxygen and Nitrogen Species

Frank B. Furnari
University of California, San Diego
PTEN

Robert Peter Gale
Center for Advanced Studies in Leukemia, Los Angeles
BCR/ABL

Susan Gapstur
Arizona Cancer Center and Southern Arizona VA Health Care System
Nutritional Supplements and Diet as Chemoprevention Agents

Lawrence B. Gardner
The Johns Hopkins University School of Medicine
c-myc Protooncogene

Harinder Garewal
Arizona Cancer Center and Southern Arizona VA Health Care System
Nutritional Supplements and Diet as Chemoprevention Agents

James E. Gervasoni, Jr.
Robert Wood Johnson Medical School
Endocrine Tumors

Pär Gerwins
Uppsala University
Anti-Vascular Endothelial Growth Factor-Based Angiostatics

Alan M. Gewirtz
University of Pennsylvania School of Medicine
Antisense Nucleic Acids: Clinical Applications

John F. Gibbs
Roswell Park Cancer Institute
Pancreas and Periampullary Tumors

Anna Giuliano
Arizona Cancer Center and Southern Arizona
VA Health Care System
*Nutritional Supplements and Diet as
Chemoprevention Agents*

R. A. Gjerset
Sidney Kimmel Cancer Center
p53 Gene Therapy

Peter S. Goedegebuure
Washington University School of Medicine,
St. Louis
T Cells against Tumors

Jason S. Gold
Memorial Sloan-Kettering Cancer Center
Cell-Mediated Immunity to Cancer

Ashwin Gollerkeri
Yale University School of Medicine
*Resistance to Inhibitor Compounds of
Thymidylate Synthase*

Jesús Gómez-Navarro
University of Alabama at Birmingham
Targeted Vectors for Cancer Gene Therapy

Ellen L. Goode
University of Washington
Genetic Predisposition to Prostate Cancer

Richard Gorlick
Memorial Sloan-Kettering Cancer Center
Bone Tumors

Kathleen Heppner Goss
University of Cincinnati College of Medicine
*APC (Adenomatous Polyposis Coli) Tumor
Suppressor*

Michael M. Gottesman
National Cancer Institute
Multidrug Resistance I: P-Glycoprotein

Joseph P. Grande
The Mayo Foundation
*Kidney, Epidemiology
Renal Cell Cancer*

Ellen Graver
Arizona Cancer Center and Southern Arizona
VA Health Care System
*Nutritional Supplements and Diet as
Chemoprevention Agents*

F. Anthony Greco
Sarah Cannon–Minnie Pearl Cancer Center
Neoplasms of Unknown Primary Site

Mark I. Greene
University of Pennsylvania
School of Medicine
Her2/neu

Peter Greenwald
National Cancer Institute
*Cancer Risk Reduction (Diet/Smoking
Cessation/Lifestyle Changes)*

John R. Griffiths
St. George's Hospital Medical School, London
*Magnetic Resonance Spectroscopy of Cancer: Clinical
Overview*

Joanna Groden
University of Cincinnati College of Medicine
*APC (Adenomatous Polyposis Coli)
Tumor Suppressor*

Jun-Lin Guan
Cornell University College of
Veterinary Medicine
Integrin Receptor Signaling Pathways

Udayan Guha
Albert Einstein Cancer Center
Transgenic Mice in Cancer Research

Parry J. Guilford
University of Otago
Gastric Cancer: Inherited Predisposition

Anjali Gupta
University of Pennsylvania Hospital
Molecular Aspects of Radiation Biology

John D. Hainsworth
Sarah Cannon–Minnie Pearl Cancer Center
Neoplasms of Unknown Primary Site

Joshua W. Hamilton
Dartmouth Medical School
Chemical Mutagenesis and Carcinogenesis

Joyce L. Hamlin
University of Virginia School of Medicine
Drug Resistance: DNA Sequence Amplification

Kenneth R. Hande
Vanderbilt University School of Medicine
Purine Antimetabolites

J. Marie Hardwick
Johns Hopkins School of Public Health
Caspases in Programmed Cell Death

Louis B. Harrison
Beth Israel Medical Center
Brachytherapy

Lynda K. Hawkins
Genetic Therapy Institute, Gaithersburg, Maryland
Replication-Selective Viruses for Cancer Treatment

Lifeng He
Albert Einstein College of Medicine
Taxol and Other Molecules That Interact with Microtubules

Stephen S. Hecht
University of Minnesota Cancer Center
Tobacco Carcinogenesis

Ingegerd Hellström
Pacific Northwest Research Institute
Tumor Antigens

Karl Erik Hellström
Pacific Northwest Research Institute
Tumor Antigens

Kurt J. Henle
University of Arkansas for Medical Sciences
Hyperthermia

Meenhard Herlyn
The Wistar Institute
Melanoma: Biology

Masao Hirose
Nagoya City University Medical School
Antioxidants: Carcinogenic and Chemopreventive Properties

Dah H. Ho
University of Texas M. D. Anderson Cancer Center
L-Asparaginase

Samuel B. Ho
University of Minnesota Medical School
Glycoproteins and Glycosylation Changes in Cancer

F. Stephen Hodi
Dana-Farber Cancer Institute
Interleukins

Kyle Holen
Memorial Sloan-Kettering Cancer Center
Colorectal Cancer: Epidemiology and Treatment

Julianne L. Holleran
Case Western Reserve University School of Medicine
Extracellular Matrix and Matrix Receptors: Alterations during Tumor Progression

Waun Ki Hong
University of Texas M. D. Anderson Cancer Center
Chemoprevention Trials

Susan Band Horwitz
Albert Einstein College of Medicine
Taxol and Other Molecules That Interact with Microtubules

Alan N. Houghton
Memorial Sloan-Kettering Cancer Center
Cell-Mediated Immunity to Cancer
DNA-Based Cancer Vaccines

Jane Houldsworth
Memorial Sloan-Kettering Cancer Center
Germ Cell Tumors

Franklyn A. Howe
St. George's Hospital Medical School, London
Magnetic Resonance Spectroscopy of Cancer: Clinical Overview

H.-J. Su Huang
University of California, San Diego
PTEN

Leaf Huang
University of Pittsburgh
Liposome-Mediated Gene Therapy

James Hulit
Albert Einstein Cancer Center
Transgenic Mice in Cancer Research

Tony Hunter
The Salk Institute
Kinase-Regulated Signal Transduction Pathways
Signal Transduction Mechanisms Initiated by Receptor Tyrosine Kinases

Mark D. Hurwitz
Harvard Medical School
Bladder Cancer: Assessment and Management

David H. Ilson
Memorial Sloan-Kettering Cancer Center
Esophageal Cancer: Treatment

Katsumi Imaida
Nagoya City University Medical School
Antioxidants: Carcinogenic and Chemopreventive Properties

Harry L. Ioachim
Lenox Hill Hospital
Immune Deficiency: Opportunistic Tumors

John T. Isaacs
Johns Hopkins University School of Medicine
Hormone Resistance in Prostate Cancer
Mark A. Israel
University of California, San Francisco
Brain Tumors: Epidemiology and Molecular and Cellular Abnormalities
Nobuyuki Ito
Nagoya City University Medical School
Antioxidants: Carcinogenic and Chemopreventive Properties
Helen A. James
University of East Anglia
Ribozymes and Their Applications
Gail P. Jarvik
University of Washington Medical Center
Genetic Predisposition to Prostate Cancer
Alan M. Jeffrey
Columbia University
Carcinogen–DNA Adducts
D. Joseph Jerry
University of Massachusetts, Amherst
TP53 Tumor Suppressor Gene: Structure and Function
Eric Johannsen
Harvard Medical School
Epstein–Barr Virus and Associated Malignancies
Ricky W. Johnstone
Peter MacCallum Cancer Institute, East Melbourne
P-Glycoprotein as a General Antiapoptotic Protein
Wilms Tumor Suppressor WT1
Douglas J. Jolly
Chiron Viagene, Inc., San Diego, California
Retroviral Vectors
Peter A. Jones
University of Southern California
DNA Methylation and Cancer
V. Craig Jordan
Northwestern University Medical School
Estrogens and Antiestrogens
Ellen D. Jorgensen
The American Health Foundation
Multistage Carcinogenesis
Jacqueline Jouanneau
Institut Curie
Tumor Cell Motility and Invasion

Raymond Judware
Case Western Reserve University School of Medicine
Extracellular Matrix and Matrix Receptors: Alterations during Tumor Progression
Joseph G. Jurcic
Memorial Sloan-Kettering Cancer Center
Monoclonal Antibodies: Leukemia and Lymphoma
Joanna Kaczynski
The Mayo Clinic
Pancreatic Cancer: Cellular and Molecular Mechanisms
William G. Kaelin, Jr.
Harvard Medical School
von Hippel–Lindau Disease
Dhananjaya V. Kalvakolanu
Greenebaum Cancer Center
Interferons: Cellular and Molecular Biology of Their Actions
Barton A. Kamen
Cancer Institute of New Jersey
Folate Antagonists
Mark P. Kamps
University of California, San Diego School of Medicine
Differentiation and Cancer: Basic Research
Gary D. Kao
University of Pennsylvania Hospital
Molecular Aspects of Radiation Biology
Johanne M. Kaplan
Genzyme Corporation, Framingham, Massachusetts
Cationic Lipid-Mediated Gene Therapy
Emmanuel Katsanis
University of Arizona
Neuroblastoma
Frederic J. Kaye
National Cancer Institute
Lung Cancer: Molecular and Cellular Abnormalities
Michael J. Keating
University of Texas M. D. Anderson Cancer Center
Chronic Lymphocytic Leukemia
David Kelsen
Cornell University Medical College
Esophageal Cancer: Treatment

Nancy Kemeny
Memorial Sloan-Kettering Cancer Center
Colorectal Cancer: Epidemiology and Treatment

Fadlo R. Khuri
University of Texas M. D. Anderson Cancer
Center
Chemoprevention Trials

Se Won Ki
University of California, San Diego
Cellular Responses to DNA Damage

Edward S. Kim
University of Texas M. D. Anderson Cancer
Center
Chemoprevention Trials

Young S. Kim
University of California, San Francisco
*Glycoproteins and Glycosylation Changes
in Cancer*

Sol Kimel
Sheba Medical Center, Israel
*Photodynamic Therapy: Basic Principles and
Applications to Skin Cancer*

Timothy Kinsella
University of Wisconsin–Madison
Radiation Resistance

John M. Kirkwood
University of Pittsburgh Cancer Institute
Melanoma: Epidemiology

David Kirn
Kirn Biopharmaceutical Consulting
*Replication-Selective Viruses for
Cancer Treatment*

Jan Kitajewski
Columbia University
Wnt Signaling

George Klein
Karolinska Institute
Tumor Suppressor Genes: Specific Classes

Priit Kogerman
Case Western Reserve University School
of Medicine
*Extracellular Matrix and Matrix Receptors:
Alterations during Tumor Progression*

Richard D. Kolodner
Ludwig Institute for Cancer Research
*Mismatch Repair: Biochemistry
and Genetics*

Genady Kostenich
Sheba Medical Center, Israel
*Photodynamic Therapy: Basic Principles and
Applications to Skin Cancer*

Robert J. Kreitman
National Cancer Institute
*Antibody–Toxin and Growth Factor–Toxin
Fusion Proteins*

J. Kurhanewicz
University of California, San Francisco
*Metabolic Diagnosis of Prostate Cancer by Magnetic
Resonance Spectroscopy*

Alexander E. Kuta
U.S. Food and Drug Administration
Gene Therapy Vectors, Safety Considerations

Mark Ladanyi
Memorial Sloan-Kettering Cancer Center
TLS-CHOP in Myxoid Liposarcoma

Michael M. C. Lai
University of Southern California Keck School
of Medicine
Hepatitis C Virus (HCV)

Wayne D. Lancaster
Wayne State University School of Medicine
Viral Agents

Jean-Baptiste Latouche
Memorial Sloan-Kettering Cancer Center
*Cancer Vaccines: Gene Therapy and Dendritic
Cell-Based Vaccines*

John S. Lazo
University of Pittsburgh
Bleomycin

Derek Le Roith
National Institutes of Health
Insulin-like Growth Factors

Jane S. Lebkowski
Applied Immune Sciences, Inc.,
Santa Clara, California
*Adeno-Associated Virus: A Vector for
High-Efficiency Gene Transduction*

Linda A. Lee
The Johns Hopkins University School
of Medicine
c-myc Protooncogene

Loïc Le Marchand
Cancer Research Center of Hawaii
Lung, Larynx, Oral Cavity, and Pharynx

Alexandra M. Levine
University of Southern California Keck School
of Medicine
*Neoplasms in Acquired
Immunodeficiency Syndrome*

Alexander Levitzki
The Hebrew University of Jerusalem
Protein Kinase Inhibitors

Jay A. Levy
University of California, San Francisco
HIV (Human Immunodeficiency Virus)

Runzhao Li
Medical University of South Carolina
ETS Family of Transcription Factors

Nicole T. Liberati
Duke University Medical Center
TGFβ Signaling Mechanisms

David C. Linehan
Washington University School of Medicine,
St. Louis
T Cells against Tumors

Stephen J. Lippard
Massachusetts Institute of Technology
Cisplatin and Related Drugs

Philip O. Livingston
Memorial Sloan-Kettering Cancer Center
Carbohydrate-Based Vaccines

Jay S. Loeffler
Harvard Medical School
Proton Beam Radiation Therapy

W. Thomas London
Fox Chase Cancer Center
Liver Cancer: Etiology and Prevention

Dan L. Longo
National Institute on Aging
Lymphoma, Non-Hodgkin's

Ti Li Loo
George Washington University Medical Center
L-Asparaginase

Michael T. Lotze
University of Pittsburgh
Cytokine Gene Therapy

Henry T. Lynch
Creighton University School of Medicine
*Colorectal Cancer: Molecular and
Cellular Abnormalities*

Wendy J. Mack
University of Southern California
Thyroid Cancer

Robert G. Maki
Memorial Sloan-Kettering Cancer Center
Sarcomas of Soft Tissue

David Malkin
University of Toronto School of Medicine
Li-Fraumeni Syndrome

Yael Mardor
Sheba Medical Center, Israel
*Magnetic Resonance Spectroscopy and Magnetic
Resonance Imaging, Introduction*

Marc M. Mareel
Ghent University Hospital
Molecular Mechanisms of Cancer Invasion

Paul A. Marks
Memorial Sloan-Kettering Cancer Center
*Differentiation and the Role of Differentiation
Inducers in Cancer Treatment*

Peter M. Mauch
Harvard Medical School
Lymphoma, Hodgkin's Disease

Harold M. Maurer
University of Nebraska Medical Center
Rhabdomyosarcoma, Early Onset

George Mavrothalassitis
University of Crete
ETS Family of Transcription Factors

William H. McBride
University of California, Los Angeles
Radiobiology, Principles of

Thomas S. McCormick
Case Western Reserve University
Steroid Hormones and Hormone Receptors

Charles J. McDonald
Brown University Medical School
Skin Cancer, Non-Melanoma

Sharon S. McDonald
Scientific Consulting Group, Inc.,
Gaithersburg, Maryland
*Cancer Risk Reduction (Diet/Smoking
Cessation/Lifestyle Changes)*

Clare H. McGowan
The Scripps Research Institute
Cell Cycle Checkpoints

Melissa S. McGrath
Memorial Sloan-Kettering Cancer Center
Resistance to Antibody Therapy

W. Gillies McKenna
University of Pennsylvania Hospital
Molecular Aspects of Radiation Biology

Paul M. J. McSheehy
St. George's Hospital Medical School, London
*Magnetic Resonance Spectroscopy of Cancer:
    Clinical Overview*

Peter W. Melera
University of Maryland School of Medicine
Resistance to Inhibitors of Dihydrofolate Reductase

Richard A. Messmann
National Cancer Institute
Targeted Toxins

Paul A. Meyers
Memorial Sloan-Kettering Cancer Center
Bone Tumors

Carson J. Miller
Case Western Reserve University School
    of Medicine
*Extracellular Matrix and Matrix Receptors:
    Alterations during Tumor Progression*

Amin Mirhadi
University of California, Los Angeles
Radiobiology, Principles of

Elizabeth Moran
Temple University School of Medicine
DNA Tumor Viruses: Adenovirus

Thomas Moritz
University of Essen Medical School
*Transfer of Drug Resistance Genes to
    Hematopoietic Precursors*

John C. Morris
National Cancer Institute
Suicide Genes

Krzysztof Mrózek
Roswell Park Cancer Institute
Chromosome Aberrations

Bijay Mukherji
University of Connecticut Health Center
Molecular Basis for Tumor Immunity

Annegret Müller
Thomas Jefferson University
*Hereditary Colon Cancer and DNA
    Mismatch Repair*

Karl Münger
Harvard Medical School
Papillomaviruses

Tatsuya Nakamura
Kimmel Cancer Center
ALL-1

Hector R. Nava
Roswell Park Cancer Institute
Pancreas and Periampullary Tumors

Andrea K. Ng
Harvard Medical School
Lymphoma, Hodgkin's Disease

Jac A. Nickoloff
University of New Mexico School of Medicine
*Recombination: Mechanisms and Roles
    in Tumorigenesis*

Garth L. Nicolson
Institute for Molecular Medicine
*Autocrine and Paracrine Growth Mechanisms in
    Cancer Progression and Metastasis*

John L. Nitiss
St. Jude Children's Research Hospital
Resistance to Topoisomerase-Targeting Agents

Karin C. Nitiss
St. Jude Children's Research Hospital
Resistance to Topoisomerase-Targeting Agents

Philip D. Noguchi
U.S. Food and Drug Administration
Gene Therapy Vectors, Safety Considerations

Shoichiro Ohta
University of California, San Francisco
*Brain Tumors: Epidemiology and Molecular and
    Cellular Abnormalities*

Arie Orenstein
Sheba Medical Center, Israel
*Photodynamic Therapy: Basic Principles and
    Applications to Skin Cancer*

George A. Orr
Albert Einstein College of Medicine
*Taxol and Other Molecules That Interact
    with Microtubules*

Keren Osman
Memorial Sloan-Kettering Cancer Center
Stem Cell Transplantation

Michelle A. Ozbun
University of New Mexico School of Medicine
*TP53 Tumor Suppressor Gene: Structure
    and Function*

Robert F. Ozols
Fox Chase Cancer Center
Ovarian Cancer: Epidemiology

Kevin W. Page
Applied Immune Sciences, Inc.,
Santa Clara, California
*Adeno-Associated Virus: A Vector for
High-Efficiency Gene Transduction*

Tej Krishan Pandita
Columbia University
Telomeres and Telomerase

Renata Pasqualini
University of Texas M. D. Anderson Cancer
Center
Vascular Targeting

Ira Pastan
National Cancer Institute
*Antibody–Toxin and Growth Factor–Toxin
Fusion Proteins*

Frederica P. Perera
Mailman School of Public Health at Columbia
University
Molecular Epidemiology and Cancer Risk

Richard G. Pestell
Albert Einstein Cancer Center
Transgenic Mice in Cancer Research

Anusch Peyman
Avetis Pharma Deutschland GmbH
Antisense: Medicinal Chemistry

Pieter Pil
Massachusetts Institute of Technology
Cisplatin and Related Drugs

Giuseppe Pizzorno
Yale University School of Medicine
Pyrimidine Antimetabolites

Miriam C. Poirier
National Cancer Institute
DNA Damage, DNA Repair, and Mutagenesis

Pamela M. Pollock
National Human Genome Research Institute
Melanoma: Molecular and Cellular Abnormalities

Randy Y. C. Poon
Hong Kong University of Science and Technology
Cell Cycle Control

Susan Preston-Martin
University of Southern California
Thyroid Cancer

Wendy Morse Pruitt
University of North Carolina at Chapel Hill
Ras Proteins

Amanda Psyrri
Yale University School of Medicine
Pyrimidine Antimetabolites

Harry Quon
Beth Israel Medical Center
Brachytherapy

Govindaswami Ragupathi
Memorial Sloan-Kettering Cancer Center
Carbohydrate-Based Vaccines

R. Beverly Raney
University of Texas M. D. Anderson Cancer
Center
Rhabdomyosarcoma, Early Onset

Ritesh Rathore
Boston University School of Medicine
Vinca Alkaloids and Epipodophyllotoxins

Bandaru S. Reddy
American Health Foundation
Animal Models for Colon Cancer Chemoprevention

E. Premkumar Reddy
Fels Institute for Cancer Research and Molecular
Biology
myb

John C. Reed
The Burnham Institute
*Bcl-2 Family Proteins and the Dysregulation of
Programmed Cell Death*

Heinz R. Reiske
Cornell University College of Veterinary Medicine
Integrin Receptor Signaling Pathways

Victoria Richon
Memorial Sloan-Kettering Cancer Center
*Differentiation and the Role of Differentiation
Inducers in Cancer Treatment*

Richard A. Rifkind
Memorial Sloan-Kettering Cancer Center
*Differentiation and the Role of Differentiation
Inducers in Cancer Treatment*

Gert Rijksen
University Hospital, Utrecht, The Netherlands
Pyruvate Kinases

Paul F. Robbins
National Cancer Institute
Cancer Vaccines: Peptide- and Protein-Based Vaccines

Leslie Robinson-Bostom
Brown University Medical School
Skin Cancer, Non-Melanoma

Sara Rockwell
Yale University School of Medicine
Hypoxia and Drug Resistance

Charles E. Rogler
Albert Einstein College of Medicine
Hepatitis B Viruses

Ronald K. Ross
University of Southern California/Norris
Comprehensive Cancer Center
Bladder Cancer: Epidemiology

Astrid A. Ruefli
Peter MacCallum Cancer Institute,
East Melbourne
P-Glycoprotein as a General Antiapoptotic Protein

N. Saadatmandi
Sidney Kimmel Cancer Center
p53 Gene Therapy

Michel Sadelain
Memorial Sloan-Kettering Cancer Center
*Cancer Vaccines: Gene Therapy and Dendritic
Cell-Based Vaccines*

Ajay Sandhu
Eastern Virginia Medical School
Late Effects of Radiation Therapy

Kapaettu Satyamoorthy
Manipal Academy of Higher Education, India
Melanoma: Biology

Edward A. Sausville
National Cancer Institute
Targeted Toxins

David A. Scheinberg
Memorial Sloan-Kettering Cancer Center
*Monoclonal Antibodies: Leukemia and Lymphoma
Resistance to Antibody Therapy*

Charles A. Schiffer
Barbara Ann Karmanos Cancer Institute
Acute Lymphoblastic Leukemia in Adults

Cornelius Schmaltz
Memorial Sloan-Kettering Cancer Center
Graft versus Leukemia and Graft versus Tumor Activity

John D. Schuetz
St. Jude Children's Research Hospital
*Genetic Basis for Quantitative and Qualitative
Changes in Drug Targets*

Nicholas T. Schulz
University of Pittsburgh School of Medicine
c-mos Protooncogene

Shelley Schwarzbaum
Weizmann Institute of Science
Antibodies in the Gene Therapy of Cancer

Andrew D. Seidman
Memorial Sloan-Kettering Cancer Center
Breast Cancer

Victor Sementchenko
Medical University of South Carolina
ETS Family of Transcription Factors

Arun Seth
University of Toronto
ETS Family of Transcription Factors

George Sgouros
Memorial Sloan-Kettering Cancer Center
Radiolabeled Antibodies, Overview

Brenda Shank
University of California, San Francisco
Total Body Irradiation

Navneet Sharda
University of Wisconsin–Madison
Radiation Resistance

Yang Shi
Harvard Medical School
Wilms Tumor Suppressor WT1

Kang Sup Shim
Thomas Jefferson University
*Hereditary Colon Cancer and DNA
Mismatch Repair*

James D. Shull
University of Nebraska Medical Center
Hormonal Carcinogenesis

William M. Siders
Genzyme Corporation, Framingham, Massachusetts
Cationic Lipid-Mediated Gene Therapy

Alfred R. Smith
Harvard Medical School
Proton Beam Radiation Therapy

Judy L. Smith
Roswell Park Cancer Institute
Pancreas and Periampullary Tumors

Thomas Smyrk
Creighton University School of Medicine
*Colorectal Cancer: Molecular and
Cellular Abnormalities*

Mark J. Smyth
Peter MacCallum Cancer Institute,
East Melbourne
P-Glycoprotein as a General Antiapoptotic Protein

Robert J. Soiffer
Dana-Farber Cancer Institute
Interleukins

Michael B. Sporn
Dartmouth Medical School
Chemoprevention, Pharmacology of

Gerard E. J. Staal
University Hospital, Utrecht, The Netherlands
Pyruvate Kinases

Patricia S. Steeg
National Cancer Institute
nm23 Metastasis Suppressor Gene

Peter G. Steinherz
Memorial Sloan-Kettering Cancer Center
Acute Lymphoblastic Leukemia in Children

M. I. Straub
Connecticut Veterans Administration
Medical Center
Carcinogen–DNA Adducts

Dwayne G. Stupack
The Scripps Research Institute
Integrin-Targeted Angiostatics

Michael Wei-Chih Su
Dana-Farber Cancer Institute
T Cells and Their Effector Functions

Hubert Szelényi
Weill Medical College of Cornell University
Multiple Myeloma

Chris H. Takimoto
University of Texas Health Science Center
Camptothecins

R. V. Tantravahi
Fels Institute for Cancer Research and Molecular
Biology
myb

Jean Paul Thiery
Institut Curie
Tumor Cell Motility and Invasion

Gian Paolo Tonini
National Institute for Cancer
Research, Genoa
Pediatric Cancers, Molecular Features

Timothy J. Triche
Keck School of Medicine at the University of
Southern California
Ewing's Sarcoma (Ewing's Family Tumors)

Donald L. Trump
University of Pittsburgh Medical Center
Prostate Cancer

Shigeki Tsuchida
Hirosaki University School of Medicine
Glutathione Transferases

Eugen Uhlmann
Aventis Pharma Deutschland GmbH
Antisense: Medicinal Chemistry

Raul Urrutia
The Mayo Clinic
*Pancreatic Cancer: Cellular and
Molecular Mechanisms*

Marcel R. M. van den Brink
Memorial Sloan-Kettering Cancer Center
*Graft versus Leukemia and Graft versus
Tumor Activity*

Catherine Van Poznak
Memorial Sloan-Kettering Cancer Center
Breast Cancer

Amelia M. Wall
St. Jude Children's Research Hospital
*Genetic Basis for Quantitative and Qualitative
Changes in Drug Targets*

Andrew D. Wallace
National Institute of Environmental Health Sciences
Corticosteroids

Fred Wang
Harvard Medical School
Epstein–Barr Virus and Associated Malignancies

Hwei-Gene Heidi Wang
Bristol Myers Squibb, Wallingford, Connecticut
DNA Tumor Viruses: Adenovirus

Jean Y. J. Wang
University of California, San Diego
Cellular Responses to DNA Damage

Xiao-Fan Wang
Duke University Medical Center
TGFβ Signaling Mechanisms

Carl F. Ware
La Jolla Institute for Allergy and Immunology
Tumor Necrosis Factors

Dennis K. Watson
Medical University of South Carolina
ETS Family of Transcription Factors

Pascal A. Oude Weernink
University Hospital, Utrecht,
The Netherlands
Pyruvate Kinases

Alan B. Weitberg
Boston University School of Medicine
Vinca Alkaloids and Epipodophyllotoxins

Haim Werner
Tel Aviv University, Israel
Insulin-like Growth Factors

Ainsley Weston
National Institute for Occupational Safety and
Health
DNA Damage, DNA Repair, and Mutagenesis

Luke Whitesell
University of Arizona
Neuroblastoma

Peter H. Wiernik
New York Medical College
Acute Myelocytic Leukemia

David W. Will
Avetis Pharma Deutschland GmbH
Antisense: Medicinal Chemistry

David A. Williams
Children's Hospital Medical Center
*Transfer of Drug Resistance Genes to
Hematopoietic Precursors*

Jacqueline Williams
University of Rochester Medical Center
Late Effects of Radiation Therapy

Brian C. Wilson
Ontario Cancer Institute
Photodynamic Therapy: Clinical Applications

D. R. Wilson
Introgen Therapeutics, Inc.
p53 Gene Therapy

Jedd D. Wolchok
Memorial Sloan-Kettering Cancer Center
DNA-Based Cancer Vaccines

Margaret Wrensch
University of California, San Francisco
Brain and Central Nervous System Cancer

Yue Xiong
University of North Carolina at Chapel Hill
p16 and ARF: Crossroads of Tumorigenesis

Yoshiya Yamada
Memorial Sloan-Kettering Cancer Center
Stereotactic Radiosurgery of Intracranial Neoplasms

Chin-Rang Yang
University of Wisconsin–Madison
Radiation Resistance

Wendell G. Yarbrough
University of North Carolina at Chapel Hill
p16 and ARF: Crossroads of Tumorigenesis

James W. Young
Memorial Sloan-Kettering Cancer Center
*Cancer Vaccines: Gene Therapy and Dendritic
Cell-Based Vaccines*

Mimi C. Yu
University of Southern California/Norris
Comprehensive Cancer Center
Bladder Cancer: Epidemiology

Brad Zerler
Locus Discovery Inc., Blue Bell,
Pennsylvania
DNA Tumor Viruses: Adenovirus

Dong-Er Zhang
The Scripps Research Institute
RUNX/CBF Transcription Factors

Foreword

Cancer, a most feared and morbid disease, is the second most common cause of mortality in the United States after cardiovascular disease. Clinical and research information with respect to cancer is expanding at an extraordinary rate. Keeping abreast of information relative to one's field, whether a clinician, researcher, student, or patient, is an increasing challenge. The *Encyclopedia of Cancer, Second Edition* organizes such information in a style that is highly effective and remarkably useful. The encyclopedia will be a source of great assistance to general practitioners, cancer specialists, and researchers and should be available in all institutional and private libraries. The editors and the contributors have been carefully selected for their outstanding credentials and should be congratulated for the excellence of the encyclopedia they produced.

Emil Frei
Director and Physician-in-Chief, Emeritus
Dana-Farber Cancer Institute
Professor of Medicine, Emeritus
Harvard Medical School

Preface

Since the last edition of the *Encyclopedia of Cancer*, there has been an amazing amount of new information published in the cancer research field. This second edition has attempted to capture these advances that have occurred in the etiology, prevention, and treatment of this disease. Accordingly, we have increased the coverage of topics, and the encyclopedia now requires four volumes instead of three volumes to accommodate the increase in articles.

Feedback about and reviews of the first edition have been positive, and this second edition builds on the format of the first edition. Our goal was to cover all aspects of cancer, from basic science to clinical application. A distinguished group of associate editors has provided topics to be covered, suggested authors for those topics, and reviewed the submitted manuscripts. Without them, this compendium would not have been possible. The authors chosen to write the articles are experts in their fields, and we are indebted to them for their contributions.

A major problem in organizing this effort was to avoid overlap of the material presented. While some redundancy is unavoidable, it also may be of interest to the reader to have a subject covered from more than one vantage point. We have limited references to a few key ones listed at the end of each article as a guide for further reading. The intent of the encyclopedia is not to provide a comprehensive, detailed review of each subject, but a concise exposition of the topic, directed toward the reader who would like information on topics outside of his or her expertise. Thus the encyclopedia should be especially useful as a reference for students, fellows in training, and educators.

I thank the many authors who made this second edition possible and the associate editors for their invaluable input. I also thank Craig Panner, Hilary Rowe, and Cindy Minor of Academic Press, who have been instrumental in bringing this effort to fruition.

Joseph R. Bertino

Guide to the Use of the Encyclopedia

The *Encyclopedia of Cancer, Second Edition* is a comprehensive summary of the field of cancer research. This reference work consists of four separate volumes and 220 different articles on various aspects of the disease of cancer, including its epidemiology, its treatment, and its molecular and genetic processes. Each article provides a comprehensive overview of the selected topic to inform a wide range of readers, from research professionals to students.

This *Encyclopedia of Cancer* is the second edition of an award-winning, widely used reference work first published six years ago. Dr. Joseph Bertino has served as Editor-in-Chief for both editions, and the Editorial Board has remained largely the same.

This new version provides a substantial revision of the first edition, reflecting the dynamic nature of cancer research. Of the 220 articles appearing here, more than 60% have been newly commissioned for this edition, and virtually all the others have been significantly rewritten, making this in effect more of an original work than a revision.

ORGANIZATION

The *Encyclopedia of Cancer* is organized to provide the maximum ease of use for its readers. All of the articles are arranged in a single alphabetical sequence by title. Articles whose titles begin with the letters A to Cm are in Volume 1, articles with titles from Co to K are in Volume 2, articles from L to Q to in Volume 3, and R to Z in Volume 4.

So that they can be easily located, article titles generally begin with the key word or phrase indicating the topic, with any descriptive terms following (e.g., "Radiobiology, Principles of" is the article title rather than "Principles of Radiobiology").

TABLE OF CONTENTS

A complete table of contents for the entire encyclopedia appears in the front of each volume. This list of article titles represents topics that have been carefully selected by Dr. Bertino and the members of the Editorial Board (see p. ii for a list of editors).

Following this list of articles by title is a second complete table of contents, in which the articles are listed alphabetically according to subject area. The *Encyclopedia of Cancer* provides coverage of twenty specific subject areas within the overall field of cancer, such as cell proliferation, drug resistance, gene therapy, oncogenes, tumor suppressor genes, and viral carcinogenesis.

INDEX

A subject index is located at the end of Volume 4. Consisting of more than 7,500 entries, this index is the most convenient way to locate a desired topic within the encyclopedia. The subjects in the index are listed alphabetically and indicate the volume and page number where information on this topic can be found.

ARTICLE FORMAT

Each new article in the *Encyclopedia of Cancer* begins at the top of a right-hand page so that it may be quickly located by the reader. The author's name and affiliation are displayed at the beginning of the article.

Each article in the encyclopedia is organized according to a standard format, as follows:

- Title and author
- Outline
- Glossary
- Defining paragraph
- Body of the article
- Cross-references
- Bibliography

OUTLINE

Each article begins with an outline indicating the content of the article to come. This outline provides a brief overview of the article so that the reader can get a sense of what is contained there without having to leaf through the pages. It also serves to highlight important subtopics that will be discussed within the article (for example, risk factors in the article "Thyroid Cancer"). The outline is intended as an overview and thus it lists only the major headings of the article. In addition, extensive second-level and third-level headings will be found within the article.

GLOSSARY

The glossary contains terms that are important to an understanding of the article and that may be unfamiliar to the reader. Each term is defined in the context of the particular article in which it is used. Thus the same term may be defined in two or more articles, with the details of the definition varying slightly from one article to another. The encyclopedia includes approximately 1,700 glossary entries.

DEFINING PARAGRAPH

The text of each article begins with a single introductory paragraph that defines the topic under discussion and summarizes the content of the article. For example, the article "Camptothecins" begins with the following defining paragraph:

Camptothecin derivatives are a novel group of antitumor agents with clinical utility in the treatment of human malignancies, including colorectal, lung, and ovarian tumors. Camptothecins uniquely target target topoisomerase I, an enzyme that catalyzes the relaxation of torsionally strained double-stranded DNA. Camptothecins stabilize the binding of topoisomerase I to DNA and, in the presence of ongoing DNA synthesis, can generate potentially lethal DNA damage.

CROSS-REFERENCES

Many of the articles in the encyclopedia have cross-references to other articles. These cross-references appear at the end of the article, following the article text and preceding the bibliography. The cross-references indicate related articles that can be consulted for further information on the same topic, or for other information on a related topic.

BIBLIOGRAPHY

The bibliography appears as the last element in an article. It lists recent secondary sources to aid the reader in locating more detailed or technical information. Review articles and research papers that are important to an understanding of the topic are also listed.

The bibliographies in this encyclopedia are for the benefit of the reader, to provide references for further research on the given topic. Thus they typically consist of a half-dozen to a dozen entries. They are not intended to represent a complete listing of all materials consulted by the author in preparing the article.

COMPANION WORKS

The *Encyclopedia of Cancer* is one of a series of multi-volume references in the life sciences published by Academic Press/Elsevier Science. Other such works include the *Encyclopedia of Human Biology, Encyclopedia of Virology, Encyclopedia of Immunology, Encyclopedia of Microbiology, Encyclopedia of Reproduction, Encyclopedia of Stress, and Encyclopedia of Genetics.*

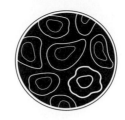

Acute Lymphoblastic Leukemia in Adults

Charles A. Schiffer

Barbara Ann Karmanos Cancer Institute and
Wayne State University School of Medicine, Detroit

I. Clinical Presentation
II. Diagnosis
III. Therapy
IV. Future Prospects

GLOSSARY

cytogenetic Having to do with the identification or analysis of chromosomal abberrations.
flow cytometry An analytical technique for sorting, selecting, or counting individual cells in a suspension as they pass through a tube, often used in cancer research.
pancytopenia A condition marked by an abnormal deficiency of all cell elements in the blood.
stem cell transplantation A technique in which undifferentiated precursor cells are introduced into a patient for the purpose of generating new specialized cells to compensate for loss through disease.

Acute lymphoblastic leukemia (ALL) occurs in individuals of all ages but is more common in children. Although the disease is morphologically similar in children and adults, there are major differences in the incidence of discrete biological subtypes and associated major differences in outcome. Whereas >95% of children achieve complete remission (CR) with initial therapy, CR rates in adults are maximally 80–90%. Long-term disease-free survival can be expected in 70+% of children overall, but in only about 30–40% of adults who enter CR and in 15–30% of adults overall. Younger children (4–10 years old) have a better prognosis than adolescents, whereas in adults, patients less than 30 years of age have an absolute survival advantage of about 20% compared to older patients, and long-term survival is infrequent in patients greater than 60 years of age (Fig. 1). This article reviews current diagnostic and therapeutic approaches to the management of adults with ALL.

I. CLINICAL PRESENTATION

Patients with ALL usually present with complications of pancytopenia, including weakness secondary to anemia, bleeding or bruising due to thrombocytopenia, or bacterial infections as a consequence of

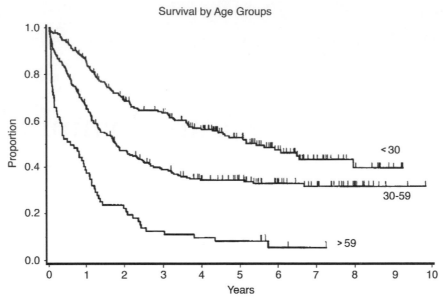

FIGURE 1   Overall survival from time of diagnosis according to age in recent CALGB studies.

neutropenia. Other complaints may include bony pain, headache, or visual disturbances in the occasional individual with central nervous system (CNS) involvement at the time of diagnosis. Physical examination may reveal signs of anemia or bleeding, findings referable to infections, as well as lymphadenopathy and splenomegaly. In general, adenopathy and organomegaly are not striking, and extramedullary leukemic involvement of skin, gingiva, or other sites is uncommon. All of these signs and symptoms are nonspecific, and further evaluation of the peripheral smear and usually the bone marrow is required for more precise diagnosis.

II. DIAGNOSIS

A. Morphology

Morphologically undifferentiated blasts can usually be identified in the peripheral blood of patients with ALL, although in patients with low white blood cell counts, it can sometimes be difficult to distinguish with certainty between leukemic cells and reactive lymphoid elements. Once leukemia has been diagnosed by the presence of blasts in the blood and/or bone marrow, it is critical to distinguish lymphoid blasts from the myeloid blasts of acute myeloid leukemia (AML). Myeloid blasts are usually larger, have more cytoplasm, which contains granules or Auer rods, and may have folded nuclei (monocytic leukemias), whereas ALL blasts have round nuclei and less cytoplasm with no granulation. The distinction is apparent on standard Wright stains in most patients, but further testing with histochemical staining and immunophenotyping by flow cytometry is generally needed to be certain of the diagnosis. Blasts from patients with AML are positive with varying combinations of peroxidase, Sudan black B, and specific or nonspecific esterases, whereas ALL cells are negative for these histochemical stains. Occasionally, these stains are not informative [FAB (French, American, British), M0 (undifferentiated AML), or M7 (megakaryocytic leukemia)] and immunophenotyping is necessary. ALL has been traditionally classified into three morphologic subgroups. FAB L1 and L2 differ primarily by the relative cell size and heterogeneity and amount of cytoplasm in the blasts. The distinction is often arbitrary and not predictive of clinical outcome, immunophenotype, or cytogenetic finding. FAB L3 is more distinctive morphologically, with blasts usually having more rarified chromatin with prominent cytoplasmic vacuolization. Large numbers of cells in mitosis and apoptotic cells are frequently seen.

B. Immunophenotype

Flow cytometry is a mandatory part of the evaluation, both in terms of establishing the diagnosis and in determining prognostic and clinical information. Blasts from the majority of adults and children with ALL derive from various stages of early B-cell lineage and express surface antigens associated with immature B cells, such as CD10 (CALLA) and CD19. Although not done routinely, immunoglobulin gene rearrangements are detected in these B lineage cells. About 15–20% of children also have cytoplasmic immunoglobulin μ chain (Cμ) detectable in at least 10% of their blasts. This phenotype, termed "pre-B cell," suggests that these blasts are somewhat more differentiated than the "early pre-B" phenotype, which lacks Cμ. The presence of Cμ confers a poorer prognosis in both children and adolescents, particularly in patients with the associated t(1;19)(q23;p13) translocation. There are no comparable evaluations of the Cμ-positive subset in adults, and the t(1;19) translocation is an uncommon finding in adults. Even less differentiated lymphoblasts [progenitor B-cell (pro-B) phenotype] are CD19$^+$, CD10-, Cμ-, often coexpress myeloid antigens and may have a rearranged MLL gene arrangement, and a t(4;11). This subtype is common in infants with ALL and is associated with high white blood cell (WBC) counts in adults, female gender, and poor outcome (Table I).

Approximately 15–25% of ALL patients of all ages have leukemia with a T-cell phenotype, which is associated with higher initial WBC counts, male gender, mediastinal masses, and probably a higher incidence of CNS involvement. Although older studies suggested a poorer prognosis for adults with T-cell ALL, recent reports using more intensive regimens indicate a very high remission rate and better overall survival than other immunologic subtypes.

Burkitt-type, mature B-cell ALL is surface immunoglobulin positive, has a FAB-L3 morphology, a high rate of leukemia cell proliferation (and thus elevated LDH and uric acid levels), a frequent occurrence of tumor lysis syndrome, a higher frequency of CNS leukemia and abdominal masses, and t(8;14) or the variant t(2;8) or t(8;22) karyotypes, which juxtapose the c-myc oncogene with different immunoglobulin gene promoter regions, resulting in overexpression of c-myc. B-cell ALL occurs as a small proportion (~5%) of cases in all age groups and, until recently, had a uniformly poor outcome (see later).

About 15–20% of childhood ALL and 25–30% of adult ALL cases will have blast cells of either B or T lineage, which coexpress antigens associated with myeloid differentiation (especially CD13 and CD33). Although many cases of ALL with t(9;22) or t(4;11) are myeloid antigen positive, this phenotype is not restricted to any particular cytogenetic subtype. Studies using intensive chemotherapy have shown that myeloid antigen expression has no effect on treatment outcome.

C. Cytogenetics

Cytogenetic analyses are a critical element of the diagnostic evaluation of all patients with acute leukemia. The frequency of different cytogenetic findings varies markedly in adults and children with ALL. For example, hyperdiploid karyotypes occur in up to 50% of children but are rare in adults. Patients with marked hyperdiploidy (greater than 50 chromosomes) have the best prognosis, whereas patients with 47–50 chromosomes or hypodiploidy have a somewhat poorer outcome. Both groups, however, have a

TABLE I
Prognostic Factors in Children and Adults with ALL[a]

Adverse
  Infancy (<1 year old)
  Increasing age in adults (especially >60 years old)
  Increased WBC count (>50,000/μl)
  FAB L2 morphology
  CNS leukemia at diagnosis
  Delay in achieving CR
  Cytogenetics
    t(4;11)
    t(9;22) [Ph+, much more common in adults]
Favorable
  t(12;22) or TEL/AML 1 [uncommon in adults]
  Hyperdiploidy (>50 chromosomes) [rare in adults]
  Mature B-cell phenotype (Burkitt-type)(FAB L3; t(8;14); SIg positive) [high cure rate in children of ~80+% with intermediate results in adults of ~40–50%]
  CALLA positivity [? effect in adults]
  T-cell immunophenotype in adults

[a]Except as noted in brackets, the incidence and effects of these factors are similar in children and adults.

substantially better outcome than patients with most detectable translocations. It is unknown why patients with numerical additions of apparently intact chromosomes have a better prognosis. Some pediatric studies suggest that the prognosis is best for patients in whom there is duplication of chromosome 10.

Some translocations are specifically associated with B lineage ALL, whereas others are associated with T lineage (often with genes encoding the T-cell antigen receptor at chromosomes 14q11 or 7q34). A cryptic translocation t(12;22) detectable only by molecular technology has been identified in 20–25% of B lineage pediatric ALL cases but in <2% of adult cases. This rearrangement involves ETV6/CBFA2 (also termed TEL-AML1) genes and has a favorable outcome with current intensive therapies. It is likely that in the future, other clinically relevant translocations will be identifiable only by molecular techniques, underscoring the importance of these molecular screening approaches. The Philadelphia chromosome [t(9;22)(q34;q11)] (Ph) is found in <3% of children with ALL, and almost always in patients with the precursor B-cell phenotype.

Although less data are available in adults, it is clear that the frequencies of both hypo- and hyperdiploidy are much lower (<5%) than in children, while some translocations, such as t(4;11) [associated with a mutation of the MLL gene (mixed lineage leukemia or ALL 1 gene) at band 11q23] and t(8;14) (associated with progenitor B ALL or Burkitt-type ALL, respectively), have approximately the same incidence in adults and children. Perhaps most importantly, the Ph chromosome is present in a much higher fraction of adults with ALL. About 20% of adults with ALL have detectable t(9;22) by cytogenetic analyses alone, whereas polymerase chain reactions techniques detect BCR/ABL, which is the hallmark of the (9;22) translocation in patients with chronic myelogenous leukemia (CML) in ~30% of adults, with higher rates with increasing patient age. Molecular abnormalities are always present in patients in whom the Ph chromosome is recognized cytogenetically, although the molecular techniques can detect the translocations in some patients with "normal" cytogenetics or inadequate preparations. The ABL oncogene from chromosome 9 can be translocated to two distinct regions of the breakpoint cluster region (BCR) gene on chromosome 22. One translocation involves the same BCR area found in classic CML and codes for a chimeric tyrosine kinase of 210 kDa, whereas the other is in the first intron of the BCR gene and produces a 190-kDa protein.

There are no distinctive clinical findings at the time of presentation in patients with either molecular variant of the t(9;22). In both adults and children, the presence of the Ph chromosome with either breakpoint confers a poor prognosis. The CR rate is somewhat decreased (~70% in adults even when using more intensive regimens), and there are virtually no long-term disease-free survivors when these patients are treated with conventional chemotherapeutic approaches.

III. THERAPY

The small number of randomized clinical trials in adults hampers comparison among different treatment programs, although certain general principles are well accepted.

A. Remission Induction Therapy

A number of different classes of chemotherapeutic agents have significant lympholytic activity and can result in rapid and substantial cytoreduction. Thus, even the relatively nonmyelosuppressive agents vincristine and prednisone can produce CR in approximately 40% of adults with ALL, albeit with a short response duration. The addition of daunorubicin to an induction regimen of vincristine, prednisone, and L-asparaginase increased the CR rate from 47 to 83% in an older randomized trial, supporting the use of an anthracycline in induction therapy. Building on this, most treatment programs now use four or five drugs during induction, including a corticosteroid (prednisone or dexamethasone), vincristine, an anthracycline (usually daunorubicin) with or without L-asparaginase, and sometimes with the addition of an alkylating agent (cyclophosphamide). ALL regimens tend to be rather complicated, and there are virtually no randomized trials addressing issues of dose and schedule of drug administration. A representative regimen is provided in Table I.

All induction programs are associated with pancytopenia, requiring red blood cell and platelet transfusions, as well as appropriate prophylaxis and treatment of infections. The prolonged use of corticosteroids also increases the infectious risk, particularly with fungal organisms. Granulocyte colony-stimulating factor (G-CSF) moderately shortens the duration of neutropenia in children and younger adults during induction therapy, but with little effect on response rate or the severity of infectious complications. Older patients >60 years of age may have more clinical benefit, but overall, although the use of growth factors can certainly be justified, they have not had the hoped for impact on the long-term treatment outcome.

In summary, 80–90% of adults with ALL should achieve CR with currently available induction therapies. Although a wide range of response rates and remission durations have been reported, the disparities relate more to differences in the age of the patients treated and the frequency of Ph chromosome positivity than to the details of the specific regimens. There is no evidence of superiority of any given regimen nor is there an inference that particular induction programs result in greater cytoreduction as deduced from their influence on remission duration. Most patients are in CR by 4 weeks after treatment is begun and CR durations are shorter in the 10–20% of patients who require a longer period of therapy to achieve CR. It is unlikely that further improvements will come from further empiric modification of existing regimens and new drugs or more targeted biologic agents are needed.

B. Postremission Treatment

Unless further treatment is given after CR, all patients will have relapse of their leukemia within weeks to months. Short-term consolidation treatment as well as more prolonged maintenance programs are used in adults with ALL in CR.

C. Postremission Consolidation

Analogous to approaches used in AML, intermittent courses of more intensive postremission chemotherapy have been given immediately after CR is achieved or inserted between courses of lower dose mainte-

nance treatment. In addition to variably myelosuppressive doses of cytarabine (ara-C) and "high-dose" methotrexate, differing drugs from the same class of compounds have been empirically used in later courses (e.g., daunorubicin/adriamycin/mitoxantrone, prednisone/dexamethasone, cyclophosphamide/ifosfamide) in the hope of overcoming "resistance" to the original agent. Because of variability in the doses, schedules, number of courses of treatment, patient population, and the absence of randomized trials, it is difficult to assess the effect of individual components of these regimens (Table I).

Although most investigators attribute the gradual improvements in overall results to intensification of postremission treatment, this has been difficult to document in controlled trials. The CALGB did not show improvement in survival or CR duration in patients receiving postremission intensification with two courses of daunorubicin and cytarabine administered in doses used in induction therapy for AML when compared to lower dose standard therapy with methotrexate, 6-MP, vincristine and prednisone. Nor could other studies evaluating the relatively intensive M-2 regimen, high-dose cytarabine, early consolidation with doxorubicin or mitoxantrone, and high-dose ara-C demonstrate an advantage on results to be expected from the regimens to which they were added. All of these studies produce long-term disease-free survival rates in approximately 30–40% of complete responders. Unfortunately, because the studies were too small, were not randomized, or did not contain sufficient patient breakdown into B/T or cytogenetic subgroups, it is not known whether intensive consolidation approaches benefit subgroups of ALL patients.

D. Maintenance Therapy

Most adult protocols have incorporated long-term, continuous postremission "maintenance" therapy using multiple drugs patterned after the experience in children. Median durations of CR are 18–24 months with 30–40% of complete responders remaining in remission, depending on the prognostic factors in the patients studied. The "backbone" of such treatment consists of variations of daily oral 6-mercaptopurine, weekly methotrexate, and intermittent "pulses" of vincristine and prednisone (Table II). This treatment

TABLE II
A Representative Treatment Program for Adult ALL[a]

	Dose	Days
Induction		
Vincristine	2 mg iv	1, 8, 15, 22
Prednisone	60 mg/m^2/day	1–21 (days 1–7 if >60 years)
Daunorubicin	45 mg/m^2 iv	1, 2, 3
L-Asparaginase (some regimens use less L-Asp)	6000 μ/m^2 sc	5, 8, 11, 15, 18, 22
Cyclophosphamide	1200 mg/m^2 iv	1
	(800 mg/m^2 if >60 years)	
Intensification (two courses each 28 days)		
Intrathecal methotrexate	15 mg	Day 1
Cyclophosphamide	1000 mg/m^2 iv	Day 1
6-Mercaptopurine	60 mg/m^2 po	1–14
Cytarabine	75 mg/m^2 day sc	1–4, 8–11
Vincristine	2 mg iv	15, 22
L-Asparaginase	6000 mg/m^2 sc	5, 8, 22, 25
CNS prophylaxis		
Cranial irradiation	2400 CGY	
Intrathecal methotrexate	15 mg	1, 8, 15, 22, 29
6-Mercaptopurine (other programs utilize combinations of high-dose systemic intrathecal methotrexate without cranial irradiation)	60 mg/m^2 po	1–70
Late intensification		
Similar to intensification		
Some programs substitute 6-thioguanine for 6-MP and add an anthracycline (daunorubicin or doxorubicin) for 3 weekly doses (days 1, 8, 15), delaying the cytarabine until days 29–32 and 36–39		
Maintenance (28-day cycle)[a]		
Vincristine	2 mg iv	Day 1 of each month
Prednisone	60 mg/m^2 po	Days 1–5 of each month
Methotrexate	20 mg/m^2 po	Days 1, 8, 15, 22
6-Mercaptopurine	60 mg/m^2 po	Days 1–28

[a]Adapted from Larson *et al.* (1998) and Hoelzer *et al.* (1988).
[b]Maintenance is generally continued to provide a total of 24 months of therapy.

is usually well tolerated and rarely requires hospitalization, although dose adjustment because of myelosuppression is frequently necessary, perhaps because of individual differences in drug metabolism, and monitoring of hepatic function is mandatory. The duration of therapy has been derived empirically, and programs providing a total of 2+ years of chemotherapy are commonly used. No randomized studies are available to help to define the ideal duration of therapy, although some studies utilizing shorter treatment programs of approximately 8–10 months noted shorter CR durations and possibly a lower fraction of long-term disease-free survivors.

Burkitt-type ALL represents an exception to the need for longer term maintenance therapy. Until recently, this group of adult patients was generally in-curable using conventional ALL or lymphoma-based chemotherapeutic approaches. Studies in children, however, have shown that >75% of patients with mature B-cell ALL or Burkitt's lymphoma enjoy long-term, event-free survival after intensive therapy based on rotating, repetitive cycles of cyclophosphamide or ifosphamide, high-dose methotrexate, and higher dose ara-C administered over a 3- to 4-month period of time. No maintenance therapy is given and all patients receive CNS prophylaxis. Studies in adults using a similar therapeutic approach produce disease-free survival in approximately 40–50% of patients with mature B-cell ALL. The regimens are highly myelosuppressive and are associated with tumor lysis syndrome during initial induction and significant mucositis, but clearly represent an improvement over older approaches. Given the differences in treatment approach, it is critical that this subtype of ALL be recognized promptly at the time of diagnosis.

E. Central Nervous System Prophylaxis

Leukemia relapse in the CNS, either in association with marrow recurrence or as an isolated finding, is quite common in patients with ALL, and prophylactic treatment of the meninges and brain is a standard part of therapy. In addition, 5–10% of patients have CNS leukemia at the time of diagnosis. Patients with higher initial blast counts and mature B- or T-cell phenotypes are at higher risk of CNS leukemia. There is no consensus about the optimal CNS prophylaxis for adults. The approach of cranial irradiation plus intrathecal methotrexate is effective and seems to be associated with fewer long-term side effects than in children. Other studies have suggested that similar results may be accomplished with high-dose systemic therapy with high-dose methotrexate and ara-C, which penetrate the CNS, or intraventricular methotrexate alone administered via an Ommaya reservoir. Finally, some clinicians have added ara-C or dexamethasone intrathecally; the latter may have an anti-inflammatory as well as an antileukemic effect. When it occurs, CNS leukemia is managed with intrathecal or intraventricular instillation of methotrexate or ara-C, in combination with cranial irradiation, particularly if there is involvement of cranial nerves. High-dose systemic therapy with these agents can also be effective.

F. Relapsed or Refractory ALL

No standard approach can be recommended for the treatment of primarily refractory or relapsed ALL. Patients who relapse off treatment have a high rate of another CR with the possibility of sustained response using the types of treatment to which they had responded previously. In contrast, patients relapsing while receiving therapy, or those with short remissions, usually do not benefit from regimens they have received in the recent past and the use of new agents should be considered. The multidrug nature of many of the ALL protocols can make the choice of new treatment difficult. A commonly used program ad-

ministers high-dose ara-C ($2 \ g/m^2$ every 12 h for 8–12 doses), sometimes in combination with an anthracycline, mitoxantrone, amsacrine, or teniposide. Subsequent remissions tend to be quite short, however, and such patients should be considered for allogeneic stem cell transplantation (SCT).

G. Stem Cell Transplantation

Allogeneic bone marrow transplantation (now more commonly done using peripheral blood stem cells) can cure a considerable fraction of patients with ALL in relapse or in second or subsequent remission. Although comparative trials have not been done, it is likely that allogeneic SCT produces a long-term benefit superior to further chemotherapy, particularly if the duration of the prior remission was short or if relapse had occurred while the patient was receiving treatment. A summary of 391 adults and children transplanted in second CR from the International Bone Marrow Transplant Registry demonstrated a leukemia-free survival of 25%, with leukemia relapse as the major cause of treatment failure. Autologous SCT can also be of some benefit in selected patients who are in second or subsequent remission, although relapse remains a major cause of failure.

Although SCT can be recommended for patients who have relapsed, the benefits of transplantation for patients in first remission are controversial. The overall results of both allogeneic and autologous SCT in ALL are inferior to those in comparable patients with AML because of an increased rate of leukemia relapse, reflecting a greater inherent resistance of the leukemia or a decreased graft vs leukemia effect. Relapse rates are appreciably higher in recipients of autologous compared to allogeneic transplants. Clearly, more effective conditioning programs are required. Critical interpretation of many of the transplantation reports is difficult because most series include small numbers of highly selected patients whose clinical characteristics and cytogenetic features are not clearly presented.

Given the invariably poor prognosis of patients with Ph chromosome-positive ALL, SCT in first CR has been evaluated in a number of small studies. Leukemia-free survival after allogeneic transplantation varies from 38 to 49% in different series. Patient selection obviously influences these results, and there are no reports of patients on a prospective trial intending to transplant all age eligible patients with available family or matched unrelated donors. However, given the uniformly poor prognosis when treated with chemotherapy alone, it is appropriate to evaluate all Ph+ ALL patients of suitable age for allogeneic bone marrow transplantation. Even less data are available on the outcome of SCT in other poor prognosis subgroups, including those with t(4;11) and those patients who do not rapidly achieve CR, as well as those failing to achieve initial CR, although most current protocols suggest consideration of allogeneic SCT in younger patients with suitable donors.

It is otherwise premature to recommend SCT in first remission as the treatment of choice for other subgroups of adults with ALL. Retrospective comparisons of results compiled by the International Bone Marrow Transplant Registry failed to show improved survival in patients receiving allogeneic transplantation in first CR compared to matched patients treated with contemporary ALL regimens in Germany. Lower relapse rates in the SCT recipients were offset by increased transplant-related mortality. Factors predicting relapse in patients treated with chemotherapy were also associated with higher relapse rates in the transplant recipients. The only randomized trial of autologous or allogeneic SCT was conducted in France. Patients <50 years of age without donors were randomized to conventional maintenance therapy or autologous SCT with a similar 3-year disease-free survival of 39 and 32%, respectively, in an intent to treat analysis. As in many transplant studies, not all patients randomized to autotransplant actually received this therapy. A disease-free survival of 43% was noted in 116 recipients <40 years of age transplanted with marrow from identical HLA siblings. Survival was 44% after allogeneic SCT for high-risk patients compared with 11% with chemotherapy ($p=0.009$), but with no difference in the standard risk patients (49% vs 39%, $p=0.3$).

IV. FUTURE PROSPECTS

It seems unlikely that additional "tinkering" with available agents will produce significant changes in overall survival. Nor is it likely that modest increases in dose intensity, such as may be permitted by hematopoietic growth factors, will overcome the intrinsic drug resistance associated with different subtypes of ALL, as suggested by the significant relapse rate even following the major increase in dosage used with SCT. There has been a dearth of new active agents for ALL. Recently, however, GW506U78, a prodrug of arabinosylguanine, has shown promising efficacy against T lineage ALL. This drug is being evaluated in a number of phase I/II studies in adults and children and likely will be intercalated into phase III studies in the future. Of greater interest is the new tyrosine kinase inhibitor STI571, which is a relatively specific inhibitor of the BCR/ABL tyrosine kinase and produces dramatic, albeit short-lived responses in PH+ ALL and lymphoid blast crisis of chronic myelogenous leukemia. Given the well-characterized surface antigens in ALL, studies with monoclonal antibodies, either alone or coupled to toxins or radioisotopes, will be evaluated in the future as well.

Minimal residual disease (MRD) can be identified and monitored serially in patients with ALL in apparent "morphologic" remission utilizing either fluorescence-activated cell sorter techniques, sometimes with multiple antibodies known to be present on specific patient's leukemia cells, or by polymerase chain reaction enhanced detection of clonal immunoglobulin gene rearrangements or translocations. Although these methods are still experimental, studies done in children suggest that they can be highly sensitive and predictive of impending relapse. It is likely, although unproved, that similar findings will be found in adults, although the higher rates of relapse might influence the sensitivity and specificity of the MRD assays. Serial monitoring of patients in remission may become practical with the identification of clonal leukemic abnormalities serving as the "signal" for initiating different therapies, including possibly SCT. Studies are in progress using a variety of quantitative methods, which should help determine at which point after induction persistence of MRD is predictive of relapse.

See Also the Following Articles

Acute Lymphoblastic Leukemia in Children • Acute Myelocytic Leukemia • ALL-1 • Chronic Lymphocytic Leukemia • Chronic Myelogenous Leukemia • Graft

VERSUS LEUKEMIAS AND GRAFT VERSUS TUMOR • MONO-CLONAL ANTIBODIES: LEUKEMIA AND LYMPHOMA • STEM CELL TRANSPLANTATION

Bibliography

Barrett, J. A., Horowitz, M. M., Gale, R. P., Biggs, J. C., Camitta, B. M., Dicke, K. A., Gluckman, E., Good, R. A., Herzig, H., Lee, M. B., Marmont, A. M., Masaoka, T., Ramsay, N. K. C., Rimm, A. A., Speck, B., Zwaan, F. E., and Bortin, M. M. (1989). Marrow transplantation for acute lymphoblastic leukemia: Factors affecting relapse and survival. *Blood* **74,** 862.

Bleyer, W. A., and Poplack, D. G. (1985). Prophylaxis and treatment of leukemia in the central nervous system and other sanctuaries. *Semin. Oncol.* **12,** 131.

Boucheix, C., David, B., Sebban, C., Racadot, E., Bene, M-C., Bernard, A., Campos, L., Louault, H., Sigaux, F., Lepage, E., Herve, P., Fiere, D., for the French Group on Therapy for Adult Acute Lymphoblastic Leukemia. (1994). Immunophenotype of adult lymphoblastic leukemia, clinical parameters and outcome: An analysis of a prospective trial including 562 tested patients (LALA87). *Blood* **84,** 1603.

Cave, H., van der Werff ten Bosch, J., Suciu, S., Guidal, C., Waterkeyn, C., Otten, J., Bakkus, M., Thielemans, K., Grandchamp, B., and Vilmer, E. (1998). Clinical significance of minimal residual disease in childhood acute lymphoblastic leukemia: European Organization for Research and Treatment of Cancer–Childhood Leukemia Cooperative Group. *N. Engl. J. Med.* **339,** 591–598.

Chao, N. J., Blume, K. G., Forman, S. J., *et al.* (1995). Long-term follow-up of allogeneic bone marrow transplants recipients for Philadelphia chromosome-positive acute lymphoblastic leukemia. *Blood* **85,** 3353.

Crist, W., Carroll, A., Shuster, J., Jackson, J., Head, D., Borowitz, M., Behm, F., Link, M., Steuber, P., Ragab, A., Hirt, A., Brock, B., Land, V., and Pullen, J. (1990). Ph chromosome positive childhood acute lymphoblastic leukemia: Clinical and cytogenetic characteristics and treatment outcome: A Pediatric Oncology Group study. *Blood* **76,** 489.

Crist, W. M, Carroll, A. J., Shuster, J. J., Behm, F. G., Whitehead, M., Vietti, T. J., Look, A. T., Mahoney, D., Ragab, A., Pullen, D. J., and Land, V. J. (1990). Poor prognosis of children with pre-B acute lymphoblastic leukemia is associated with the t(1;19)(q23;p13): A Pediatric Oncology Group Study. *Blood* **76,** 117.

Czuczman, M. S., Dodge, R. K., Stewart, C. C., Frankel, S. R., Davey, F. R., Powell, B. L., Szatrowski, T. P., Schiffer, C. A., Larson, R. A., and Bloomfield, C. D. (1999). Value of immunophenotype in intensively treated adult acute lymphoblastic leukemia: Cancer and Leukemia Group B Study 8364. *Blood* **93,** 3931–3939.

Druker, B. J., Sawyers, C. L., Kantarjian, H., Resta, D. J., Reese, S. F., Ford, J. M., Capdeville, R., and Talpaz, M. (2001). Activity of a specific inhibitor of the BCR-ABL ty-rosine kinase in the blastcrisis of chronic myeloid leukemia and acute lymphoblastic leukemia with the Philadelphia chromosome. *N. Engl. J. Med.* **344,** 1038–1042.

Ellison, R. R., Mick, R., Cuttner, J., Schiffer, C. A., Silver, R. T., Henderson, E. S., Woliver, T., Royston, I., Davey, F. R., Glicksman, A. S., Bloomfield, C. D., and Holland, J. F. (1991). The effects of postinduction intensification treatment with cytarabine and daunorubicin in acute lymphocytic leukemia: A prospective randomized clinical trial by Cancer and Leukemia Group B. *J. Clin. Oncol.* **9,** 2002.

Faderl, S., Kantarjian, H. M., Talpaz, M., and Estrov, Z. (1998). Clinical significance of cytogenetic abnormalities in adult acute lymphoblastic leukemia. *Blood* **91,** 3995–4019.

Finiewicz, K. J., and Larson, R. A. (1997). Dose-intensive therapy for adult acute lymphoblastic leukemia. *Semin. Oncol.* **24,** 70–82.

Gandhi, V., Plunkett, W., Rodriguez, C. O., Jr., Nowak, B. J., Du, M., Ayres, M., Kisor, D. F., Mitchell, B. S., Kurtzberg, J., and Keating, M. J. (1998). Compound GW506U78 in refractory hematologic malignancies: Relationship between cellular pharmacokinetics and clinical response. *J. Clin. Oncol.* **16,** 3607–3615.

Gottlieb, A. J., Weinberg, V., Ellison, R. R., Henderson, E. S., Terebelo, H., Rafla, S., Cuttner, J., Silver, R. T., Carey, R. W., Levy, R. N., Hutchinson, J. L., Raich, P., Cooper, M. R., Wiernik, P., Anderson, J. R., and Holland, J. F. (1984). Efficacy of daunorubicin in the therapy of adult acute lymphocytic leukemia: A prospective randomized trial by Cancer and Leukemia Group. *Blood* **4,** 267.

Groupe Francais de Cytogénétique Hématologique (1996). Cytogenetic abnormalities in adult acute lymphoblastic leukemia: Correlations with hematologic findings and outcome. *Blood* **87,** 3135–3142.

Hiddemann, W., Kreutzmann, H., Straif, K., Ludwig, W. D., Mertelsmann, R., Planker, M., Donhuijsen-Ant, R., Lengfelder, E., Arlin, Z., and Buchner, T. (1987). High-dose cytosine arabinoside in combination with mitoxantrone for the treatment of refractory acute myeloid and lymphoblastic leukemia. *Semin. Oncol.* **2,** 73.

Hoelzer, D., Ludwig, W., Thiel, E., Gassmann, W., Loffler, H., Fonatsch, C., Rieder, H., Heil, G., Heinze, B., Arnold, R., Hossfeld, D., Buchner, T., Koch, P., Freund, M., Hiddemann, W., Machmeyer, G., Heyll, A., Aul, C., Raak, T., Kuse, R., Ittel, T., Gramatzki, M., Diedrich, H., Kolbe, K., Fuhr, H., Fischer, K., Schadeck-Gressel, C., Weiss, A., Strohscheer, I., Metzner, B., Fabry, U., Gokbuget, N., Volkers, B., Messerer, D., and Oberla, K. (1996). Improved outcome in adult B-cell acute lymphoblastic leukemia. *Blood* **87,** 495–508.

Hoelzer, D., Thiel, E., Lauoffler, H., Buchner, T., Ganser, A., Heil, G., Koch, P., Freund, M., Diedrich, H., Ruhl, H., Maschmeyer, G., Lipp, T., Nowrousian, M. R., Burkert, M., Gerecke, D., Pralle, H., Müller, U., Lunscken, C. H., Fulle, H., Ho, A. D., Kuchler, R., Busch, F. W., Schneider, W., Görg, C. H., Emmerich, B., Braumann, D., Vaupel, H. A., von Paleske, A., Bartels, H., Neiss, A., and

Messerer, D. (1988). Prognostic factors in multicenter study for treatment of acute lymphoblastic leukemia in adults. *Blood* **71,** 123.

Horowitz, M. M., Messerer, D., Hoelzer, D., Gale, R. P., Neiss, A., Atkinson, K., Barrett, A. J., Buchner, T., Freund, M., Heil, G., Hiddemann, W., Kolb, H.-J., Loffler, H., Marmont, A. M., Maschmeyer, G., Rimm, A. A., Rozman, C., Sobocinski, K. A., Speck, B., Thiel, E., Weisdorf, D. J., Zqaan, F. E., and Bortin, M. M. (1991). Chemotherapy compared with bone marrow transplantation for adults with acute lymphoblastic leukemia in first remission. *Ann. Int. Med.* **115,** 13.

Laport, G. F., and Larson, R. A. (1997). Treatment of adult acute lymphoblastic leukemia. *Semin Oncol.* **24,** 70–82.

Larson, R. A., Dodge, R. K., Linker, C. A., Stone, R. M., Powell, B. L., Lee, E. J., Schulman, P., Davey, F. R., Frankel, S. R., Bloomfield, C. D., George, S. L., and Schiffer, C. A. (1998). A randomized controlled trial of filgrastrim during remission induction and consolidation chemotherapy for adults with acute lymphoblastic leukemia: CALGB study 9111. *Blood* **92,** 1556.

Ludwig, W. D., Rieder, H., Bartram, C. R., *et al.* (1998). Immunophenotype and genotypic features, clinical characteristics, and treatment outcome of adult pro-B acute lymphoblastic leukemia: Results of the German multicenter trials GMALL 03/87 and 04/89. *Blood* **94,** 1898–1909.

Mandelli, F., Annio, L., Vegna, M. L., Camera, A., Ciolla, S., Deplano, W., Fabiano, F., Ferrara, F., Ladogana, S., Muti, G., Peta, A., Recchia, A., Sica, S., Stasi, R., Tabilio, A., Visani, G., Baccarani, M. for the GIMEMA group (1992). GIMEMA ALL 0288: A multicentric study on adult acute lymphoblastic leukemia: Preliminary results. *Leukemia* **6,** 182.

Omura, G. A., Moffitt, S., Vogler, W. R., and Salter, M. M. (1980). Combination chemotherapy of adult acute lymphoblastic leukemia with randomized central nervous system prophylaxis. *Blood* **55,** 199.

Patte, C., Philip, T., Rodary, C., Zucker, J. M., Behrendt, H., Gentet, J. C., Lamagnagere, J. P., Otten, J., Dufillot, D., Pein, F., Caillou, B., and Lemerle, J. (1991). High survival rate in advanced-stage B-cell lymphomas and leukemias without CNS involvement with a short intensive polychemotherapy: Results from the French Pediatric Oncology Society of a randomized trial of 216 children. *J. Clin. Oncol.* **9,** 123.

Pui, C.-H., and Evans, W. E. (1998). Acute lymphoblastic leukemia. *N. Engl. J. Med.* **339,** 605–615.

Radich, J. P., Kopecky, K. J., Boldt, D. H., Head, D., Slovak, M. L., Babu, R., Kirk, J., Lee, A., Kessler, P., Appelbaum, F., and Gehly, G. (1994). Detection of BCR-ABL fusion genes in adult acute lymphoblastic leukemia by the polymerase chain reaction. *Leukemia* **8,** 1688.

Reiter, A., Schrappe, M., Ludwig, W.-D., Hiddemann, W., Sauter, S., Henze, G., Zimmermann, M., Lampert F., Havers, W., Niethammer, D., Odenwald, E., Ritter, J., Mann, G., Welte, K., Gadner, H., and Riehm, H. (1994). Chemotherapy in 998 unselected childhood acute lymphoblastic leukemia patients: Results and conclusions of the multicenter trial ALL-BFM 86. *Blood* **84,** 3122.

Roberts, W. M., Rivera, G. K., Raimondi, S. C., Santana, V. M., Sandlund, J. T., Crist, W. M., and Pui, C-H. (1994). Intensive chemotherapy for Philadelphia-chromosome-positive acute lymphoblastic leukaemia. *Lancet* **343,** 331.

Rubnitz, J. E., Pui, C.-H., and Downing, J. R. (1999). The role of *TEL* fusion genes in pediatric leukemias. *Leukemia* **13,** 6–13.

Thiebaut, A., Vernant, J. P., Degos, L., Huguet, F. R., Reiffers, J., Sebban, C., Lepage, E., Thomas, X., and Fiere, D. (2000). Adult acute lymphocytic leukemia study testing chemotherapy and autologous and allogeneic transplantation: A follow-up report of the French protocol LALA 87. *Hematol. Oncol. Clin. North Am.* **14,** 1353–1366.

Thomas, D. A., Cortes, J., O'Brien, S., Pierce, S., Faderl, S., Albitar, M., Hagemeister, F. B., Cabanillas, F. F., Murphy, S., Keating, M. J., and Kantarjian, H. (1999). Hyper-CVAD program in Burkitt's-type adult acute lymphoblastic leukemia. *J. Clin. Oncol.* **17,** 2461–2470.

Wetzler, M., Dodge, R. K., Mrózek, K., Carroll, A. J., Tantravahi, R., Block, A. M. W., Pettenati, M. J., Frankel, S. R., Stewart, C. C., Szatrowski, T. P., Schiffer, C. A., Larson, R. A., and Bloomfield, C. D. (1999). Prospective karyotype analysis in adult acute lymphoblastic leukemia: The Cancer and Leukemia Group B Experience. *Blood* **93,** 3983–3993.

Williams, D. L., Harber, J., Murphy, S. B., Look, A. T., Kalwinksy, D. K., Rivera, G., Melvin, S. L., Stass, S., and Dahl, G. V. (1986). Chromosomal translocations play a unique role in influencing prognosis in childhood acute lymphoblastic leukemia. *Blood* **68,** 205.

Acute Lymphoblastic Leukemia in Children

Peter G. Steinherz

Memorial Sloan-Kettering Cancer Center

GLOSSARY

central nervous system (CNS) prophylaxis Therapy directed at eliminating subclinical CNS leukemia by intrathecal chemotherapy, cranial irradiation, or both modalities.

complete remission Reduction of lymphoblasts in the bone marrow to less than 5% with return of normal hematopoiesis in the marrow and normalization of peripheral blood counts.

consolidation therapy Chemotherapy phase after remission induction aimed at further reducing the body leukemic burden.

higher risk patient Patient whose prognostic factors indi-cate a high risk of leukemic recurrence after remission induction.

immunophenotype Protein clusters on the surface membrane of leukemic cells indicating the lineage of the cell's origin, i.e., pre-B, B, pre-T, and T cells.

induction therapy The first phase of chemotherapy after diagnosis, aimed at achieving remission of the disease.

maintenance therapy Therapy after achieving remission with combination of chemotherapy agents aimed at eliminating residual disease still present in the body.

ploidy The number of chromosomes present in cells: diploid, 46; aneuploid, more or less than 46; hypodiploid, <46; hyperdiploid, >46; and pseudodiploid, 46 with translocation or other abnormality within one or more chromosomes.

prognostic factor A clinical or biologic feature of the patient or the leukemic cell that predicts for a better or worse outcome for those that possess it as compared to those that do not have it.

rapid early response Reduction of the blast percentage in the bone marrow to <25% by day 7 or to <5% by day 14 of treatment.

sanctuary sites Areas of the body not reached by adequate concentrations of chemotherapeutic agents where leukemic cells can be sequestered and survive, i.e., CNS, testis, and anterior chamber of the eye.

slow early responders Patients who achieve remission by day 28 of treatment but who did not have a rapid early response in the marrow on day 7 or 14.

standard risk Patients who are between 2 and 10 years of age with a presenting white blood cell count <50,000/mm³ at diagnosis.

Acute lymphoblastic leukemia (ALL) is a biologically and clinically heterogeneous malignancy of the lymphoid cells. It is the most frequent pediatric cancer.

I. ETIOLOGY

Leukemia is believed to begin as a random clonal change in a single cell. Once the malignant change occurs, the cells proliferate without response to normal growth inhibition mechanisms, fail to undergo apoptotic changes, and gradually replace the normal marrow. The cells compete with normal hematopoietic elements and eventually inhibit the growth of normal precursors either by mass effect or by liberating humoral inhibitory factors. The immature cells leave the marrow and infiltrate normal organs. If untreated, the disease leads to pancytopenia and organ failure. Death usually results from infection or bleeding within 9 months.

II. EPIDEMIOLOGY

Thirty-one percent of pediatric malignancies are leukemias. Eighty-six percent of all pediatric leukemias are acute lymphoblastic leukemia. ALL occurs in approximately 2500 new cases in the United States in children under 15 years of age. The annual incidence is 31 cases per one million children. It is slightly more frequent in males (57%) than in females. The rate in Caucasians is twice that of the black population. Eighty-nine percent of children with leukemia in the United States are Caucasian. Peak age at diagnosis is between 2 and 3 years of age. Seventy-seven percent are diagnosed between the age of 1 and 9, 3% under 1 year of age, and 20% of the cases are first seen in children over 10 years.

III. PATHOPHYSIOLOGY

Random mutations are believed to cause most of the cases with at least two mutations necessary around the regular gene or an oncogene in proliferating lymphoid cells. The usual first event is a genetic rearrangement or mutation, and the second event is the loss of heterozygosity of the involved site. Interactions of the host, the environment, and genetic factors may play a significant role in the development of some of the cases. However, known increased risk factors account only for about 1% of the cases. These risk factors include the following.

A. Genetic Predisposition

There is a concordance in the occurrence of acute lymphoblastic leukemia in monozygotic twins. If one of the twins develops acute lymphoblastic leukemia, the risk of the second twin developing leukemia is 20% within months of the index case. There is also a slight increase incidence of ALL in siblings, in infants of mothers with leukemia, and in children of consanguineous union.

B. Host Factors

Incidence of leukemia is higher in patients with pre-existing bone marrow damage such as aplastic anemia. Patients with chromosome fragility syndromes (Bloom syndrome, Fanconi's anemia, and ataxia telangiectasia) have a high incidence of developing acute lymphoblastic leukemia (8 to 12 times the expected rate). Children with Down's syndrome have a very high incidence (1 in 200) of leukemia. The incidence of leukemia is also higher in patients with neurofibromatosis, in the various kinds of immunodeficiencies, in congenital neutropenia, and with Wiscott–Aldrich syndrome.

C. Environmental Risk Factors

Exposure to radiation, alkylating agents, hydrocarbons and solvents, and viral disease (EBV, HTLV) increases the risk of leukemia. There is some evidence that parental occupation in hydrocarbon-, chemical-, or solvent-related industries increases the risk of their children developing leukemia. There is contradictory evidence whether maternal smoking contributes to an increased risk of developing leukemia.

IV. CLASSIFICATION

A. Morphologic

ALL can be subclassified according to the appearance of cells on right Wright–Giemsa stain under light microscopy. There are three different morphologic appearances to lymphoblasts according to the French/American/British (FAB) classification.

1. L_1 lymphoblasts have variable cell size, little cytoplasm with occasional granules, vacuoles, nuclear clefts, and rare nucleolii.
2. L_2 lymphoblasts are usually larger in size with abundant cytoplasm, prominent nucleolii, and irregular nuclear outline. These cells are very difficult to distinguish under light microscopy from M_0/M_1 myeloblasts.
3. L_3 lymphoblasts can be either large or small in size with a small amount of very basophilic cytoplasm with prominent vacuoles.

Most of the patients do not have pure L_1 or L_2 or L_3 lymphoblasts, but a mixture of multiple cell types: 78% of the cases have over 90% L_1 lymphoblasts, 12% have L_1 morphology with 10–25% L_2 blasts, and 6% have 26–50% L_2, whereas only 3% have more than 50% L_2 cells and 1% have 1–25% L_3 lymphoblasts.

B. Immunophenotypic

Leukemias can be classified based on protein clusters on their membrane surface. These markers can indicate the lineage of the cell's origin. There are markers for B cells, T cells, myeloid precursors, and some antigens are nonlineage specific. The nomenclature of these antigens is by cluster designation (CD) number. B lineage markers are CD19, CD20, and CD22; T lineage markers are CD2, CD4, CD5, CD7, and CD8; and myeloid markers are CD13, CD14, and CD33. Markers that are frequently seen but are non-lineage specific are CD10 (CALLA), CD34, and HLA-DR.

The most frequent immunophenotype (64%) in childhood leukemia is an early pre-B cell that is CD19 positive and, in addition, may have CD10 positivity. Next in frequency is the pre-B cell, which is CD10, CD19, and CD20 positive and occurs in about 14% of the cases. A slightly more mature, transitional pre-B cell that has cytoplasmic immunoglobulin positivity in addition to CD19 and CD20 and the mature B-cell phenotype, which also has surface immunoglobulin expression, occurs in about 1% of patients each. Fifteen percent of patients have a T-cell immunophenotype exhibiting various combinations of CD2, CD4, CD5, CD7, and CD8. Five percent of the cases have either mixed lineage or biphenotypic features or are unclassifiable into a specific category.

C. Cytogenetic

Acute lymphoblastic leukemias can be divided into prognostic groups based on the number of chromosomes and other cytogenetic features of the leukemia cell. Forty-two percent of the patients have the normal complement of 46 chromosomes, but they are pseudodiploid containing various translocation or other abnormalities. Only 8% of patients are diploid with no other abnormalities. Twenty-seven percent of the patients are hyperdiploid with over 50 chromosomes. An additional 15% have hyperdiploidy with only 1 to 3 additional chromosomes. Seven percent of the patients are hypodiploid with less than the normal complement of 46 chromosomes.

Many of the pseudodiploid patients have nonrandom chromosomal translocations that are associated with specific cell lines. B-cell leukemias frequently have t(8;14), t(8;22), or t(2;8). T-cell leukemias are associated with t(11;14), t(10;14), t(1;14), t(8;14), t(7;9), t(7;19), or t(1;7). In pre-B or early B-cell leukemia, the most frequent chromosome abnormality is t(12;21) involving the TEL-AML-1 gene (22%). Translocation among t(1;19), t(4;11), t(5;14), t(11;19), t(9;11), or t(17;19) has also been reported. Philadelphia chromosome [t(9;22)] can be seen in all lineages. The mixed lineage leukemia (MLL) chromosome abnormality t(4;11) is frequently seen in infants with both lymphoid and myeloid leukemia.

V. CLINICAL FINDINGS

Children with leukemia usually present with fairly nonspecific symptomology. Over 90% complain of fatigue or malaise. Almost 80% of the patients have bone pain. This pain may be migratory and intermittent and persist for a long period of time. Any unexplained bone pain in a child should raise the suspicion of possible disease in the bone marrow. Young children frequently cannot complain of specific pain. The presence of bone pain may only be manifested by limping or refusal to walk. Two-thirds of the patients with leukemia at presentation will have a history of fever for various durations with no apparent cause. About one-half the patients will have signs of bleeding with ecchymotic areas or petechiae.

On physical examination, more than 75% of patients will have various degrees of hepatosplenomegaly and lymphadenopathy. Bone tenderness and petechiae or achymosis are the other frequent findings.

An abnormal blood count is the key clue to diagnosis. However, the possibility of leukemia should be entertained even when the CBC seems to be within normal limits if sufficient suspicion is raised by the history or physical examination. Although the word leukemia means "white blood" and is suggestive of a very high blood count, the majority of children presenting with ALL have a near normal blood count with a white count under 10,000/μl. Studies of large numbers of children with ALL showed that 35% of the patients had a white count between 10,000 and 50,000/μl and only 7% of the patients had a white count that was higher than 100,000/μl. Eighty percent of the patients will present with various degrees of anemia with hemoglobin <10 g/dl. The platelet count is abnormal in a majority of patients. Twenty-eight percent have a <20,000/μl platelet count at diagnosis. Another 47% have a platelet count between 20,000 and 100,000/μl. Central nervous system involvement is the most frequent site of extramedullary disease and occurs in about 4% of patients at diagnosis.

The diagnosis is established through a bone marrow aspirate. This is best accomplished in children under brief general anesthesia to avoid traumatizing the child, who will need to establish a trusting relationship with the physician over multiple future years of therapy. The bone marrow aspirate should be done at a medical center with facilities to perform all the diagnostic tests necessary, not only to establish the diagnosis, but also to perform the various studies necessary to properly categorize the patient's leukemia and identify the important prognostic factors. To establish a diagnosis of leukemia, the patient must have over 25% immature cells in the marrow aspirate.

VI. DIFFERENTIAL DIAGNOSIS

Leukemia in a child is a very rare event. It has been estimated that an average pediatrician sees a new case of childhood leukemia about once every 10 years of their practice. The pediatrician will see many cases of lymphadenopathy, fever of unknown origin, or malaise before seeing a child with leukemia. Therefore, the index of suspicion must be high not to miss the diagnosis. Prompt institution of effective therapy is crucial to achieve optimal outcome.

Various nonmalignant conditions that can mimic leukemia include (1) viral infections, (2) mononucleosis/Epstein–Barr virus, (3) AIDS, (4) congenital infections (TORCH, syphilis), (5) rheumatoid arthritis, (6) multiple iron/vitamin deficiency, (7) immune cytopenia, (8) congenital cytopenia, (9) bone marrow hypoplasia/aplasia (postinfectious, drug, toxin), (10) pertussis, (11) infectious lymphocytosis, (12) leukemoid reaction (Down's syndrome), (13) osteopetrosis, and (14) hypereosinophilia.

The best way to exclude leukemia from the differential diagnosis is to perform a bone marrow examination. Delays due to prolonged evaluation searching for other causes should be avoided. Nonmalignant etiologies can be pursued after a bone marrow aspirate reassures that there is no replacement of marrow by immature cells. Once immature cells are identified, the origin of these cells must be established. Non-Hodgkin's lymphoma, neuroblastoma, rhabdomyosarcoma, Ewing sarcoma, primitive neuroectodermal tumor, retinoblastoma, and medulloblastoma are all malignancies that can metastasize the marrow and can have features resembling acute lymphoblastic leukemia. If these entities cannot be differentiated on light microscopy, histochemistry, cytogenetics, and immunophenotypic studies are usually helpful. Lymphoblastic leukemia also has to be differentiated from myelodysplastic syndrome and nonlymphoid leukemias, which present in a very similar fashion.

VII. PROGNOSTIC FACTORS

When all patients with ALL were treated similarly, it was apparent that some groups of patients had better prognosis than others. Evaluation of the outcome of thousands of patients has revealed a number of prognostic factors at diagnosis that can predict the likelihood of a favorable response to treatment in achieving remission and long-term remission duration. These factors are listed in Table I. Identification of these prognostic factors permits selection of appropriate intensity of treatment based on the patient's likelihood of a long-term outcome. Patients who are likely to have a good outcome are treated less intensively with fewer side effects, whereas patients who are at high risk of disease recurrence need to be treated more intensively to try to improve on prognosis. The predictive value of prognostic features at diagnosis on future

TABLE I
Prognostic Factors at Diagnosis of ALL

	Favorable	Unfavorable
At diagnosis		
WBC	<10,000/μl	>10,000/μl
Age	2–10 years	<1 year, >10 years
Sex	Female	Male
Hemoglobin	<10 g/dl	>10 g/dl
Platelet count	Normal	<100,000/μl
Organomegaly	Minimal	Marked
Mediastinal mass	None	Present
Lymphadenopathy	Minimal	Marked
Extramedullary disease	Absent	Present
FAB morphology	L_1	L_2, L_3
Immunoglobulins	Normal	Depressed
Surface immunoglobulin	Absent	Present
CALLA	Positive	Negative
Diploidy	Hyperdiploid	Hypo/pseudodiploid
DNA index	>1.16	<1.16
Translocation	None	t(4–11), t(8–14), t(9–22)
Race	Caucasian	Black
Infection	Absent	Present
Hemorrhage	Absent	Present
Response to therapy		
Marrow day 7	<25% blasts	>25% blasts
Marrow day 14	<5% blasts	>5% blasts

events becomes less and less the longer the patient stays in remission. By 18 months after diagnosis, even the height of the initial white count (the most significant prognostic factor at diagnosis) loses its predictive value. At that point, patients with less than a 10,000/mm^3 and patients with over a 100,000/mm^3 white blood count at diagnosis have the same chance of subsequently staying in remission. The only factor that is still prognostic for late relapse is the speed of response to therapy. Patients who are slow to go into remission, with more than 25% blasts remaining on day 7 or day 14, have a higher rate of relapse even after discontinuation of 2 or 3 years of chemotherapy than patients who respond much more rapidly.

VIII. TREATMENT

A. Strategy for Disease Control

1. Complete remission must be achieved as promptly as possible. Combination chemotherapy must be used to avoid the emergence of drug-resistant cells.

2. During remission induction therapy, intensive supportive care must be administered to prevent electrolyte and renal abnormalities due to tumor lysis and hemorrhagic and infectious complications.

3. After achieving remission, when circulating lymphoblasts are no longer present, the central nervous system must be prophylaxed. This is done either with intrathecal methotrexate alone or in combination with cranial irradiation depending on the patient's risk of central nervous system leukemia. Local treatment of any other proven extramedullary disease also needs to be addressed.

4. Maintenance therapy with combination of chemotherapy agents must then continue for a sufficient time to allow for the eradication of all disease with time to allow for the dormant leukemic cells to also go into the cell cycle in order to be eliminated. The intensity of this chemotherapy needs to be tailored to the severity of the initial prognostic factors and to the rapidity of the early response to therapy.

5. While the therapy needs to be of sufficient duration to minimize the risk of posttherapy relapse, its intensity and duration must be optimized to reduce therapy-induced complications.

6. During therapy the patient's organ functions must be monitored and therapy adjusted to minimize toxicities.

B. Risk Group Categories

Uniform age and white count criteria have been established for separating patients with B-cell precursor ALL into two cohorts based on their likelihood of disease recurrence. Criteria for standard risk and high-risk cohorts adopted by the CTEP/NCI workshop are shown in Table II. Standard risk patients are those between 1 and 10 years of age with an initial white count $<50,000/mm^3$. These patients comprise approximately 68% of the children with ALL with an 80% 4-year event-free survival. High-risk patients are infants (less than 1 year of age), patients over 10 years of age, or patients with a white count at diagnosis that was $>50,000/mm^3$. This group has about a 64% long-term event-free survival. There is no uniform risk group definition for the 15% of the patients with T-cell immunophenotype. The Children's Cancer Group considers these patients the same way as those with the B-cell precursor phenotype, dividing them into standard and high-risk groups. There are other centers who consider and treat all T-cell patients as a high risk of disease recurrence.

C. Specific Disease Control Steps

Treatment of children with leukemia should be undertaken only by a certified pediatric oncologist experienced with the various current studies at a medical center that has all the necessary supportive care staff and facilities available.

Leukemia therapy is a constantly evolving undertaking. New therapies are developed constantly, building on the best currently available therapy. These new treatments then need to be compared in a randomized prospective study to see if the anticipated better results have been achieved. Only general principles will be discussed here. These should not be used for specific treatment.

1. Remission Induction Therapy

Four weeks of vincristine, a glucocorticoid and asparaginase therapy are the minimum remission induction therapy for any patient with ALL. This will put 97 to 98% of patients into remission. Patients with a higher risk of postremission relapse are also given daunorubicin and/or adriamycin with or without cyclophosphamide during remission induction.

2. Supportive Care

See Table III.

3. Sanctuaries, Prophylaxis, and Therapy

The most frequent sanctuary site involved with leukemia is the central nervous system (5%), followed by the testes. An occasional patient may also have

TABLE II

Risk Categories For B-Cell Precursor ALL Patients

Risk	Definition	4-year EFS[a] (%)	B-cell precursor Patients (%)
Standard	WBC <50,000 and age 1.00–9.99 years	80.3	68
High	WBC ≥ 50,000 or age ≥ 10.00 years	63.9	32

[a]EFS, adverse event free survival.

TABLE III

Supportive Therapy for Complications of ALL

Complication	Therapy
Metabolic	
Hyperuricemia	Allopurinol, hydration, alkalinization
Hyperkalemia	No IV K+, alkalinization, glucose/insulin, Kayexalate, dialysis
Hyperphosphatemia	Low-phosphate diet, Amphojel
Hypocalcemia	Replacement
Hypercalcemia	Fluids, calcitonin, pamidronate
Lactic acidosis	Fluids, electrolyte replacement
Hematologic	
Hyperleukocytosis	Hydration, do not correct anemia, leukophoresis/exchange transfusion
Anemia	Transfusion (all blood products should be filtered and irradiated)
Thrombocytopenia	Platelets, aminocaproic acid
Hypofibrinogenemia	Fresh frozen plasma, cryoprecipitate
Prolonged PT	Vitamin K, factor replacement
Granulocytopenia	Broad-spectrum antibiotics if febrile
Thrombosis	Heparin, fresh frozen plasma
Infectious	
Bacterial	Broad-spectrum antibiotics if febrile
Fungal	Nystatin, fluconazole, amphotericin
Viral (VZ)	Acyclovir, zoster immune globulin
Opportunistic	Trimethoprim/sulfa, pentamidine

leukemic involvement of the anterior chamber of the eye or have skin infiltration with leukemic cells. All these sanctuaries need local irradiation therapy because systemic chemotherapy does not adequately penetrate these sites to reliably eradicate the leukemic cells.

Even when the spinal fluid is clear of leukemic cells at diagnosis, the CNS must receive prophylactic therapy. When this is not done, over 50% of the patients will have disease recurrence in the CNS.

4. Central Nervous System Prophylaxis

Patients with no evidence of meningeal leukemia at diagnosis are given intrathecal methotrexate on days 0, 7 and 28 of induction; after remission is achieved, four weekly intrathecal doses are given during the next month of treatment. The dose of intrathecal methotrexate needs to be adjusted for the volume of the spinal fluid, which varies with the age of the patient. Some groups, in addition to intrathecal methotrexate, will add intrathecal cytarabine and hydrocortisone in similar frequency and age-adjusted doses. Attempts to prophylaxis the central nervous system with moderate to high doses of methotrexate have not been successful. Patients at very high risk of CNS recurrence need cranial irradiation in addition to intrathecal methotrexate for adequate prophylaxis. Cranial irradiation needs to be reserved for the very highest risk group because of its potential neurotoxicity and other late effects.

CNS prophylaxis must be repeated after each bone marrow relapse because of the potential reseeding of the meninges after each disease recurrence.

5. Continuation of Treatment for Standard Risk Patients

Remission maintenance chemotherapy for 2 to 3 years is administered with daily oral 6-mercaptopurine. Weekly methotrexate is also given orally, intravenously, or intramuscularly. Every 4 weeks a dose of intravenous vincristine accompanied by 5 days of oral glucocorticoids is administered. This treatment is interrupted after 2 months for one or two cycles of reinduction–reintensification therapy.

The duration of continuation treatment recommended for boys is 3 years and is 2 years for girls.

6. Additional Treatment for High-Risk Patients

Remission induction and consolidation are followed for 4 to 7 weeks with four to eight drugs. This is followed by central nervous system prophylaxis with an age-adjusted dose schedule of methotrexate or triple therapy during induction and consolidation with a minimum of seven doses over the first 2 months of treatment. Periodic intrathecal therapy during the remission maintenance treatment has an added benefit. Cranial irradiation is given to those at very high risk of CNS disease.

Cycles of remission consolidation and periodic reinduction reintensification therapy similar to induction treatment follow remission induction for the first 6 to 12 months of treatment. Continuation treatment of high-risk patients must include intensive multiagent chemotherapy with rotation of drugs with different modes of action and with agents to which leukemic cells show different patterns of potential resistance. Treatment lasting 2 years for girls and 3 years for boys postremission induction is recommended. For boys, 2 years may be sufficient with very intensive treatment. Assessment of response to therapy should be done 7 to 14 days after initiation of therapy. Fast early responders will have less than 25% remaining lymphoblasts by day 7 of treatment. By day 14 there should be less than 5% blasts in the marrow. Patients who clear their lymphoblasts slower need more intensive treatment. Only these patients, those with WBC over 200,000/mm^3 at diagnosis, and those with adverse cytogenetics should be considered for possible bone marrow transplant in first remission and only if they have a matched sibling donor identified.

IX. FUTURE DIRECTIONS

Over the last 30 to 40 years the outlook of children with ALL has improved from having a uniformly fatal disease to an overall long-term disease-free survival of close to 80%. We still need to improve our ability to detect minimal residual disease, determine if there are any drug-resistant cells in the body and their location, and identify patients who are destined to relapse so that we can change their therapy and eradicate their disease. Therapies need to be tailored with more precision to the expected prognosis of the patient to maximize effectiveness while minimizing the short- and long-term consequences of treatment.

See Also the Following Articles

ACUTE MYELOCYTIC LEUKEMIA • ALL-1 • CHRONIC MYELOGENOUS LEUKEMIA • LYMPHOMA, HODGKIN'S DISEASE • LYMPHOMA, NON-HODGKIN'S • MONOCLONAL ANTIBODIES: LEUKEMIA AND LYMPHOMA

Bibliography

Childhood ALL Collaborative Group (1996). Duration and intensity of maintenance chemotherapy in acute lymphoblastic leukemia: Overview of 42 trials involving 12,000 randomised children. *Lancet* **347,** 1783–1788.

Dunsmore, K. P. (1999). Acute lymphoblastic leukemia in the adolescent: Diagnosis, treatment, and outcome. *Adolesc. Med.* **10**(3), 407–417.

Felix, C. A., and Lange, B. J. (1999). Leukemia in infants. *Oncologist* **4**(3), 225–240.

Gaynon, P., Qu, R. P., Chappell, R. J., Willoughby, M., Tubergen, D., Steinherz, P. G., and Trigg, M. (1998). Survival after relapse in childhood acute lymphoblastic leukemia: Impact of time to first relapse, the Children's Cancer Group Experience. *Cancer* **82,** 1387–1395.

Poplock, D. G. (1997). Acute Lymphoblastic Leukemia in Principles and Practice of Pediatric Oncology (P. Pizzo and P. G. Poplock, eds.), pp. 409–463. Lippicott-Raven, New York.

Pui, C. H. (2000). Acute lymphoblastic leukemia in children. *Curr. Opin. Oncol.* **12**(1), 3–12.

Pui, C. H., and Evans, W. E. (1998). Acute lymphoblastic leukemia. *N. Engl. J. Med.* **339**(9), 605–615.

Radich, J. P. (2000). Clinical applicability of the evaluation of minimal residual disease in acute leukemia. *Curr. Opin. Oncol.* **12**(1), 3–12.

Smith, M., Arthur, D., Camitta, B., *et al.* (1996). Uniform approach to risk classification and treatment assignment for children with acute lymphoblastic leukemia. *J. Clin. Oncol.* **14,** 18–24.

Steinherz, P. G., Gaynon, P. S., Breneman, J. C., Cherlow, J. M., Grossman, N. J., Kersey, J. H., Johnstone, H. S., Sather, H. N., Trigg, M. E., Hammond, D., and Bleyer, W. A. (1996). Cytoreduction and prognosis in acute lymphoblastic leukemia: The importance of rapid early response. Report from the Childrens Cancer Group. *J. Clin. Oncol.* **14,** 389–398.

Steinherz, P. G., Gaynon, P. S., Breneman, J. C., Cherlow, J. M., Grossman, N. J., Kersey, J. H., Johnstone, H. S., Sather, H. N., Trigg, M. E., Uckun, F., and Bleyer, W. A. (1998). Treatment of acute lymphoblastic leukemia with bulky extramedullary disease and T cell phenotype or other poor prognostic features, Randomized Controlled Trial from the Childrens Cancer Group. *Cancer* **82,** 600–612.

Steinherz, P. G., Redner, A., Steinherz, L., Meyers, P., Tan, C., and Heller, G. (1993). Development of a new intensive therapy for the treatment of acute lymphoblastic leukemia in children at increased risk of early relapse: The MSK New York II protocol. *Cancer* **72,** 3120–3130.

Uckun, F. M., Sensel, M. G., Waddick, K. G., Steinherz, P. G., Trigg, M. E., Heerema, N. A., Sather, H. N., Reaman, G. H., and Gaynon, P. S. (1998). Biology and treatment of childhood T-lineage acute lymphoblastic leukemia. *Blood* **91,** 735–747.

Acute Myelocytic Leukemia

Peter H. Wiernik

Our Lady of Mercy Comprehensive Cancer Center, New York Medical College

I. Etiology
II. Clinical Presentation
III. Treatment

GLOSSARY

allogeneic bone marrow transplantation The donor of marrow cells is an individual other than the recipient.

autologous bone marrow transplantation Marrow cells are obtained from a donor and stored frozen. After the donor is treated, he or she becomes the recipient of the marrow cells when they are reinfused intravenously.

bone marrow aspirate Marrow material obtained by negative pressure on a syringe attached to a needle that has been introduced into the bone marrow cavity.

bone marrow biopsy A surgical specimen obtained by cutting through bone consisting of bone and bone marrow.

cytogenetic translocation A section of one arm of a chromosome is physically attached to another, usually in reciprocal fashion.

A cute myelocytic leukemia (AML) is a neoplasm of the bone marrow of largely unknown etiology that occurs primarily in adults. It is usually a rapidly progressive disease if not treated. Proliferation of malignant cells within the bone marrow compromises normal marrow function and results in susceptibility to infection due to progressive granulocytopenia and bleeding secondary to thrombocytopenia, as well as lassitude due to anemia.

A number of gene rearrangements have been identified in certain subtypes of AML (Table I) that have prognostic import and may dictate therapy. With proper supportive care to prevent and treat infection and hemorrhage, treatment will render the majority of patients disease free, and cure will be obtained in approximately one-third of patients who respond to treatment with a complete remission.

I. ETIOLOGY

A. Environmental Factors

Acute myelocytic leukemia is the most common acute leukemia in the immediate postnatal period, but the vast majority of cases occur in adults in which the

TABLE I
Abbreviated French–American–British (FAB) Classification of AML

Subtype	Morphology	Cytochemistry[a]	Cytogenetics	Immunophenotype
M0	No cytoplasmic granules	POX−	Abnormal, variable	POX+, CD33+ CD34+, HLA-DR+
M1	Occasional cytoplasmic granules	Few cells POX+	−7 or t(9;22) or other abnormalities	Same as M0
M2	Most cells granulated. Many immature cells beyond the promyelocyte stage. Auer rods may be seen	Strongly POX+	t(8;21) frequent	Same as M0
M3	Most cells are hypergranulated	Strongly POX+	t(15;17)	CD34− HLA-DR−
M4	Immature myeloid and monocytic precursors. Abnormal eosinophils may be seen	Strongly POX+ May be PAS+	11q23 abnormalities inv(16) or t(16;16) if eosinophils involved	CD11b+, POX+
M5	Immature monocytes predominate	Same as M4, plus nonspecific esterase+	11q3 abnormalities	CD11b+ POX− CD34−
M6	Megaloblastoid erythroid precursors predominate	PAS+, ringed sideroblasts	Abnormal, complex	CD34− HLA-DR− Glycophorin A+
M7	Variable morphology	Platelet POX+ by electron microscopy	T(1;22)	CD41+ CD42+ CD36+

[a]POX, myeloperoxidase; PAS, periodic acid–Schiff reagent.

incidence increases with each decade of life. AML occurs with roughly equal frequency (approximately two to three cases per 100,000 population) throughout the world, but is more common in urban and industrialized areas. Its cause is largely unknown, but ionizing radiation can be an etiologic factor, as evidenced by the increased and dose-related incidence of AML in Japan after the atomic bomb blasts. The increased incidence of AML in jet cockpit crew members with extensive flying hours is thought to result from exposure to cosmic irradiation. Exposure to high concentrations of benzene in the air for prolonged periods of time has been demonstrated to be a cause of AML among certain unprotected workers. Smoking is associated with a higher incidence of AML, possibly due to increased benzene exposure. Some drugs used to treat cancer, such as alkylating agents and topoisomerase II inhibitors, have been associated with a small but definite increased incidence of AML in cancer survivors.

B. Genetic Factors

Certain hereditary factors are known to be associated with an increased risk for acute leukemia. The sibling of a child with acute leukemia has a slightly increased relative risk of developing acute leukemia, but an identical twin of a child with acute leukemia has a relative risk on the order of 350. The relative risk for a child with Down's syndrome is a log less, and half the cases are AML. Other rare diseases with characteristic cytogenetic abnormalities, such as Fanconi's anemia, ataxia telangiectasia, and Bloom's syndrome, are associated with relative risks for acute leukemia of approximately 2000, 25,000, and >30,000, respectively.

C. Genetic Alterations and Chromosome Rearrangements

A large number of chromosome deletions, balanced translocations, and other alterations occur in AML.

In some cases, known genes are fused and produce unique products that play a role in the pathogenesis of AML. Many translocations and deletions are associated with a specific prognosis, primarily because they confer increased sensitivity to certain antileukemic agents. Indeed, some treatments are only effective in patients with certain specific cytogenetic alterations.

Monosomy 5 or 7 and deletions of those chromosomes are associated with a poor prognosis and are frequently found in patients with AML secondary to prior treatment with alkylating agents for a previous neoplasm. In del(5q), the arm of chromosome 5 on which the genes for a number of hematopoietic growth factors and their receptors are located is deleted. The absence of those genes is thought to be relevant to the pathogenesis of the disease and its poor response to treatment. AML associated with exposure to topoisomerase II inhibitors frequently harbor 11q23 abnormalities.

Several important balanced cytogenetic translocations that influence prognosis and response to therapy in patients with AML have been identified. Approximately 10% of patients with the M2 subtype, which is found in 35–40% of all patients with AML, have t(8;21)(q22;q22), which results in a fusion gene formed by AML1 and MTG8. Most, but not all, patients with this translocation are adolescents or young adults and have an excellent response to chemotherapy. Molecular quantitation of minimal residual disease by reverse transcription polymerase chain reaction methods in patients with t(8;21) can identify those destined to relapse after a complete response to initial treatment. Such information is useful in determining when to discontinue therapy in apparent complete responders.

Patients with acute promyelocytic leukemia (M3) have the t(15;17)(q24;q21) translocation, which involves the retinoic acid receptor-α gene and the PML gene. Two new fusion genes result from the translocation: PML/RARα on chromosome 15 and RARα/PML on chromosome 17. Patients with t(15;17) are extremely responsive to treatment with all-*trans* retinoic acid, which induces maturation and differentiation in leukemic cells with this translocation. M3 patients are also highly sensitive to anthracycline antibiotics commonly used in the treatment of acute leukemia and therefore have an excellent prognosis in general. Reverse transcription polymerase chain reaction techniques are also used in this form of AML to determine the quality of the response to treatment and detect early relapse at the molecular level.

Translocation t(16;16)(p13;q22) or inv(16)(p13;q22) is found in patients with acute myelomonocytic leukemia (M4) and abnormal eosinophils in blood and bone marrow. M4 accounts for less than 10% of AML and is most commonly found in patients aged 35 to 50 years. This translocation or inversion involves MYH11 and CBFβ genes. The latter codes for the β subunit of core-binding factor and is a known important transcription factor in murine leukemogenesis. Patients with inv(16) or t(16;16) have an excellent response to therapy, primarily because they are especially sensitive to cytosine arabinoside, a standard agent for the treatment of AML. Such patients do, however, have an increased incidence of central nervous system leukemic infiltration.

Many other chromosomal translocations and other aberrations are known to occur in patients with AML, but less is known about them at the molecular level, and their influence on prognosis is less clear due to their infrequent occurrence.

II. CLINICAL PRESENTATION

A. Physical Findings

The two major reasons why patients with AML seek medical attention are bleeding and/or bacterial infection. Hemorrhage is usually minor, consisting of capillary bleeding (petechiae) on dependent body parts, secondary to thrombocytopenia. However, nose bleeds, gingival bleeding while brushing the teeth, or more serious bleeding may be present. On occasion, life-threatening hemorrhage may occur, especially with the M3 subtype in which a disseminated intravascular coagulopathy commonly occurs principally due to production of a clotting factor V-like substance by the leukemic cells. Bacterial pneumonia, pharyngitis, or perirectal abscess may be present at diagnosis due to severe granulocytopenia. There are usually few additional findings on physical examination. Lymphadenopathy and splenomegaly, common in acute lymphocytic leukemia (ALL), are uncommon in AML. Small, raised painless leukemic infiltrates (leukemia cutis) may be found, and patients with a monocytic subtype of AML (M4 or M5) may have gingival hypertrophy secondary to leukemic infiltration, which may be of such magnitude as to virtually obscure the teeth.

B. Laboratory Diagnosis

Routine blood counts reveal a normal, low, or elevated white blood cell count in an equal number of patients. Anemia is usually moderate unless significant bleeding has occurred, in which case it may be severe. The platelet count is usually severely reduced. Immature myeloid blast cells diagnostic of AML are almost always seen on routinely stained peripheral blood smears, but occasionally none are evident. Such patients are usually leukopenic and, like all others with AML, usually have reduced numbers of normal granulocytes on blood smears. Leukemic cells vary considerably from cell to cell in size, shape, and nuclear and cytoplasmic characteristics in AML, unlike the cells of ALL. Myeloid leukemic blasts are usually larger than the blast cells of ALL, and their abundant cytoplasm usually contains granules (lysosomes) readily identified with routine stains under the microscope (M1, M2, or M3). Rarely, such granules may not be visible on routine smears and found only with flow cytometric techniques employing a monoclonal antibody to myeloperoxidase, or electron microscopy (M0). Such patients have a poor response to treatment. On occasion, dense cytoplasmic granulation characteristic of M3 will be seen. In a minority of patients, abnormal granulation in the form of elongated rods (Auer rods) will be detected, especially in patients with M2 or M3 (Fig. 1), and such patients have a relatively good response to treatment. Typically the cytoplasm of leukemic cells in AML does not stain with the periodic acid–Schiff reagent, which usually stains the cytoplasm of leukemia cells in ALL, whereas Sudan black B usually stains the cytoplasm of leukemic cells in AML but not in ALL. Leukemic cells with morphologic features of a monocytic lineage (such as twisted or folded nuclei) are designated M4 or M5, depending on the maturity of the cells, and leukemic cells of erythroid lineage are designated M6. A rare

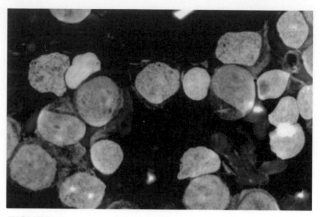

FIGURE 1 Wright's stained bone marrow aspirate from a patient with AML M2. The red, elongated structures in the cytoplasm of many cells are Auer rods, which are sometimes seen in patients with M2 or M3. Auer rods are elongated lysosomes. They are never seen in acute lymphocytic leukemia, but may be found in mature granulocytes of fetal blood.

megakaryocytic form of the disease (M7) cannot be identified morphologically and requires immunophenotyping for diagnosis. Such patients have an extremely poor prognosis.

Blood chemistry studies usually indicate mild or moderate hyperuricemia due to increased cell turnover, and patients with monocytic morphology (M4 or M5) usually have elevated serum lactic dehydrogenase and lysozyme activity.

The surface antigen HLA-DR and the transmembrane molecule, p-glycoprotein (which interferes with the accumulation of certain antileukemic agents within the leukemic cell), are rarely found in M3. HLA-DR is common in virtually all other AML subtypes. P-glycoprotein is present in approximately one-third of newly diagnosed and two-thirds of previously treated AML patients with other than M3.

In patients with AML, immunophenotyping discloses that the leukemic cells are usually devoid of terminal deoxynucleotidyl transferase (found in ALL) and have myeloid antigens on the cell surface and no lymphoid antigens. Results of cytogenetic and immunophenotyping studies establish the diagnosis of leukemia, allow for the distinction between AML and other forms of leukemia, which may not be possible on the basis of morphology alone, and are essential in determining the subtype of AML.

C. Bone Marrow Examination

It is necessary to examine the bone marrow in all patients with AML at the time of diagnosis whether or not blast forms are present in the peripheral blood. This is done by introducing a special needle percutaneously into the bone marrow cavity of the posterior iliac crest or of the sternum. A few drops of marrow can usually be aspirated by negative pressure into a syringe attached to the needle and then thinly smeared on glass slides. The slides are air dried and then stained with certain dyes that facilitate morphologic and histochemical assessment of individual cells and their components under the microscope. Aspirated marrow is superior to blood for cytogenetic and immunophenotyping studies.

In addition to a marrow aspirate, a bone marrow core biopsy is obtained to determine the cellularity of the marrow and whether marrow fibrosis or necrosis is present. Usually the marrow is hypercellular in AML with little normal marrow fat dispersed among hematopoietic elements. However, in older patients or in those whose leukemia is radiation or chemically induced, the marrow is often hypocellular.

III. TREATMENT

A. General

The treatment of hematologic malignancies includes relatively specific antineoplastic treatment and supportive care. Supportive care includes antiemetics for the prevention of nausea and vomiting that frequently result from chemotherapy. Empiric broad-spectrum antibiotic therapy is frequently required for fever and granulocytopenia, with the latter due to leukemia and/or intensive cytotoxic therapy. Recombinant human hematopoietic growth factors such as erythropoietin, granulocyte–macrophage colony-stimulating factor, or granulocyte colony-stimulating factor are frequently given for chronic anemia or acute granulocytopenia, respectively. Recombinant human thrombopoietin is currently in clinical trials. Erythropoietin administration will, in some patients, reduce the need for blood transfusion during treatment, and granulocyte or granulocyte–macrophage colony-stimulating factor will often accelerate recovery of the peripheral blood granulocyte count to a safe level ($>500/\mu$l). A xanthine oxidase inhibitor such as allopurinol is given prior to and during chemotherapy to prevent urate nephropathy, which may result from rapid cell kill with effective therapy. Prophylactic platelet transfusions are administered frequently during treatment and recovery to maintain the blood platelet count at a level sufficient to prevent thrombocytopenic hemorrhage, usually above 15,000–20,000/μl. Packed red blood cell transfusions are given to maintain a hematocrit above 25%. Granulocytes may be transfused from a compatible donor when the patient has a serious infection with an identified organism that is not responding to appropriate antibiotics and, because of leukemia or its treatment, bone marrow recovery is not imminent.

B. Chemotherapy

Initial (induction) therapy for AML other than subtype M3 usually consists of the synthetic pyrimidine nucleoside, cytosine arabinoside, given as a continuous 7-day infusion and an anthracycline antibiotic such as daunorubicin or idarubicin given daily for the first 3 days of the 7-day treatment. Approximately 65% of all adults and 75% of children will achieve a complete remission with this regimen, defined as a normalization of the blood, bone marrow, karyotype, and physical examination. As discussed earlier, studies at the molecular level may disclose minimal residual disease not otherwise detectable at this point. Clinical trials are underway to determine how best to deal with positive molecular tests during clinical, hematologic, and cytogenetic remission.

After complete remission is achieved, further treatment (consolidation therapy) is given in an effort to treat residual disease that cannot be detected clinically. Cytosine arabinoside in doses 20- to 30-fold higher than those used during induction therapy is usually given alone in this phase in bolus doses twice a day, every other day for a total of 12 doses. Such courses may be repeated at intervals of 1 or 2 months, several times. The median disease-free survival with this regimen is approximately 18 months, and at least 30% of adults and 40% of children who achieve complete remission are cured.

Allogeneic or autologous bone marrow transplantation with high-dose chemotherapy alone or with total body irradiation is considered for patients with poor prognostic factors for long-term disease-free survival, such as those with the M0, M6, or M7 subtype and those with cytogenetic abnormalities other than t(8;21), t(16;16), inv(16), or t(15;17). Transplantation is also considered for relapsed patients who have obtained a second complete remission with chemotherapy, as such patients are rarely cured with additional conventional treatment. However, bone marrow transplantation is usually not feasible for patients over the age of 60 years because of its toxicity. An additional impediment to allogeneic transplantation is the fact that results are best with an HLA-compatible sibling donor, although transplants utilizing matched, unrelated donors are being employed by some centers with limited success.

Central nervous system (CNS) leukemia occasionally complicates the presentation of patients with AML subtype M4 and t(16;16) or inv(16). Specific treatment is usually not necessary, as therapeutic levels of cytosine arabinoside are achieved in the central nervous system when the drug is given intravenously during induction therapy. On occasion, central nervous system involvement occurs before or during systemic relapse. This problem is more common in ALL than in AML and in children with AML than in adults. It responds to direct injection of antileukemic drugs into the cerebrospinal fluid because the disease is usually confined to the meninges. Methotrexate, a dihydrofolate reductase inhibitor, or cytosine arabinoside is used for this purpose. Although CNS relapse is likely, intrathecal administration of chemotherapeutic agents usually eradicates signs and symptoms of CNS leukemia for several months or more. On the rare occasion when CNS leukemia may occur deep in the brain, cranial irradiation may be required for its control.

For patients with acute promyelocytic leukemia (M3), induction therapy usually consists of an anthracycline antibiotic and the differentiation-inducing agent, all-*trans* retinoic acid. This type of AML is highly sensitive to anthracyclines, and the gene rearrangements that characterize it are specifically treated with the retinoid. After complete remission is achieved, consolidation therapy similar to that employed for other subtypes of AML is given. In addition, all-*trans* retinoic acid treatment is continued, usually for years. At least 70% of patients with M3 AML will achieve a complete remission with this treatment, and the median duration of complete remission is in excess of 2 years in recent studies. At least 40% of patients are cured. However, unlike other patients with AML, 10–15% of patients with the M3 subtype will die of hemorrhage shortly after the diagnosis as a result of clotting factor deficiencies. Most fatal hemorrhages are intracerebral, for unknown reasons. Some authorities recommend prophylactic heparinization immediately after the diagnosis in those patients with low plasma fibrinogen levels to prevent further consumption of coagulation factors.

It may be possible to discontinue postremission therapy in patients with M3 AML if a sensitive reverse transcription polymerase chain reaction technique cannot detect the PML/RARα fusion gene product in a bone marrow aspirate.

Patients with M3 AML who relapse usually achieve a second complete remission with arsenic trioxide. Once a second remission is confirmed, bone marrow transplantation may be offered to appropriate candidates.

See Also the Following Articles

Acute Lymphoblastic Leukemia in Adults • Acute Lymphoblastic Leukemia in Children • Chronic Lymphocytic Leukemia • Chronic Myelogenous Leukemia • Monoclonal Antibodies: Leukemia and Lymphoma

Bibliography

Hoffman, R., Benz, E. J., Jr., Shattil, S. J., *et al.* (2000). "Hematology Basic Principles and Practice," 3rd Ed. Churchill Livingstone, New York.

Holland, J. F., and Frei, E., III (2000). "Cancer Medicine," 5th Ed. Decker, Hamilton.

Lee, R. G., Foerster, J., and Lukens, J., *et al.* (1999). "Wintrobe's Clinical Hematology," 10th Ed. Lippincott Williams and Wilkins, Philadelphia.

Pecham, M., Pinedo, H. M., and Veronesi, U. (1995). "Oxford Text Book of Oncology." Oxford Univ. Press, Oxford.

Wiernik, P. H., Canellos, G. P., Dutcher, J. P., and Kyle, R. A. (1996). "Neoplastic Diseases of the Blood." Churchill Livingstone, New York.

Adeno-Associated Virus: A Vector for High-Efficiency Gene Transduction

Kevin W. Page
Jane S. Lebkowski

Applied Immune Sciences, Inc., Santa Clara, California

GLOSSARY

helicase An enzyme that is able to unwind the DNA α-helix.

immunogenicity The property that endows a substance with the capacity to provoke an immune response.

intron A noncoding intervening sequence within a gene.

Numerous gene therapy strategies and protocols have been devised for the treatment of cancer. These strategies involve the augmentation of immune function, the repression of tumors with anti-oncogenes, and the induction of specific immune responses through vaccination and other therapeutic modalities. For each of these approaches, efficient transfer of the therapeutic gene into the target cells is required. Adeno-associated virus (AAV) is a small DNA virus which can be genetically manipulated to deliver genes into a variety of cells including cancer cells and cells of the immune system. This review details the research and potential clinical utility of AAV as a general transducing vector for the modification of cells for the treatment of a variety of disease states including globin disorders, AIDS, and some cancers.

I. INTRODUCTION

AAV was observed initially by electron microscopy as a contaminant in preparations of adenovirus in the late 1950s and was thought to be either a precursor or breakdown product of adenovirus replication. By the mid 1960s several researchers had determined AAV to be a distinct, but defective, virus where coinfection with a helper virus was necessary for viable AAV production. Although Herpes simplex virus (HSV) has been used successfully as a helper virus in the laboratory, AAV has only been isolated from people and animals suffering adenovirus infections. It remains to be shown if herpes viruses act as helpers in nature.

AAV has a very wide host range and to date has infected every cell line tested. The virus will replicate if coinfected with an adenovirus specific to the cell and species type used. For instance, human AAV will replicate in canine cells infected with canine adenovirus. AAV infection is widespread; 85% of Americans are seropositive for AAV. However, the virus has never been associated with any pathological effect and may even have positive benefits to the human host (see Section III).

II. AAV BIOLOGY

AAV is a member of the Parvoviridae virus family. It is a small single-stranded DNA virus 20–24 nm in di-

ameter. The type 2 AAV genome has been completely sequenced and is 4682 base pairs (bp) in length. Both minus and sense strands are packaged into virions. The genome structure and messenger RNA (mRNA) transcription units are shown in Fig. 1. At each end of the genome is a 145-bp inverted terminal repeat (ITR), of which the 5′ 125 bp form a palindrome. These sequences contain two 21-bp palindromes at bases 41–84, which give a predicted T-shaped structure when maximum base pairing occurs. At least one cis-acting ITR is required for the priming of AAV viral DNA replication.

The AAV genome has a very efficient protein coding strategy; mRNA synthesis is initiated at three internal promoters at map positions 5, 19, and 40. Because of different mRNA splicing patterns due to the presence of two overlapping introns, seven mature mRNAs and protein products have been identified (Fig. 1). The left-hand end of the genome codes for four protein products (collectively known as Rep) with molecular masses of 78, 68, 52, and 40 kDa. These proteins are involved in the replication of the AAV genome. Studies have shown that Rep78 and Rep68 bind to the AAV ITR, and mutations in the Rep gene that inhibit ITR binding have been mapped to the amino-terminal portion of the gene. Other ac-

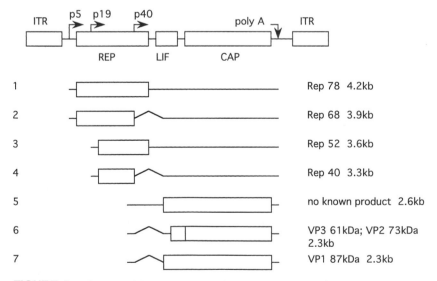

FIGURE 1 Schematic of the AAV genome. (Top) The viral open reading frames. Bent arrows show the position of the promoters and the downward bent arrow indicates the common polyadenylation sites. (Bottom) The mRNA species are represented with the coding sequence boxed. The protein products are listed on the right, as are the mRNA lengths. mRNA 6 encodes both VP3 and VP2, which is initiated from an ACG start codon located upstream of VP3.

tivities attributed to Rep are helicase activity and site-specific endonuclease activity at the terminal resolution site (trs) on the AAV genome (Fig. 2). This procedure is an essential step in DNA replication where the AAV origin of DNA replication is nicked at a specific site in an ATP-dependent manner. Endonuclease activity of Rep68 has been shown to depend on ITR secondary structure and on specific sequence elements at the trs. Recent evidence shows that Rep binds to a sequence within the locus for AAV DNA integration on human chromosome 19, and is required for site-specific integration. Rep also appears to auto-downregulate its own expression from promoters p5 and p19; however, infection with the adenovirus helper overcomes this effect and allows production of larger amounts of Rep which is then able to transactivate the capsid gene p40 promoter and thereby allow a productive AAV infection. Rep has also been shown to mediate suppression of cellu-

lar proliferation during an AAV infection. Rep52 and Rep40 do not appear to function in AAV DNA replication, but do have other *in vitro* effects, including the inhibition of heterologous promoters and the generation of single-stranded progeny.

Proteins from several regions of the obligate helper adenovirus are also involved in AAV replication. The adenovirus E1A region is required for AAV transcription as the E1A gene products bind to sequence elements near the AAV p5 promoter. The adenovirus major late transcription factor also binds in this same region and, together with E1A, increases p5 gene product expression. The E2A 72-kDa DNA-binding protein (DBP) is involved in posttranslational expression of AAV as absence of DBP greatly reduces the amounts of Rep and Cap synthesized and the yield of infectious AAV. The E1B 55-kDa protein and the E4 region 34-kDa protein are required for the efficient accumulation of AAV mRNA, proteins, and DNA. The E1B 55-kDa protein is also required for the rescue of integrated AAV genomes in infected cell lines. Adenovirus RNA VAI and VAII sequences help stimulate translation of AAV mRNA. In conjunction with DBP, they regulate capsid protein synthesis by increasing the steady-state level of transcripts in the cytoplasm, especially the spliced species, and by enhancing translation. None of the adenovirus gene products seem to function in actual AAV DNA replication, but appear involved at the transcription and translation level. Much of the detail of how these and other proteins interact to stimulate and regulate virus production remains to be elucidated. Cellular gene products may play a role in AAV replication and production. Cells treated with chemical carcinogens can replicate AAV DNA at low levels without the presence of helper virus.

The 3' half of the AAV genome contains the Capsid (Cap) gene. By making use of various spliced and unspliced mRNA species and alternative initiation codons (Fig. 1), this sequence encodes the proteins VP1, VP2, and VP3 with molecular masses of 90, 72, and 60 kDa, respectively. These three proteins are the structural proteins and form the icosahedral capsid which encapsulates the AAV genome.

The current model for AAV DNA replication is presented in Fig. 2. The ITRs act as primers to initiate DNA synthesis, followed by a series of successive

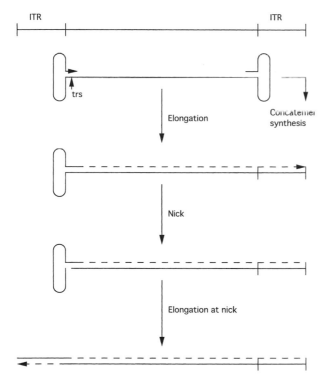

FIGURE 2 Schematic of AAV DNA replications. Solid lines represent the parental viral genome and the newly synthesized DNA is shown as hatched lines. The terminal resolution site (trs), where nicking occurs, is marked with an arrow. This is a simplified model as the parental genome can assume several initial structural forms and concatemers can also be synthesized.

elongation, nicking, and helicase steps. First the terminal palindrome acts as a primer for the synthesis of the linear duplex with one end open and the other covalently closed. The Rep protein nicks the parental strand at the trs and the strand is repaired using the palindrome as a template. This step is accomplished by an inversion of the orientation of the palindrome and extension of the 3′ strand. This process resolves the closed end and can proceed in the absence of adenovirus helper functions. The end of the double strand is denatured with a double hairpin generated followed by strand displacement, separation, and packaging of the single-strand progeny. As the ITRs have common sequences, extensive repair of deleted and mutated sequences is possible and has been observed.

If no helper virus is present, AAV enters a latent infection cycle where the viral genome integrates into the host cellular DNA. Once integrated, no AAV DNA synthesis can be detected. The AAV genome integrates at its molecular ends in the form of a tandem repeat often in head to head or tail to tail orientations by a process of illegitimate recombination. This process is not totally accurate; mutations sometimes occur at the virus–cellular junctions. Therefore, the tandem structure may be a mechanism for ensuring that a correct ITR is present. Under certain conditions in some cell types, the site of integration is not a random process; a high percentage of genomes integrate in the Iq region of chromosome 19. It appears that this process is controlled by Rep which has binding specificities for both the ITR and the chromosome 19 integration site. However, in other studies using AAV-infected Hela cells the site of integration appears to be on chromosome 17. To fully understand the integration strategies of AAV, more work is necessary to completely elucidate the mechanism and targeting of the recombination events. After integration, latent infection in tissue culture can persist for many months and viable AAV can be rescued by superinfection with adenovirus.

III. NATURAL INHIBITION OF TUMORIGENESIS

In a study done in the 1970s, serum antibody titers were determined for HSV type II and AAV in pa-

tients suffering carcinoma of either the cervix or the prostate, both epidemiologically linked to HSV type II. The normal controls were >85% seropositive for both viruses. However, the cancer patients were still >85% seropositive for HSV type II but only 14% seropositive for AAV. These epidemiological data suggest that latent AAV could be directly or indirectly protective for virally induced oncogenesis.

Most further evidence for this inhibition comes from *in vitro* and clinical studies. Early work showed that AAV could inhibit adenovirus transformation in rodents. In 1968, experiments using neonatal Syrian hamsters showed that AAV could inhibit adenovirus oncogenicity. In control animals injected with Ad 12, animals developed tumors in 26 out of 43 cases, with a mean latent period of 45 days. Animals receiving a mixture of Ad 12 and AAV had an increased mean latent period of over 60 days and only 12 out of 58 animals developed tumors. In another experiment, AAV infection was shown to reduce HSV amplification of SV40 DNA in SV40-transformed cell lines. In addition, the transforming ability of bovine papilloma virus was inhibited by AAV and this activity was mapped to Rep78. The oncosuppression function of Rep78 was investigated further using mutant Rep78 and was shown to be associated with the amino third of this protein.

Cellular transformation can also be inhibited by AAV infection. NIH 3T3 cells, a mouse fibroblast line, were transfected with the ras gene causing transformation. The subsequent cell growth rate was measured. If these transformed cells were infected with AAV, the growth rate was reduced. Furthermore, Hela cells were found to be more sensitive to gamma rays when infected with AAV, suggesting a suppressive effect of AAV on transformation. Wild-type AAV infection of HL60 cells, a leukemia line, was shown to upregulate differentiation-associated antigen and downregulate c-myc and c-myb oncogenes, suggesting a possible mechanism for AAV oncosuppression. Similar effects of AAV latent infection were highlighted by several reports which indicate that AAV could inhibit HIV-1 replication *in vitro* by Rep binding to the transactivating Tat protein. AAV through Rep gene mediation has been shown to downregulate the expression of heterologous sequences driven by the HIV LTR in the absence of Tat and also the inhibition of an HIV proviral clone as measured by reverse transcriptase activity and HIV p24 levels. HIV transcription levels were also decreased when the Rep gene was transfected into HIV-infected cells. Interestingly, human herpes virus 6, a common coinfection in HIV-infected CD4$^+$ T cells, has been shown to incorporate the AAV Rep gene into its own genome by heterologous recombination.

IV. GENE TRANSDUCTION

AAV has several features that make it an attractive candidate as a viral gene transduction vector. AAV is endogenous to humans and has never been associated with disease. As most humans are seropositive for AAV, severe viremia is unlikely, in contrast to other vectors such as vaccinia virus. The virus uncoats in the nucleus so its genome is protected from degradative lysosomal enzymes in the cytoplasm. If no helper virus is present, AAV will stably integrate into the host cellular DNA, therefore expression should be long term and not transient as in the case of vectors such as adenovirus. AAV uses host machinery for its replication and does not require the use of low fidelity enzymes like the retrovirus reverse transcriptase. Most of the AAV genome can be replaced in the recombinant genome. Only the ITRs are necessary in cis for recombinant viral production, as they appear to contain the signals necessary for replication, packaging, and integration. The AAV ITR has not been documented to inhibit other downstream promoters, unlike the retrovirus LTRs. Disadvantages of the AAV system do exist, including DNA size, as packaging occurs very inefficiently when the recombinant vector is greater than 5.2 kb in size, a cumbersome packaging protocol, and a lack of information about long-term effects of recombinant AAV infection.

The pioneer work on AAV gene transduction vectors began in the early 1980s. Initial constructs involved removing the Cap gene and replacing it with a selectable gene marker, the neomycin resistance gene, under the control of the SV40 early promoter. The native p40 promoter was also used in this way and G418 (a neomycin analog)-resistant colonies were selected. Other constructs quickly followed where both the Rep and Cap genes were removed al-

lowing larger inserts. It was found that this modification improved transduction frequencies as Rep seems to inhibit heterologous gene expression. Many different promoters have been used to express genes in AAV constructs, including the cytomegalovirus (CMV) immediate early 1 promoter, the thymidine kinase promoter, the heat shock protein promoter, and the murine sarcoma virus LTR. As the field has developed, more tissue-specific promoter, enhancer, and control sequences have been utilized as constructed with therapeutic uses.

The size of DNA inserts in recombinant AAV can vary greatly and still have reasonably efficient packaging and relatively high virus titers. Genomes ranging from 50 to 110% of the wild-type genome length with inserts of up to 4.7 kb have been used. Viral genomes in excess of the 110% wild-type size did not package efficiently. When smaller, 50% genomes were packaged, the resultant virus particles contained predominately inverted dimers, tandem dimers, and two monomers packaged in the same virus particle, producing virions of a very similar density to wild type. There appears to be no size restraint for the adenovirus-mediated rescue and replication of recombinant AAV DNA. Studies have shown that as much as 24 kb of DNA can be rescued from a recombinant plasmid.

To maximize insert DNA size it is important to determine what cis-acting elements are necessary for efficient AAV DNA replication, packaging, integration, and rescue. Vectors have been constructed which contain only the left ITR, right ITR, and 45 bp of unique sequence adjacent to the right ITR. This vector produced recombinant AAV efficiently, suggesting that the only sequences necessary are the ITRs and possibly a short unique sequence near the right ITR.

Since AAV is a DNA virus replicating in the nucleus, the virus has the ability to stably carry introns in the foreign gene cassette of the recombinant AAV genome. It has been shown that splicing of mRNA can improve expression of a gene product by a poorly understood mechanism that involves better transport of the mRNA through the nuclear membrane to the protein factories (polysomes) in the cell cytoplasm.

Conventional methods for rAAV production yield titers of 10^4–10^6 virus particles/ml. Figure 3 shows a schematic of the conventional protocol for the

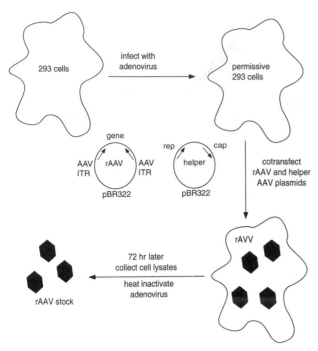

FIGURE 3 Conventional propagation of recombinant AAV. Details are presented in the text.

manufacture of these vectors. Three factors are necessary for AAV production: adenovirus-infected cells, the recombinant AAV plasmid containing the foreign gene cassette contained within AAV ITRs, and a second plasmid which supplies in trans the essential Rep and Cap functions. Optimally, this second plasmid should not contain the AAV ITRs or AAV sequences which overlap the recombinant AAV genome, therefore minimizing recombination and wild-type AAV contamination. In these schemes, the Rep/Cap helper plasmid has no ITRs and will not replicate. This lack of replication may contribute to low concentrations of Rep/Cap and may be one of the factors effecting titer. The two plasmids are cotransfected into the adenovirus-infected cells by standard DNA transfection methods, e.g., calcium phosphate precipitation or lipofection.

After a suitable incubation period, normally 2 or 3 days, the virus supernatant is collected. The supernatant is a mixture of recombinant AAV and adenovirus. The adenovirus can be inactivated by a 1-hr 55°C incubation as AAV is very heat resistant. A physical separation is also possible as the two viruses have very different buoyant densities and can be separately banded by ultracentrifugation on cesium chloride gradients.

The number of cell types transduced successfully by AAV has grown steadily over the years. These include established transformed cell lines (Hela, KB, D6, 293), human T cell lines (CEM, H9), leukemia lines (K562, KG1a, HEL, HL60, U937), human colon cancer lines (HT29, LIM, CaCo), and a normal lymphoblastoid line (NC37).

It has been shown that wild-type AAV integrates at a specific region of chromosome 19 in at least 68% of infected clones. However, when recombinant viral vectors lacking Rep were used, eight out of eight clones showed no chromosome 19 integration. Two of these integrants have been mapped by *in situ* hybridization to chromosomes 22 and 12. Recent studies suggest that Rep functions are necessary for site-specific integration, and research to understand the mechanism of Rep targeting is underway in several laboratories.

In recent years, AAV vectors have been used to transduce primary cells and tissues. The primary cells tested include human liver hepatocytes and nasal polyp cells from cystic fibrosis (CF) patients. Cells from the immune system, including primary T cells and stem cells from peripheral blood, bone marrow, and umbilical cord blood, have also been targets. Studies using the luciferase firefly (luc) reporter gene showed that murine bone marrow stem cells could be infected by recombinant AAV carrying luc under the control of the SV40 promoter and the neomycin phosphotransferase gene driven by the thymidine kinase promoter. These infected stem cells were used to reconstitute a mouse, and neomycin DNA fragments could be detected by polymerase chain reaction (PCR) from DNA isolated from peripheral blood cells 8 weeks after transplantation; no luc activity could be detected.

In experiments using β-galactosidase as a reporter gene, CD34$^+$ selected human bone marrow stem cells infected at a multiplicity of infection (moi) of 1–10 expressed β-galactosidase in 60–70% of the cells. In similar experiments, rhesus hematopoietic progenitors infected with the β-galactosidase expressing AAV showed that approximately 30% of derived colonies gave a positive signal for β-galatosidase by PCR.

When integration of AAV into human stem cells was investigated, incorporation into chromosome 19 occurred when wild-type AAV was used but appeared to be a relatively rare event. Preliminary results from *in vivo* mouse reconstitution experiments after lethal irradiation using rAAV-infected stem cells indicate that vector sequences can be detected in peripheral blood, spleen, bone marrow, and thymus for greater than 6 months posttransplant.

The ability of AAV to infect a nondividing cell type has great potential in the area of mammalian nervous system gene therapy. It has recently been shown that a recombinant AAV containing the β-galactosidase gene injected stereotactically into various regions of the rat brain expressed for up to 3 months with no toxicity to the animals. Vectors are now being developed to express human tyrosine hydroxylase which may have potential for the treatment of Parkinson's disease.

V. RECOMBINANT AAV PRODUCTION

One of the major problems in AAV gene transduction is the complex and inefficient protocol used to produce recombinant AAV. Over the past few years a major effort has been made to simplify the process, making it more amenable to large-scale manufacture and improving efficiency, thereby increasing the present low viral titers of 10^4–10^6 transducing virus particles/ml.

One strategy is to remove the need for the co-transfection of two plasmids. Epstein–Barr virus (EBV)-based plasmids are available that contain the regulatory sequences necessary for replication in bacteria, together with the EBV EBNA gene and the latent origin of replication which allow stable episomal replication in the nucleus of mammalian cells. The gene of interest flanked by AAV ITRs can be cloned into the EBV plasmid in bacteria followed by transfection into mammalian cells. Transformants are selected by hygromycin resistance which is encoded on the plasmid. To produce recombinant AAV, the transformed cells are adenovirus infected and transfected with the Rep/Cap helper plasmid. This technology has been shown to produce virus; however, a stable Rep/Cap producer cell line needs to be developed to make this system truly efficient.

Attempts to make AAV package lines analogous to those of the retroviruses have been disappointing to date. Constitutive production of the capsid proteins has been accomplished in several cell types, including 293, KB, and Hela cells; however, expression of the Rep functions has proven problematic. The main difficulty appears to be Rep toxicity. Many attempts have been made using inducible eukaryotic gene promoters to drive Rep expression. New strategies include the use of tightly controlled inducible promoters or bacterial gene promoters to express Rep and the use of new base cell lines, more resistant to Rep toxicity, for the construction of packaging lines. In one case, 293 cells which inducibly express the Rep elements have been described. Upon induction, the cells will support the replication of Rep vectors. The permanent expression of the Capsid proteins in these cells has yet to be achieved. Preliminary studies of Hela-based packaging lines have been reported; however, further investigation will be required to determine the utility of these systems for the production of therapeutic recombinant virus. Other strategies to efficiently manufacture rAAV include novel methods for the efficient introduction of plasmid DNA into producer cells and the use of specialized procedures for the concentration and purification of recombinant viruses.

VI. THERAPEUTIC USES OF AAV

Many gene therapy strategies and protocols are being developed using recombinant AAV vectors. In one of the most exciting areas of gene therapy research, AAV vectors will be used for globin gene replacement for the treatment of hemoglobinopathies. The molecular defects for diseases like sickle cell anemia and β-thalassemia are well characterized and have the potential to be corrected by the introduction of the normal β-globin gene. AAV is an ideal vector as it has the ability to infect very early progenitor stem cells. The inclusion of the hypersensitivity site 2 (HS2) from the locus control region, which normally flanks the human globin gene cluster, in the AAV vector markedly increased expression of both β-globin and γ-globin in K562 cells. Investigations continue to explore which control regions are important in globin expression and to determine the duration of globin gene expression in animal models.

Another approach for the treatment of β-thalassemia involves the inhibition of α-globin expression using an antisense RNA protocol. One of the problems in β-thalassemia patients is an overproduction of α-globin which reduces the lifespan of red blood cells. Experiments were carried out in K562 cells, which constitutively overexpress α-globin. AAV vectors expressing an antisense RNA α-globin sequence were able to inhibit α-globin production by up to 91%. Although still at the research stage, this type of antisense RNA approach could be used to treat many diseases where overexpression of a gene product has clinical significance.

Another single gene disorder that may be amenable to treatment by AAV gene transduction is cystic fibrosis. The main symptom of the disease is a defect in cyclic AMP (cAMP)-mediated chloride secretion in the airway epithelium causing a thick mucus in the lung which cannot be cleared by cilia action, leading to many lung infections. The condition is caused by mutations in the CF transmembrane conductance regulator (CFTR) protein. AAV vectors have been shown to infect and integrate into a CF bronchial epithelial cell line at high frequency and that AAV expressing the normal CFTR gene could complement the chloride transport defect in this cell line. In these experiments, the CFTR gene was efficiently driven by the AAV p5 promoter. Recent animal studies in rabbits have shown that CFTR RNA and protein could be detected for up to 6 months in the airway epithelium cells of a AAV/CFTR-infected rabbit lung lobe. These findings suggest the potential utility of *in vivo* administration of recombinant AAV vectors for the treatment of human diseases.

Several groups are now devising protocols using recombinant AAV vectors to protect CD4$^+$ and other susceptible cells from HIV infection and replication. Most protocols involve using sense or antisense RNA to inhibit HIV replication. One group has used an AAV construct which contains antisense RNA complementary to two separate regions of the HIV genome. Region 1 is from the 5′-untranslated HIV LTR (bases 13 to 75). This includes the TAR sequence which binds the HIV Tat protein, a transactivator of HIV replication. Region 2 is from bases 9096

to 9160 which contain the common poly(A) signal of all HIV mRNA species. The TAR sequence is on both LTRs and on all mRNA species; it has been shown that the sequence and secondary structure are essential for Tat binding and replication activation, therefore, any escape mutants should be nonviable. If viable virus can escape the antisense RNA blockage of Tat then they should be inhibited by the disruption of the poly(A) signal which should make the RNA transcripts less stable. The neomycin resistance gene was also included in the AAV construct so that clones could be selected from CD4$^+$ recombinant AAV-infected cell lines. When such cell lines were challenged with HIV the amount of viable HIV replicated was reduced by 99.99% when compared to non-AAV-transduced CD4$^+$ cell lines. The incubation time for these experiments was 20 days and protection continued for that time period.

Strategies using sense RNA molecules have also been developed. Initially, TAR decoys expressed in AAV vectors have been used where RNA sequences with the same sequence as the TAR region have been introduced into cells. Tat protein binds to these molecules and hence these overproduced "decoys" act to scavenge available Tat and prevent Tat transactivation. Eventually, however, HIV viral breakthrough occurred and it was found that the TAR decoys bound essential cellular factors whose loss could be potentially toxic if used in humans.

Interest has switched to inhibiting another regulatory HIV protein, Rev. This protein is made later in HIV replication and its function is to bind to an area within the env gene known as the Rev-response element (RRE). This allows efficient transport of the viral RNA out of the nucleus. Rev, along with Tat, is also involved in the inhibition of mRNA splicing, so full-length transcripts can be synthesized which encode the virion structural proteins. Again, sense RNAs with the same sequence as the RRE can be stably introduced in AAV vectors so that Rev binds to these molecules and transcription of spliced mRNA continues, inhibiting translation of the viral structural proteins and the spread of the virus.

The use of AAV vectors for the treatment of cancer is still in its infancy. One group is, however, pursuing two strategies. The first is to use AAV to express human granulocyte–macrophage colony-stimulating factor (GM-CSF) stably in transformed cells, using an

AAV vector. GM-CSF is a hematopoietic growth factor that drives stem cell differentiation toward the granulocyte, macrophage, and eosinophil lineage and has been shown to be effective in clinical trials to increase blood cell production in patients with various cancers. This study showed that the recombinant AAV could infect COS-1 cells, a monkey kidney line, and express high levels of biologically active GM-CSF, suggesting this approach may have potential in malignant disorders.

The second, more novel, approach is a potential treatment for multiple myeloma which is incurable with today's chemotherapy protocols. Myeloma precursor cells are surface immunoglobin positive and are targets for the low affinity Fcγ receptor III (CD16) which causes tumor lysis through a myc-signaling pathway. An AAV vector expressing CD16 has been constructed which stably infects KB and K562 cell lines. Supernatants from these infected cells contain soluble CD16 which could inhibit the growth of ARH-77 myeloma cells, reducing DNA synthesis by >90% and loss in viability to <2% of controls. If safety studies in an animal model and infection of primary myeloma cells show positive results, this system could be an excellent candidate for human gene therapy trials.

VII. NEW APPLICATIONS

To overcome the problem of low AAV virus titers, studies were initiated to use AAV recombinant plasmids together with physical or chemical means of gene transfer to yield high expression of transfected genes. It was found that the recombinant plasmid containing the gene cassette of interest flanked by AAV ITRs gave higher and longer expression in primary T lymphocytes and cultured tumor cells than the gene cassette in a standard plasmid backbone lacking the ITRs. These experiments were carried out *ex vivo* using cationic liposome/DNA complexes as the method of transfection. Expression of a reporter gene chloramphenicol acetyltransferase (Cat) was demonstrated for 30 days. The presence of transfected gene and plasmid DNA was shown by Southern blot analysis for at least 25 days; the standard plasmid DNA was degraded after 5–10 days. Random integration of the gene cassette has been demonstrated;

however, the efficiency and site of integration have yet to be determined. This procedure is now being scaled up for therapeutic application in the generation of tumor vaccines and modified T cells.

VIII. CONCLUSIONS

AAV has potential applications in several areas for gene therapy. It is a nonpathogenic DNA virus that stably integrates into cells, allowing long-term expression of recombinant gene cDNA. Because two wild-type viruses are necessary to rescue recombinant virions, it is relatively safe compared to vectors requiring a single complementing virus. The virus genome can carry introns and replicates in the nucleus, reducing the risk of degradation. Low titers are a difficulty at present, but increasingly higher titer stocks are being reported. Depending on the application, the use of recombinant AAV plasmid transfections could help remove this problem for *ex vivo* gene therapy of primary cells with a finite lifespan.

Acknowledgments

The authors thank Drs. B. J. Carter, A. Srivastava, A. N. Shelling, and R. J. Samulski for allowing details of unpublished results to be discussed in the review article. Our thanks also to Drs. C. Smith and T. B. Okarma, whose input was greatly valued during the writing of this article.

See Also the Following Articles

Antibodies in the Gene Therapy of Cancer • DNA Tumor Viruses: Adenovirus • Cell-Mediated Immunity to Cancer • Recombination: Mechanisms and Roles in Tumorigenesis • Targeted Vectors for Cancer Gene Therapy

Bibliography

Berns, K. I., and Bohenzky, R. A. (1987). Adeno-associated virus: An update. *Adv. Virus. Res.* **32,** 243–306.

Carter, B. J. (1990). Parvoviruses as vectors. *In* "Handbook of Parvoviruses" (P. Tijssen, ed.), Vol. II, pp. 247–284. CRC Press, Boca Raton, FL.

Muzyczka, M. (1992). Use of adeno-associated virus as a general transduction vector for mammalian cells. *Curr. Top. Microbiol. Immunol.* **158,** 97–129.

Alkylating Agents

O. Michael Colvin

Duke University

I. Types of Alkylating Agents: Mechanisms of Cytotoxicity and Uses
II. Cellular Mechanisms of Cytoxicity and Resistance
III. Toxicities

Alkylating agents were the first chemical agents to demonstrate significant clinical regressions of tumors. These initial alkylating agents were nitrogen mustards, derived from a vesicant war gas, sulfur mustard, utilized in World War I. Sulfur mustard was found to be toxic to proliferating tissues, and the less volatile nitrogen mustard compounds were found to have antitumor activity in animals and patients. Agents of this type, which have been and continue to be utilized in the treatment of cancer, are different chemically, but have in common the feature that they covalently bind to (alkylate) the nucleic acid bases of DNA and produce cellular death unless the damage is repaired. Monofunctional alkylating agents appear to produce cell death by a cellular reaction to the presence of the lesion, whereas bifunctional agents covalently bind the two complementary strands of a DNA molecule, preventing effective cell division and producing cell death unless the cross-link is repaired. Alkylating agents are still used extensively in the treatment of cancer, usually in combination with other types of antitumor agents. The major toxicity of alkylating agents is bone marrow and gastrointestinal toxicity. They also produce a significant incidence of second cancers in patients, as do other classes of antitumor agents.

I. TYPES OF ALKYLATING AGENTS: MECHANISMS OF CYTOTOXICITY

A. Monofunctional Alkylating Agents

These agents react with nucleotides in DNA bases to methylate them. While many nucleotides can be methylated, the effective target is deoxyguanylate. There is now convincing evidence that the cell death produced by these agents is due to the action of the DNA mismatch repair and other enzymes, which recognize the presence of the abnormal DNA base and attempt to repair or remove it.

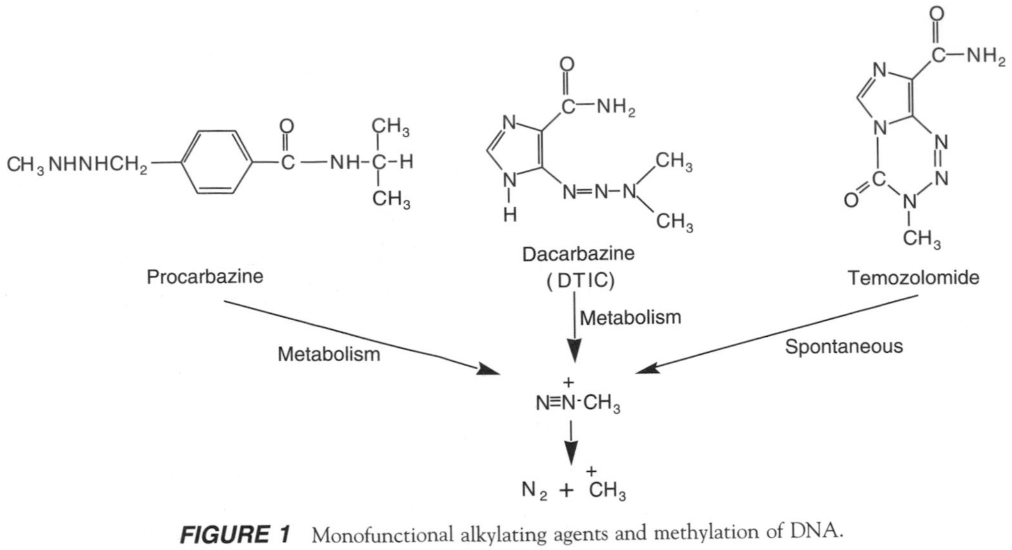

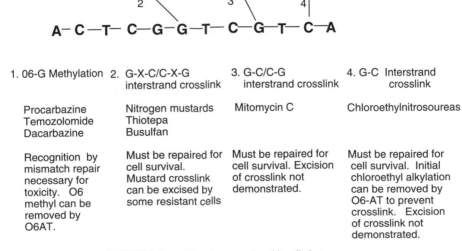

FIGURE 1 Monofunctional alkylating agents and methylation of DNA.

The two most frequently used monofunctional alkylating agents are procarbazine and dacarbazine (Fig. 1). Both of these compounds are metabolized to produce a very reactive methyl diazonium, which methylates the O6 position of guanylate in DNA (Fig. 2). Temozolomide (Fig. 1) is an analog of dacarbazine, which spontaneously degrades to produce methyl diazonium. Attempts of the mismatch repair enzymes to repair the methylated guanylate appear to be the major mechanism of cellular damage produced by these compounds, and cells deficient in DNA mismatch repair enzymes are resistant to these agents.

Procarbazine and dacarbazine continue to be used in the treatment of Hodgkin's disease in MOPP and ABVD regimens. Procarbazine is also used in the treatment of brain tumors, and dacarbazine is used in the treatment of malignant melanoma. Temozolomide has shown activity in the treatment of brain tumors

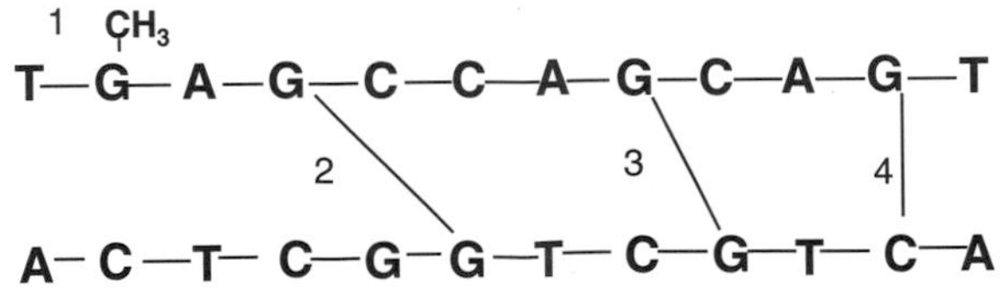

FIGURE 2 content:

T—G—A—G—C—C—A—G—C—A—G—T
(position 1 with CH₃ on G)

A—C—T—C—G—G—T—C—G—T—C—A

1. O6-G Methylation	2. G-X-C/C-X-G interstrand crosslink	3. G-C/C-G interstrand crosslink	4. G-C Interstrand crosslink
Procarbazine Temozolomide Dacarbazine	Nitrogen mustards Thiotepa Busulfan	Mitomycin C	Chloroethylnitrosoureas
Recognition by mismatch repair necessary for toxicity. O6 methyl can be removed by O6AT.	Must be repaired for cell survival. Mustard crosslink can be excised by some resistant cells	Must be repaired for cell survival. Excision of crosslink not demonstrated.	Must be repaired for cell survival. Initial chloroethyl alkylation can be removed by O6-AT to prevent crosslink. Excision of crosslink not demonstrated.

FIGURE 2 DNA lesions produced by alkylating agents.

and other malignancies. This compound is administered orally and appears to have a higher therapeutic index in animal models and less toxicity in patients than the two older compounds.

B. Bifunctional Alkylating Agents

These agents react with a nucleotide on each strand of DNA to produce an interstrand cross-link, which prevents the two strands from separating, and one such cross-link will prevent the cell from successfully replicating, unless the cross-link is repaired. The presence of the interstrand cross-link may also initiate ineffective attempts at repair by the cell, leading to death by apoptosis or necrosis. Cross-links produced by these agents differ structurally (Fig. 2), and these differences result in different effects on cells, which are probably mediated by the different cellular responses to the structural changes in DNA.

1. Nitrogen Mustards

The original nitrogen mustard used clinically, mustargen, is still used today in the MOPP regimen for Hodgkin's disease, but four nitrogen mustards—chlorambucil, melphalan, cyclophosphamide, and ifosfamide (Fig. 3)—are used more extensively, usually in

combination with other antitumor agents. These compounds cross-link DNA (Fig. 4) between the N7 atoms of guanylate nucleotides in a G-X-C/C-Y-G sequence (Fig. 2).

Cyclophosphamide and ifosfamide are structurally related compounds, which share the property of requiring activation by hepatic microsomal P450 enzymes (Fig. 5). The initial activated product of both compounds can be inactivated by the enzyme aldehyde dehydrogenase, which is present in cells with proliferative potential in both the bone marrow and the gastrointestinal tract. For this reason, these two compounds have relatively less bone marrow and gastrointestinal toxicity than the other nitrogen mustards. Because the metabolism of ifosfamide is more variable than that of cyclophosphamide, higher doses are required, and renal toxicity and neurotoxicity are associated with ifosfamide, but are rare with cyclophosphamide.

Cyclophosphamide is used in the treatment of breast cancer, usually in combination with adriamycin, in the treatment of lymphomas in the CHOP and other regimens and for the treatment of sarcomas and pediatric tumors. Ifosfamide is particularly used for the treatment of sarcomas. Cyclophosphamide is a potent immunosuppressant, and for this reason is

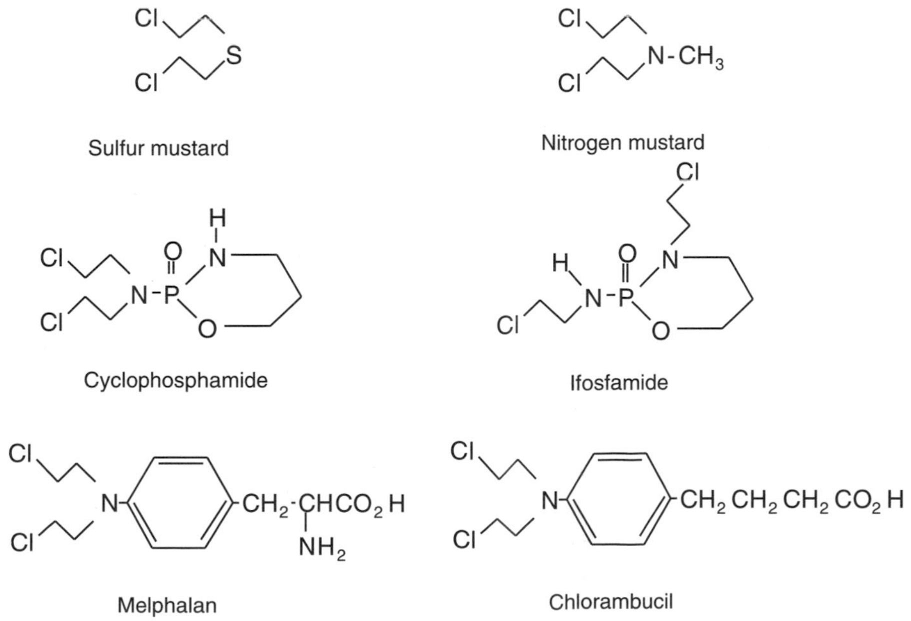

FIGURE 3 Sulfur mustard and nitrogen mustards.

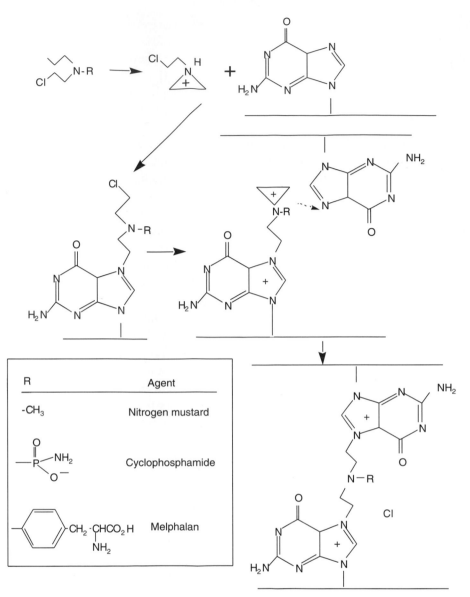

FIGURE 4 Cross-linking of DNA by nitrogen mustards.

extensively used for bone marrow transplantation and for the treatment of autoimmune diseases. Melphalan is used in the treatment of multiple myeloma, usually in combination with prednisone, and is also used in high doses for bone marrow transplantation.'

2. Aziridines

Aziridine alkylating agents are structurally similar to the nitrogen mustards, but react with DNA through uncharged aziridine rings, which are less reactive than

the aziridinium intermediates through which the nitrogen mustards alkyate DNA. The aziridine alkylating agents, which are used significantly in cancer therapy, are thiotepa and mitomycin C (Fig. 6). These compounds are both bifunctional agents, which produce interstrand DNA cross-links. The cross-link formed by thiotepa appears to be similar to that of the nitrogen mustards, with two aziridine carbons reacting with the N7 of guanylates in complementary strands in the G-X-C/C-Y-G sequence (Fig. 2).

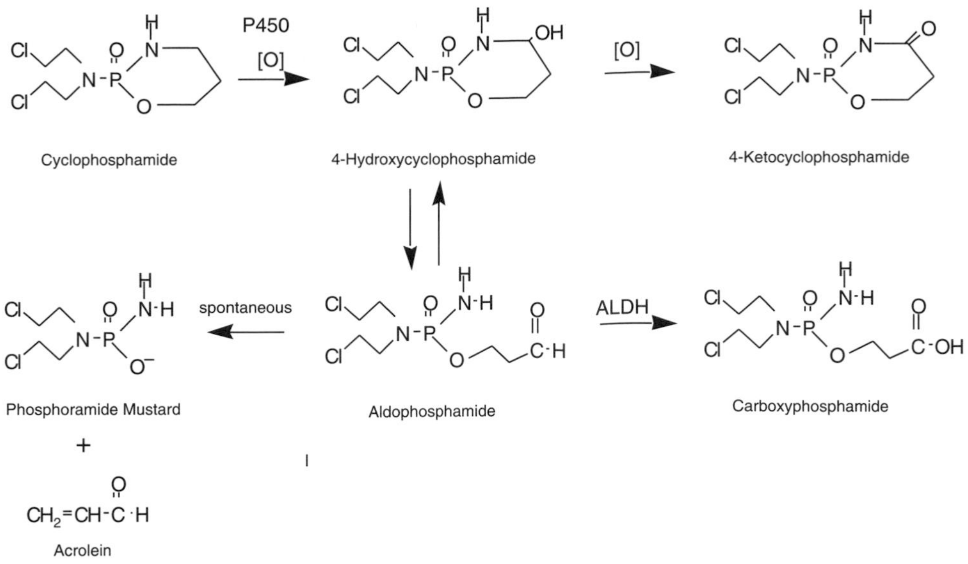

FIGURE 5 Metabolism of cyclophosphamide.

Mitomycin C has a unique mode of cross-linking. The molecule is reduced, particularly under hypoxic conditions, and the activated C1 position reacts with the extracyclic N2 of guanylate in the minor groove of DNA. This event approximates the C10 of the carbamate moiety to the N2 of a guanylate in the complementary DNA strand to produce a cross-link in the minor groove (Fig. 2).

Thiotepa has been particularly used in the high-dose treatment of breast cancer, but this practice is declining. Mitomycin C, an antibiotic extracted from a microorganism, is used in the treatment of breast, esophageal, and stomach cancer.

3. Alkyl Sulfonates

Busulfan (Fig. 7) is the alkyl sulfonate that is currently used clinically. This compound produces a DNA cross-link similar to that produced by the nitrogen mustards, but has very different biological and clinical effects. The compound has the interesting property of having much less effect on lymphoid cells than the immunosuppressive nitrogen mustards. The basis for this sparing of lymphoid cells is not understood.

Busulfan was introduced in 1953 for the treatment of chronic mylegenous leukemia. The drug is still used

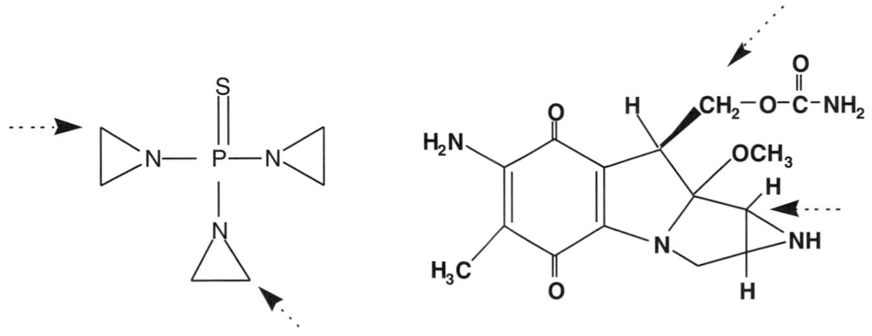

FIGURE 6 Structures of thiotepa and mitocycin C. Arrows indicate the sites of N7 guanylate alkylation and DNA cross-linking.

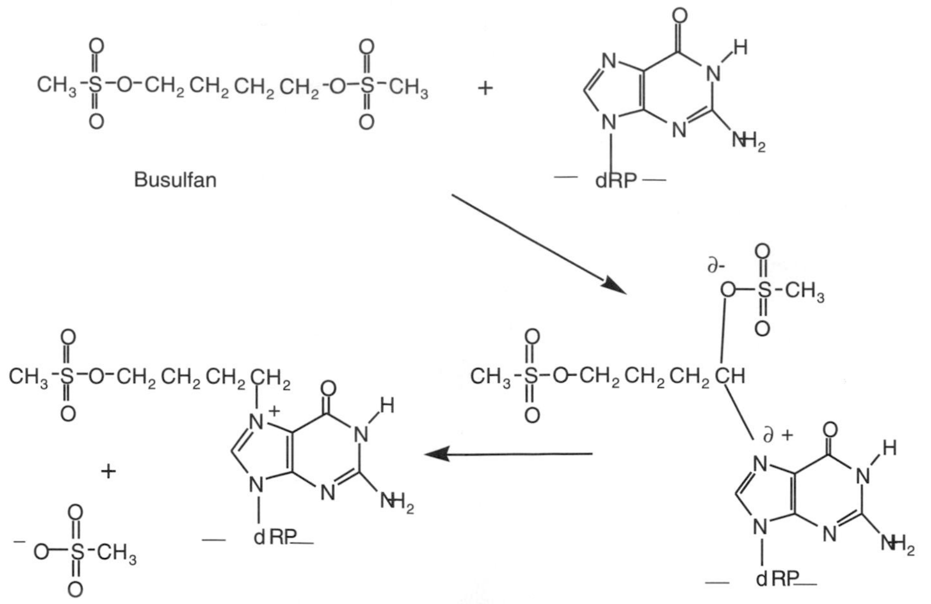

FIGURE 7 Alkylation of guanylate in DNA by busulfan. A second reaction with the N7 of a guanylate on the complementary DNA strand produces an interstrand cross-link.

for this purpose, but usually after interferon or hydroxyurea, and now, the oncogene targeted agent Gleevac. Busulfan is used in combination with cyclophosphamide and other agents at high doses in preparative regimens for bone marrow transplantation.

4. Nitrosoureas

Bischlorethylnitrosourea (BCNU, Fig. 8) is used in the treatment of brain tumors and in high-dose combination therapy for bone marrow transplantation. Bifunctional nitrosoureas spontaneously decompose under physiologic conditions to a chlorethyl diazonium moiety, which alkylates the O6 position of guanylate in DNA. This adduct then alkylates the N2 of the based paired cytosine on the other strand of DNA to produce a C-G interstrand cross-link (Fig. 8).

II. CELLULAR MECHANISMS OF CYTOXICITY AND RESISTANCE

Because the alkylating agents are potent electrophiles, they can react with electron-rich cellular molecules to be inactivated before they can react with DNA. Glutathione (GSH), a tripeptide molecule with a free

cyteine sulfhydryl atom, is present in millimolar concentrations in cells, and increased cellular concentrations of GSH are associated with cellular resistance to alkylating agents. The protective effect of GSH appears to be enhanced by increased cellular concentrations of the glutathione S-transferase in tumor cells. The enzyme has been demonstrated to catalyze the reaction of akylating agents with GSH. Increased cellular concentrations of the sulfhydryl-rich protein metallothionine has also been demonstrated to be associated with cellular resistance to alkylating agents.

As described earlier, toxicity of the monofunctional antitumor agents appears to be due to the recognition of the cell of the alteration of the DNA bases and the attempts by cellular mechanisms to repair these highly mutagenic lesions. An extensive amount of information indicates that the activities of the mismatch repair system are the principal mechanisms through which cytoxicity occurs, as tumor cells deficient in mismatch repair are resistant to these agents. Another mechanism of resistance to these agents is the enzyme O6-alkylguanine-alkyltransferase, which removes methyl and other alkyl groups from the O6 position of guanine.

Figure 2 illustrates the DNA cross-links that are

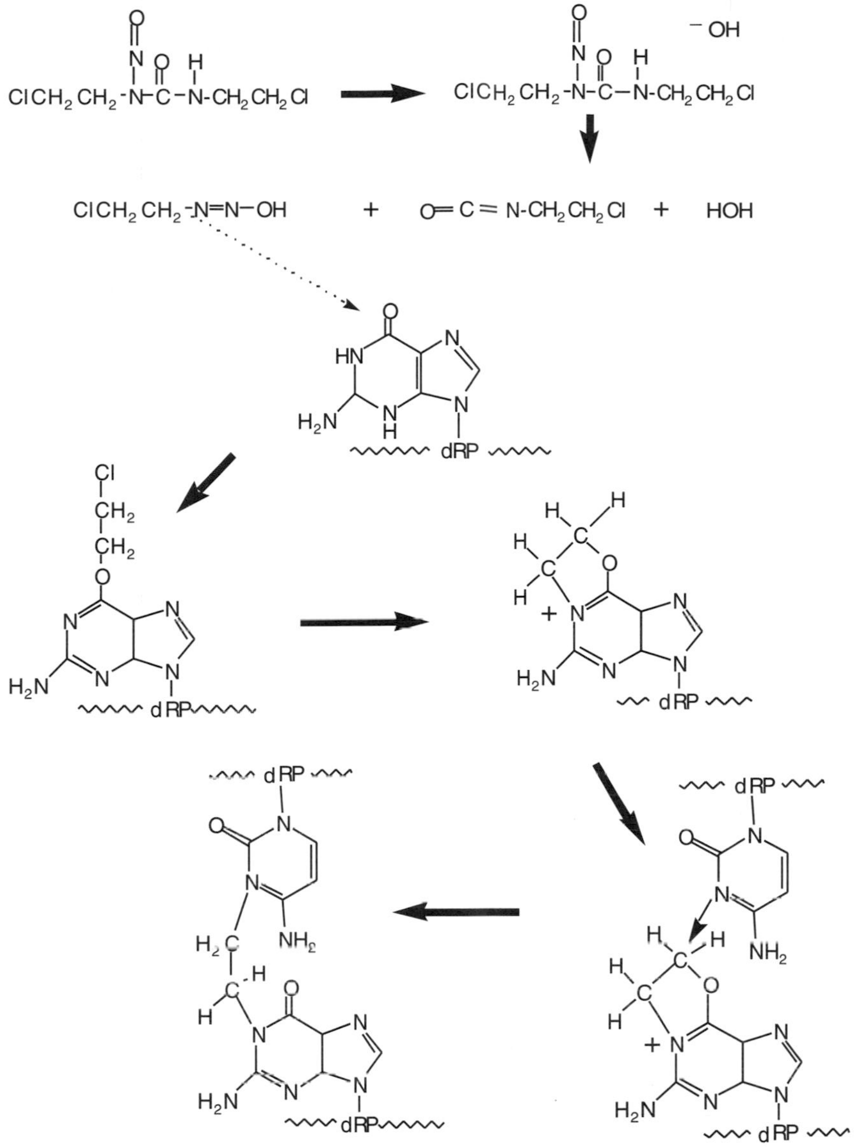

FIGURE 8 Reaction of BCNU with DNA to produce a G-C interstrand cross-link.

produced by the bifunctional alkylating agents. The major mechanism of resistance to BCNU appears to be elevated O6-alkylguanine-alkyltransferase, which removes an initial O6 alkylation before cross-linking can occur. While it appears that the cross-links produced by the other bifunctional agents are repaired, the cellular mechanisms through which this repair occurs are poorly understood. The repair of the cross-link produced by phosphoramide mustard (the cross-linking moiety of cyclophosphamide) has been demonstrated in a cell-free system and does not ap-

pear to utilize the more characterized excision repair enzymes.

III. TOXICITIES

Hematopoietic and gastrointestinal toxicity in the form of mucositis, stomatitis, and diarrhea are common side effects of alkylating agents. However, there are remarkable differences in the toxicities of the different agents. Cyclophosphamide is relatively sparing of

TABLE I
Toxicities of Alkylating Agents

Hematopoietic depression
Gastrointestinal toxicity
Gonadal damage: amenorrhea and oligospermia
Teratogenesis: when administered in first trimester
Secondary malignancy

hematopoietic cells, especially platelets, and produces little direct gastrointestinal toxicity. This property of cyclophosphamide is due to the presence of the detoxifying enzyme aldehyde dehydrogenase in hematopoietic precursors and in the repopulating cells of the small intestine. The nausea and vomiting produced by alkylating agents are mediated in large part by direct effects on the central nervous system. These side effects can now be controlled much more effectively in the new generation of antiemetics currently used in conjunction with chemotherapy.

Alkylating agents produce significant gonadal toxicity, with depletion of testicular germ cells, oligospermia, or aspermia in men and amenorrhea in women. Treatment of women with an alkylating agent during the first trimester of pregnancy has a risk that may be as high as 15% of having a malformed infant. Administration of alkylating agents during the second and third trimesters has not been associated with increased fetal malformations.

Because alkylating agents damage DNA, an increased incidence of secondary malignancies would be expected and occurs. In certain cohorts of patients treated with intensive alkylating agent therapy, this incidence has been as high as 30%, but the overall incidence appears to be 5% or lower. There also is an increased incidence of secondary solid tumors after alkylating agent therapy, but it is less than the incidence of leukemia (Table I).

All of the alkylating agents probably produce some degree of immunosuppression, but there is no evidence that this effect contributes to posttherapy infections or is otherwise clinically detrimental. Cyclophosphamide is one of the most potent immunosuppressants and is used to treat autoimmune diseases, as is chlorambucil.

See Also the Following Articles

BLEOMYCIN • CHRONIC MYELOGENOUS LEUKEMIA • LYMPHOMA, HODGKIN'S DISEASE • MISMATCH REPAIR: BIOCHEMISTRY AND GENETICS • TRANSFER OF DRUG RESISTANCE GENES TO HEMATOPOIETIC PRECURSORS

Bibliography

Colvin, O. M. (2000–2001). Antitumor alkylating agents. *In* "Cancer: Principles and Practice (V. T. DeVita, S. Hellman, and S. A. Rosenberg, eds.) p. 363. Lippincott Williams & Wilkins, Philadelphia.

Colvin, O. M. (2000). Alklating agents and platinum antitumor compounds. *In* "Cancer Medicine" (R. C. Bast, Jr., D. W. Kufe, R. E. Pollock, R. R. Weichselbaum, J. F. Holland, and E. Frei, III, eds.) p. 648. Decker, Hamilton and London.

Ludeman, S. M. (1999). Cyclophosphamide. *In* "Current Pharmaceutical Design," Vol. 5, pp. 555–665.

Rhoads, C. (1946). Nitrogen mustards in treatment of neoplastic disease. *JAMA* **131,** 6568.

Rhodes, R. (1986). "The Making of the Atomic Bomb." Simon & Shuster, New York.

Russo, J. E., Hilton, J., and Colvin, O. M. (1989). The role of aldehyde dehydrogenase isozymes in cellular resistance to the alkylating agent cyclophosphamide. *Prog. Clin. Biol. Res.* **290,** 65.

ALL-1

Tatsuya Nakamura
Carlo M. Croce
Kimmel Cancer Center and Thomas Jefferson University

Eli Canaani
Kimmel Cancer Center and The Weizmann Institute of Science

GLOSSARY

ALL-1 The gene located at chromosome band 11q23 and rearranges through chromosome translocations.

chimeric proteins Products of fused genes generated by chromosome translocations.

chromatin alterations Modification of proteins associated with DNA, most commonly histones, resulting in activation or repression of transcription.

infant acute leukemia Diagnosed in children of less than 1 year old and usually associated with ALL-1 rearrangements.

secondary acute leukemia Resulting from therapy with anticancer drugs and frequently involving ALL-1 rearrangements.

Nonrandom, somatically acquired chromosomal translocations or inversions have been identified in the majority of human acute leukemias and lymphomas. These rearrangements lead to the overexpression of critical genes positioned near the breakpoints or to the incorporation of coding exons derived from two genes disrupted by the translocation into a fusion gene encoding a chimeric protein. Expression of the latter undermines normal cellular programs of proliferation and/or survival and eventually leads to malignant transformation. Frequent targets of these chromosomal translocations are genes encoding transcription factors. The modular nature of these factors enables a translocation-mediated exchange of domains, resulting in altered function of the affected protein. The target genes for chromosomal transloca-tions are highly conserved in evolution and act at early stages of regulatory cascades. The specificity of these translocations to hematopoietic lineages and to distinct precursor cells suggests that the affected genes are oncogenic only in the setting of specific tran-scriptional programs. One of the striking examples of a transcription factor involved in acute leukemia is ALL-1, also termed HRX, MLL, or HTRX. ALL-1 is located at chromosome band 11q23 involved in mul-tiple chromosome abnormalities associated with both acute lymphocytic (ALL) and acute myeloid (AML) leukemia. ALL-1 is the human homologue of *Drosophila trithorax (trx)*, which acts to regulate the expression of homeotic genes by modifying the struc-ture of chromatin. The unique clinical and biological characteristics of ALL-1-associated leukemias, the large number of ALL-1 translocation partners, the important role of ALL-1 in development, and the epigenetic mechanism by which it acts make this pro-tein and its leukemic derivatives attractive subjects for investigation.

I. CYTOGENETICS OF 11q23 ABNORMALITIES AND INVOLVEMENT OF ALL-1

Karyotypic alterations in band 11q23, mostly reciprocal chromosomal translocations, are associated with 5–10% of children and adults with ALL, AML, biphe-notypic leukemias, or myeloplastic syndromes. Two groups of patients with acute leukemia who show high concordance (60–90%) with 11q23 abberations are children under the age of 12 months and children or adults with secondary (therapy-related) leukemia. The most common translocations are t(4:11) and t(9:11), which account for 40 and 27% of 11q23 transloca-tions, respectively; t(11:19) associated with 12% of the aberrations; and t(6:11) and t(10:11), each in-volving around 5% of the total. Currently, more than 30 different chromosome translocations have been as-sociated with 11q23, pointing ALL-1 as unusually promiscuous in recombination with partner genes. There is a marked association between the type of the translocation and the disease phenotype. Thus, the vast majority of t(4:11) cases are ALL, 80–90% of the t(9:11) are AML, and nearly all cases of t(6:11) and t(10:11) are AML. The t(11:19)(q23:p13.1) is found in AML patients, whereas the t(11:19)(q23:p13.3) is distributed equally between AML and ALL patients. Most cases of AML with 11q23 abnormalities are of the M4 or M5 subtypes. The correlation between spe-cific ALL-1 translocations and disease phenotype might reflect the existence of different windows throughout the differentiation of hematopoietic cells, during which only specific translocation products can act to initiate the malignant process. A similar kind of reasoning can be applied to explain the detection by sensitive molecular methodologies of minute num-ber of cells with the t(4:11) abnormality in normal bone marrows and in leukemic patients with no evi-dence of 11q23 aberrations.

In all chromosome translocations involving ALL-1, the gene is cleaved between exons 5 and 11, and the region 3′ of the breakpoint is replaced by the translocation partner. The critical product of the translocation is located on the derivative of chromo-some 11. It contains the ALL-1 promoter and the 5′ five to eleven exons (depending on the translocation breakpoint) linked upstream to the 3′ segment of the partner gene. Transcript of the fused gene encodes a chimeric protein. In some AMLs, particularly those with trisomy 11, ALL-1 undergoes a different type of rearrangement—partial tandem duplication of exons 2-8, 2-6, or 4-6, resulting in production of a longer protein. Not a single case of ALL-1 truncation was re-ported. This suggests that the modified proteins—chimeric or partially duplicated—play an active role in the pathogenesis. Therefore, a simple model of loss of function is not compatible with these features of ALL-1 rearrangements.

II. CLINICAL AND BIOLOGICAL CHARACTERISTICS OF ALL-1-ASSOCIATED LEUKEMIAS

Some properties of ALL-1-associated leukemias make them unique and have provided some insights to the pathogenesis. ALL of infancy with ALL-1 rearrange-ments are of immature prepre-B lineage. They are negative for CD10, but express some myeloid-associated markers. These biphenotypic features suggest that the leukemic cells originate from a precursor cell not fully committed to lymphoid differentiation. The presence of ALL-1 rearrangements in ALL has a clear adverse prognostic impact. These patients initially respond to therapy but usually relapse after a short duration. The rate for 5 years event-free survival for children with ALL and ALL-1 translocations is around 11%. In AML, the presence of 11q23 abnormalities does not appear to have an extreme adverse effect as in ALL, but prognosis is still inferior in comparison to many other types of AML.

Both infant leukemias and secondary leukemias associated with ALL-1 rearrangements show a very short latency period of only a few months. Remarkably, several studies utilizing molecular techniques indicate that many, or perhaps all, infant leukemias arise *in utero*. The short latency period strongly suggests that a very limited number of additional mutations are required for the emergence of these malignancies.

The association of ALL-1 rearrangement with secondary leukemias is instructive because these diseases arise in most cases in patients treated with drugs such as epipodophyllotoxin or anthyacycline, which inhibit topoisomerase II. This enzyme acts during replication or transcription. It binds to consensus sites distributed across the DNA and facilitates unwinding of the latter by nicking and resealing. Inhibition of the enzyme will result in accumulation of double stranded DNA ends. The nicked DNA could be repaired by cellular ligases involved in nonhomologous recombination, which will result in DNA rearrangements. The breakpoint cluster region within ALL-1 contains a number of sequences closely related to topoisomerase II-binding sites. In addition, mapping of the breakpoints in secondary leukemias (as well as in infant ALL) indicated congregation near these sites. This is consistent with the idea that treatment with inhibitors of the enzyme promotes ALL-1 rearrangements. Such inhibitors are also found in the environment and include flavonoids, catechines, benzene metabolites, estrogens, and quinolone antibiotics. Therefore, these materials could be considered mutagenic, particularly for fetuses.

III. THE ALL-1 GENE AND PROTEIN

Sequence analysis indicated several regions of homology between ALL-1 and the *Drosophila trithorax* gene. The latter is a member of the *trithorax/polycomb* gene family. These genes function as activators or repressors of the homeotic gene clusters (HOM/HOX) during embryogenesis. Hometic genes act in setting up the body structures along the anterior–posterior axis. Once the pattern of expression of homeotic genes is initially established in individual cells, it has to be maintained during subsequent cell divisions. The maintenance function is carried out by the proteins encoded by *trithorax* and *Polycomb* genes, which act by altering the chromatin through nucleosome displacement, histone acetylation, deacetylation, and so on. Gene disruption experiments in the mouse showed functional similarity between ALL-1 and *trithorax*. This was clearly indicated by a posterior shift in HOX gene expression and consequent homeotic transformation of the skeleton in ALL-1 heterozygotes.

ALL-1 encodes a protein, All1, of 3968 residues. Several structural/functional domains have been identified in the protein (Fig. 1). The C-terminal 130 amino acids SET domain is shared with *trithorax*, as well as with dozens of other proteins from yeast to human. These proteins are usually associated with chromatin and have diverse functions, such as maintenance of the transcriptional state, silencing of genes located at telomeres or centromeres, and silencing of heterochromatin regions. The function of the SET domain itself might vary between proteins. Thus, SET of SUV39H1 methylates histone H3 and All1 SET was found to physically interact with the Ini1 protein, a component of the SWI/SNF chromatin remodeling complex. Another interaction of All1 SET is with the dual antiphosphatase Sbf1. This association suggested that the function of All1 is dependent on the phosphorylation state of a particular serine or tyrosine within the SET domain. A second domain, highly conserved between All1 and *trithorax*, is composed of several zinc fingers termed PHD fingers. This domain has been identified in a number of chromatin proteins and is thought to be involved in protein–protein interactions. A partial bromodomain is present within the PHD fingers of All1 and *trithorax*. In

Motifs within the ALL-1 Protein

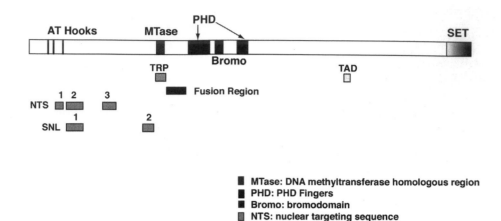

FIGURE 1 Motifs within the ALL-1 proteins.

several proteins, this motif was found to bind to acetylated lysine 9 within histone H3. All1, as well as its leukemic derivatives, is present within the cell nucleus in hundreds of small dots whose function is not known. Several polypeptides within the N-terminal portion were found to confer nuclear location, and two sequences (conserved with *trithorax*) conferred distribution in speckles. All1 contains three N-terminal AT hook motifs. These sequences bind to the minor groove of DNA in AT-rich regions. An All1 sequence with homology to DNA methyl transferase exhibits transcriptional repression activity in transfection assays, suggesting a role in repression. Finally, a polypeptide at the C terminus of All1 was initially identified as conferring transcriptional activation and subsequently demonstrated to act through binding to the coactivator acetylase CBP.

In summary, the position and content of the different domains indicate that the N-terminal 1300–1400 residues of All1, retained within the leukemic derivatives, act in transporting the protein into the nucleus, binding it to target DNAs, and endowing it with the ability to repress transcription. The C-terminal portion of All1 confers transcriptional activation capacity to the protein and is likely to be involved in regulation of the protein activity through interaction of the SET domain with Sbf1. The latter

domain appears to also have a function in nucleosome remodeling.

IV. ALL-1 PARTNER PROTEINS AND LEUKEMOGENICITY OF FUSION PROTEINS

Twenty-four partner proteins have been described (Fig. 2). Eleven of these are nuclear, 5 are cytoplasmic, and the rest are of unknown localization. Although the proteins are a diverse lot, several pairs (AF4 and AF5, AF9 and ENL, AF10 and AF17, MSF and hCDrel, CBP and p300) show strong or moderate homology. A number of the partner proteins contain protein–protein interaction domains such as leucine zipper, α-helical coil, PDZ, and SH3. Although the diversity of the partner proteins is puzzling, their indispensable role in to the leukemogenicity of the chimeric proteins is well established. This was shown in two mouse models. In the first, ALL-1/AF-9 or truncated ALL-1 was inserted by a "knock-in" methodology into the germline of mice to replace one allele of ALL-1. Mice expressing ALL-1/AF9 but not truncated ALL-1 developed AML with a median latency of 8 months. Another methodology applied was to retroviral transduce ALL-1/ENL and truncated

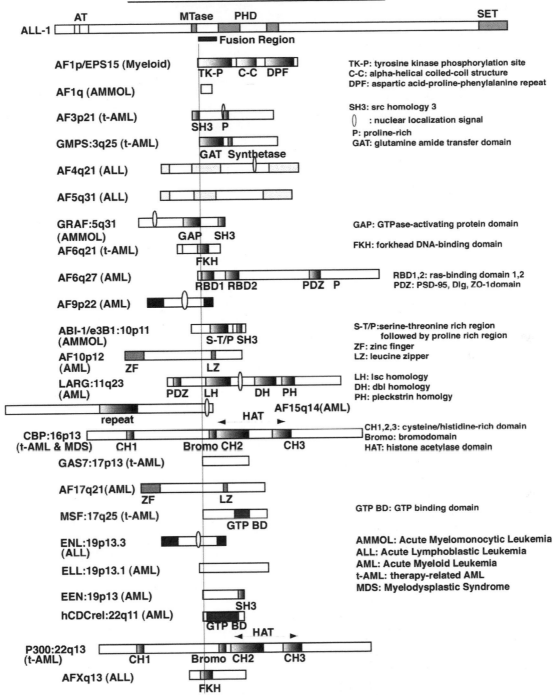

PARTNER PROTEINS FUSED TO ALL-1

FIGURE 2 Partner proteins fused to ALL-1.

ALL-1 into murine bone marrow cells. Serial plating in methylcellulose indicated continuous proliferation/immortalization of cells expressing the fusion protein but not of cells expressing other protein species. Injection of the former cells into syngenic or SCID mice induced leukemia. Moreover, point mutations introduced into the ENL portion of the fusion protein abolished immortalization/leukemogenicity.

V. UNRESOLVED ISSUES AND FUTURE DIRECTIONS

The most interesting questions related to ALL-1 are (1) Does the protein function both as transcriptional activator and repressor? (2) How does All1 alter the structure of chromatin? (3) How is All1 led to target genes? (4) What are All1 target genes? (5) Is the function of All1 modulated by cellular pathways? (6) What is the function of PHD fingers, SET domain, methyl transferase homology domain, and the motifs conferring speckles distribution? (7) How do ALL-1 rearrangement products trigger leukemia? What is the critical difference in function between the normal protein and its leukemic derivatives? What is the role of the partner proteins?

Some of the experimental directions to be applied for resolving these issue will be the purification and characterization of multiprotein complexes containing All1 and its derivatives; comparing transcription profiles of normal cells, cells lacking All1, and cells expressing All1 leukemic proteins, by microarray methodology; and identifying specific DNA sequences directing All1 to gene targets by coimmunoprecipitation techniques.

See Also the Following Articles

EWS/ETS Fusion Genes • PAX3-FKHR and PAX7-FKHR Gene Fusions in Alveolar Rhabdomyosarcoma • RUNX/CBF Transcription Factors • TLS-CHOP

Bibliography

Cimino, G., Rapanotti, M. C., Biondi, A., Elia, L., LoCoco, F., Price, C., Rossi, V., Rivolta, A., Canaani, E., Croce, C. M., Mandelli, F., and Greaves, M. (1997). Infant acute leukemias show the same biased distribution of ALL-1 gene breaks as topoisomerase II related secondary leukemias. *Cancer Res.* **57**, 2879–2883.

Corral, J., Lavenir, I., Impey, H., Warren, A. J., Forster, A., Larson, T. A., Bell, S., McKenzie, A. N. J., King, G., and Rabbits, T. H. (1996). An MLL-AF9 fusion gene made by homologous recombination causes acute leukemia in chimeric mice: A method to create fusion oncogenes. *Cell* **85**, 853–861.

Cu, X., DeVivo, I., Slany, R., Miyamoto, A., Finestein, R., and Cleary, M. L. (1998). Association of SET domain and myotubularin-related proteins modulates growth control. *Nature Genet.* **18**, 331–337.

Ernst, P., Wang, J., Huang, M., Goodman, R. H., and Korsmeyer, S. J. (2001). MLL and CREB bind cooperatively to the nuclear coactivator CREB-binding protein. *Mol. Cell. Biol.* **21**, 2249–2258.

Ford, A. M., Ridge, S. A., Cabrera, M. E., Mahmoud, H., Steel, C. M., Chan, L. C., and Greaves, M. (1993) *In utero* rearrangements in the trithorax-related oncogene in human leukemias. *Nature* **363**, 358–360.

Gu, Y., Nakamura, T., Adler, H., Prasad, R., Canaani, O., Cimino, G., Croce, C. M., and Canaani, E. (1992). The t(4:11) chromosome translocation of human acute leukemias fuses the ALL-1 gene, related to *Drosophila trithorax*, to the AF-4 gene. *Cell* **71**, 701–708.

Lavau, C., Szilvassy, S. J., Slany, R., Tsukamoto, A., and Cleary, M. L. (1997). Immortalization and leukemic transformation of a myelomonocytic precursor by retrovirally-transduced HRX-ENL. *EMBO J.* **16**, 4226–4237.

Prasad, R., Yano, T., Sorio, C., Nakamura, T., Rallapalli, R., Gu, Y., Leshkowitz, D., Croce, C. M., and Canaani, E. (1995). Domains with transcriptional regulatory activity within the ALL-1 and AF-4 proteins involved in acute leukemia. *Proc. Natl. Acad. Sci. USA* **92**, 12160–12164.

Rubnitz, J. E., Behm, F. G., Pui, C.-H., Evans, W. E., Relling, M. V., Raimondi, S. C., Harrison, P. L., Sandland, I. T., Ribeiro, R. C., Grosveld, G., and Downing, J. R. (1997). Genetic studies of childhood ALL with emphasis on p16, MLL and ETV6 gene abnormalities: Results of St. Jude total therapy study XII. *Leukemia* **11**, 1201–1206.

Schichman, S. A., Canaani, E., and Croce, C. M. (1995). Self fusion of the ALL-1 gene, a new genetic mechanism for acute leukemia. *J. Am. Med. Assoc.* **273**, 571–576.

Secker-Walker, L. M. (1998). General report on the European Union Concerted Action Workshop on 11q23, London, U.K. May 1997. *Leukemia* **12**, 776–778.

Tkachuk, D. C., Kohler, S., and Cleary, M. L. (1992). Involvement of a homolog of *Drosophila trithorax* by 11q23 chromosomal translocations in acute leukemias. *Cell* **71**, 691–670.

Yu, B. D., Hanson, R. D., Hess, J. L., Horning, S. E., and Korsmeyer, S. J. (1998). MLL, a mammalian trithorax group gene functions as a transcriptional maintenance factor in morphogenesis. *Proc. Natl. Acad. Sci. USA* **95**, 10632–10636.

Animal Models for Colon Cancer Chemoprevention

Bandaru S. Reddy

American Health Foundation, Valhalla, New York

GLOSSARY

cancer chemoprevention Intervention with chemical agents that may block the tumor initiation and promotion events that are the sequential stages of cancer development or delay the carcinogenic process.

preclinical efficacy Studies involving the evaluation of agents in a realistic laboratory animal model for cancer indicating the inhibition of carcinogenesis

Colorectal cancer is a tumor of colon and rectum, which occurs with high frequency in both men and women in Western countries. Most cases of colorectal cancers arise in a benign adenoma; some evidence suggests that some cancers arise directly from the mucosal cells. With regard to genetic mechanisms of colorectal cancer, the disease appears to result from an increase in the number of genetic mutations, mostly acquired, that accumulate in the genome of the evolving cancer cell. The histopathologic changes associated with the development of colorectal cancer are driven by the progressive accumulation of definable genetic changes, including the activation of one or more oncogenes plus the inactivation of several tumor suppressor genes and by endogenous and exogenous promoting agents. These genetic changes proceed from cellular hyperproliferation to small, benign adenomas to more dysplastic, larger adenomas and then can become cancer and ultimately metastasize. Identification and removal of these premalignant lesions are considered important in order to design a rational approach to reduce the incidence and mortality of colon cancer.

I. INTRODUCTION

In studies of various human diseases, it is critical that reliable animal models both chemically induced and transgenic are developed that demonstrate similarity to the human disease. Animal models are extremely valuable in our understanding of the human disease, but one has to be familiar with the limitations of the model system that is being used to study the human disease. Animal models should bear relevance to human colorectal cancer with similarities not only in terms of histopathology and molecular and genetic lesions during early and promotion/progression stages of carcinogenesis, but also adequacy of the model for prevention studies. The animal models should also reflect the efficacy of both effective and ineffective nutritional and chemopreventive agents that have been evaluated in humans. It should also be recognized that extrapolation of data obtained in animal model systems entails inherent sources of uncertainty that must be taken into account in predicting human responsiveness. This brief article discusses the carcinogen-induced colon cancer model to study the relationship between chemopreventive agents and colon carcinogenesis.

II. PRECLINICAL MODELS FOR COLON CANCER

Animal models have been developed to study the multiple environmental factors involved in the pathogenesis of cancer of the colon. These animal models are (a) induction of colon tumors in rats through aromatic amines such as 3,2'-dimethyl-4-aminobi-phenyl (DMBA); (b) derivatives and analogs of cycacin such as methyazoxymethanol (MAM), 1,2-dimethylhydrazine (DMH), and azoxymethane (AOM) in rats and mice of selected strains; (c) direct-acting carcinogens of the type of alkylureas, such as methylnitrosourea (MNU) or *N*-methyl-*N*`nitro-*N*-nitrosoguanidine (MNNG); and (d) heterocyclic amines such as 2-amino-3-methylimidazo[4,5-*f*]quinoline (IQ) and 2-amino-1-methyl-6-phenylimidazo[4,5-*b*]pyridine (PhIP). The spectrum of epithelial lesions induced in the colon by these carcinogens is similar to various types of neoplastic lesions observed in the colorectum of humans. Several studies have utilized these relevant animal models to investigate the modulation of colon carcinogenesis by nutritional and chemopreventive agents.

A. Alkylnitrosoureido Compounds

MNNG and MNU are direct alkylating agents, which do not require metabolic activation, and thus they are topical and potent carcinogens. Intrarectal instillation of NMU or MNNG induced colorectal tumors in rodent models. Because of the fact that biochemical activation is not required for these carcinogens, it is an ideal way of inducing colon tumors in animals and of studying modifying effects during the postinitiation stage of colon carcinogenesis without involving metabolism of the genotoxic, initiating carcinogen. Intrarectal administration of MNNG at a dose rate of 1–3 mg/rat/week for 20 weeks induced colon tumors in 100% of male F344 rats of which 43% tumors were adenocarcinomas and 57% were adenomas. The neoplasms were all located in the distal colon and rectum, as MNNG and MNU are locally acting carcinogens. No metastatic lesions were usually observed. Although MNNG and MNU given intrarectally provided the most reliable model for the topical and selective production of tumors in the distal colon and rectum, the major weakness of this model is that the technique of intrarectal injection requires highly skilled technicians and quantification of carcinogens instilled intrarectally is difficult.

B. Heterocyclic Amines

2-Amino-3,8-dimethylimidazo[4,5-f]quiniline (IQ), a heterocyclic aromatic amine produced from food pyrolysis, was first isolated from a variety of broiled or cooked fish and meat. Among a number of heterocyclic amines that have been demonstrated to be highly mutagenic and tumorigenic in rodent models, IQ and 2-amino-1-methyl-6-phenylimidazo[4,5-*b*]pyridine (PhIP) have attracted a lot of attention because they demonstrate a multitarget organospecificity with specific cancer induction in Zymbal gland, skin, colon, oral cavity, and mammary gland of rodents. Colon tumors were induced in male F344 rats by administering PhIP daily in the diet at 100 and 400 ppm for 52 and 104 weeks. Although the colon tumor incidences were about 43 and 55% in animals given PhIP at 100 and 400 ppm, respectively, there was severe toxicity due to PhIP. We have also utilized heterocyclic amines such as IQ and PhIP to induce colon tumors. Results of these studies from our laboratory indicate that when these agents were administered daily in the diet for 52 weeks, the tumor incidence was very low, ranging between 5 and 28%.

C. 1,2-Dimethylhydrazine

1,2-Dimethylhydrazine is an effective carcinogen for the induction of tumors of the colon and rectum in rats and mice by systemic subcutaneous or intraperitoneal injections. The usefulness of this organospecific carcinogen, which induces selectively tumors in the colon, was confirmed by several laboratories. Despite the differences in doses, schedules, and animal strains used by different investigators, there is some consistency in their results in using DMH as a colon carcinogen. Subcutaneous injection of DMH at a dose rate of 20 mg/kg body weight, once weekly for 20 weeks induces colon adenomas and adenocarcinomas in about 60% of male F344 rats. However, the major weakness of this model is that multiple injections of DMH are required to induce colon tumors in the laboratory rodents.

D. Azoxymethane

Azoxymethane, a metabolite of DMH, has been used extensively by many investigators to induce colon tumors and to study the effects of nutritional factors and chemopreventive agents in colon carcinogenesis. AOM is a potent inducer of carcinomas of the large intestine in various strains of male and female rats. We have used a two-dose (15 mg/kg body weight, once weekly for 2 weeks sc) regimen in all our chemoprevention and nutritional studies since mid-1985. Our results and those of others indicate that the just-mentioned dose regimen in male F344 rats induced colon tumors in about 80% of animals with a mean of three tumors/rat after 40–50 weeks following the second AOM treatment. Endoscopic examination of animals revealed that the first endoscopically visible colonic tumor can be detected 15 weeks after the AOM treatment and that the mean latency period of such tumors is about 20 weeks.

Of all the model systems, use of Fischer (F344) rats and AOM seem to be appropriate because rat colons have light and electron microscopic morphology as well as histochemical properties that are quite similar to that of humans and biological behaviors of AOM-induced rat colon carcinomas have close similarity to those of human colon carcinomas. AOM-induced carcinomas metastasize to regional lymph nodes and liver, and these carcinomas are transplantable. Epithelial neoplasms of colon induced by AOM in F344 rats include both adenomas and adenocarcinomas. Based on our past experience with this model, about 70% of colon tumors are adenocarcinomas and the rest are adenomas. Histologically, adenomas of the colon are benign, with mild or moderate epithelial atypia. Malignant neoplasms of the colon (epithelial origin) are adenocarcinomas, the majority of which are well-differentiated, frank malignant tumors showing invasion across the line of the muscularis mucosa. Some of these are poorly differentiated, which are highly infiltrative, and often reach the intestinal wall and the serosa and may even invade the neighboring organs. In our past experience with this model, the extension of lesions into the adjacent peritoneal tissues can occur, and metastic lesions, if present, can be seen in the mesenteric lymph nodes, lung, or liver.

Similar to the regional distribution of tumors in human colon, AOM treatment induces colonic tumors predominantly in the distal colon. AOM treatment also induces *ras* oncogene mutations at codon 12 of K- and H-*ras* and increases the expression of the *ras* family of protooncogenes that have been causally associated with colon tumor development. Enhanced *ras* oncogene expression has been observed in a variety of human colon tumors. AOM-induced colon tumors also demonstrate enhanced cyclooxygenase-2 and inducible nitric oxide synthase expression similar to human colonic tumors. Mutations in the tumor suppression gene, APC, are known to be early events in the colon cancer process in humans. APC gene mutations have been identified in patients with familial adenomatous polyposis, who have germline mutation in one of the APC alleles, and in sporadic colorectal cancer. Evidence in humans thus implicates the APC suppressor gene as causal in large bowel carcinogenesis. Studies indicating the presence of APC mutation in AOM-induced colon tumors in mice strengthens the concept that these models are appropriate for human colon cancer studies.

III. CHEMOPREVENTION STUDIES UTILIZING PRECLINICAL MODELS

The developmental strategies for chemoprevention have been markedly facilitated by the use of relevant animal models mimicking the neoplastic process that occurs in humans. The F344 rat model for AOM-induced colon cancer has been used extensively to obtain critical information on the chemopreventive efficacy of several agents.

A. Phytochemicals

Several studies have demonstrated that generous consumption of vegetables reduces the risk of colon cancer. Although the nature of the constituents of these vegetables and other food items that are responsible for reduced risk has not been fully elucidated, it is clear that the plant foods contain chemopreventive agents, including several micronutrients, such as vitamins, and minerals and also contain nonnutrients, such as organosulfur compounds, polyphenols, and isoflavones, to cite a few. The diversity of these compounds is a positive feature, indicating that a variety of approaches to cancer prevention by these agents may be made so that the optimal selection will emerge. Mechanisms of chemopreventive activity of these

agents range from inhibition of carcinogen activation to detoxification of the carcinogen, blockage of binding of critical carcinogen metabolites to DNA, scavenging reactive electrophiles, and inhibiting arachidonic acid (AA) metabolism. Phytochemicals and their substituted and synthetic analogs tested for their efficacy in the AOM colon cancer model assay included anethole trithione, oltipraz [5-(2-pyrazinyl)-4-methyl-1,2-dithiole-3-thione], diallyl sulfide, and curcumin, to cite a few.

Administration of organosulfur compounds such as diallyl sulfide, oltipraz, or anethole trithione during the initiation and/or postinitiation stage significantly suppressed the incidence and multiplicity of AOM-induced colonic adenocarcinomas in male F344 rats (Table I). The inhibition of colon carcinogenesis by these agents was associated with an increase in the activities of detoxifying enzymes, such as glutathione S-transferase, quinone reductase, and UDP-glutathione transferase in the colonic mucosa and tumors.

Curcumin [diferuloylmethane; 1,7-bis-(4-hydroxy-3-methoxyphenyl)-1,6-heptadiene-3,5-dione)], which has been identified as the major pigment in turmeric, the powdered rhizome of *Curcuma longa* Lim, possesses both anti-inflammatory and antioxidant properties. Importantly, dietary administration of curcumin inhibited AOM-induced colon tumor incidence and multiplicity in a dose-dependent manner (Table I). Curcumin, given as a dietary supplement during the promotion/progression period, dramati-

TABLE I

Chemopreventive Efficacy of Naturally Occurring and Synthetic Agents against Azoxymethane-Induced Colon Carcinogenesis in F344 Rats

Chemopreventive agent	Dosage μg/g diet (ppm)	% Inhibition
Oltipraz	200	35
Curcumin	2000	42
Aspirin	200	32
Ibuprofen	400	45
Sulindac	320	55
Piroxicam	400	64
Celecoxib	1500	96
Piroxicam + DL-difluoromethylornithine	150 + 1000	80
1,4-Phenylenebis(methylene)selenocyanate	20	42

cally inhibited colon tumorigenesis, suggesting that curcumin may retard growth and/or the development of existing neoplastic lesions in the colon and that this agent may be an effective chemopreventive agent for individuals at high risk for colon cancer development, such as patients with polyps.

B. Nonsteroidal Anti-inflammatory Drugs

In recent years, attention has been drawn to the potential chemopreventive properties of nonsteroidal anti-inflammatory drugs (NSAIDs). Several case-control and cohort studies have provided unequivocal evidence for the inverse relationship between colon cancer and the use of NSAIDs, specifically aspirin. There has been ample and consistent experimental evidence from laboratory animal model studies to indicate that NSAIDs, including indomethacin, piroxicam, sulindac, aspirin, ibuprofen, and ketoprofen, inhibit chemically induced colon cancer (Table I). More importantly, piroxicam and sulindac administered during the promotion/progression stage significantly inhibit colon tumorigenesis. Results generated in this preclinical model assay provided baseline information for eventual clinical evaluation of the efficacy of NSAIDs in the late intervention/prevention protocols of colonic tumors in high-risk individuals, such as patients with sporadic colonic polyps of familial adenomatous polyposis (FAP).

One of the mechanisms by which NSAIDs inhibit colon cancer is through the modulation of cyclooxygenase 1 and 2 (COX-1 and COX-2), which leads to a reduction of eicosanoid production, which in turn affects cell proliferation and tumor growth. However, these drugs can cause unwanted side effects, including gastrointestinal ulceration, bleeding, and renal toxicity, through the inhibition of constitutive COX-1 activity. Overexpression of COX-2 has been observed in colon tumors, and many commonly used NSAIDs have very little selectivity for COX-1 or COX-2; therefore, more specific yet minimally toxic inhibitors of COX-2 were developed and tested for chemopreventive efficacy. Celecoxib, a selective COX-2 inhibitor that induces very few toxic side effects, has been found to be significantly more effective than the commonly used NSAIDs in the chemoprevention of colon carcinogenesis in laboratory animal models; it

may thus be an effective chemopreventive agent against colon cancer (Table I). A recent clinical trial has shown a reduction in adenomas in patients with FAP-administered celecoxib.

C. Combinations of Low Doses of Various Chemopreventive Agents

There is increasing interest in the use of combinations of low doses of chemopreventive agents that differ in mode of action, rather than administering single agents as a means of obtaining increased efficacy and minimized toxicity. This approach is extremely important when a promising chemopreventive agent demonstrates apparent efficacy but may produce toxic effects at higher doses. An example of combination of agents producing positive results in laboratory animal models has been a study in which the NSAID piroxicam and DFMO, a specific irreversible enzyme-activated or suicide inhibitor of ornithine decarboxylase (ODC), were evaluated for their chemopreventive efficacy. An important finding of the study was that the lowest dose levels of piroxicam (100 ppm) and DFMO (1000 ppm), when administered together, were more effective in inhibiting the incidence and multiplicity of colon adenocarcinomas than administration of these compounds as single agents, even at higher levels. These data strongly support the view that the use of combinations of chemopreventive agents having diverse actions should have beneficial applications in human cancer chemoprevention trials. This should be one of the approaches used in future research and human intervention trials.

D. Organoselenium

Epidemiological studies have also pointed to an inverse association between dietary selenium intake and colon cancer risk in humans. A randomized clinical trial demonstrated that supplementation of selenium-enriched brewer's yeast reduced the incidence and mortality from cancer of the colon. This finding was corroborated by studies with selenium supplementation of the diet in chemically induced colon carcinogenesis in laboratory animals. Humans ingest primarily organic forms of selenium, such as selenomethionine and selenocysteine, by eating grains, vegetables, and animal products. Chronic feeding of inorganic and certain organic forms of selenium at levels >5 ppm produced toxic effects. Therefore, substantial efforts were made to find and/or develop forms of organic selenium compounds that have the maximal chemopreventive efficacy and lowest possible toxicity. Studies in our laboratory have indicated that certain synthetic organoselenium compounds, such as 1,4-phenyulenebis(methylene)selenocyanate (p-XSC), hold great promise as chemopreventive agents because they have been found to be superior to historically used selenium compounds, such as sodium selenite and selenomethionine. More importantly, the chemopreventive efficacy of this agent is more pronounced when given along with a low-fat diet, thus making a strong case for the use of low-fat dietary regimens along with a chemopreventive agent as a desirable approach for primary prevention in the general population and for secondary prevention of colon cancer in high-risk individuals.

IV. CONCLUSION

An impressive body of observation supports the concept that chemoprevention has the potential to be a major component of colon cancer prevention and control. Accumulating evidence indicates that several NSAIDs, including aspirin, piroxicam, and sulindac, can reduce the incidence of colon cancer in laboratory animals and in humans. Celecoxib, a selective COX-2 inhibitor that induces very few toxic side effects as compared to traditional NSAIDs, has been found to be more effective than the commonly used NSAIDs against colon carcinogenesis in laboratory animal models. Studies have also indicated that the synthetic organoselenium compound p-XSC holds great promise as a chemopreventive agent because its chemopreventive index is higher than inorganic and naturally occurring organic forms of selenium. Growing knowledge of the mechanisms by which chemopreventive agents act offers opportunities to use combinations of specific chemopreventive agents, the aggregate action of which would be clinically beneficial while toxicity would be minimal. How to best use such knowledge toward prevention and control of colorectal cancer is a primary challenge for the future.

See Also the Following Articles

Bibliography

Clark, L. C., Combs, G. F., Turnbull, B. W., State, E. H., Chalker, D. K., Chow, J., Gover, R. A., Graham, G. F., Gross, E. G., Krongard, A., Lesher, J. L., Park, K., Sanders, B. S., Smith, C. L., and Taylor, J. R. (1996). Effect of selenium supplementation for cancer prevention in patients with carcinoma of the skin: A randomized controlled trial. *J. Am. Med. Assoc.* **276,** 1957–1963.

Dubois, R. N., Radhika, A., Reddy, B. S., and Entingh, A. J. (1996). Increased cycloozygenase-2 levels in carcinogen-induced rat colonic tumors. *Gastroenterology* **110,** 1259–1262.

Elwell, M. R., and McConnell, E. S. (1990). Small and large intestine. *In* "Pathology of Fischer Rat" (G. A. Boorman, S. L. Eustis, M. R. Wlwell, C. A. Montgomer, and Mackenzie, eds.), p. 43 Academic Press, San Diego.

Holt, P. R., Mokuolu, A. O., Distler, P., Liu, T., and Reddy, B. S. (1996). Regional distribution of carcinogen-induced colon neoplasia in the rat. *Nutr. Cancer* **25,** 129–135.

Ito, N., Hasegawa, R., Sano, S., Tamano, S., Esumi, H., Takayama, S., and Sugimura, T. (1991). A new colon and mammary carcinogen in cooked food, 2-amino-1-methyl-6-phenylimidazo-[4,5-b]pyridine (PhIP). *Carcinogenesis* **12,** 1503–1506.

Kawamori, T., Lubet, R., Steele, V. E., Kelloff, G. J., Kaskey, R. B., Rao, C. V., and Reddy, B. S. (1999). Chemopreventive effect of curcumin, a naturally-occurring anti-inflammatory agent, during the promotion/progression stages of colon cancer. *Cancer Res.* **59,** 597–601.

Kawamori, T., Rao, C. V., Siebert, K., and Reddy, B. S. (1998). Chemopreventive activity of celecoxib, a specific cyclooxygenase-2 inhibitor, against colon carcinogenesis. *Cancer Res.* **58,** 409–412.

Kensler, T. W., Tsuda, H., and Wogan, G. N. (1999). United States–Japan workshop on new rodent models for the analysis and prevention of carcinogenesis. *Cancer Epidemiol. Biomark. Prevent.* **8,** 1033–1037.

Kune, G. A., Kune, S., and Watson, L. F. (1988). Colorectal cancer risk, chronic illness, operations and mediations: Case-control results from the Melbourne Colorectal Cancer Study. *Cancer Res.* **48,** 4399–4404.

Pozharisski, K. M. (1990). Tumors of the intestines. *In* "Pathology of Tumors in Laboratory Animals" (V. Turuso, and U. Mohr, Eds.), Vol. 1, pp. 159–198. IARC Scientific Publication No. 99, Lyon, France.

Rao, C. V., Rivenson, A., Simi, B., and Reddy, B. S. (1995). Chemoprevention of colon carcinogenesis by dietary curcumin, a naturally occurring plant phenolic compound. *Cancer Res.* **55**, 2219–2225.

Rao, C. V., Rivenson, A., Simi, B., Zang, E., Kelloff, G., Steele, V., and Reddy, B. S. (1995). Chemoprevention of colon carcinogenesis by sulindac, a non-steroidal antiinflammatory agent. *Cancer Res.* **55**, 1464–1472.

Rao, C. V., Tokumo, K., Kelloff, G., and Reddy, B. S. (1991). Inhibition by dietary oltipraz of experimental intestinal carcinogenesis induced by azoxymethane in male F344 rats. *Carcinogen. (Lond.)* **12**, 1051–1056.

Reddy, B. S., Hirose, Y., Lubet, R. A., Steele, V. E., Kelloff, G. J., Paulson, S., Siebert, K., and Rao, C. V. (2000). Chemoprevention of colon cancer by specific cyclooxygenase-2 inhibitor, celecoxib, administered during different stages of carcinogenesis. *Cancer Res.* **60**, 293–297.

Reddy, B. S., Maruyama, H., and Kelloff, G. J. (1987). Dose-related inhibition of colon carcinogenesis by dietary piroxicam, a nonsteroidal anti-inflammatory drug, during different stages of rat colon tumor development. *Cancer Res.* **47**, 5340–5346.

Reddy, B. S., Narisawa, T., Maronpot, R., and Weisburger, J. (1975). Animal models for the study of dietary factors and cancer of the large bowel. *Cancer Res.* **35**, 3421–3426.

Reddy, B. S., Nayini, J., Tokumo, K., Rigotty, J., Zange, E., and Kelloff, G. (1990). Chemoprevention of colon carcinogenesis by concurrent administration of piroxicam, a nonsteroidal antiinflammatory drug, with D,L-α-difluoromethylornithine, an ornithine decarboxylase inhibitor in diet. *Cancer Res.* **50**, 2562–2568.

Reddy, B. S., Rao, C. V., Rivenson, A., and Kelloff, G. J. (1993). Inhibitory effect of aspirin on azoxymethane-induced colon carcinogenesis in F344 rats. *Carcinogen. (Lond.)* **14**, 1493–1497.

Reddy, B. S., Rao, C. V., Rivenson, A., and Kelloff, G. (1997). Chemoprevention of colon carcinogenesis by organosulfur compounds. *Cancer Res.* **53**, 3494–3498.

Reddy, B. S., and Rivenson, A. (1993). Inhibitory effect of *Bifidobacterium longum* on colon, mammary, and liver carcinogenesis induced by 2-amino-3-methylimidazo[4,5-*f*] quinoline, a food mutagen. *Cancer Res.* **53**, 3914–3918.

Reddy, B. S., Rivenson, A., El-Bayoumy, K., Upadhyaya, P., Pittman, B., and Rao, C. V. (1997). Chemoprevention of colon cancer by synthetic organoselenium compounds, 1,4-phenylenebis(methylene)selenocyanate and *p*-methoxy benzyl selenocyanate, in low and/or high fat fed F344 rats. *J. Natl. Cancer Inst.* **89**, 506–516.

Reddy, B. S., Tokumo, K., Kulkarni, N., Aliga, C., and Kelloff, G. (1992). Inhibition of colon carcinogenesis by prostaglandin synthesis inhibitors and related compounds. *Carcinogenesis* **13**, 1019–1023.

Reddy, B. S., Wantanabe, K., and Weisburger, J. H. (1997). Effect of high-fat diet on colon carcinogenesis in F344 rats treated with 1,2-dimethylhydrazine, methylazoxymethanol acetate, or methylnitrosourea. *Cancer Res.* **37**, 4156–4158.

Singh, J., Hamid, R., and Reddy, B. S. (1997). Dietary fat and colon cancer: Modulation of cyclooxygenase-2 by types and amount of dietary fat during the postinitiation stage of colon carcinogenesis. *Cancer Res.* **57**, 3465–3470.

Singh, J., Kulkarni, N., Kelloff, G., and Reddy, B. S. (1994). Modulation of azoxymethane-induced mutational activation of *ras* protooncogens of chemopreventive agents in colon carcinogenesis. *Carcinogenesis* **15**, 1317–1323.

Thun, M. H., Namboodiri, M. M., and Heath, C. W. (1991). Aspirin use and reduced risk of fatal colon cancer. *N. Engl. J. Med.* **325**, 1593–1596.

Anthracyclines

Nicholas R. Bachur

University of Maryland Cancer Center

This family of anticancer antibiotics includes the clinically important doxorubicin, daunorubicin, epidoxorubicin, idarubicin and others. Found primarily as natural products of the family *Streptomyces* and other fungi of the Actinomycetalis order, these antibiotics have provided significant clinical utility as well as a stimulus for research advances since their first use as anticancer agents in the 1960s.

I. HISTORY

Although discovered in 1939 by Krassilnikov and Koreniako, the first systematic separation and chemical identification of anthracyclines from Streptomyces purpurascens occurred in the 1950s by Brockmann and co-workers. In 1963, DiMarco's group at Farmilia described the new antibiotic, daunomycin, from *Streptomyces peucetius* and DuBost and co-workers at Rhone-Poulenc described rubidomycin from *Streptomyces coerubleorubidus*. These two compounds were found to have the same structure, and their original names were combined to daunorubicin, indicating the dual discovery. Initial clinical trials in Italy, primarily on solid tumors, showed only modest clinical responses with significant toxicities. However, by 1967, clinical trials in France on adult acute leukemia and childhood acute leukemias yielded dramatic complete remissions of these leukemias. These clinical responses produced considerable excitement and launched new investigations on the anthracycline family of structures. Led by Arcamone, the scientists at Farmitalia, utilizing a mutated variant named S. *peucetius* var. *caesius*, isolated a new anthracycline, adriamycin, which was later changed to the generic name, doxorubicin. Doxorubicin proved to be unusually effective in animal studies, and in clinical trials by Bonnadona and co-workers, the new agent displayed unusual efficacy against several groups of solid tumors.

This second jolt of discovery shook the scientific and clinical communities with the new anthracycline, doxorubicin, that was effective against solid tumors and complemented daunorubicin, which was more effective against leukemias. These discoveries stimulated the search for less toxic and more effective anthracyclines through chemical modifications of the original compounds and *de novo* synthesis of anthracyclines, as well as the search of the biosphere for new members of the family. Carminomycin, the 4-demethyl analog of daunomycin isolated from *Actinomadura carminata* in 1973 by Gause and co-workers in the U.S.S.R., had significant anticancer activity. Other anthracyclines, ruticulomycins, were isolated by Mitcher and colleagues at Lederle Laboratories in 1964, and nogalamycin was reported by Bhuyan and associates at the Upjohn Company in 1965. In 1975, aclacinomycins A and B were isolated from *Streptomycin galilaeus* by Oki and co-workers at Sanraku-Ocean Company. Nettleton and associates at Bristol Laboratories isolated a new group of anthracyclines they named the bohemic complex: musettamycin, marcellomycin, and others based on pyromycinone as the anthracycline core. Since then, hundreds of native, chemically modified and synthesized anthracyclines have been described and investigated for pharmacologic activity. Several have advanced to clinical trials and a few to ultimate clinical utility. Scientific interest in the chemistry of anthracyclines and their impact in their pharmacodynamics and pharmacokinetics has led to important collatoral discoveries and observations.

II. CHEMISTRY

Anthracycline antibiotic structures are based on the anthracyclinone (anthraquinone) or (naphthaquinone) core with quinones, phenolic groups, and other substitutents on the reasonating ring structure A, B, and C and on the saturated D ring. Water solubility is provided to the water-insoluble anthracyclinone ring system by mono- or multisaccharide substitutions on the D ring system, most frequently at the 7 position (Fig. 1).

Important functional characteristics of the anthracycline antibiotics, daunorubicin and doxorubicin, are (1) the planar anthraquinone ring system, (2) quinone groups on the unsaturated rings, (3) stereochemistry of the D ring substitution at position 9, and (4) the amino sugar, daunosamine, which provides water solubility and chemical architecture for stabilizing DNA binding.

III. CLINICAL ACTIVITIES

Since their first clinical trials, several anthracyclines have become and remain mainstays as cancer chemotherapeutic agents. Daunorubicin is important for induction in treating acute leukemias. Doxorubicin and epirubicin are primary therapeutic agents in combination regimens for the treatment of lymphomas and solid tumors. Idarubicin is used in the treatment of leukemias.

Although most of the anthracyclines possess significant anticancer activities as single agents, they are now used in combination chemotherapy to improve therapeutics efficacy and to reduce toxicities. The types of malignancies that are treated with the various anthracyclines range from acute myelogenous leukemia to lymphoma to solid tumors of the breast, lung, gastrointestinal tract, and genitourinary system.

IV. PHARMACOLOGY

Anthracycline antibiotics are administered intravenously because these molecules do not survive oral administration. They are rapidly absorbed by tissues where the highest concentrations are detected in lungs, liver, marrow cells, and spleen. These agents do not pass the blood–brain barrier except idarubicin, which will pass the barrier in pediatric patients.

The long plasma half-life for most anthracyclines generally exceeds 24 h showing extensive tissue absorption with slow multiphasic release. These agents are rapidly metabolized by both phase 1 and phase 2 enzymes so that the plasma components of the drugs are composed heavily of drug metabolites as well, which complicates the pharmacokinetic factors.

Excretion of the parent drug and metabolites is primarily through biliary excretion (60 to 80%) with

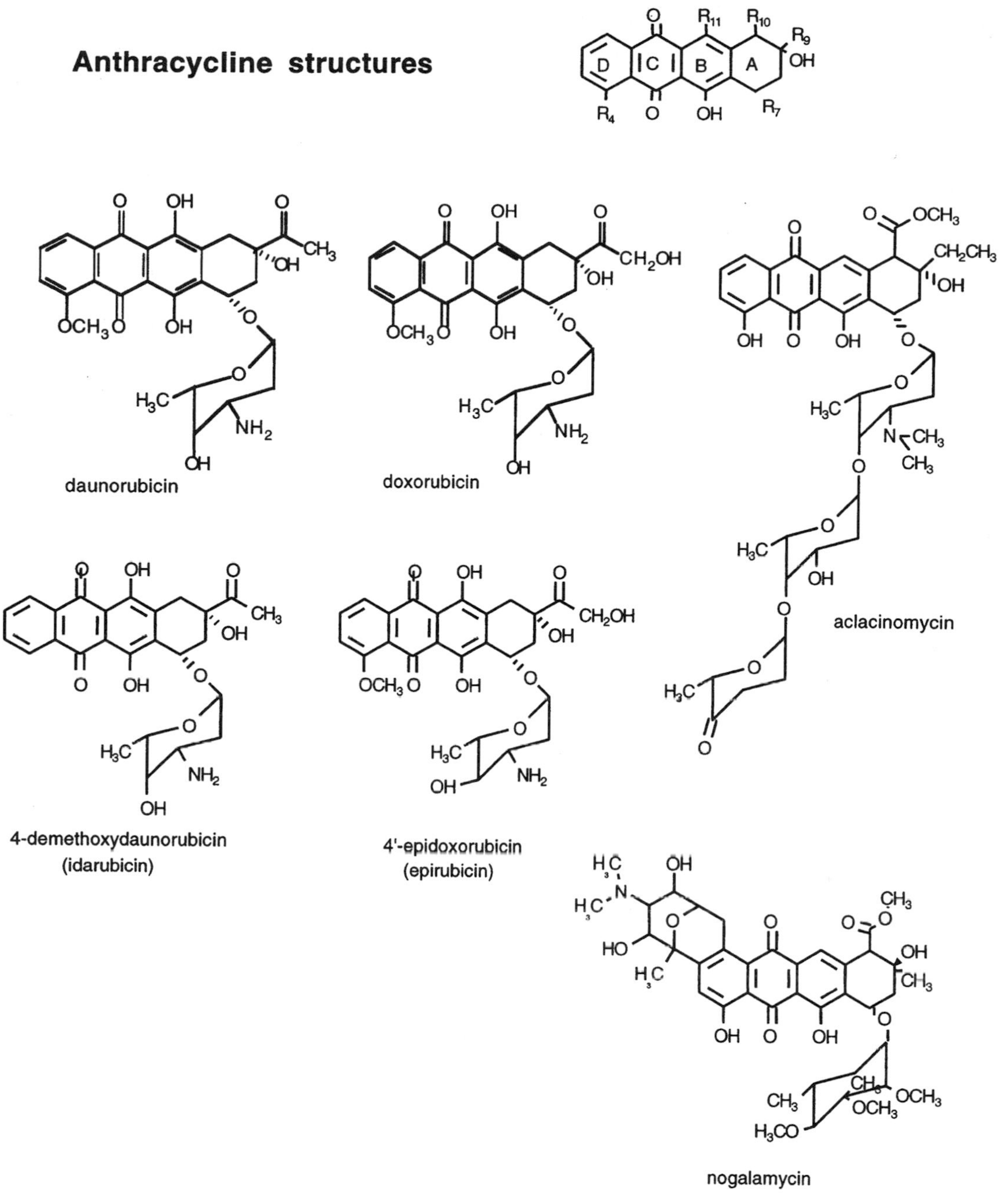

Anthracycline structures

daunorubicin

doxorubicin

aclacinomycin

4-demethoxydaunorubicin
(idarubicin)

4'-epidoxorubicin
(epirubicin)

nogalamycin

FIGURE 1 Anthracycline structures.

urinary excretion accounting for most of the remainder (40–20%). Because of the predominent biliary excretion, normal doses may produce increased toxicity in patients with hepatic impairment. In addition, several examples of drug–drug interaction are reported causing delayed biliary excretion and increased toxicities.

The organs and systems most affected by anthracyclines that lead to toxicities are (1) suppression of bone marrow regeneration, (2) suppression of gastrointestinal regeneration with concomitent mucositis and necrotizing colitis, and (3) myocardial toxicity upon total cumulative doses exceeding 300 mg/m^2.

Another important toxicity related to the administration mechanics is extravasation necrosis. This potentially highly tissue destructive toxicity occurs when the parenterally administered anthracycline escapes outside the receiving vein into the local tissues. The tissue cells contacted by drug are killed and the affected tissues necrose, often requiring extensive surgery and debridement.

V. MECHANISM OF ACTION

In the early studies of daunorubicin and other anthracycline antibiotics, investigators recognized the rapid intracellular binding of these agents to nuclear DNA. This phenomenon is conveniently observable in the fluorescence microscope when living cells are placed in anthracycline-containing media. The cells rapidly take up the drug, and the drug can be seen under fluorescence throughout the nucleus. The binding of anthracyclines to duplex DNA and other nucleic acid structures has been studied by many investigators who have developed detailed structural assemblies of these molecules and duplex DNA. The primary type of anthracycline binding to Watson–Crick base pairs is by minor groove intercalation. The hydrophobic aromatic D ring inserts between and perpendicular to base pairs while the substituted A ring and amino sugar are positioned at the minor groove. The daunosamine sugar completes hydrogen binding in the minor groove to stabilize the binding. Macroscopic DNA-binding constants approximate $10^6 \, M^{-1}$, although there are reports that some DNA base sequences and configurations have higher binding constants of $10^8 \, M^{-1}$.

Basically, several actions occur through this specific binding to DNA: DNA synthesis, RNA synthesis, and DNA repair are inhibited. As the complexity of DNA interactions with proteins and other molecules is resolved, modes and effects of anthracycline binding to DNA have shown more specificity. DNA base sequence has an important effect on the anthracycline-binding affinity, and the base sequence AGCT appears to have the highest affinity for doxorubicin and daunomycin.

DNA helicases, enzymes responsible for the separation of duplex DNA strands for DNA processing, are dramatically inhibited by anthracycline binding. This process is rapid, highly effective, and can account for the secondary inhibition of DNA and RNA synthesis, as well as inhibition of DNA repair. Because of the multiple specific DNA helicases in the eucaryotic cell, a wide range of actions and specificities of the anthracyclines is expected. Production of an irreversible ternary complex of anthracycline–DNA helicase is probably lethal to the cell.

Topoisomerase II is well studied as a target of anthracycline action. Anthracycline, the enzyme, topoisomerase II, and DNA develop into a "cleavable complex," which results in DNA double strand breakage and ultimately cell death.

Free radical generation in cells by anthracyclines occurs because of the quinone structure of the anthracycline chromophore. Anthracycline quinones are reducible by cellular enzymes and can produce free radicals. The action of these free radicals can be destructive to cellular DNA and other macromolecules. Experimental evidence has supported the free radical formation as another mechanism of action of the anthracycline antibiotics.

Several other cellular actions by anthracyclines have been described, which may also play a part in the anticancer and cytotoxic activities of these agents.

VI. RECENT DEVELOPMENTS

Anthracyclines have been the focus of many novel attempts to improve their actions against cancer and to reduce their toxicities. Anthracyclines have been incorporated into liposomes and utilized for therapy. Anthracyclines have been combined with antibodies to direct their actions against specific cell types and locations. They have been linked to carrier molecules such as specific proteins for release at specific cell targets.

See Also the Following Articles

Acute Lymphoblastic Leukemia in Adults • Acute Lymphoblastic Leukemia in Children • Acute Myelocytic Leukemia • Bleomycin • Camptothecins • Folate Antagonists • L-Asparaginase

Bibliography

Arcamone, F. (1981). "Doxorubicin: Anthracycline Antibiotics," Vol. 17. Academic Press, New York.

Bachur, N. R. (1995). Anthracycline antihelicase action. *In* "Anthracycline Antibiotics: New Analogues, Methods of Delivery, and Mechanisms of Action" (W. Priebe, ed.), pp. 204–221. American Chemical Society, Washington, DC.

Chaires, J. B. (1996). Molecular recognition of DNA by daunorubicin. *In* "Advances in DNA Sequence Specific Agents." (L. H. Hurley, and J. B. Chaires, eds.), Vol. 2, pp. 141–167. JAI Press, Greenwich, TC.

Priebe, W. (1995). "Anthracycline Antibiotics: New Analogues, Methods of Delivery, and Mechanisms of Action." American Chemical Society, Washington, DC.

Remers, W. A. (1979). Anthracycline antibiotics. *In* "The Chemistry of Antitumore Antibiotics," Vol. 1. Wiley, New York.

Antibodies in the Gene Therapy of Cancer

Zelig Eshhar
Shelley Schwarzbaum
The Weizmann Institute of Science, Israel

GLOSSARY

intrabodies Antibody fragments (usually in the scFv configuration, see later and Fig. 1) expressed intracellularly. Such antibodies bind a target molecule and are used to inhibit a specific cellular function or pathology.

phage display technology An *in vitro* technique for the artificial selection and maturation of antibody molecules from libraries of phage particles expressing antibody V regions.

scFv A single chain antibody fragment, usually composed of the two variable regions (V_H and V_L) joined with an artificial flexible peptide linker (see Fig. 1A). The scFv construct can include immunoglobulin constant chain regions, which confer greater stability, and/or various targeting peptides to control intracellular localization.

T body A construct containing an immunoglobulin variable region (usually in the form of an scFv) linked to a signaling molecule, such as the ζ chain derived from the CD3/T-cell receptor complex. This construct, when transduced into and expressed by immune effector cells, is able to redirect the (cytotoxic) effector function of these cells to antibody-determined specificity (Fig. 1B).

viral vector targeting Inclusion of antibody-derived recognition elements as part of the viral envelope in order to alter the species or cell type specificity of viral vectors. This technique should enable highly efficient and cell type-specific gene transfer (Fig. 1C).

Antibodies have long been envisioned as potential "magic bullets," able to identify and destroy tumors and other diseased tissues. In gene therapy, foreign genes are expressed in a predetermined cell population for therapeutic purposes. Antibodies have been incorporated as specific recognition elements in a number of gene therapy approaches to cancer treatment. These include the intrabodies, in which antibody fragments are expressed intracellularly (inside the cell) in an attempt to modify a specific cell function or pathology; the use of antibodies expressed on the viral envelope to target viral vector-mediated gene transfer to specific cell types or to tissue expressing a particular disease marker; and the T-body approach, in which immune effector cells are retargeted using antibody-containing receptors to recognize and kill target cells expressing a particular surface marker, such as a tumor-associated antigen.

I. RATIONALE AND ADVANTAGES OF USING ANTIBODIES AS A TARGETING MEANS IN GENE THERAPY

Gene therapy, while still in its infancy, represents a revolutionary approach to cancer therapy. Conventional cancer therapy involves treating patients with surgery, high doses of radiation, or toxic drugs, which are not particularly specific for the tumor cells. Such nonspecific conventional treatment is often accompanied by unpleasant and dose-limiting side effects, and many tumors are able to escape these therapies. In gene therapy, a DNA construct encoding a gene of interest, usually aimed at inducing cell demise or increasing the immunogenicity of tumor cells, is expressed specifically in the diseased tissue or, alternatively, in an effector cell population to promote its antitumor potential. These approaches all require that the transferred gene be expressed in a particular population of cells. In addition, gene therapy may involve the inhibition of an intracellularly expressed protein by its binding and inactivation at the RNA or protein level.

Antibodies, specific binding proteins produced by the humeral immune response, are ideally suited for the cell type and protein targeting required by many gene therapy approaches. Antibody molecules are composed of two heavy and two light chains, which join to form a tetrameric structure. Each pair of heavy and light chains associates to form a variable region, responsible for antigen binding, and a constant region, which mediates or recruits effector functions. The variable region domains, consisting of the first 100–110 amino-terminal residues of both heavy and light chains, are highly diverse and are generated by

a complex mechanism of gene rearrangement, recombination, and point mutations. The huge number of variable region genes, the mechanism of heavy and light chain recombination, and the process of somatic mutation ensure that an antibody can be produced that can specifically recognize virtually any target molecule. While antibodies do have effector functions mediated by their constant regions, modern therapeutic approaches utilizing antibodies have relied on the variable regions of antibodies for target recognition, with the addition of powerful artificial effector mechanisms. For targeting in gene therapy, the variable region of the antibody molecule is also the region of interest. For a more detailed description of antibody structure, see our article in the first edition of this encyclopedia and references therein.

The variable region to be used in gene therapy may come from several sources. The classic source is from a monoclonal antibody, which is produced by immortalization, using cell fusion, of antibody-producing mouse spleen cells, followed by screening for the required specificity. The V region sequences from such an antibody-producing cell can then be cloned, altered, and incorporated into various configurations (Fig. 1). Several manipulations are used to render the cloned antibody suitable for use in gene therapy. Often, if only a variable region is required, a single chain Fv (scFv) fragment can be made. This configuration contains the variable regions derived from the heavy and light antibody chains, connected by a synthetic linker peptide (see Fig. 1A). These fragments have been shown to recognize antigen similarly to intact antibodies, but are much smaller, and may be easily linked to other effector molecules. Other alterations in the antibody structure are also possible. To reduce immunogenicity when used in therapy, mouse-derived monoclonal antibodies are often "humanized." This is accomplished by using recombinant DNA techniques to "graft" the antigen recognition sequences derived from the murine antibody of interest onto a human variable region backbone. A recent significant advance was the development of a transgenic strain of mouse that was engineered to contain most of the human loci encoding the antibody variable regions. The corresponding genes in these mice were inactivated by "knock out," resulting in mice whose antibodies are

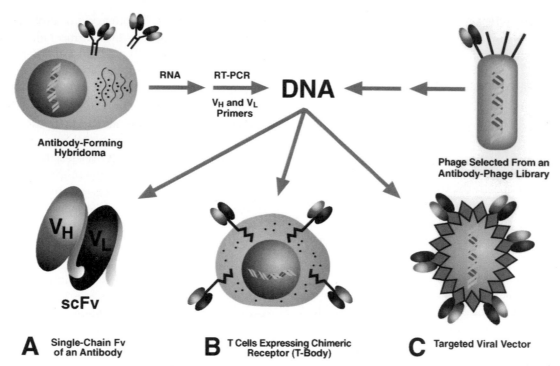

FIGURE 1 Sources of antibody-derived V region constructs and their use in gene therapy. Antibodies are selected by screening of monoclonal antibody-producing B-cell hybridomas (top left) or by phage display technology (top right), and the DNA encoding the variable regions is used in the configurations shown below. (A) Single chain Fv (scFv) consisting of heavy chain and light chain variable regions (V_H and V_L) expressed in a single construct and connected by a peptide linker sequence. scFv may be expressed intracellularly in the cytoplasm or nucleus and used to modulate the expression or function of specific proteins to which they bind. (B) Single chain antibody constructs can be linked to a T-cell activation chain and transduced into patient-derived effector cells to produce "T bodies." The antibody-derived recognition element redirects the specificity of the cytotoxic effector cell to a tumor marker of choice. (C) Antibodies may also be used as recognition elements to control the specificity of the viral vectors used to deliver gene therapy. Such modified viral envelopes may have broadened specificity, enabling a virus that previously infected only rodent cells to now infect human cells, or they may be used to limit infection to a specific cell lineage or to cells expressing a tumor marker. See color insert in this volume.

of human origin. These mice can be immunized (e.g., with human tumors) and their B cells then fused to murine myeloma cell lines to create human monoclonal antibodies.

Sometimes, standard monoclonal antibody technology is unable to generate an antibody of desired specificity or of sufficient affinity. In this case, artificial selection methodologies such as phage display technology are used. In this technique, phage expressing a large repertoire of random recombinant variable region fragments are selected for adhesion to a surface coated with the antigen of interest (Fig. 1). The selected phage are then expanded, and the variable region sequence is characterized and used simi-

larly to an antibody derived by conventional cell fusion techniques (see article by Winter *et al.* in the bibliography).

Once an antibody with the desired properties has been obtained, it may be used as a recognition element in some of the gene therapy configurations described later. These include intrabodies, in which the antibodies act as intracellular binding agents and inhibitors, the T-body approach, in which antibody-derived sequences act to redirect the specificity of immune effector cells, and the targeting of retroviral tropism to specific cell populations for targeted gene therapy. These three approaches are each described in more detail in the following sections.

II. INTRABODIES

A. Technical Considerations

One approach to the gene therapy of cancer is to regulate gene expression in tumor cells. This could involve targeting gene products that determine the transformed phenotype of these cells or of housekeeping genes that are necessary for cell survival. Early attempts at downregulating gene expression in selected cells relied on the transfection of "antisense" DNA. This gene fragment would be transcribed to form an RNA species opposite in sequence to the gene of interest. It was expected that such sequences would hybridize with and inactivate the RNA encoding the gene whose expression was to be blocked. Unfortunately, it was found that expression levels of antisense RNA were not sufficient to completely block the expression of most genes. Intracellularly expressed antibodies, or intrabodies, usually in the form of an scFv (Fig. 1A), have been designed to similarly block the expression of certain genes, but at the level of their specific protein end products.

The intracellular expression of functional, antigen-binding antibody fragments is hindered by several technical problems. The folding of antibodies into the "correct" antigen-binding configuration requires an oxidizing environment for the formation of intramolecular disulfide bonds, which serve to stabilize their three-dimensional structure. The reducing environment inside the cell does not support disulfide bond formation. This problem has been circumvented by the preselection of certain V region framework sequences that are naturally hyperstable or by manipulations designed to increase antibody stability. These include expression of modified scFv fragments that include a single constant region domain, which has been shown to stabilize correct folding. Other studies have utilized directed mutations of specific variable region framework residues that have been shown to increase antibody stability, even in the reducing environment of the cytoplasm.

Intrabody fragments of mouse origin can appear on the cell surface following processing and presentation by the MHC class I transplantation antigen pathway. Thus, the use of such variable region sequences could result in an immune response against mouse-derived antibody sequences. To prevent this problem, the antibody sequences destined for intracellular expression are often "humanized," as described earlier.

The intracellularly expressed antibody fragment may also be targeted to specific intracellular compartments by the use of specific targeting sequences, such as an endoplasmic reticulum (ER) retention signal, or a nuclear localization signal (NLS) that can direct the scFv to the nucleus. The nuclear localization signal could be useful when targeting nuclear proteins such as transcriptional activators, which may regulate the abnormal proliferation of tumor cells.

B. Examples

To date, several intracellular antibodies have been shown to inhibit gene expression both *in vivo* and *in vitro*. Intrabodies have been functionally expressed in bacteria, yeast, xenopus oocytes, and plant cells. Several successful attempts at modulating cell function in mammalian cells have been reported. Intrabodies have been produced against the IL-2 receptor, which are able to block IL-2-mediated T-cell proliferation. An engineered antibody directed against the HIV Tat regulatory protein was expressed intracellularly as an scFv fragment. HIV-infected cell lines expressing this intrabody were found to exhibit decreased HIV virus production, and intrabody expression inhibited the ability of HIV to infect intrabody-transduced primary T cells.

In other studies, intrabodies against p53 have been shown to inhibit the transactivation function of the p53 protein in cells expressing this construct. Surprisingly, in both HIV and p53 systems, while the targeted protein has a nuclear function, the cytoplasmic intrabody version was a more effective competitor than the intrabody construct containing a nuclear localization signal. This could be due to superior folding of the intrabody or to more efficient antigen binding in the cytoplasm versus the nucleus.

C. Intrabodies for Cancer Therapy

For cancer therapy, intrabodies could be used to block any cellular function involved in the proliferation of these cells. These could include functions or growth factor receptors that are expressed uniquely or predominantly in the tumor, such as the EGF receptor (EGF-R). Jannot *et al.* (1996) introduced intracellularly expressed anti EGF-R scFv fragments and showed that the growth of cells expressing these antibodies was partially inhibited. Alternatively, the intrabody could be designed to target and interfere with a cellular housekeeping function if the intrabody gene is designed to be preferentially transfected into or expressed only in cancer cells. Tumor specificity can be determined by the use of a retroviral vector for transfection, which specifically targets a surface-expressed tumor antigen (see Section IV).

III. T BODIES

A. Methodology

Another approach to combining gene therapy with the use of antibody specificity is the "T-body" methodology, pioneered by our group. This approach seeks to genetically alter and redirect cytotoxic effector cells rather than the diseased tissue or tumor. The transfection of immune effector cells rather than target tissues is advantageous, as this method does not require the transfection of the entire population of tumor cells, but rather can modify cells of the immune system in a way that they will selectively recognize and reject cancerous cells. Immune effector cells [cytotoxic T cells or "natural killer" (NK) cells] are removed from a patient and transduced with a chimeric construct encoding an activation molecule (usually the T-cell receptor ζ chain or the Fc receptor γ chain) linked to an antibody-derived scFv with antitumor specificity (Fig. 1B). The transfected cells are expanded *in vitro* and then returned to the patient, where they are expected to home to and kill tumor cells expressing the antigen of choice. Proof of concept has been demonstrated using an *in vitro* coculture of tumor cells and immune effector cells and using human tumor explants in immunodeficient murine *in vivo* systems. Several groups have initiated phase I clinical trials using protocols based on this methodology.

The advantages of this technique over other attempts at recruiting cytotoxic antitumor effector cells is that recognition of tumor antigens using an antibody-derived element is not genetically restricted to an individual patient. Thus, a panel of T-body constructs can be prepared as a universal reagent, with the only requirement being that the target tumor express a tumor-specific antigen against which a T-body construct is available.

TABLE I
Specificity of Antitumor Antibodies Used in Chimeric Receptors

Antigen	Tumor target	Group (year)
Folate receptor	Ovarian carcinoma	Hwu and Eshhar (1995)
Her2/Neu	Adenocarcinomas (breast)[a]	Eshhar (1993), Groner (1994)
Lewis^y glycolipid	Lung and other carcinomas	Mezzanzanica and Eshhar (1998)
CD19,20,22	B-cell lymphomas	Jensen (1998)
EGP40	Colorectal carcinoma	Eshhar and Hwu (2000)
G250	Renal carcinoma	Bolhuis (1998)
CEA	Colorectal carcinoma	Smyth (1998), Junghans (1999, 2000), Abken (1999, 2000)
GD-2	Melanoma	Sadelain (1998)
HMW-Mei.Ag	Melanoma	Abken (1999)
TAG-72, Mucin	Adenocarcinomas (colon)	Abken (1998), McArthur (1999)
CD30	Hodgkin's lymphoma	Abken (1999)
EGP-2	Various carcinomas	Trevor (2000)

[a]Overexpression of Her/Neu has been reported in several types of tumors, including breast, ovarian, lung, gastric, and oral cancers.

B. Preliminary Results in Tumor Therapy

The T-body approach has been used to target several tumor types in preclinical studies and in phase I clinical trials. Table I summarizes the specificities of the chimeric receptors that have been made against tumor-associated antigens and the tumors targeted by them. As can be seen, a large repertoire of tumors can be targeted by the T-body approach. The feasibility of T bodies in tumor therapy has been demonstrated in animal models and it is currently being evaluated in several clinical trials. Obviously, the therapeutic potency of this approach is dependent on the functional expression of the chimeric genes in the immune effector cells and the ability of these genetically engineered cells to seek and home to their tumor targets and eventually eliminate them. Recent advances in vector design and gene delivery and expression in T lymphocytes have increased the chances of bringing this promising approach to the clinic.

IV. RETROVIRAL TARGETING

A. Description

One of the main factors limiting the application of T bodies, and other gene therapy modalities, are limitations in the vectors available for the specific, safe, and efficient transfection of human cells. Only a small proportion of the viruses that are able to infect human cells can be used safely and effectively for gene delivery, and even fewer are capable of lineage-specific gene transfer. In modalities such as the T-body approach, which involve *ex vivo* transduction of a defined population of cells, the retrovectors used need not be cell type specific. However, many gene therapy approaches require high efficiency *in situ* transduction of the tumor cells themselves (such as the intrabody approach described earlier). Thus, vectors are required that can be administered to the patient, with the expectation of infection and gene transfer only in a defined population of cells. To this end, several laboratories, including the groups of Ralph Dornberg and David Curiel, have attempted to add antibody-derived recognition elements to the viral envelope protein (Fig. 1C). This has enabled the

generation of viral vectors specific for a predetermined cell lineage (such as T-cell leukemia, using an antibody directed against a T-cell specific marker) or a vector that specifically infects cells expressing a particular tumor antigen.

Most of the viral vectors used today for gene therapy either naturally infect a broad spectrum of human cells due to their native tropism (such as adenovirus) or represent modified animal retroviruses (such as the Moloney murine leukemia virus) whose envelope protein, responsible for their binding and penetration into the infected cells, is replaced by a protein with a broad tropism toward human cells, a procedure named xenotyping. A recent example is the use of lentiviruses such as the Simian (monkey) immunodeficiency virus (SIV) or even the human immunodeficiency virus (HIV) that have been engineered by removal of their hazardous elements to serve as efficient, and hopefully safe, lentivectors. To confer on these vectors a broad tropism to human cells, they were pseudotyped with the envelope of the vesicular stomatitis virus (VSV).

Two possible approaches may be taken in retroviral targeting. The first utilizes an ecotropic virus, which is species specific, and does not normally infect human cells. Adding an antibody-derived recognition unit to the viral envelope enables cross-species infection of cells expressing the appropriate surface antigen. In the studies published to date, the wild-type envelope enhances the otherwise poor infectivity of such redirected recombinant envelopes. Alternatively, viruses that are already able to infect human cells may be used, including adenoviruses or retroviruses with amphotropic envelopes. Adding specific recognition elements (such as the scFv of an antibody) enables the specific targeting of cells expressing a predetermined surface marker. The main challenge limiting widespread application of this approach is the difficulty in restricting the general infectivity of these viruses for human cells while maintaining the ability of the viral vectors to penetrate and infect cells expressing a surface marker of choice. The specific targeting of tumor cells is enhanced by the selective transfection by retrovectors of dividing cells; tumor or cell type specificity can be further increased by the use of tissue-specific promoters included in the transduced gene.

B. Examples

Early studies used antibodies against small immunogenic haptens (such as dinitrophenol) as a model system and demonstrated specific targeting of retroviruses containing antibody/env fusion proteins to hapten-coupled cells. More recent studies have combined several of the techniques and approaches described in this article. For example, scFv sequences derived using phage display technology were incorporated into the viral envelope of spleen necrosis virus to retarget the resulting vector specifically to cells of the T-cell lineage. Such a vector could be used for specific transduction of patient-derived T cells with a tumor-specific T-body construct. Other retrovectors have been targeted to melanoma-specific antigens and to the tumor antigen her2/neu. Curiel's group (2000) conducted a phase I trial of an scFv recognition element directed against the tumor antigen erbB-2 on the surface of ovarian cancer cells. This study, which used an adenovirus-based vector, demonstrated that the approach is safe and provided some preliminary evidence for efficacy.

Such vectors could permit gene transfer to specific tumor or effector cell populations, possibly following direct systemic administration of the vector. This would eliminate the need for the removal of tissue and *ex vivo* expansion and would allow transfection of tumors that are not accessible to biopsy. Studies that will further elucidate the mechanism of retroviral envelope fusion with the host membrane should enable improved control of retroviral host tropism.

V. CONCLUSIONS

Gene therapy represents a series of therapeutic modalities that involve the transfer of genetic material into patient tissue. Limitations of these techniques include the difficulty of specifically targeting gene transfer or cytotoxic functions to defined cell populations and to selected cellular processes. The ability to generate antibodies that recognize virtually any chosen determinant is expected to enhance both the cell-specific targeting of such therapy and the ability to inhibit or modulate particular cellular functions in the targeted cell population.

See Also the Following Articles

ANTIBODY-TOXIN AND GROWTH FACTOR-TOXIN FUSION PROTEINS • ANTI-IDIOTYPIC ANTIBODY VACCINES • MONOCLONAL ANTIBODIES AGAINST SOLID TUMORS • MONOCLONAL ANTIBODIES: LEUKEMIA AND LYMPHOMA • RADIOLABELED ANTIBODIES, OVERVIEW • RESISTANCE TO ANTIBODY THERAPY • TARGETED VECTORS FOR CANCER GENE THERAPY • TUMOR ANTIGENS

Bibliography

Bitton, N., Gorochov, G., Debre, P., and Eshhar, Z. (1999). Gene therapy approaches to HIV-infection: Immunological strategies: Use of T bodies and universal receptors to redirect cytolytic T-cells. *Front. Biosci.* **4,** 386–393.

Cosset, F. L., and Russell, S. J. (1996). Targeting retrovirus entry. *Gene Ther.* **3,** 946–956.

Eshhar, Z., Bach, N., Fitzer-Attas, C. J., Gross, G., Lustgarten, J., Waks, T., and Schindler, D. G. (1996). The T-body approach: Potential for cancer immunotherapy. *Spring. Semin. Immunopathol.* **18,** 199–209.

Eshhar, Z., and Schwarzbaum, S. (1996). Genetically engineered antibodies in cancer therapy. *In* "Encyclopedia of Cancer. Academic Press, San Diego.

Marasco, W. A., LaVecchio, J., and Winkler, A. (1999). Human anti-HIV-1 tat scFv intrabodies for gene therapy of advanced HIV-1-infection and AIDS. *J. Immunol. Methods* **231,** 223–238.

Russell, S. J., and Cosset, F. L. (1999). Modifying the host range properties of retroviral vectors. *J. Gene Med.* **1,** 300–311.

Winter, G., Griffiths, A. D., Hawkins, R. E., and Hoogenboom, H. R. (1994). Making antibodies by phage display technology. *Annu. Rev. Immunol.* **12,** 433–455.

Antibody–Toxin and Growth Factor–Toxin Fusion Proteins

David FitzGerald
Robert J. Kreitman
Ira Pastan
National Cancer Institute, Bethesda, Maryland

GLOSSARY

endoplasmic reticulum (ER) retention sequence Specific amino acids located at the C termini of proteins that retain them in, and/or retrieve them to, the ER.

Fv fragment The portion of a monoclonal activity that is composed of the variable domain of the heavy chain linked with the variable domain of the light chain.

immunotoxin An antibody–toxin or a ligand–toxin hybrid protein.

ligand Either a growth factor or a cytokine that binds to a cell surface receptor.

recombinant Signifying that molecules have been expressed in *Escherichia coli*.

translocation Toxins have the unusual property of being able to move from one side of a cell membrane to the other side. This movement is called translocation.

The goal of cancer treatment is the elimination of tumor cells while inflicting the least amount of harm to normal cells. Because approximately half of all cancers are not cured using conventional therapies, new strategies are needed. One emerging therapeutic approach is the targeted delivery of highly toxic substances.

I. INTRODUCTION

Certain bacterial and plant toxins [e.g., diphtheria toxin, ricin, and pseudomonas exotoxin (PE)] are among the most toxic substances known. Because these toxins bind to cell surface receptors that are expressed on many normal cell types, they would, unmodified, be useless as therapeutics. Therefore, to convert toxins into useful agents, their binding to normal tissues has to be eliminated and replaced with tumor-selective binding. The strategies for modifying toxin activity and engineering novel binding specificities are discussed. The combination of a modified toxin with a binding ligand is often called an immunotoxin or chimeric toxin and the term "recombinant" usually signifies that molecules have been expressed in *E. coli*.

II. IMMUNOTOXIN DESIGN AND TESTING

The genes for diphtheria toxin, ricin, and PE have been cloned and sequenced. In addition, structural data are available from protein crystals of each toxin. Structure–function studies have indicated which part of each gene encodes sequences of a particular function. Based on this knowledge, recombinant immunotoxins have been generated by deleting the DNA encoding the binding portion of the toxin and replacing it with an antibody, growth factor, or other ligand that will bind selectively to cancer cells. Once the immunotoxin is made, its usefulness is assessed in a series of preclinical tests. A favorable outcome leads to the initiation of clinical trials, which determine the properties of immunotoxins in cancer patients.

Conventional DNA cloning techniques are used to delete the sequences in toxin genes that are responsible for toxin binding. cDNA sequences encoding tumor-binding ligands are then inserted in place of these sequences. Immunotoxin sequences are cloned in an expression plasmid downstream of the T7 promoter. Plasmids are transformed into an expression host, typically *E. coli* stain BL21 (λDE3), developed by Studier. This strain produces T7 polymerase in response to induction of the lactose operon. BL21 (λDE3), transformed with the appropriate plasmid, is grown in Luria-Bertani broth with ampicillin (100 μg/ml). At an absorbance of 0.5–2.0 (600 nm), the culture is induced with isopropyl-β-D-thiogalactopyranoside to bring about high-level expression. Recombinant immunotoxins are usually produced within the *E. coli* cell and are later recovered from inclusion bodies by denaturation and renaturation.

The renatured material is then typically purified by Q Sepharose, Mono Q, and HPLC size-exclusion chromatography.

Purified immunotoxins are tested for cytotoxicity by measuring their ability to inhibit protein synthesis. Typically, immunotoxins in the range of 0.1–100 ng/ml are added to both target and nontarget cells. After an overnight incubation at 37°C, protein synthesis is measured by incubating cells for 1 hr with [³H]leucine. Immunotoxins that exhibit IC_{50} values below 10 ng/ml for target cells and above 1000 ng/ml for nontarget cells are considered potent and selective enough for testing in tumor models. Mice are injected with the appropriate tumor xenograft. After several days to allow the tumor to get established, immunotoxin treatments are given (immunotoxin injections on days 5, 7, and 9 are typical). Antitumor activity and toxicity to mice are assessed. A therapeutic window is established whereby the therapeutic dose is compared with the toxic dose (the LD_{50} is divided by the dose giving complete regressions of tumor).

Immunotoxins with a good therapeutic window are then evaluated in monkeys for toxicity to normal primate tissue. On completion of these preclinical evaluations, compounds with an acceptable therapeutic profile go forward to phase I trials in patients harboring cancers that have failed to respond adequately to conventional treatment.

III. PSEUDOMONAS EXOTOXIN: STRUCTURE–FUNCTION

Because our group has worked almost exclusively with PE, most working examples are drawn from that experience. PE, which is a three-domain protein (Fig. 1), binds and enters cells by receptor-mediated endocytosis (Fig. 2). Specifically, PE binds via its N-terminal domain (termed domain I) to the heavy chain of the low-density lipoprotein receptor-related protein (LRP). LRP carries the toxin to the endocytic compartment. Once there, the toxin is cleaved by a furin-like protease. Cleavage, which is necessary for toxicity, has an optimum of pH 5.5 and because of this it most likely occurs in the endosomal compartment. The cleavage site is located in the middle domain (termed domain II) between arginine 279 and glycine

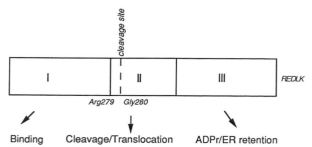

FIGURE 1 PE structure–function. PE is composed of three structural domains. Domain I encodes the binding domain. Domain II has translocating activity and contains the site of proteolytic processing. Cleavage is between arginine 279 and glycine 280. Domain III has ADP-ribosylating activity and a ER retention sequence at the C terminus.

280 (see Figs. 1 and 2). Proteolytic cleavage followed by the reduction of the disulfide bond that joins cysteines 265 and 287 produces a N-terminal fragment of 28 kDa and a C-terminal fragment of 37 kDa (Fig. 2). The 28-kDa fragment is composed of all of domain I and a small portion of domain II. The 37-kDa fragment is composed of most of domain II and all of domain III. Besides serving as the site of cleavage, domain II has sequences necessary to translocate domain III to the cell cytosol. Domain III, which is located at the C terminus, has ADP-ribosylating activity and it is this activity that mediates cell killing. Specifically, once in the cell cytosol, domain III ADP ribosylates elongation factor 2 and shuts down the synthesis of new cellular protein (Fig. 2). Domain III also has an endoplasmic reticulum retention sequence that is located at the very C terminus of PE and is

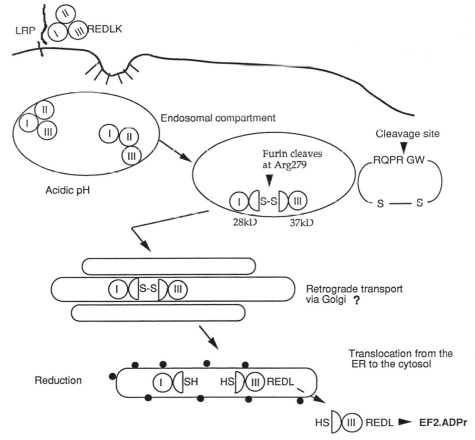

FIGURE 2 Pathway for PE as it enters the cell cytosol of mammalian cells. Binding is followed by internalization to the endosomal compartment. Cleavage by a furin-like enzyme is essential for toxicity. A C-terminal fragment of 37 kDa is generated, which translocates from the ER to the cell cytosol where it inactivates protein synthesis by ADP-ribosylating elongation factor 2.

composed of the following five amino acids:REDLK. The terminal lysine is probably removed by carboxy peptidases, leaving REDL as the last four amino acids of PE. This sequence closely resembles KDEL, which is the authentic ER retention sequence. An ER retention sequence is necessary for toxin-mediated inhibition of protein synthesis, presumably because it directs PE to the ER where it can translocate to the cytosol (Fig. 2).

IV. CONSTRUCTION OF RECOMBINANT IMMUNOTOXINS

Because it binds LRP, which is present on the surface of most cells and tissues, native PE exhibits no selective cytotoxic activity for tumor cells. However, selective binding can be engineered by eliminating toxin binding to LRP and redirecting domains II and III to the surface of tumor cells. Routinely, the DNA encoding domain I is deleted and replaced with cDNAs encoding binding ligands such as tumor growth factor α (TGFα), interleukin (IL)-2, IL-4, IL-6, and single chain antibodies that bind surface determinants on various human malignancies (Fig. 3). Ligand–toxin and single chain antibody–toxin fusion proteins are expressed in *E. coli*, purified, and tested for cytotoxic activity on appropriate target lines. A similar strategy can be used to construct ligand–toxin fusion proteins with diphtheria toxin (DT). For DT, the sequences encoding toxin binding are located at the 3' end of the structural gene of the toxin. Many of the same ligands that have been fused to the 5' end of PE have also been fused to the 3' end of DT.

Most ligand–toxin fusions exhibit potent toxicity for target cell lines and little or no cytotoxicity for nontarget lines. The activity of TGFαPE38 (PE38 is a truncated version of PE that is composed of domains II and III) for a variety of target lines is provided in Table I. TGFα binds to and is internalized by the epidermal growth factor (EGF) receptor. TGFαPE38 is not toxic for CHO cells, which express no EGF receptors on their cell surface. Like native PE, TGFαPE38 is cleaved within cells by a furin-like protease (data not shown). The mutation of arginine 279 to glycine makes this chimeric toxin refractory to cleavage and nontoxic for cells (Table I). Similar

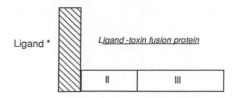

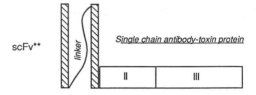

* ligands include growth factors and cytokines

**scFV is the single chain Fv of a monoclonal Ab. The variable portion of light and heavy chains are joined by a flexible peptide linker

FIGURE 3 Construction of fusion proteins with domains II and III of PE. The binding domain of PE is removed and replaced with binding ligands to direct the remainder of the toxin to cancer cells expressing particular antigens or receptors. Usually, the targeting ligand is placed at the N terminus of the PE fusion protein. The single asterisk represents ligands that include growth factors and cytokines. The single chain Fv of a monoclonal Ab is shown by the double asterisk. The variable portion of light and heavy chains is joined by a flexible peptide linker.

kinds of results were obtained when key basic residues at the DT cleavage site were mutated to nonbasic amino acids.

Because recombinant immunotoxins are made by gene fusion technology, certain constraints are inherent in their construction. A ligand fused with domains II and III of PE has to be placed at the N ter-

TABLE I
Cytotoxic Activity of TGFα-Toxins for Various Cell Lines

Cell line	Type	IC$_{50}$ (ng/ml)	
		TGFαPE38	TGFαPE38 Gly279
MCF7	Breast	1.1	>1000
HT29	Colon	2.4	~2000
KB	Epidermoid	0.1	310
A431[a]	Epidermoid	0.28	10
CHO	Ovary	>1000	>1000

[a]A431 IC$_{50}$ (PE) = 5 ng/ml. IC$_{50}$ (PEGly279) > 1000 ng/ml.

minus of the construction. This means that the C terminus of the ligand is joined via a peptide bond with the N terminus of domain II. If the ligand requires a free C terminus to mediate receptor binding, this kind of construction is likely to exhibit diminished binding activity. Another problem that can arise stems from the need for toxin cleavage at the Arg279–Gly280 bond. If the ligand does not transport domains II and III of PE into a furin-containing compartment, there will be little or no cleavage, the 37-kDa fragment will not be generated, and there will be no toxicity. Similarly, if cells fail to express sufficient furin, there will be no cleavage and no toxicity. Single chain antibodies are composed of the variable light and variable heavy chains of a monoclonal antibody. Routinely, to hold these two chains together, a 15 amino acid peptide is used to tether the C terminus of one chain with the N terminus of the second chain. While this approach facilitates the expression of the recombinant antibody from a single transcript, the product is not always stable and binding activity may be reduced.

To address each of the three problems mentioned earlier, novel engineering strategies had to be developed. The placement of the binding ligand in the immunotoxin construction can be modified in one of two ways. The ligand can be moved from its N-terminal location and inserted near the C terminus of domain III of PE (Figs. 4A and 4B). Unfortunately, the KDEL sequence must still be placed C-terminal to the ligand, but at least there are fewer structural constraints than when the ligand is placed in front of domain II. This kind of construct has been made with TGFα (Fig. 4B). Another strategy is used to deal with molecules such as human IL-4, which retain very little binding activity when placed N-terminal to domain II (Fig. 5). Because the N and C termini of human IL-4 are close together, it was possible to link them with a flexible peptide linker. Then new termini were generated artificially by "opening up" the molecule at one of two different loops that are not involved in ligand binding (Fig. 5). This strategy generates circularly permuted molecules. Circularly permuted IL-4 beginning at either residue 38 or residue 105 and fused to domains II and III of PE exhibited much better binding activity than the same construct with the linear version of IL-4 (Fig. 5).

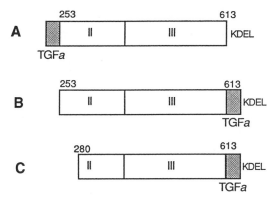

FIGURE 4 Possible ligand placements. The binding ligand (e.g., TGFα) is placed routinely at the N terminus of domains II and III. It can, however, be placed near the C terminus. This only produces an active cytotoxic agent if the ER retention sequence is present as the last four amino acids. The need for furin-mediated cleavage can be bypassed by initiating translation of domain II at residue 280 (glycine is replaced by methionine). (A) TGFα is placed at the N terminus and cell-mediated cleavage is required. (B) TGFα is placed near the C terminus and cleavage is required. (C) TGFα is placed near the C terminus with no cleavage necessary.

The need for furin-mediated proteolysis can be overcome by initiating translation of the recombinant immunotoxin at residue 280 and placing the ligand near the end of domain III (Fig. 4C). The example given is of TGFα. When assayed on a number of different cell lines, this construct proved more active than the conventional chimeric toxin shown in Fig. 4A. From this we concluded that furin cleavage can be rate limiting and that strategies to bypass this step may prove useful in the design of more potent molecules.

Finally, unstable single chain antibodies can be stabilized by the introduction of novel disulfide bonds into the framework segments of the variable chains (Fig. 6). Residues that are opposed and separated by the appropriate distance were modified to create novel cysteine residues, one each in the light and heavy chains. The light chain with a free sulfhydryl could then be linked by a disulfide bond with a heavy chain construct to form a disulfide-stabilized Fv immunotoxin. Such an approach has been used successfully to generate several very stable recombinant immunotoxins.

Experiments in nude mice have been performed to test the antitumor activity of many PE-derived recombinant immunotoxins. For example, TGFα–toxin and B3Fv–toxin were both shown to inhibit the

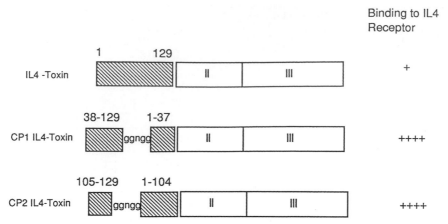

FIGURE 5 Circularly permuted (CP) IL-4-toxin. Circular permutation can be used to modify ligands that lose most of their binding activity when placed at the N terminus of domains II and III.

growth of human A431 tumors. (B3Fc is derived from the B3 monoclonal antibody, which binds to carbohydrate antigens displayed on the surface of many human adenocarcinomas.) TGFα–toxin caused a profound reduction in the rate of tumor growth but did not produce complete regressions. B3Fv–toxin had a larger therapeutic window and, at dose levels of 0.75 mg/kg × 3, caused complete regression of tumors and produced long-lasting cures. Variants of both of these immunotoxins are currently in clinical trials.

V. CONCLUSION

It is possible to design and produce wholly recombinant immunotoxins composed of truncated toxin molecules joined with tumor-targeting agents that exhibit cytotoxic activity for target cell lines and antitumor activity in model systems. Results of ongoing clinical trials will determine the utility of these agents.

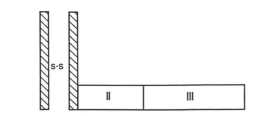

FIGURE 6 Disulfide-stabilized Fv antibody–toxin constructs.

See Also the Following Articles

Anti-Vascular Endothelial Growth Factor-Based Angiostatics • Hematopoietic Growth Factors • Insulin-like Growth Factors • Targeted Toxins

Bibliography

Brinkman, U., Pai, L. H., FitzGerald, D. J., Willingham, M. C., and Pastan, I. (1991). B3(Fv)-PE38KDEL, a single chain immunotoxin that causes complete regression of a human carcinoma in mice. *Proc. Natl. Acad. Sci. USA* **88**, 8616–8620.

Chaudhary, V. K., Jinno, Y., FitzGerald, D., and Pastan, I. (1990). Pseudomonas exotoxin contains a specific sequence at the carboxyl terminus that is required for cytotoxicity. *Proc. Natl. Acad. Sci. USA* **87**(1), 308–312.

Chiron, M. F., Fryling, C. M., and FitzGerald, D. J. (1994). Cleavage of pseudomonas exotoxin and diphtheria toxin by a furin-like protease prepared from beef liver. *J. Biol. Chem.* **269**, 18167–18176.

Jung, S. H., Pastan, I., and Lee, B. (1994). Design of interchain disulfide bonds in the framework region of the Fv fragment of the monoclonal antibody B3. *Proteins* **19**(1), 35–47.

Kounnas, M. Z., Morris, R. E., Thompson, M. R., FitzGerald, D. J., Strickland, D. K., and Saelinger, C. B. (1992). The alpha 2-macroglobulin receptor/low density lipoprotein receptor-related protein binds and internalizes pseudomonas exotoxin A. *J. Biol. Chem.* **267**, 12420–12423.

Kreitman, R. J., Puri, R. K., and Pastan, I. (1994). A circularly permuted recombinant interleukin 4 toxin with increased activity. *Proc. Natl. Acad. Sci. USA* **91**(15), 6889–6893.

Murphy, J. R. (1988). Diphtheria-related peptide hormone

gene fusions: A molecular genetic approach to chimeric toxin development. *Cancer Treat. Res.* **37**(123), 123–140.

Ogata, M., Fryling, C. M., Pastan, I., and FitzGerald, D. J. (1992). Cell-mediated cleavage of pseudomonas exotoxin between Arg279 and Gly280 generates the enzymatically active fragment which translocates to the cytosol. *J. Biol. Chem.* **267**(35), 25396–25401.

Pai, L. H., Gallo, M. G., FitzGerald, D. J., and Pastan, I. (1991). Anti-tumor activity of a transforming growth factor α-Pseudomonas exotoxin fusion protein (TGFα-PE40). *Cancer Res.* **51**, 2808–2812.

Pai, L. H., and Pastan, I. (1993). Immunotoxin therapy for cancer. *JAMA* **269**(1), 78–81.

Pastan, I., Chaudhary, V., and FitzGerald, D. J. (1992). Recombinant toxins as novel therapeutic agents. *Annu. Rev. Biochem.* **61**(331), 331–354.

Reiter, Y., Brinkmann, U., Jung, S. H., Lee, B., Kasprzyk, P. G., King, C. R., and Pastan, I. (1994). Improved binding and antitumor activity of a recombinant anti-erbB2 immunotoxin by disulfide stabilization of the Fv fragment. *J. Biol. Chem.* **269**(28), 18327–18331.

Reiter, Y., Brinkmann, U., Kreitman, R. J., Jung, S. H., Lee, B., and Pastan, I. (1994). Stabilization of the Fv fragments in recombinant immunotoxins by disulfide bonds engineered into conserved framework regions. *Biochemistry* **33**(18), 5451–5459.

Strom, T. B., Anderson, P. L., Rubin, K. V., Williams, D. P., Kiyokawa, T., and Murphy, J. R. (1990). Immunotoxins and cytokine toxin fusion proteins. *Semin. Immunol.* **2**(6), 467–479.

Studier, F. W., and Moffatt, B. A. (1986). Use of bacteriophage T7 polymerase to direct selective expression of cloned gene. *J. Mol. Biol.* **189**, 113–130.

Theuer, C. P., FitzGerald, D., and Pastan, I. (1992). A recombinant form of pseudomonas exotoxin directed at the epidermal growth factor receptor that is cytotoxic without requiring proteolytic processing. *J. Biol. Chem.* **267**, 16872–16877.

Theuer, C. P., FitzGerald, D. J., and Pastan, I. (1993). A recombinant form of *Pseudomonas* exotoxin A containing transforming growth factor alpha near its carboxyl terminus for the treatment of bladder cancer. *J. Urol.* **149**(6), 1626–1632.

Williams, D. P., Wen, Z., Watson, R. S., Boyd, J., Strom, T. B., and Murphy, J. R. (1990). Cellular processing of the interleukin-2 fusion toxin DAB486-IL-2 and efficient delivery of diphtheria fragment A to the cytosol of target cells requires Arg194. *J. Biol. Chem.* **265**(33), 20673–20677.

Anti-idiotypic Antibody Vaccines

Paul B. Chapman

Memorial Sloan-Kettering Cancer Center

GLOSSARY

adjuvant A substance used to boost an immune response against a specific antigen.

complementarity-determining regions (CDRs) Hypervariable regions within the heavy and light chain variable domains of an immunoglobulin molecule. CDRs are generally involved in contacting antigen and so are critical in determining the specificity of an antibody.

differentiation antigen An antigen expressed on a normal cell as part of its differentiation program. The antigen may be lineage specific and may be expressed only at a certain stage of cellular differentiation.

epitope The region on an antigen molecule recognized by a specific antibody or T-cell clone.

idiotope A unique epitope on an immunoglobulin molecule.

By definition, idiotopes lie within the variable domains of the immunoglobulin molecule.

idiotype The set of idiotopes expressed by a given immunoglobulin molecule.

isotype Refers to the type of heavy chain in an antibody molecule. There are nine antibody isotypes identified in humans (IgM, IgD, IgG1, IgG2, IgG3, IgG4, IgA1, IgA2, IgE), each of which is encoded by a separate gene. The isotype can be identified serologically, as isotype-specific antibodies can be raised.

tolerance A state of immunological unresponsiveness toward a given antigen.

Anti-idiotypic antibodies bind to unique regions on other antibody molecules. One of the central hypotheses of modern immunology is that the immune system is regulated through a network of antibody–anti-idiotypic antibody interactions. One consequence of this theory is the idea that a specific B- or T-cell clone can be specifically activated by the appropriate anti-idiotypic antibody. In this way, anti-idiotypic antibodies may be used as vaccines to induce active immunity against a foreign antigen.

Using animal models, it has been possible to demonstrate that anti-idiotypic antibody vaccines can induce specific protective immunity against a variety of infectious agents and tumor antigens. Based on these types of studies, anti-idiotypic vaccines are being tested in patient trials in an attempt to induce specific immunity against human cancers.

I. INTRODUCTION

The last two decades have seen a frenzy of activity in the search for tumor-specific antigens. With few exceptions, all tumor antigens defined to date are differentiation antigens, molecules expressed on selected normal cell populations during differentiation, or molecules found on several types of tumors as well as normal testes. These antigens may be abundantly expressed by certain tumor cells but they are also found on some normal tissues, although perhaps at a much lower level of expression. This difficulty in identifying tumor-restricted antigens has led to two approaches toward immunizing patients against tumors. The first approach uses whole cell or cell extract vaccines consisting of mixtures of undefined antigens with the theory being that, even if we cannot identify them, tumor-specific antigens probably exist and can be recognized by the immune system if administered correctly. The second approach attempts to immunize patients against defined tumor antigens that have been identified as potential targets due to the presence of either naturally occurring antibodies or T lymphocytes that recognize these molecules. Among these immune targets are both carbohydrate antigens (e.g., gangliosides, TF, Tn) and proteins. The majority of antigens identified so far are autoantigens, i.e., they are nonmutated molecules present on certain normal cells, as well as on tumor cells. As a result, the host is generally tolerant toward these antigens and it is often difficult to induce a specific immune response. Several strategies designed to break tolerance against these antigens are being pursued, including chemical modification of the antigen, addition of carrier proteins with T-cell epitopes, and addition of potent immune adjuvants.

This article focuses on a different strategy to immunize against defined tumor antigens—the use of anti-idiotypic antibody vaccines. Anti-idiotypic antibodies can be used as surrogate antigens and can induce immune responses against the native antigen. Further, anti-idiotypic antibodies offer certain potential advantages over vaccines using native antigen.

II. WHAT ARE ANTI-IDIOTYPIC ANTIBODIES?

The basic antibody (immunoglobulin) structure consists of two heavy chains and two light chains covalently linked by disulfide bonds (Fig. 1). Each heavy and light chain is made up of a variable domain and one (light chain) or three (heavy chains) constant domains. Within a given species, the amino acid sequences of the constant domains are largely conserved between antibodies of the same isotype and are not directly involved in antibody binding to antigen. In contrast, three-dimensional interactions of the

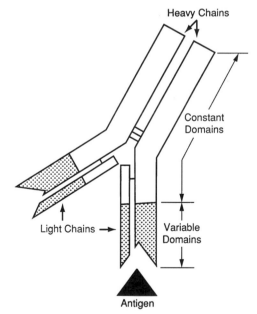

FIGURE 1 Structure of an IgG antibody molecule. The IgG molecule consists of two heavy chains and two light chains covalently linked through disulfide bonds. The variable domains (shaded), which contain regions unique to the individual heavy and light chains, form the antigen-binding site of the antibody. The constant domains (open) determine antibody functions such as complement fixation. From Chapman, P. B., and Houghton, A. N. (1992). Anti-idiotypic vaccines. *Biol. Ther. Cancer Updates* **2**(5).

variable domains of the heavy and light chains form the antigen-binding site of the antibody.

Although a detailed description of the basis of antibody diversity is beyond the scope of this article, it is useful to remember that the DNA encoding the variable domain of a heavy chain (V_H) is assembled from three genomic segments; variable (V), diversity (D), and joining (J). For human heavy chains, it is estimated that there are 100–200 V segments, at least 4 D segments, and at least 6 J segments. DNA encoding light chains is assembled from a large number of V and 5 J segments (there is no D segment for light chains). In addition to this recombinatorial diversity for both heavy and light chains, somatic hypermutation also occurs within the V_H and V_L DNA. It has been estimated that, in mice, this diversity would generate approximately 2.7×10^8 different antibody molecules. Thus, the potential number of unique antibody molecules is enormous. Within each V_H and V_L domain are three hypervariable regions, also called complementarity-determining regions (CDRs). Association of the heavy and light chains in three dimensions forms the antigen-binding site, and the amino acid residues of the CDRs are usually critical in forming hydrogen bonds, van der Waal forces, and salt bridges with which the antibody binds antigen.

Each mature B cell makes an antibody with a unique antigen-binding specificity determined by a unique set of V_H and V_L domains. This means that each antibody contains unique regions within its variable domains. These unique regions are termed "idiotopes" and the set of idiotopes expressed by a given antibody defines the "idiotype" of the antibody. Because idiotopes are unique epitopes, it is possible to raise antibodies against idiotopes; in fact, idiotopes are defined by the antibodies raised against them. These antibodies are "anti-idiotypic" antibodies because they bind to an idiotope expressed by another antibody molecule. Anti-idiotypic antibodies can recognize idiotopes expressed entirely on the variable domain of either the heavy or the light chain, or anti-idiotypic antibodies can recognize idiotopes defined by amino acids from both heavy and light chain variable domains (Fig. 2). Some anti-idiotypic antibodies bind to the actual antigen-binding site of the target antibody, as discussed later.

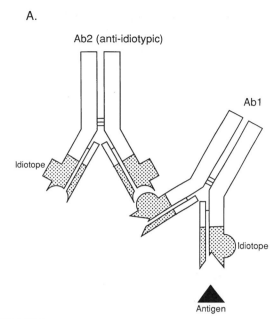

FIGURE 2 Interactions between an antibody and an anti-idiotypic antibody. An antibody (Ab1) recognizing an antigen (solid triangle) is itself recognized by Ab2 antibodies. Because the antigen-binding sites of antibodies are also unique epitopes (i.e., idiotopes), the Ab1–Ab2 relationship is reciprocal, i.e., the Ab1 is also an anti-idiotypic antibody with relation to the Ab2. From Chapman, P. B., and Houghton, A. N. (1992). Anti-idiotypic vaccines. *Biol. Ther. Cancer Updates* 2(5).

III. MODULATION OF THE IMMUNE RESPONSE BY ANTI-IDIOTYPIC ANTIBODIES

A. The Jerne Hypothesis

Anti-idiotypic antibodies were initially described in 1963 by Henry Kunkel and Jacques Oudin working independently. They observed that an animal immunized with an antigen produced an antibody response (Ab1). If this Ab1 were isolated and injected into a second, naive animal, antibodies (Ab2) were produced that bound specifically to the Ab1. These Ab2 antibodies were termed anti-idiotypic antibodies because they recognized an epitope on the Ab1 that was unique to the Ab1. Oudin also observed that the antigenic specificity of the Ab1 tended to correlate with the idiotopes expressed by the Ab1. In other words, different Ab1 antibodies recognizing the same antigen tended to express the same idiotopes. Anti-idiotypic antibodies were defined as antibodies with specificity for an Ab1, or group of Ab1 antibodies, elicited by a specific antigen. Later, Alfred Nisonoff and others described two types of Ab2 antibodies—Ab2α and Ab2β—based on whether the Ab2 could bind to Ab1 in the presence of antigen. Ab2β anti-idiotypic antibodies do not bind to Ab1 in the presence of excess antigen, presumably because Ab2β antibodies bind to the antigen-binding site of the Ab1. Ab2α anti-idiotypic antibodies, however, bind to idiotopes distinct from the antigen-binding site of the Ab1.

In 1974, Niels Jerne hypothesized that the immune system (both B and T cells) was regulated by a network of idiotype–anti-idiotype interactions. Jerne envisioned that for every antibody, there were corresponding Ab2α and Ab2β anti-idiotypic antibodies encoded by the genome (Fig. 3). Binding of soluble Ab2α to Ab1 on the surface of a B cell resulted in inhibition of the B-cell clone, whereas binding by soluble Ab2β resulted in stimulation. A curious aspect of idiotype—anti-idiotype interactions as envisioned by Jerne is that every Ab1-Ab2α interaction is reciprocally an Ab1–Ab2β interaction. For example, in Fig. 3, if the Ab2α antibody were considered the Ab1, then the antibody labeled Ab1 (solid) becomes an Ab2β because its idiotope (solid rectangle) is recognized by the antigen-binding site of the other antibody. Jerne proposed that introduction of a foreign antigen resulted in an initial elimination of circulating Ab1. This would release the inhibitory effect on Ab2β B cells, leading to the production of Ab2β and stimulation of the Ab1 B cell. Elimination of Ab1 by the foreign antigen would also eliminate the stimulatory effect of Ab1 on B cells, making Ab2α anti-idiotypic antibodies, resulting in less of the inhibitory Ab2α antibodies in the circulation. Therefore, the overall effect would be more Ab1 production. As the antigen is cleared, the network would return to its previous homeostatic steady state. Through this interconnecting, dynamic network of idiotypic–anti-idiotypic interactions, the immune system was hypothesized to be self-regulating. It is important to remember that Jerne hypothesized that this idiotype network would also regulate T-cell reactivities.

A special feature of the Ab2β anti-idiotypic antibodies was that they could functionally mimic the foreign antigen. This was first suggested by Alfred Nisonoff and Edmundo Lamoyi and independently by Ivan Roitt. Because of this, it should be possible to induce immunity against a foreign antigen by using an appropriate anti-idiotypic antibody as a surrogate immunogen. This was confirmed in the early 1980s when several investigators demonstrated that it was possible to induce specific and protective immunity in rodents against a variety of infectious agents using anti-idiotypic monoclonal antibodies (MAb). Not only could antibodies be induced against protein antigens, but anti-idiotypic antibodies mimicking nonprotein antigens were effective immunogens. As predicted by the Jerne hypothesis, it was possible to demonstrate the induction of T-cell immunity as well as humoral immunity.

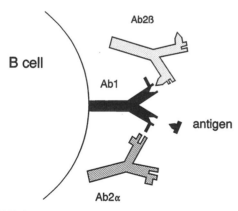

FIGURE 3 Possible mechanism of immune regulation through a network of idiotype–anti-idiotype interactions. A B cell expresses surface antibody (Ab1) with specificity for a particular antigen. This Ab1 also expresses an idiotope outside of its antigen-binding region (depicted as rectangles). An anti-idiotypic antibody (Ab2α) can recognize this idiotope, and the interaction results in the suppression of the Ab1 B-cell clone. At the same time, this interaction also occurs between soluble Ab1 and cell surface Ab2α (not shown), resulting in the activation of the Ab2α B cell and further secretion of the Ab2α antibody. The Ab2β anti-idiotypic antibody expresses an idiotope that binds to the antigen-binding domain of Ab1 and mimics the antigen. Interactions between soluble Ab2β and cell surface Ab1 result in activation of the Ab1 B cell and enhanced secretion of the Ab1 antibody. Reciprocally, Ab1 binds to an idiotope.

B. Structural Basis for Antigen Mimicry

There are at least three potential mechanisms by which anti-idiotypic antibodies can induce antibody against a foreign antigen. Some anti-idiotypic antibodies appear to reproduce the antigenic epitope within one of its CDRs. Anti-idiotypic antibodies that induced antibodies against the GAT antigen (a random synthetic terpolymer made up of glutamic acid[60] alanine[30] tyrosine[10]) contain "GAT-like" sequences within the V_H CDR3 domains (corresponding to the D segment at the DNA level). These antibodies contained either Glu-Glu-Tyr or Tyr-Tyr-Glu sequences, and it has been hypothesized that this is the basis for their ability to mimic the GAT antigen. In the hepatitis B surface antigen (HBsAg) system, an anti-idiotypic MAb, designated 2F10, can induce antibodies against HBsAg and can prime HBsAg-specific helper T cells (T_H) in mice. A 15 amino acid sequence within the V_H CDR3 was identified that was homologous with a region on HBsAg representing a common immunogenic determinant. In fact, CD4[+] T cells from patients immunized against hepatitis B could be stimulated using only this 15 amino acid peptide. Mark Greene's laboratory showed that a 16 amino acid epitope of reovirus type 3 hemagglutinin is mimicked by an anti-idiotypic MAb. CDR2 regions from both V_H and V_L contribute to form a homologous epitope. These examples demonstrate one mechanism of antigenic mimicry by anti-idiotypic MAb, which is expression of the original antigenic epitope within the variable domains of the anti-idiotypic MAb. This is not the only mechanism

of antigenic mimicry and certainly cannot explain anti-idiotypic antibody mimicry of nonprotein antigens.

Some anti-idiotypic antibodies may recapitulate the conformation and charge of the antigen sufficiently to activate the appropriate B-cell clone. Perhaps the best studied example is MAb E225, an anti-idiotypic MAb that mimics an epitope on lysozyme recognized by the Ab1 MAb D1.3. Bentley and colleagues at the Institut Pasteur were able to determine the crystal structure of E225–D1.3 complexes and compare how D1.3 binds to E225 with how D1.3 binds to lysozyme. This analysis showed that E225 does not form an image of the lysozyme epitope on the atomic level. Thirteen amino acids within the D1.3 variable domains directly contacted E225. Of these 13 amino acids, only 7 also served as contact residues in D1.3 binding to lysozyme. Further, these 7 amino acids interacted with E225 differently than with lysozyme (Table I). These data suggest that an anti-idiotypic MAb does not need to mimic the antigen at the atomic level in order to induce antibodies that cross-react with the antigen. This may be how an anti-idiotypic MAb (which is a protein) can mimic a nonprotein antigen such as a carbohydrate.

Although not entirely consistent with Jerne's first approximation of his network theory, an anti-idiotypic antibody might be able to activate a specific

TABLE I

Atomic Interactions Involving Amino Acid Residues of MAb D1.3 That Contact Both Antigen (Lysozyme) and Anti-idiotypic MAb (E225)[a]

	Amino acid within the D1.3 idiotope	Intactions with lysozyme	Interactions with anti-idiotypic MAb E225
V_L	Tyr32	van der Waal	H bond
	Tyr50	H bond	H bond
	Trp92	van der Waal	H bond
V_H	Trp52	van der Waal	van der Wall
	Asp54	H bond	One salt bridge, one H bond
	Asp100	Five H bonds	van der Waal
	Tyr101	H bond	van der Waal

[a]Seven amino acid residues within the variable domains of MAb D1.3 are involved in binding to both antigen (lysozyme) and anti-idiotype MAb E225. For five of the seven amino acids, the nature of the atomic interaction with antigen differs from the interactions with anti-idiotypic MAb. Adapted from Bentley, G.A., Boulot G., Riottot, M. M., and Poljak, R.J. (1990) Three-dimensional structure of an idiotope–anti-idiotope complex. *Nature* **348**; 254–257.

B-cell clone without providing a true internal image of the antigen. One example is an Ab2 antibody raised by Oosterlaken and colleagues in the Netherlands against an Ab1 that neutralizes Semliki forest virus (SFV). Although this Ab2 could immunize BALB/c mice, the same mouse strain from which the Ab2 was made, mice from other strains did not respond. This suggests that the Ab2 does not provide a pure internal image of the SFV antigen, as internal image anti-idiotypic antibodies should immunize across strain and species barriers. It is conceivable that this Ab2 activates a B-cell clone in BALB/c mice that produces an antibody with significant affinity for SFV without providing a true internal image.

Despite these complexities, it is apparent that anti-idiotypic antibodies can induce immunity against protein and nonprotein antigens and, in certain circumstances, can induce T-cell immunity. Further, studies in infectious disease animal models have shown that this immunity can be protective. These beneficial effects are not limited to rodents; Ronald Kennedy and colleagues have demonstrated that an anti-idiotypic antibody vaccine can be used to induce protective immunity against hepatitis B in chimpanzees. Because of these encouraging results, investigators have applied the concept of anti-idiotypic vaccines to the problem of cancer.

IV. USE OF ANTI-IDIOTYPIC ANTIBODIES AS TUMOR VACCINES

A. Potential Advantages of Anti-idiotypic Antibody Tumor Vaccines

A practical question arises: Why use an anti-idiotypic MAb vaccine? Given that they can be quite difficult to generate, clone, and characterize, it is reasonable to consider that there are at least two potential advantages of an anti-idiotypic MAb vaccine. The first is that the antigen of interest may be difficult to obtain in sufficient quantity or may be dangerous to handle (infectious, tumorigenic). An anti-idiotypic MAb mimicking the antigen circumvents these problems. The second advantage is that anti-idiotypic MAb can be more effective immunogens than some native antigens. In some cases, it has been possible to

demonstrate that anti-idiotypic MAb vaccines can break immunological tolerance against the native antigen. One example, reported by Stein and Soderstrom, used neonatal mice incapable of mounting an immune response to bacterial capsular polysaccharide. If mice were primed with anti-idiotypic antibody, they were able to respond to antigen and develop protective immunity. Because most tumor antigens are differentiation antigens and are expressed on selected normal tissues, the host is usually tolerant to these molecules. Therefore, the ability to break tolerance may be an important feature of anti-idiotypic MAb vaccines.

Anti-idiotypic MAbs offer a similar advantage in immunizing against nonprotein tumor antigens. B-cell responses to nonprotein antigens (T-cell independent) are generally low-titer, transient IgM responses. Anti-idiotypic MAbs that mimic nonprotein antigens represent a xenogeneic protein mimic that can be more immunogenic than the original nonprotein antigen. Presumably, one of the ways this could occur is that the anti-idiotypic MAb can provide T_H cell epitopes, which the B cell can present to T_H cells through its MHC class II molecules. Indeed, in the reovirus system, the V_H domain of an anti-idiotypic MAb was demonstrated to contain a T_H determinant. As noted earlier, evidence from animal studies shows that anti-idiotypic MAb mimicking carbohydrate bacterial antigens can be more effective than the antigens themselves in inducing immunity.

These theoretical and actual advantages of anti-idiotypic antibody vaccines have provided a rationale for developing antitumor vaccines using anti-idiotypic antibodies.

B. Anti-idiotypic Monoclonal Antibodies Can Be Used to Immunize Animals against Tumors

Anti-idiotypic antibodies have been used to induce immune responses in rodents against a variety of antigens expressed by tumor cells. In all cases, the antitumor immune response was characterized by the induction of antibodies against the tumor antigen. In a few cases, it was possible to demonstrate a delayed-type hypersensitivity (DTH) reaction against tumor cells, suggesting recruitment of T_H cells, although more detailed T-cell studies have not been reported. Only a very few studies have assessed whether the antitumor immune response induced by the anti-idiotypic antibody provided any protective effect; in the few studies reporting tumor protection, the effect was incomplete.

Studies using anti-idiotypic MAb raised against Ab1 recognizing nonprotein tumor antigens have confirmed previous observations in other systems that immune responses against nonprotein antigens can be induced by anti-idiotypic MAb. Tumor responses have been induced against both carbohydrate and ganglioside (acidic glycolipids) tumor antigens. This is of particular importance for several reasons. First, it is clear that carbohydrates and gangliosides represent potentially important antigenic targets for the immunotherapy of tumors. Second, for nonprotein antigens, the anti-idiotypic vaccine approach holds special potential advantages over immunization with native antigen, as discussed earlier.

C. Anti-idiotypic Antibody Vaccines in Cancer Trials

Several clinical trials have been completed in which anti-idiotypic MAbs were used to immunize cancer patients against tumor antigens (Table II). In these early trials, the primary goal was to see if immunization resulted in a detectable immune response against the antigen expressed by the tumor cell. As a result, investigators have explored different doses and schedules of anti-idiotypic MAb, as well as trying to increase

TABLE II
Clinical Trails Using Anti-idiotypic Antibodies to Immunize Patients against Tumor Antigens[a]

Antigen	Tumor	Anti-idiotypic vaccines	Results
HMW-MAA	Melanoma	MF2-23 conjugated to KLH, BCG adjuvant; MF11-30; Melimmune-1 and −2	14/23 patients immunized with MF2-23 vaccine developed antibodies to antigen-positive melanoma. Three partial tumor responses. No anti-HMW-MAA responses induced by the other anti-id vaccines
GD3	Melanoma, SCLC	BEC2 + BCG adjuvant	In a series of trials, 20–30% of patients developed detectable anti-GD3 antibodies. In SCLC after a major response to chemotherapy, vaccination associated with prolonged survival compared to historical experience
GD2	Melanoma, stage IV	1A7 + QS21 adjuvant	Anti-GD2 and antibodies detectable in 40/47 patients. One CR noted
CEA	Colon carcinoma (advanced), lung adenocarcinoma	3H1 + alum adjuvant	Approximately 50% of patients developed detectable anti-CEA antibodies. Also, 50% developed proliferative T-cell responses against CEA. No clinical responses observed
791 Typ72	Colon carcinoma (advanced)	105AD7	After immunization with 105AD7, it was possible to detect enhanced IL-2 release in response to antigen-expressing cells and cytotoxicity against autologous tumor cells. Anti-791Typ72 antibodies have not been detected. No clinical responses observed
gp37	T-cell lymphoma		One of four patients developed anti-gp37 antibodies. One patient had a dramatic clinical response lasting 11 months
CA125	Ovarian carcinoma	ACA125	9/16 patients developed anti-CA125 antibodies. 9/16 also developed CA125-specific PBMC responses
GA733-2	Colon	Anti-idiotypic MAb against MAb 17-1A	Induced a proliferative T-cell response against antigen. Three different peptides recognized.

[a]HMW-MAA, high molecular weight melanoma-associated antigen; PBMC, peripheral blood mononuclear cells; KLH, keyhole limpet hemocyanin; BCG, bacille Calmette–Guérin; HMFG, human milk fat globulin; CEA, carcinoembryonic antigen; SCLC, small cell lung carcinoma; CR, complete response.

their immunogenicity by adding immune adjuvants. Triggering antitumor effects has generally not been an end point of these early trials and, in fact, many of the trials (although not all) were conducted in patients who were free of disease after surgery or chemotherapy but who were at high risk for recurrence.

Monoclonal anti-idiotypic antibodies were first used to immunize melanoma patients against the high molecular weight proteoglycan–melanoma-associated antigen (HMW-MAA). Several anti-idiotypic MAbs have been produced against HMW-MAA, but only one particular one so far—MK2-23—appears to induce antibodies against the HMW-MAA itself. Mittelman immunized patients with MK2-23 conjugated to KLH as a carrier protein and mixed with BCG adjuvant and found that 14/23 patients developed antibodies to HMW-MAA and 3 patients actually had partial shrinkage of their tumors.

Anti-idiotypic MAb vaccines are also being used to immunize cancer patients against nonprotein tumor antigens. 1A7 is an anti-idiotypic MAb that mimics the ganglioside GD2. In stage IV melanoma patients immunized with 1A7 + alum, it was possible to detect anti-GD2 antibodies in 40/47 patients, although it required that the sera be partially purified and concentrated. One of the patients had complete shrinkage of the melanoma tumors as a result of immunization.

BEC2, another example of an anti-idiotypic mouse MAb that mimics a ganglioside antigen, in this case GD3, is being used to immunize both melanoma and small cell lung cancer (SCLC) patients. Immunizing with BEC2 mixed with BCG, it is possible to detect the induction of anti-GD3 antibodies in the serum of 20–30% of patients. An intriguing observation was made in a pilot trial in which BEC2 was used to immunize patients with SCLC who had had a partial or complete response to chemotherapy. Among the seven patients with limited stage disease, only one patient relapsed with SCLC. This has led to a multicenter randomized phase III trial testing BEC2 in limited stage SCLC.

Another phase III randomized trial conducted to test an anti-idiotypic MAb vaccine was conducted in advanced colon carcinoma patients to test 105AD7, a human anti-idiotypic MAb that mimics a protein designated 791Typ72, also known as decay-accelerating factor. Initial nonrandomized results were promising, but the randomized trial did not show a survival advantage in patients receiving 105AD7. The trial design may have been too stringent to detect a modest effect of the vaccine, however.

These studies support previous animal studies that showed that anti-idiotypic MAb can be used to immunize against both protein and nonprotein antigens. Also, it appears that the use of immune adjuvants (such as BCG) will be needed to optimize immunogenicity. To date, significant toxicity has not been observed in patients immunized with anti-idiotypic MAb. One randomized phase III trial is underway and others are planned in order to test whether these vaccines can make an impact on the natural history of cancer.

V. FUTURE DIRECTIONS OF ANTI-IDIOTYPIC ANTIBODY CANCER VACCINES

There have now been several pilot trials and one phase III trial testing anti-idiotypic antibody vaccines in cancer patients. The studies so far have shown that it is possible to induce antibodies against specific self-antigens, although the antibody titers are low. The success of anti-idiotypic vaccine therapy depends not only on the identification of appropriate tumor antigen targets, but also on whether relevant titers of antibodies can be induced. It is not surprising that it is more difficult to induce an immune response against an autoantigen, such as a tumor antigen, than against a foreign antigen, such as a viral antigen. For this reason, parameters such as vaccine dose, route, schedule, and use of immune adjuvants will be critical for optimization of anti-idiotypic antibody vaccines. It is also possible that modification of the anti-idiotypic antibody molecule can improve its immunogenicity. Such modifications may include removal of the Fc region by creating Fab or F(ab′)$_2$ fragments, chimerization of the molecule to replacing the mouse constant regions with homologous human regions, and attaching carrier molecules with known T-cell epitopes. Once optimized, it could turn out that anti-idiotypic antibody vaccines are best used to prime patients for an immune response against the native antigen.

One question that arises is: Do anti-idiotypic MAb

vaccines offer any real advantage over immunizing with antigen? With regard to protein antigens, the answer may be "no." As we come to a better understanding of how to activate T cells against tumor antigens, and as we explore newer immunization techniques, such as peptide constructs or DNA immunization, it seems that immunizing with some form of the antigen itself will be more likely to result in an effective immune response than immunizing with an anti-idiotypic MAb. However, the situation may be quite different in the case of a nonprotein antigen. These antigens also tend to be poorly immunogenic but we cannot easily manipulate these molecules to circumvent this poor immunogenicity the way we can manipulate proteins. In this case, anti-idiotypic MAb vaccines represent a strategy to induce an immune response against a poorly immunogenic antigen.

Once an anti-idiotypic MAb vaccine is shown to induce a specific immune response against an appropriate tumor antigen convincingly and reproducibly, it is necessary to test the *real* question in a well-designed phase III trial: Can an effective antitumor immune response be induced in patients?

See Also the Following Articles

ANTIBODIES IN THE GENE THERAPY OF CANCER • CANCER VACCINES: GENE THERAPY AND DENDRITIC CELL BASED VACCINES • CANCER VACCINES: PEPTIDE- AND PROTEIN-BASED VACCINES • CARBOHYDRATE-BASED VACCINES • DNA-BASED CANCER VACCINES • TARGETED TOXINS • TUMOR ANTIGENS

Bibliography

Bhattacharya-Chatterjee, M., and Foon, K. A. (1998). Anti-idiotype antibody vaccine therapies of cancer. *Cancer Treat. Res.* **94,** 51–68.

Chapman, P. B., and Houghton, A. N. (1991). Induction of IgG antibodies against GD3 in rabbits by an anti-idiotypic monoclonal antibody. *J. Clin. Invest.* **88,** 186–192.

Foon, K. A., John, W. J., Chakraborty, M., *et al.* (1997). Clinical and immune responses in advanced colorectal cancer patients treated with anti-idiotype monoclonal antibody vaccine that mimics the carcinoembryonic antigen. *Clin. Cancer Res.* **3,** 1267–1276.

Foon, K. A., Lutzky, J., Baral, R. N., *et al.* (2000). Clinical and immune responses in advanced melanoma patients immunized with an anti-idiotype antibody mimicking disialoganglioside GD2. *J. Clin. Oncol.* **18,** 376–384.

Grant, S. C., Kris, M. G., Houghton, A. N., and Chapman, P. B. (1999). Long survival of patients with small cell lung cancer after adjuvant treatment with the anti-idiotypic antibody BEC2 plus BCG. *Clin. Cancer Res.* **5,** 1319–1324.

Greenspan, N. S., and Bona, C. A. (1993). Idiotypes: Structure and immunogenicity. *FASEB J.* **7,** 437–444.

Jerne, N. K. (1974). Towards a network theory of the immune system. *Ann. Immunol. (Inst. Pasteur)* **125,** 373–389.

Kennedy, R. C., Melnick, J. L., and Dreesman, G. R. (1986) Anti-idiotypics and immunity. *Sci. Am.* **255,** 48–56.

Antioxidants: Carcinogenic and Chemopreventive Properties

Nobuyoki Ito
Masao Hirose
Katsumi Imaida
Nagoya City University Medical School, Nagoya, Japan

GLOSSARY

chemoprevention The primary prevention of carcinogenesis by chemicals. Any chemical agent that inhibits initiation, promotion, or progression, or more than one of these steps, is considered to be a chemopreventor.

forestomach The proximal part of the rodent stomach, situated between the esophagus and glandular part of the stomach and lined by squamous epithelium. Occupying about half of the stomach and separated from the glandular stomach by a limiting ridge, the forestomach is found in rats, mice, and hamsters.

initiation An irreversible alteration in the heritable material of target cells caused by carcinogens; this is considered the first step of the carcinogenesis process.

progression The process by which benign tumors or premalignant lesions progress to increasing malignant behavior.

promotion The process by which initiated cells grow to form benign tumors or precancerous lesions.

squamous cell carcinoma A malignant tumor originating from squamous epithelium and demonstrating squamous differentiation such as cornification and intercellular bridges. Characteristics include frequent invasion of adjacent tissues.

squamous cell papilloma A benign papillary tumor originating from squamous epithelium with fine or abundant connective tissue stroma. Structural and cellular atypia, or invasive growth, is absent.

Chemical carcinogens, which are present widely in our environment, are considered to play an important role in the causation of most human cancers. They may be classified into genotoxic and nongenotoxic types, the former including nitrosamines,

aromatic hydrocarbons, aromatic amines, and nitro-
furans, and the latter being exemplified by peroxi-
some proliferators, antioxidants, chlorinated pesticides, uracil, and D-limonene. For primary prevention
of human cancer, it is essential that we eliminate carcinogens as far as possible and ingest possible chemopreventors. One problem with eliminating carcinogens is the existence of nongenotoxic compounds
which escape detection in short-term assays. The development of chemopreventors therefore assumes particular importance in approaches to the prevention of
cancer. Since antioxidants possess both carcinogenic
and chemopreventive properties, a detailed analysis
of this group of agents should contribute to their
introduction.

I. INTRODUCTION

Antioxidants have been used widely in the food industry to prevent or retard autooxidation of fats, oils,
and fat-soluble compounds. Some water-soluble antioxidants prevent oxidation in aqueous material.
Apart from foodstuffs, they are contained in various
cosmetics, medicines, plastics, and rubbers. They may
be synthetic or naturally occurring; the latter type of
antioxidants are widely distributed in plants. Humans
may thus be exposed to mixtures of synthetic and naturally occurring antioxidants orally from foodstuffs or
through the skin from cosmetics. Generally, antioxidants can be classified into five types:

1. Primary antioxidants which terminate free radical
   chain reactions (phenolic compounds,
   tocopherols, tertiary amines, flavonoids)
2. Oxygen scavengers which react with oxygen and
   remove it (ascorbic acid and its derivatives)
3. Secondary antioxidants which decompose lipid
   peroxides into stable products (sulfur compounds,
   seleno-compounds)
4. Enzymic antioxidants which remove highly
   oxidative species (superoxide dismutase, catalase,
   glutathione peroxidase)
5. Chelating agents which chelate metallic ions
   such as copper and iron (citric acid, phytic acid)

Of these antioxidants, ascorbic acid and chelating

agents are able to enhance the antioxidant action of
tocopherols or phenolic compounds, and are therefore called synergists. Antioxidants are generally not
mutagenic as evaluated by the Ames test and may
even inhibit the mutagenic activity of mutagens.
Moreover, they inhibit chemical carcinogenesis in
various organs of rodents when they are given prior to
and/or simultaneously with certain carcinogens.
Therefore, antioxidants may have potential applications as potent chemopreventors in man. However,
some of them have been shown to enhance second-
stage chemical carcinogenesis in rodents when administered after exposure to carcinogens. In addition,
the synthetic antioxidant BHA, which is commonly
used throughout the world as a food additive, was
demonstrated to induce forestomach carcinomas in
F344 rats of both sexes and in male Syrian golden
hamsters. Subsequently, modifying effects of antioxidants and the mechanism(s) underlying antioxidant
induction of tumors have been the focus of extensive
investigations.

In addition to their antioxidant effects, many antioxidants possess various kinds of biological activities
such as enzyme induction, interference with the immune response, anti-viral activity, anti-inflammatory
activity, interference with prostaglandin synthesis, inhibition of platelet aggregation, and protection against
reperfusion injury. Some of these properties are closely
linked to chemical carcinogenesis.

The present review article covers the latest results
of research on antioxidants, especially in relation to
neoplastic and chemopreventive properties.

II. ANTIOXIDANT CARCINOGENICITY

Carcinogenicity studies of antioxidants have been extensive since the demonstration of forestomach carcinogenicity for the synthetic antioxidant BHA in
1983. Before then, BHA had been used widely in the
world as a safe food antioxidant and was generally regarded to be beneficial to humans due to its lack of
mutagenicity and its inhibition of rodent carcinogenesis induced by several carcinogens.

In the first examination of long-term BHA exposure, male and female F344 rats were continuously

administered 2% (maximum tolerable dose) or 0.4% BHA in the diet for 2 years. Histopathological examination showed that the high dose of BHA induced forestomach squamous cell carcinomas at incidences of 34.6% in males and 29.4% in females. No neoplastic lesions which could be attributed to BHA administration were observed in any other organs. This was the first report that antioxidants could induce tumors in rodents. Subsequently, BHA was also shown to be carcinogenic to make Syrian golden hamster forestomach at doses at 1 and 2% in the diet, although the results were equivocal when male $B6C3F_1$ mice received doses of 0.5 and 1%. In a dose–response study using F344 male rats at levels of 0.125 to 2%, only the highest dose caused squamous cell carcinomas while 1% induced only a low incidence of squamous cell papillomas; no tumors were observed at doses lower than 0.5%.

Since the carcinogenicity of BHA appeared limited to the forestomach which humans do not possess, it was necessary to examine its effects on other animals without a forestomach for the evaluation of human hazard potential. Continuous oral treatment with BHA at doses lower than 1% of 20 months in guinea pigs, daily intragastric doses of 500 mg/kg body weight of BHA for 20 days and then 250 mg/kg body weight 5 times/week until 84 days in cynomolgus monkeys, or 0–100 mg/kg/days or dietary 0.25–1% BHA for up to 1 year in beagle dogs did not cause any histopathological changes in any tissue. Therefore it has been concluded that the carcinogenic potential of BHA is limited to forestomach epithelium.

The carcinogenicity of butylated hydroxytoluene (BHT), which is as potent as BHA as an antioxidant and is commonly used in cosmetics or as a food additive, has also been extensively studied. Wistar rats and $B6C3F_1$ mice of both sexes were treated with BHT at dose levels of 0.25 or 1.0%, and 0.02, 0.1, or 0.5% in the diet, respectively, for up to 104 weeks. However, no tumors were induced that could be attributed to the treatment. On the other hand, administration of 1 or 2% BHT in the diet to male $B6C3F_1$ mice for 104 weeks was associated with an increased incidence of hepatocellular adenomas or foci of alteration in a clear dose-dependent manner. Although there was an inverse dose relationship, male C3H mice fed diets containing 0.5 or 0.05% of BHT

for 10 months also had significantly increased incidences of liver tumors as compared to those kept on basal diet alone. Olsen *et al.* also reported weak tumorigenicity for BHT in the rat liver in a two-generation study. However, none of the evidence to date is unequivocal and the question of BHT carcinogenicity in rodents remains open.

Although no standard carcinogenic bioassays have been reported for *tert*-butylhydroquinone (TBHQ), continuous feeding of this antioxidant for <20 months at doses of 0–0.5% did not result in any compound-related gross or microscopic lesions. Propyl gallate was also studied in F344 rats and $B6C3F_1$ mice by feeding at dietary levels of 5000–20,000 mg/kg, but no dose-related increases in incidences of tumors or differences in survival were found. The potential carcinogenicity of other gallates has not been fully evaluated.

Since BHA was found to induce pronounced forestomach hyperplasia in a short period and forestomach squamous cell carcinoma in rats and hamsters in the long term, many other structurally related phenolic antioxidants were examined for associated proliferative activity in the forestomach epithelium as an aid to prediction of potential to induce forestomach tumors. Among these are TBHQ, 4-methoxyphenol, 1,4-dimethoxybenzene, catechol, resorcinol, hydroquinone, 3-methoxyphenol, 2-methoxyphenol, anisole, 4-cresol, phenol, 4-hydroxybenzoic acid *n*-alkyl esters (alkyl parabenes), 4-hydroxybenzoic acid esters, gallic acid, caffeic acid, sesamol, chlorogenic acid, syringic acid, ferulic acid, eugenol, esculin, 4-methylphenol, 4-*tert*-buthylphenol, pyrogallor, methylhydroquinone, 2-*tert*-butyl-4-methylphenol, and BHT tested in short-term feeding studies in rats or hamsters at a dose of 0.7–2% in diet; 4-methoxyphenol and sesamol were found to be as active as BHA in the induction of forestomach hyperplasia and, in addition, they caused a circular deep ulceration parallel to the limiting ridge. Caffeic acid, 2-*tert*-butyl-4-methylphenol, and 4-*tert*-butylphenol also induced pronounced hyperplasia in the forestomach epithelium. The labeling index in the glandular stomach was also significantly increased in animals fed catechol and 4-methoxyphenol. This prompted investigation in long-term experiments. Chemical structures and the results of carcinogenicity studies of

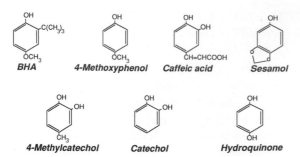

FIGURE 1   Chemical structures of carcinogenic antioxidants.

antioxidants are presented in Fig. 1 and Table I, respectively.

When male and female F344 rats were treated with caffeic acid, sesamol, 4-methoxyphenol, or 4-methylcatechol at a dose of 2% or catechol at a dose of 0.8% in the diet for 2 years, the agents except catechol induced significantly increased incidences of forestomach squamous cell carcinomas. Females were less sensitive than males. In addition, 4-methylcatechol induced carcinomas in glandular stomach epithelium. Although catechol did not induce tumors in the forestomach, it did induce glandular stomach carcinomas. In a dose–response study, even 0.16% cate-

chol in the diet induced adenomas at a low incidence. Since this demonstration of catechol (1,2-dihydroxybenzene) carcinogenicity, hydroquinone (1,4-dihydroxybenzene), one of its isomers, was further examined in male and female rats at a dose of 0.8% in diet. Whereas it was not found to be carcinogenic for either the forestomach or glandular stomach, it induced a 46.6% incidence of kidney adenomas, predominantly in male rats. 1,2,4-Benzenetriol, protocatechuic acid, protocatechualdehyde, dopamine, and DL-dopa, all dihydroxybenzene derivatives like caffeic acid and catechol, were examined for their potency to induce cell proliferation in the rat forestomach and glandular stomach epithelium. However, only 1,2,4-benzenetriol and dopamine, each at 1.5% in the diet, were effective in increasing the BrdU-labeling index in the forestomach epithelium. 2-Methoxyphenol, with one hydroxy substituent replaced by a methoxy substituent, also lacked any effects on cell proliferation in either forestomach or glandular stomach epithelium. Therefore, the *ortho*-dihydroxy structure appears important, but substituents actually determine cell proliferation on stimulus.

Many phenolic compounds that do not show stim-

TABLE I
Incidences of Tumors in the Stomach and Kidney

Chemicals	Sex	No. of rats	Squamous cell carcinoma (forestomach)	Adenocarcinoma (Gl stomach)	Adenoma (kidney)
BHA	M	52	18 (35)***	0	0
	F	51	15 (29)***	0	0
4-Methoxyphenol	M	30	23 (77)***	0	0
	F	30	4 (13)	0	0
Caffeic acid	M	30	17 (57)***	0	4 (13)
	F	30	15 (50)***	0	6 (20)*
Sesamol	M	29	9 (31) ***	0	0
	F	30	3 (10)	0	0
Catechol	M	28	0	15 (54)***	0
	F	28	0	12 (43)***	0
4-Methylcatechol	M	30	17 (57)***	17 (57)***	0
	F	30	12 (40)	14 (47)***	0
Hydroquinone	M	30	0	0	14 (47)***
	F	30	0	0	0
Control	M	30	0	0	0
	F	30	0	0	0

*P < 0.02.
***P < 0.001 vs control group value.

ulation activity per se on the forestomach epithelium cause very strong cell proliferation or tumorigenicity when they are combined with sodium nitrite ($NaNO_2$). For example, continuous oral treatment with 0.8% catechol alone in the diet for 51 weeks induced mild forestomach hyperplasia. The grade of forestomach hyperplasia considerably increased and papillomas were also found in 4 of 15 rats with a simultaneous administration of catechol and $NaNO_2$. When the combined effects of various phenolic compounds and $NaNO_2$ on rat forestomach cell proliferation were further examined in a 4-week experiment, the cell proliferative response to known forestomach carcinogens such as sesamol, 4-methoxyphenol, and 4-methylcatechol was further enhanced by simultaneous treatment with $NaNO_2$. In addition, markedly increased cell proliferation was found when 2% hydroquinone, 2% pyrogallol, 2% gallic acid, or 2% TBHQ in the diet was combined with 0.3% $NaNO_2$ in the drinking water, although individual phenolic compounds or $NaNO_2$ did not stimulate any proliferating activity or only mild hyperplasia. It has been known that mutagenic diazocompounds are formed by the reaction of phenols and $NaNO_2$ under acidic conditions. Such compounds could be responsible for the cell proliferation. Cell proliferation induced by these phenolic compounds and $NaNO_2$ in combination was much more pronounced than with the known forestomach carcinogens caffeic acid, sesamol, 4-methoxyphenol, and 4-methycatechol. Similar effects were observed when the nonphenolic antioxidant sodium ascorbate (NaASA) or ascorbic acid (ASA) was given to rats simultaneously with $NaNO_2$. Therefore, many phenolic compounds as well as NaASA and ASA may possess carcinogenic activity for the rat forestomach epithelium in the presence of $NaNO_2$.

III. MECHANISTIC APPROACHES TO ANTIOXIDANT CARCINOGENICITY

Since the carcinogenicity of antioxidants was found to be mostly limited to the forestomach epithelium except in the catechol, 4-methylcatechol, and hydroquinone cases, approaches to elucidating mechanisms have been primarily directed toward this tissue.

All of the carcinogenic phenolic antioxidants

which target the forestomach were shown to induce cytotoxicity as well as hyperplasia. To examine whether the observed hyperplasia was due to excess regeneration associated with cytotoxicity or due to primary mitogenic effects, early forestomach lesions induced by BHA, caffeic acid, or 4-methoxyphenol in rats were investigated.

DNA synthesis of the forestomach epithelium, expressed as the number of BrdU-labeled cells per 100 basal cells (labeling index), increased 12 hr after treatment with caffeic acid or 4-methoxyphenol. In the case of BHA, an increase in the labeling index was apparent 3 days after treatment. After 7 days of continuous antioxidant administration, the labeling index increased or continued to be high, especially in the groups treated with 4-methoxyphenol followed by caffeic acid and BHA (Fig. 2). Hyperplasia was observed 3 days after treatment with caffeic acid, but this change first became evident only later in the cases of BHA, sesamol, and 4-methoxyphenol. Evidence of toxicity, such as erosion or ulceration, developed in animals treated with caffeic acid or 4-methoxyphenol for 7 days, but were not found in those treated with BHA. A strongly elevated expression of cell proliferation-related *c-fos* oncogene expression in the forestomach epithelium was demonstrated 15 min after beginning treatment with BHA, but rapidly decreased thereafter. Another cell proliferation-related *c-myc* expression was similarly observed after 15 min of treatment, then decreased

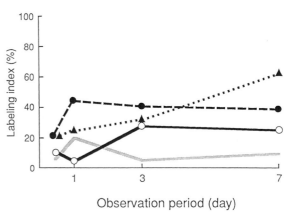

FIGURE 2 Sequential observation of labeling indices in rat forestomach epithelium treated with antioxidants. ○, 2% BHA; ●, 2% caffeic acid; ▲, 2% 4-methoxyphenol; —, basal diet.

slowly. By the electron microscopical observation, the initial changes observed in the forestomach epithelial cells are the enlargement of nucleous and an increase in free ribosomes and polysomes in the basal layer. These changes are observed 24 hr after treatment with caffeic acid and 72 hr after treatment with BHA, without any cytotoxicity. These results strongly suggest that antioxidants primarily induce cell proliferation by direct stimulation and that cell proliferation is probably further enhanced by regeneration subsequent to cytotoxicity.

Strong cell proliferation, however, does not always correlate with occurrence of carcinomas. It takes a long time (usually more than 1 year) for the development of forestomach carcinomas, and induced hyperplasia regresses after cessation of chemical treatment. We compared reversibility of rat forestomach lesions induced by an intragastric dose of 20 mg/kg body weight N-nitroso-N'-nitro-N-nitrosoguanidine (MMNG) once a week, 20 ppm N-methylnitrosourethane (MNUR) in the drinking water as genotoxic forestomach carcinogens, 2% BHA, 2% caffeic acid, or 2% 4-methoxyphenol in the diet as nongenotoxic carcinogens for 24 weeks.

Forestomach lesions induced by genotoxic carcinogens did not regress 24 weeks after the removal of the carcinogen stimulus. In contrast, hyperplasia induced by nongenotoxic carcinogens clearly regressed after the cessation of insult. Preneoplastic atypical hyperplasia, observed at high incidences in rats treated with genotoxic carcinogens, was also evident in animals receiving nongenotoxic agents, even after their withdrawal, albeit at low incidences. These results indicate that even with nongenotoxic carcinogens, a heritable alteration at the DNA level could occur during strong cell proliferation and result in atypical hyperplasia development. This preneoplastic lesion might then progress to produce carcinomas. Indeed, weak forestomach genotoxic carcinogens show potent carcinogenicity under cell-proliferating conditions induced by BHA. Thus, when animals were treated with 2% BHA and given sc injections of 50 mg/kg body weight of the weak forestomach carcinogen 3,2'-dimethyl-4-aminobiphenyl (DMAB) once a week or an ip injection of 15 mg/kg body weight of N-methylnitrosourea (MNU) once every 2 weeks for 22

weeks, the carcinogenic response was amplified. At week 24 the BHA treatment was associated with significant papilloma induction in the forestomach (40%), while no lesions were observed in the group given only DMAB. MNU alone did not induce forestomach carcinomas, but carcinomas were found in 75% of rats receiving BHA in combination with either of the genotoxic agents.

Although antioxidant forestomach carcinogens are generally negative in the Ames test and in several in vitro and in vivo mutagenesis assays, they can show weak genotoxic activity under certain conditions. Three hours after a single intragastric administration of 40 mg BHA, no detectable DNA damage was present in the forestomach epithelium, but the oxidative metabolite tert-butylquinone (TBQ) did cause DNA damage at 1/1000 of the parent concentration level. Other oxidative BHA metabolites, 3-tert-butyl-4,5-dihydroxyanisole and 3-tert-butylanisole-4,5-quinone, also showed DNA-damaging activity but were weaker than with TBQ. In vitro incubation of BHA with calf thymus DNA in the presence of an S9 mixture under acidic conditions results in DNA adducts as evaluated by a ^{32}P-postlabeling assay. Quinone metabolites of BHA form DNA adducts without the presence of an S9 mixture. Recently, low levels of DNA adducts were demonstrated in the forestomach epithelium of animals treated with 2% BHA for 2 weeks. During prostaglandin H synthase-mediated oxidative metabolism of phenolic compounds, active oxygen species could be produced. This finding was supported by the clear inhibition by aspirin of BHA-induced rat forestomach hyperplasia and ESR analyses which showed that prostaglandin H synthase administration resulted in a substantially accelerated metabolism of TBHQ into TBQ, which is accompanied by the formation of superoxide anion, hydroxy radical, and hydrogen peroxide. Thus, it is conceivable that active oxygen species are responsible for antioxidant-induced cytotoxicity or carcinogenesis. However, the results of investigation of 8-hydroxyguanosine (8-OH-dG), which is a reliable marker of oxidative DNA damage by reactive oxygen species, in the forestomach epithelium in vivo have been equivocal. Caffeic acid also causes metal-dependent DNA damage through H_2O_2 formation in

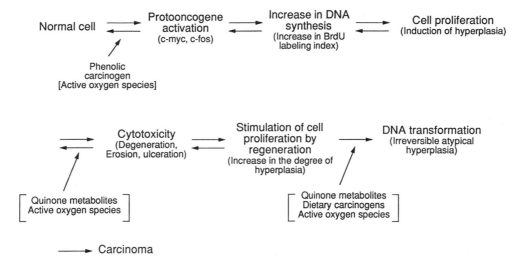

FIGURE 3 Putative pathway of rat forestomach carcinogenesis induced by phenolic antioxidants. Possible contributing factors are indicated by brackets. Observed changes in the forestomach epithelium are shown to parentheses.

vitro. In addition, food-derived mutagenic compounds could be formed in the stomach by interaction of amines and nitrite, or nitrite and phenolic compounds. Therefore, oxidative metabolites, active oxygen species, and food-derived mutagens might contribute weak genotoxicity which could act in concert with strong cell proliferation. The putative carcinogenic process driven by phenolic compounds in the forestomach epithelium is summarized schematically in Fig. 3.

IV. MODIFICATION OF CARCINOGENESIS BY ANTIOXIDANTS IN TWO-STEP CARCINOGENESIS MODELS

Many antioxidants are capable of modifying chemical or ultraviolet carcinogenesis in a broad spectrum of organs. In addition to direct effects on the initiation and/or postinitiation neoplastic process, they can also exert an influence by blocking nitrosamine formation or reducing the activity of promoters such as 12-O-tetradecanoylphorbol-13-acetate (TPA) in mouse skin carcinogenesis. The mechanisms underlying modification appear to vary with the stage of carcinogenesis and with the carcinogen.

A. Modification of Carcinogenesis by Antioxidants in the Initiation Stage

In this stage, antioxidants could modify carcinogenesis by (1) altering the metabolic activation of procarcinogens, (2) altering detoxifying enzymes, (3) direct interaction with the proximate carcinogenic species, (4) trapping active oxygen species, or (5) influencing absorption of carcinogens from the gastrointestinal tract. BHA inhibits benzo[a]pyrene (BP)- or its proximate carcinogen ($\pm$)-*trans*-7,8-dihydrobenzo[a]pyrene-induced mouse forestomach and lung carcinogenesis in the initiation stage. In this case, inhibition of the cytochrome P450-dependent monooxygenase, which metabolizes BP via 7,8-dihydrodiol to the ultimate carcinogen 7,8-diol-9,10-epoxide, and induction of phase II enzymes, such as glutathione S-transferase, which detoxify the proximate carcinogen, eventually resulted in the decreased formation of diol epoxide–DNA adducts. The plant flavonoid ellagic acid inhibits BP-induced mouse lung carcinogenesis by intraperitoneal and/or oral administration. It also reduces the mutagenic activity of BP 7,8-diol-9,10-epoxide and 7,8-diol-9,10-epoxide-induced mouse pulmonary tumor formation when administered prior to carcinogen. The observed inhibition may be due to ellagic acid decreasing hepatic and pulmonary cytochrome P450 levels, increasing hepatic glutathione S-transferase activity, and directly interacting with ultimate carcinogen. Many phenolic antioxidants, flavonoids, and seleno-compounds are thought to inhibit carcinogenesis by modifying metabolic pathways. On the other hand, BHA was found to enhance dibutylnitrosamine (DBN)-induced hepatocarcinogenesis, possibly due to enhancing cytochrome P450-mediated oxidation of DBN to proximate carcinogenic studies.

In cases of active oxygen-mediated carcinogenesis, some antioxidants lower the tumor yield or cytotoxicity induced by carcinogens, but protective effects are not general. Continuous oral treatment with 500 ppm potassium bromate ($KBrO_3$) induces renal cell tumors in 90% of rats when given for up to 2 years. Intraperitoneal or intragastric administration of $KBrO_3$ induces cytotoxicity, lipid peroxidation, and increases in 8-hydroxydeoxyguanosine (8-OH-dG) formation at the target site of carcinogenesis, and therefore active oxygen might be involved in its carcinogenic action. Combined treatment with glutathione, cystein, or ascorbic acid, but not superoxide dismutase or vitamin E, protected against its associated oxidative DNA damage and nephrotoxicity. On the other hand, ferric nitrilotriacetate-induced nephrotoxicity and lipid peroxidation were protected against by vitamin E. It is known that this renal carcinogen generates hydroxy radicals in the presence of H_2O_2 in vitro, which cause DNA cleavage and base damage. It produces 8-OH-dG in the kidney DNA and causes lipid peroxidation and nephrotoxicity in the proximal tubules. Hepatocarcinogenesis induced by peroxisomal proliferators, in which excess production of H_2O_2 may be responsible, is also blocked by BHA and ethoxyquine, and the ascorbic acid derivative (CV 3611), N,N'-diphenyl-p-phenylenediamine, or BHT protect against liver tumor induction by a choline-deficient diet in which lipid peroxidation and formation of 8-OH-dG are thought to be involved.

Chlorophyllin inhibits mutagenesis by several carcinogens, such as the heterocyclic amine Trp-P-2, in the Ames test by absorbing carcinogens to form carcinogen–chlorophyllin complexes. In the rat, chlorophyllin accelerates the excretion of Trp-P-2 into feces. Although an inhibition action for chlorophillin in in vivo carcinogenesis has not been demonstrated to date, this chemical might be expected to exert beneficial effects.

B. Modification of Carcinogenesis by Antioxidants on the Promotion/Progression Stage

The modifying effects of antioxidants on carcinogenesis when administered after carcinogen treatment have been examined in various organs by a large number of investigators. Both promoting and inhibitory effects in various organs have been documented, dependent on the organ site and agent, as shown in Table II. Carcinogenic antioxidants usually strongly enhance carcinogenesis in their target organs. Thus BHA, caffeic acid, and 4-methylcatechol promote forestomach carcinogenesis, and catechol and 4-methylcatechol enhance both forestomach and glandular stomach carcinogenesis after pretreatment with MNNG. Both BHA and BHT promote rat urinary bladder carcinogenesis initiated with N-butyl-N-(4-hydroxybutyl)nitrosamine (BBN), and BHT enhances rat urinary bladder, esophagus, and thyroid carcinogenesis in animals pretreated with BBN, DBN, and DHPN, respectively. Without carcinogen pretreatment, they induce hyperplasia or increase the BrdU-labeling index in their target organs. Therefore, promotion effects appear closely related to their potency in inducing cell proliferation.

On the positive side, BHA was found to inhibit DHPN-initiated lung carcinogenesis, 7,12-dimethylbenz[a]anthracene (DMBA)-initiated mammary carcinogenesis, and diethylnitrosamine (DEN)-induced hepatocarcinogenesis. BHT also inhibits colon, kidney, and mammary carcinogenesis, and similar findings have been widely gained for synthetic as well as naturally occurring antioxidants. Modulation of ornithine decarboxylase (ODC) activity, generation of active oxygen species, interaction with calcium- and phospholipid-dependent protein kinase C, altered prostaglandin synthesis, and influence on intercellular communication are all factors that might play a role in antioxidant effects on cell proliferation and/or modulation of carcinogenesis.

C. Antipromoting Activity of Antioxidants

Antipromotion effects have been primarily demonstrated in the two-stage mouse skin carcinogenesis model. In this system, mice are given a single topical

TABLE II
Modifying Effects of Antioxidants on Rat Carcinogenesis after Carcinogen Exposure

| | Antioxidant | | | | | | | |
| | Synthetic | | | | Naturally occurring | | | |
Target organ	BHA	BHT	TBHQ	PG	SA	α-TOC	PA	DDS
Esophagus	→	→	↑	→	→	→	→	→
Forestomach	↑	→	↑	→	↑	→	→	→
Glandular stomach	→	→	→	→	→	↑	→	→
Colon	→	↓	↓	→	↑	→	→	↓
Liver	↓	→	→	→	→	→	↓	→
Lung	↓	↓	→	→	→	↓	→	→
Kidney	→	↓	↓	→	→	↓	→	↓
Urinary bladder	↑	↑	↑	→	↑	→	↑	→
Mammary gland	↓	↓	↓	↓	→	→	NE	NE
Thyroid	→	↑	→	→	→	→	→	→

Note: TBHQ, *t*-butylhydroquinone; PG, propyl gallate; SA, sodium ascorbate; α-TOC, α-tocopherol; PA, phytic acid; DDS, diallyldisulfide. ↑, enhancement; →, no effect; ↓, inhibition, NE, not examined.

application of DMBA, 3-methylcholanthrene, BP, or BP-7,8-diol-9,10-epoxide as an initiator, then receive a continuous topical treatment with TPA or teleocidin together with synthetic antioxidants such as BHA, BHT, α-tocophenol, or other naturally occurring antioxidants such as green tea polyphenols, curcumin, chlorogenic acid, caffeic acid, and ferulic acid. The observed inhibition of TPA-induced skin promotion may be partly due to a scavenging action of these antioxidants against TPA-induced active oxygens. TPA induces superoxide anion radicals and H_2O_2 release in human peripheral leukocytes *in vitro* and H_2O_2 and 8-OH-dG in mouse skin *in vivo*. These phenomena can be strongly inhibited by copper(II)-(3,5-disopropylsalicylate)$_2$ (CuDIPS) and by nordihydroguaiaretic acid (NDGA), which are superoxide anion radical scavengers and detoxifiers. In an *in vivo* experiment, CuDIPS and NDGA significantly inhibited TPA-induced skin tumor promotion in mice initiated with DMBA. Induction of ODC in mouse epidermis also appears to be an important factor for TPA-induced skin tumor promotion. This TPA-induced ODC increase could be inhibited by lipoxygenase inhibitors NDGA, morin, fisetin, kaempferol, propyl gallate, esculetin, and BHA. In addition, morin or esculetin treatment was associated with significant inhibition of skin tumor promotion. Thus, the in-

hibitory effects of flavonoids on TPA-induced ODC induction and tumor promotion roughly paralleled their lipoxygenase inhibition. These results therefore suggest that antioxidants act by scavenging the superoxide anion radicals that are responsible for tumor promotion or by interfering with lipoxygenase in the epidermis induced by TPA.

D. Modification by Blocking Nitrosamine Formation

From the epidemiological viewpoint, a number of studies have suggested that an intake of nitrite and nitrate correlates with a high incidence of human gastric cancer and that this was due to formation of carcinogenic *N*-nitroso compounds in the stomach by the reaction of nitrite with amines present in foods and certain drugs. Some antioxidants have been shown to prevent nitrosation *in vitro* and tumor formation in animals by preventing this reaction between nitrite and amines to form *N*-nitroso compounds. Ascorbic acid and α-tocophenol are well-known inhibitors of nitrosation. For example, they significantly inhibit *in vitro* nitrosation of secondary amines such as morpholine, piperazine, diethylamine, and *N*-methylurea. The reaction of ascorbic acid with nitrite proceeds with the reduction of 2 mol of nitrite to nonnitrosating nitric oxide per mole of ascorbic acid, which is oxidized to dehydroascorbic acid. However, the nonnitrosating nitric oxide can, in the presence of oxygen, give rise to higher oxides of nitrogen, which are themselves powerful nitrosating species. Therefore, under certain conditions ascorbic acid can catalyze nitrosation. Nevertheless, sodium ascorbate at 11.5 or 23 g/kg in the diet gave 89–98% inhibition of lung adenoma induction when $NaNO_2$ was applied with a piperazine, morpholine, or methylurea system. Inhibition of nitrosation by ascorbic acid can be observed by examination of human urine following sequential oral doses of nitrite and proline. However, the dose of antioxidant required to return the N-nitrosoproline excretion to basal levels was far in excess of the proline administered. Phenolic antioxidants and flavonoids are also capable of blocking nitrosamine formation. In one carcinogenesis study, gallic acid strongly inhibited adenoma induction in mouse lung by morpholine plus $NaNO_2$. The mechanisms by which phenolic compounds inhibit nitrosation involve reduction of nitrite to nitric oxide, or formation of C-nitroso compounds and mutagenic diazoquinone. Therefore, the possibility remains that the C-nitroso compounds or diazoquinone formed could exert carcinogenic activity. Recently, continuous oral administration of ascorbic acid or some phenolic compounds, including catechol, hydroquinone, and gallic acid, and $NaNO_2$ in combination induced strong cell proliferation or papillomas in rat forestomach epithelium. Therefore, much care and attention should be given to this type of cancer prevention.

V. CHEMOPREVENTION OF CARCINOGENESIS BY ANTIOXIDANTS

Antioxidants that have demonstrated an inhibitory effect in experimental chemical carcinogenesis have been proposed as possible chemopreventors in man. However, this has been suggested primarily on the basis of epidemiological findings, and the existence of adverse effects in different experimental models has indicated that care must be taken in application of antioxidants as chemopreventors.

Necessary characteristics for an ideal chemopreventor include (1) ability to inhibit initiation activity, (2) ability to inhibit promotion or progression activity, (3) ability to block nitrosamine formation, (4) lack of genotoxicity, (5) lack of carcinogenicity, (6) not a carcinogen precursor, (7) lack of enhancing activity at any stage of carcinogenesis, (8) lack of toxicity, and (9) commercially available. Factors (5) to (8) might, however, be ignored if hazardous effects are only evident at doses much higher than the chemopreventive dose.

Nevertheless, it may still be difficult to find chemopreventors which satisfy all these requirements. For example, sodium ascorbate can satisfy requirements 1, 2, 3, 5, 8, and 9, but not 4, 6, and 7, whereas α-tocopherol satisfies 1–6, 8, and 9 but not 7. The fact that antioxidants may show opposite effects in different organs, particularly in the promotion stage, means, furthermore, that a total body approach using different carcinogenic initiators is necessary for the reliable assessment of second-stage effects.

Recently we established a multiorgan carcinogenesis model in which five different carcinogens were used as initiators. In this model, not only the enhancing but also the inhibitory effects of chemicals on carcinogenesis either in the initiating or in the promoting stage on major organs (liver, forestomach, small intestine, large intestine, lung, kidney, urinary bladder, and thyroid gland) can be examined in a single experiment, and its application for examining chemopreventive effects of several naturally occurring antioxidants suggested that green tea catechins (GTC) may be in fact possible chemopreventors. Significant decreases in the incidences of small intestinal tumors (adenomas and adenocarcinomas) were evident in the group treated with 1% GTC (content of catechins >91%, of these (−)-epigallocatechin gallate >54%) during carcinogen exposure (13%) as compared with the carcinogen alone control value (57%). Multiplicities (average no. per rat) were also lower in groups treated with GTC both during (0.13 ± 0.35) and after (0.13 ± 0.48) carcinogen exposure than in the carcinogen alone case (1.07 ± 1.21). No significant differences in esophagus, forestomach, colon, liver, kidney, urinary bladder, lung, and thyroid gland lesion induction were observed. Subsequent treatment with 1.0% GTC also inhibited rat mammary tumor development and consequently increased the survival rate (93% vs. 33.3% in DMBA alone) after a single intragastric administration of 50 mg/kg body weight of DMBA. GTC potently lowers the hepatocarcinogenicity of glutamic acid pyrolisate 2-amino-6-methyldipyridol[1,2-a:3',2'-d] imidazole (Glu-P-1) as assessed in terms of number and areas of preneoplastic glutathione S-transferase placental form (GTC-P) positive foci in our medium term liver bioassay. Green tea extracts or green tea polyphenols also inhibit benzo[a]pyrene (BP)-, DMBA, 3-methylcholanthrene-, or ultraviolet light-induced tumor initiation and complete carcinogenesis in mouse skin, 12-O-tetradecanoylphbol-13-acetate caused tumor promotion in mouse skin, N-ethyl-N'-nitro-N-nitrosoguanidine (ENNG)-induced mouse duodenal carcinogenesis, azoxymethane-induced rat colon carcinogenesis, BP- and diethylnitrosamine-induced mouse lung and forestomach carcinogenesis, and 4-(methylnitrosamino)-1-(3-pyridyl)-1-butanone-induced mouse lung carcinogenesis. These inhibitory effects were observed not only in the initiation stage but also in the promotion or progression stage in some cases. The lowest effective dose for protection to occur was 0.005% (−)-epigallocatechin gallate in the ENNG case and this dose is almost comparable with the daily intake of GTC in green tea drinkers. The mechanism(s) underlying how GTC inhibits carcinogenesis is not fully understood, but inhibition of ornithine decarboxylase and lipoxygenese activities, enhancement of Phase II enzymes, inhibition of oxidative stress induced by promoters or carcinogens, direct interaction between GTC and ultimate carcinogens, inhibition of promoter-induced protein kinase C, reduction of activating enzymes, and stimulation of immunity in the target organs may all play roles. In addition, some epidemiological data indicate a reduced risk of colon tumors and gastric cancers among populations with high levels of green tea consumption.

1-O-2,3,5-Trimethylhydroquinone (HTHQ) is a strong phenolic antioxidant. In the medium term liver bioassay for the detection of hepatocarcinogens or hepatopromoters in F344 male rats, treatment with Glu-P-1 alone was associated with a significant increase in the number (per cm^2 liver) and area (mm^2 per cm^2 liver) of preneoplastic GST-P-positive foci (47.5 ± 8.9 and 11.1 ± 4.7, respectively). Combined treat-

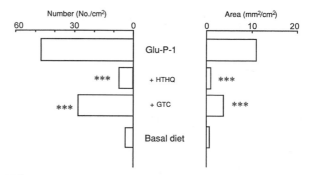

FIGURE 4 Quantitative analyses of the effects of antioxidants on Glu-P-1-induced GST-P positive foci in the medium term liver bioassay. HTHQ, 1-O-2,3,5-trimethylhydroquinone; GTC, green tea catechin. Significantly different from the Glu-P-1 group at ***$P < 0.001$.

ment with 1.0% HTHQ significantly reduced the number and area of GST-P-positive foci (to 8.1 ± 2.1 and 0.6 ± 0.2), almost to control level values without chemicals (3.6 ± 1.6 and 0.3 ± 0.1). HTHQ is therefore expected to be a selective potent chemopreventor which could reduce the carcinogenicity of heterocyclic amines such as Glu-P-1 (Fig. 4).

Since chemopreventors exert their actions in different organs, in different stages of carcinogenesis, and dependent on the carcinogen, intake of different chemopreventors in combination may prove to be important for the prevention of human cancer.

VI. EVALUATION OF ANTIOXIDANTS AS HUMAN HAZARDS

There are many synthetic and naturally occurring antioxidants in our environment. Humans may ingest considerable amounts of such compounds in foodstuffs, medicines such as vitamins C and E, and γ-oryzanol, or by absorption through the skin of antioxidant additives in cosmetics, antiseptics, disinfectants, and industrial chemicals. It is therefore possible that these antioxidants may indeed play a role in human carcinogenesis. Although there are some epidemiological and case control studies suggesting that high intake of antioxidants such as ascorbic acid, α-tocopherol, selenium, β-carotene, and vegetables that contain vitamins A, C, and E may lower the mortality rate for certain cancer types in humans, no such studies have been performed for phenolic antioxidants.

For human risk assessment of phenolic antioxidant exposure, and extrapolation from experimental data, it is of importance to take into account the target organ, dose level, and route of administration. BHA is carcinogenic for the rat, hamster, and possibly mouse forestomach epithelium, but this activity is strictly limited to this tissue, and no carcinogenic potential for other squamous epithelia, such as those lining the esophagus and oral cavity, or for glandular stomach has been found. Since humans do not have a forestomach, it appears most likely that such limited forestomach carcinogens would lack effects on human gastric epithelium. Moreover, the threshold carcinogenic dose of BHA in rats is 2% in the diet (only a small incidence of benign papillomas was induced at lower dose levels), a level that is exceedingly high as compared with the possible human exposure. The estimated daily dietary intake of BHA was reported to be less than 7 mg/person in a Canadian study and therefore the carcinogenic dose in animals is nearly 10,000 times higher than the likely human exposure level.

On the other hand, catechol, which is present in certain foods (e.g., fruits, vegetables, coffee), in tobacco, in cosmetics such as hair dye, in film developers, and in wood smoke, promotes glandular stomach carcinogenesis and induces adenocarcinomas in the rat glandular stomach, which is anatomically and biologically similar to human gastric epithelium at a dose of 0.8% in diet. Catechol at a dose of 0.16% for 2 years also caused glandular stomach adenomas to develop at low incidence. A 0.16% dose level is equivalent to 5–7.5 g catechol per person per day. The amount of catechol and its conjugates actually excreted in urine in humans was reported to be 1.1–30 mg/day, but although the carcinogenic dose in rats is 250–6250 times higher than the estimated human exposure, this chemical might still be a factor for enhancing human gastric cancer.

Thus, the promotion potential of antioxidants may be far more important for human environmental carcinogenesis than any complete carcinogen action. Experiments have shown that effective enhancement can be achieved at much lower levels than the carcinogenic dose, and since antioxidants can exert promoting potential in various organs that are not necessarily targets for carcinogenicity, as shown in Table II, this must be taken into account. Moreover, clear synergistic effects regarding promotion have been reported; that is, combined treatment with 0.5% caffeic acid, 0.16% catechol, 0.5% BHA, and 0.25% 2-tert-butyl-4-methylphenol in rats for 51 weeks in rats pretreated with MNNG induced an 80% incidence of forestomach squamous cell carcinomas, whereas the individual treatments resulted in only 13–27% incidences. In a long-term carcinogenicity study, rats were treated with 0.4% caffeic acid, 0.4% sesamol, 0.16% catechol, 0.4% BHA, and 0.4% 4-methoxyphenol either alone or in combination for 104 weeks. Although papillomas were found in 0–15.8% of the individual treatment groups, the incidence increased to 42.9% with the combined treatment. Such synergistic or additive effects in carcinogenicity or promotion of carcinogenesis have been observed not only in the forestomach. Moreover, the carcinogenic or hyperplasiagenic activity of BHA was enhanced by concurrent treatment with sodium ascorbate or vitamin A, but was inhibited by concomitant treatment with diethylmaleate, a glutathione-depleting agent, or aspirin, and some antioxidants potentiate carcinogenicity of genotoxic carcinogens possibly through metabolic activation. $NaNO_2$ also is a factor that can greatly modify carcinogenicity of phenolic compounds.

Therefore antioxidant effects may be considerably altered by changes in environmental or physiological conditions. Endogenous factors such as age, immunological condition, and other diseases in target organs will also influence the effective dose for promotion of carcinogenesis or carcinogenicity. Available data thus indicate that low concentrations of carcinogens or promoters, even if they do not show activity per se, may indeed be important for human environmental carcinogenesis.

See Also the Following Articles

Animal Models for Colon Cancer Chemoprevention • Cancer Risk Reduction (Diet/Smoking Cessation/Lifestyle Changes) • Chemoprevention, Pharmacology of • Molecular Epidemiology and Cancer Risk • Nutritional Supplements and Diet as Chemopreventive Agents

Bibliography

Hirose, M., Imaida, K., Tamano, S., and Ito, N. (1994). Cancer chemoprevention by antioxidants. In "Food Phytochemicals for Cancer Prevention" (C.-T. Ho, M.-T. Huang, R. T. Rosen, and T. Osawa, eds.), Vol. 547, p. 122, ACS Books, Washington, DC.

Hirose, M., Tanaka, H., Takahashi, S., Futakuchi, M., Fukushima, S., and Ito, N. (1993). Effects of sodium nitrite and catechol, 3-methoxycatechol, or butylated hydroxyanisole in combination in a rat multiorgan carcinogenesis. *Cancer Res.* **53,** 32.

Ito, N., Hirose, M., and Shirai, T. (1992). Carcinogenicity and modification of carcinogenic response by plant phenols. In "Phenolic Compounds in Food and Their Effects on Health II" (M.-T. Huang, C.-T. Ho, and C.-Y. Lee, eds.), Vol. 507, p. 270. ACS Books, Washington, DC.

Ito, N., Shirai, T., and Hasegawa, R. (1992). Medium-term bioassays for carcinogens. In "Mechanisms of Carcinogenesis in Risk Identification" (H. Vainio, P. N. Magee, D. B. McGregor, and A. J. McMichael, eds.), p. 353. International Agency for Research on Cancer, Lyon.

Ito, N., and Imaida, K. (1992). Strategy of research for cancer-chemoprevention. *Teratog. Carcinog. Mutag.* **12,** 79.

Ito, N., and Hirose, M. (1989). Antioxidants-carcinogenic and chemopreventive properties. *Adv. Cancer Res.* **53,** 247.

Ito, N., Hirose, M., and Takahashi, S. (1993). Cell proliferation and forestomach carcinogenesis. *Environ. Health Perspect.* **101,** Suppl. 5, 69.

Nera, E. A., Lok, E., Iverson, F., Ormsby, E., Karpinski, K. F., and Clayton, D. B. (1984). Short-term pathological and proliferative effects of butylated hydroxyanisole and other phenolic antioxidants in the forestomach of Fischer 344 rats. *Toxicology* **32,** 197.

Rodrigues, C., Lok, E., Nera, E., Iverson, F., Page, D., Karpinski, K., and Clayton, D. B. (1984). Short-term effects of various phenols and acids on the Fischer 344 male rat forestomach epithelium. *Toxicology* **38,** 103.

Schiderman, P. A. E. L., van Maanen, J. M. S., ten Vaarwerk, F. J., Lafleur, M. V. M., Westmijze, E. J., ten Hoor, F., and Kleinjans, J. C. S. (1993). The role of prostaglandin H synthase-mediated metabolism in the induction of oxidative DNA-damage by BHA metabolites. *Carcinogenesis* **14,** 1297.

Antisense: Medicinal Chemistry

Eugen Uhlmann
Anusch Peyman
David W. Will
Aventis Pharma Deutschland GmbH

I. Introduction
II. Unmodified Oligonucleotides
III. Minimal Modification of the Internucleoside Phosphodiester Bridge
IV. Modifications of the Internucleoside Phosphodiester Linkage
V. Replacement of the Internucleoside Linkage and the Sugar
VI. Sugar-Modified Oligonucleotides
VII. Modification of Nucleobases
VIII. Oligonucleotide Conjugates
IX. Design Considerations for Antisense Oligonucleotides

GLOSSARY

antisense oligonucleotide A synthetic single-stranded nucleic acid of about 12 to 30 mononucleotide units in length capable of binding via Watson–Crick base pairing to complementary ("sense") regions on mRNA, resulting in inhibition of protein synthesis.

binding affinity Strength of binding of an oligonucleotide to its single-stranded or double-stranded target nucleic acid. The melting temperature T_m, the temperature at which 50% of the double strand has dissociated into its single strands, is commonly used as a measure for binding affinity.

cellular uptake Overall uptake of an oligonucleotide after incubation for a specified period of time in cell culture, usually encompassing all cell-associated oligonucleotides without discriminating nuclear, cytosolic, or membrane fractions.

modified antisense oligonucleotide An antisense oligonucleotide whose chemical structure has been altered relative to the naturally occurring nucleic acids in order to improve its biophysical or biological properties.

nuclease stability Stability of oligonucleotides against degrading enzymes present in serum and within cells, including exonucleases and endonucleases.

RNase H A cellular enzyme that recognizes a hybrid duplex between DNA and RNA, while cleaving the RNA strand of this duplex. The capability of stimulating RNase H strongly depends on the type of chemical modification of the antisense oligonucleotide.

T he medicinal chemistry of antisense oligonucleotides has developed rapidly in recent years mainly due to their potential use as a major class of novel pharmaceuticals. Sequence-specific recognition of target nucleic acids using synthetic oligonucleotides is aimed at rationally designed therapeutics that inhibit gene expression rather than the corresponding gene products (proteins). In order to put the antisense principle into action, issues such as nuclease stability, cellular uptake, binding affinity, specificity, pharmacokinetics, and toxicity, as well as *in vivo* efficacy, have to be addressed. Suitable chemical modification of the natural nucleic acid structure is necessary to meet all these requirements. The scope of this article is to summarize the structural chemistry and properties of the major classes of antisense oligonucleotide modifications that are currently under investigation for use as antisense therapeutics.

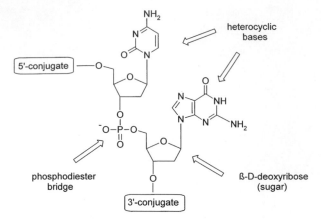

FIGURE 1 Possibilities for the modification of oligonucleotides.

I. INTRODUCTION

In recent years, the development of compounds that bind in a sequence-specific way to RNA or DNA aimed at the inhibition of gene expression has been the focus of intensive research. Already in 1978, Zamecnik and Stephenson proposed the use of synthetic antisense oligonucleotides for therapeutic purposes. By using a tridecamer oligonucleotide that was complementary to the RNA of Rous sarcoma virus, they were able to inhibit the growth of this virus in cell culture. This novel strategy, which has become known as "antisense," opened up new possibilities in research into the molecular biology of cancer and drug development.

In the last decade, around a dozen antisense oligonucleotides were put into advanced stages of clinical development, and the first antisense drug (Vitravene; Isis Pharmaceuticals) is now marketed. Vitravene and most of the antisense oligonucleotides in clinical trials are based on phosphorothioate modification. In addition to phosphorothioates, a vast number of novel oligonucleotide modifications have been created and investigated aimed at antisense drugs with improved activity and specificity.

This article focuses on the structural chemistry and properties of antisense oligonucleotide derivatives (Fig. 1). Chemical variation of the natural oligonucleotide structure becomes necessary to render these

compounds useful in biological systems: (1) They must be sufficiently stable in serum and inside the cell. (2) They must be able to penetrate cellular membranes and they should enter the various organs of the body to reach their site of action. (3) They should form stable Watson–Crick complexes with complementary target sequences under physiological conditions. (4) The interaction of the oligonucleotide with its target sequence should be sequence specific.

II. UNMODIFIED OLIGONUCLEOTIDES

Unmodified oligonucleotides have been widely used as tools for mechanistic studies in molecular biology and as lead compounds in the development of gene expression-inhibiting antisense therapeutics. In these experiments, one has to take into account that these oligonucleotides with a natural phosphodiester internucleoside linkage are degraded in serum within minutes, mainly by the action of 3′-exonucleases. Once the oligonucleotides are located intracellularly, they are further degraded by endonucleases, and in some tissues, significant 5′-exonuclease activity is observed. In addition to chemical derivatization as described in the following sections, oligonucleotides can be protected against nucleolytic cleavage by packaging into liposomes or nanoparticles, which at the same time serve as carriers for *in vivo* application of these compounds.

Although unmodified oligonucleotides are of polyanionic nature, they are taken up to a substantial extent by cells in a time- and energy-dependent endocytotic or pinocytic process. Using fluorescence microscopy, a punctate intracellular distribution of fluorescence has been observed. The current view of the uptake process therefore is that a significant fraction of the oligonucleotides are trapped in endosomes or lysosomes, resulting in a comparatively low concentration of "free" hybridizable oligonucleotide in the cytoplasm or in the nucleus. For mechanistic studies, this problem can be overcome by microinjection of the antisense oligonucleotides into the cytosol from which they rapidly penetrate into the nucleus. The cellular uptake of oligonucleotides can be enhanced by administration with cationic lipids, such as lipofectin or cellfectin, which concomitantly seem to alter intracellular distribution of the oligonucleotide. The ratio of free to trapped oligonucleotide is influenced in a positive way by using these penetration enhancers, which in turn leads to improved nuclear uptake. The overall cellular uptake of oligonucleotides can be improved by covalently attaching lipophilic groups, specific carrier peptides, or poly-L-lysine or by packaging into antibody-targeted liposomes.

The efficacy of unmodified oligonucleotides may best be explained by an antisense oligonucleotide-stimulated degradation of the target mRNA. This pseudo-catalytic mRNA cleavage is brought about by the cellular enzyme RNase H, which recognizes a duplex between DNA and RNA. The RNase H mechanism has also been called upon as an explanation why certain oligonucleotide derivatives, such as α-oligonucleotides or 2′-O-methyl oligoribonucleotides, are relatively poor inhibitors of translation despite their excellent binding properties if they are targeted to the coding part of mRNA. Duplexes of RNA with these derivatives are not substrates for RNase H. However, RNase H-mediated cleavage of mRNA was suggested as being responsible for the nonsequence-dependent effects observed in oocytes. In our opinion, this side effect is only a problem at a high oligonucleotide concentration or in rapidly dividing cells with high levels of RNase H. There is now growing evidence that by choosing the right region of the target mRNA sequence, e.g., in the 5′-nontranslated part, oligonucleotides working by a RNase H-independent mechanism can efficiently compete with RNase H-competent oligomers.

III. MINIMAL MODIFICATION OF THE INTERNUCLEOSIDE PHOSPHODIESTER BRIDGE

Minimal modification of the phosphodiester bridge encompasses oligonucleotide analogs that differ from the naturally occurring 3′,5′-phosphodiester compounds only by changes in the linkage, but do not include new chemical entities as other derivatives discussed in later sections of this article. The essential structural moieties of these minimally modified oligonucleotide analogs (Fig. 2) also appear in nature. Antisense oligonucleotides with 3′,3′- or 5′,5′-end inversions are very stable against exonucleases, and their half-life in human serum is about 30 hr. Because Watson–Crick base pairing of the antiparallel portion of the oligonucleotide is not disturbed by the inverted termini, this type of oligonucleotide analog is capable of inhibiting gene expression *in vitro*, as well as in tissue culture experiments at 10 to 30 μM concentration. Synthesis of these analogs is straightforward by using the corresponding "inverted" nucleoside-5′-O-phosphoramidites or nucleoside-5′-O-succinyl supports combined with standard phosphoramidite chemistry.

Because exonucleases need a terminal hydroxyl function for efficient cleavage of terminal internucleoside linkages, cyclic oligonucleotides are not degraded by these enzymes. Thus, cyclic oligonucleotide analogs involving nonnucleotidic oligo-ether linkages show no cleavage after 2 days of incubation in human serum at 37°C, whereas the linear variants are already partially digested within 30 min. The cyclic oligonucleotide sequence can be designed so as to allow triplex formation on a single-stranded nucleic acid target. Thereby, one part of the cyclo-oligonucleotide binds via Watson–Crick base pairing and another part binds via Hoogsteen base pairing to a single-stranded target nucleic acid, resulting in a triple helical structure.

Naturally occurring 2′,5′-oligoadenylates play an important role in the stimulation of RNase L, which cleaves single-stranded RNA adjacent to

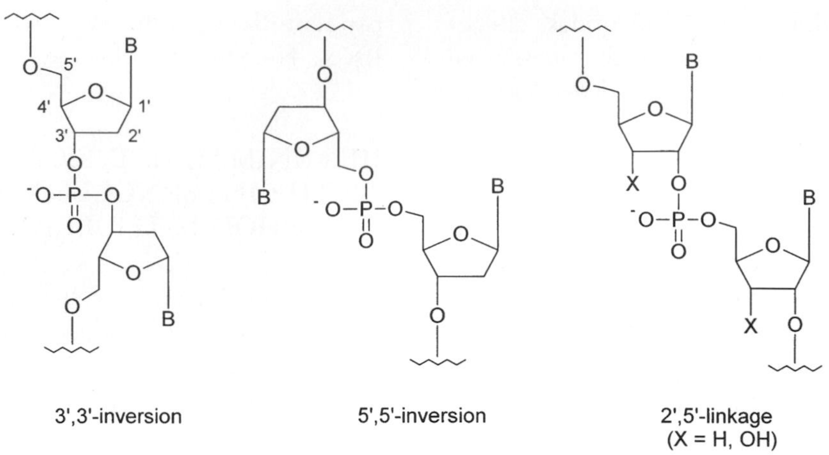

| 3',3'-inversion | 5',5'-inversion | 2',5'-linkage (X = H, OH) |

FIGURE 2 Structural elements of minimally modified oligonucleotides.

double-stranded RNA in response to interferon treatment. Self-complementary 2',5'-linked oligoribonucleotides of mixed sequence form duplexes that melt at lower temperatures as compared to their 3',5'-linked analogs. Furthermore, the 2',5'-linked oligoribonucleotides are not stable in serum, but they can be substantially stabilized by modification of the phosphate backbone and by removal of the 3'-hydroxyl group. Interestingly, 2'5'-linked 3'-deoxyoligonucleotides (Fig. 2, X = H) bind with higher affinity to RNA than their 3'5'-linked counterparts, whereas they do not bind to complementary DNA. Chimeric molecules having 5'-phosphorylated 2',5'-triadenylate (Fig. 2, X = OH) conjugated to a normal 3',5'-linked antisense oligonucleotide have been successfully used to cleave target RNA by activation of 2',5'-adenylate-dependent RNase L. Because 2',5'-adenylate-dependent RNase L is present in most mammalian cells, this strategy is of use when applied in combination with antisense oligonucleotide derivatives that do not stimulate RNase H cleavage, such as peptide nucleic acids (PNA).

IV. MODIFICATIONS OF THE INTERNUCLEOSIDE PHOSPHODIESTER LINKAGE

The easiest way to make oligonucleotides resistant against nucleases is modification of the chemical group that is cleaved during degradation, meaning modification of the internucleotide phosphodiester linkage. Replacement of one or both nonbonding phosphate oxygens also allows the alteration of other properties of oligonucleotides and may allow for enhanced affinity or increased cellular permeation. The most common types of modification are depicted in Figs. 3 and 4. In addition, oligonucleotides have been synthesized in which the entire phosphodiester backbone has been replaced with novel linkages. These are discussed in Section V.

A. Phosphorothioates

Phosphorothioates, in which one oxygen is replaced by a sulfur, are among the most obvious and thus probably the earliest used analogs of naturally occurring phosphodiesters. Phosphorothioate-containing oligonucleotides are easy to synthesize; the same synthons used for "natural" oligonucleotide synthesis (phosphoramidite or H-phosphonate chemistry) can be used, as it is only in the oxidation step where sulfur is introduced instead of oxygen. From standard solid-phase synthesis, phosphorothioates usually result in a mixture of $2n$ diastereoisomers of S_P or R_P configuration, respectively (Fig. 3). This is why compounds in clinical trials are a mixture of $2n$ diastereoisomers, where n is the number of phosphorothioate linkages.

The hybridization properties of phosphorothioates

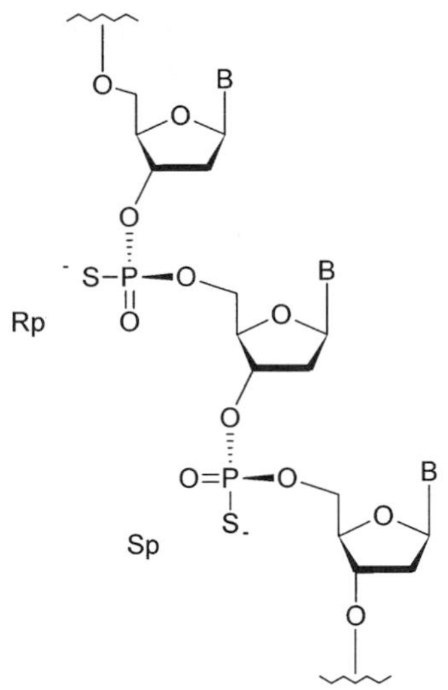

FIGURE 3 Structure of phosphorothioates of R_P and S_P configurations.

are reasonably good, although there is an average loss of $-0.5\ °C/P{=}S$ bond in the melting temperature for the racemic mixture. Duplexes consisting of oligoribonucleotides and all-R_P phosphorothioates are more stable than duplexes formed with all-S_P phosphorothioates or with the random mixture of diastereoisomers. Furthermore, a PS·RNA duplex containing the phosphorothioate in all-R_P configuration is a better substrate of RNase H than the corresponding hybrid with all-S_P linkages or the random mixture of diastereoisomers. Finally, phosphorothioates of R_P configuration are much better substrates of 3'-exonucleases present in human serum than phosphorothioates of S_P configuration. Degradation of a 25-mer PS oligonucleotide having a S_P-phosphorothioate linkage at the 3' terminus has been reported to be more than 300 times slower than an analog with a 3'-terminal PS linkage of R_P configuration.

The uptake of phosphorothioate oligonucleotides has been described to be similar to "natural" oligonucleotides. In our hands, they seem to be taken up to a somewhat lesser extent, depending on the phosphorothioate content of the DNA. A serious drawback of uniformly phosphorothioate-modified oligonucleotides, however, is their propensity for nonspecific effects, which results mainly from their interaction with cellular proteins. Oligonucleotides containing a mixture of phosphorothioate and phos-

phodiester bridges do show much less undesirable side effects. Nonetheless, phosphorothioates remain the most widely used class of derivatives for antisense experiments primarily due to their ease of synthesis, their ability to stimulate RNase H, and their favorable solubility characteristics.

B. Alkyl- and Arylphosphonates

One of the earliest and most intensively studied oligonucleotide analogs are the methylphosphonates, in which the negatively charged oxygen atom in the phosphodiester link is replaced by a neutral methyl group. Like the phosphorothioate group, the methylphosphonate group is chiral, meaning that under standard synthesis conditions, methylphosphonate oligonucleotides are obtained as a mixture of 2^n diastereoisomers. Using special synthesis conditions, short diastereomerically pure methylphosphonate oligomers have been synthesized, and it was found that methylphosphonates with an all-Rp backbone had a higher binding affinity than the random diastereomeric mixture, and even the corresponding phosphodiester oligonucleotide. Although methylphosphonates are highly stable to nuclease degradation and methods for their synthesis are well established, they have a number of disadvantages compared to phosphorothioates. First, their cellular uptake characteristics are poorer than those of phosphodiester or phosphorothioate oligonucleotides. The mechanism of uptake of nonionic methylphosphonates is apparently different than that of their negatively charged counterparts. Second, duplexes formed between methylphosphonate oligomers and RNA are not substrates for RNase H. This has been overcome by synthesizing chimeric oligomers consisting of a "window" of at least five to seven phosphodiester-linked nucleotides, which activate RNase H, flanked by methylphosphonates, which provide nuclease stability to the chimera. These chimeric oligomers also have an overall negative charge and are thus much more water soluble than the nonionic and poorly soluble uniform methylphosphonate-modified oligonucleotides.

The use of oligomers consisting of 2'-O-methyl RNA oligomers (see Section VI A) containing alternating methylphosphonate and phosphodiester linkages in antisense experiments has been reported. These oligomers had very favorable binding affinities compared to uniform methylphosphonates.

Finally, it should be mentioned that oligonucleotides containing octyl- and phenylphosphonate linkages, in which the negatively charged oxygen atom in the phosphodiester link is replaced by an eight carbon alkyl chain and a phenyl ring, respectively, have also been synthesized. The binding affinity of octylphosphonate-containing oligonucleotides was reduced considerably and that of phenylphosphonates was highly sequence dependent.

C. Phosphotriesters

Phosphotriesters, in which one of the nonbridging oxygen atoms in the phosphodiester internucleotide bridge carries an alkyl chain, were one of the earliest oligonucleotide analogs to be investigated for their potential as antisense agents. Like methylphosphonates, they are nonionic; however, the lability of the phosphotriester group, especially of P-methoxy phosphotriester oligonucleotides to basic aqueous conditions, makes their synthesis challenging. Furthermore, the potential of P-methoxy phosphotriester (Fig. 4, R = CH$_3$) oligonucleotides to act as alkylating agents has considerably reduced interest in their use as anti-

sense agents. However, the more stable P-ethoxy phosphotriester oligonucleotides (Fig. 4, R = CH$_2$CH$_3$) have been shown to specifically downregulate gene expression and to cause no significant toxicity over 6 weeks in rodents.

D. Phosphoramidates

A more recent and very promising addition to phosphate bridge-modified oligonucleotide analogs consists of the N3'-P5' phosphoramidates, in which the 3'-bridging oxygen of the phosphodiester link is replaced by NH. These zwitterionic analogs form very stable duplexes with complementary DNA and RNA, and also with themselves, following the Watson–Crick base pairing rules. The synthesis of N3'-P5' phosphoramidates is, however, nontrivial compared to many other phosphate bridge-modified oligonucleotide analogs. The N-alkylphosphoramidate linkage 3'-O-P(O)(NH-alkyl)O-5', in which one of the nonbridging oxygen atoms of the phosphodiester linkage is replaced by an NH-alkyl group, is synthesized much more readily using H phosphonate chemistry. Unfortunately, this modification results in a considerably reduced binding affinity to complementary DNA. One limitation of both N3'-P5' phosphoramidates and N-alkylphosphoramidates is the lability of the P-N bond to acid hydrolysis.

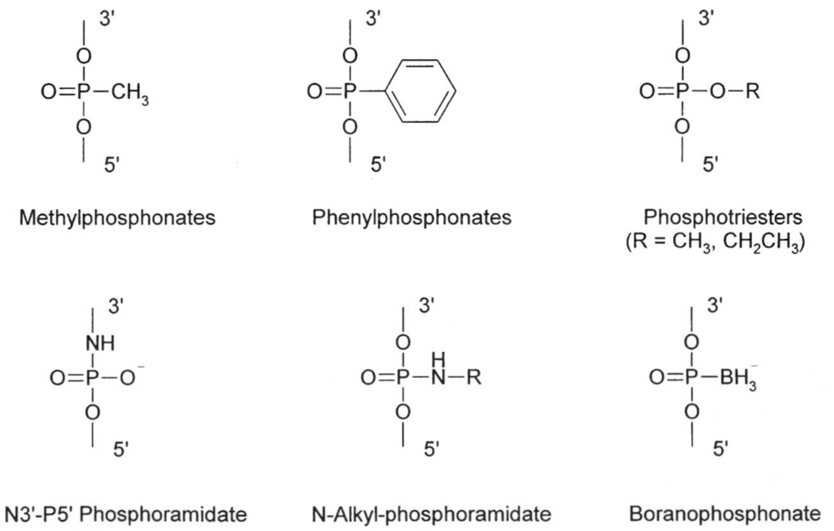

FIGURE 4 Examples of modifications of the internucleoside phosphodiester bridge.

E. Boranophosphonates

Boron-containing oligonucleotides were originally developed as spin offs from research into boron neutron capture therapy. Boranophosphonate-linked oligonucleotides, in which one of the nonbridging oxygen atoms in the phosphodiester internucleotide bridge is replaced by a negatively charged BH_3^- group, have especially interesting properties. They are isoelectronic and isoionic to DNA and phosphorothioates, but isostructural to methylphosphonates. Remarkably, and in contrast to methylphosphonates, the duplex formed between boranophosphonates and RNA is a substrate for RNase H. As would be expected, they are highly resistant to nuclease degradation; however, their binding affinity is reduced compared to DNA or even phosphorothioates.

More recently, oligonucleotides containing carbon–boron clusters attached to the internucleoside link, the carboranylmethyl phosphonates, have been synthesized.

F. Dephospho Analogs

Modifications to the internucleoside linkage described in Section IV are deliberately rather conservative in their scope in an effort to mimic the physical and structural properties of natural DNA as closely as possible, while at the same time introducing additional desirable properties, such as nuclease resistance. Unfortunately, most of these modifications also result in oligonucleotide analogs with undesirable properties, such as reduced binding affinity, poor cellular uptake, sequence-nonspecific biological activity, or stereochemical problems. One approach to overcome these difficulties is the synthesis of oligonucleotide analogs containing achiral, uncharged, phosphorus-free internucleoside linkages—the so-called dephospho analogs (Fig. 5). A remarkable variety of different linkages have been synthesized, including carbonate, carboxymethyl, acetamidate, carbamate, thioether, sulfonate, sulfonamide, oxime, methyleneimino, methylene methylimino (MMI), methylene dimethylhydrazo (MDH), methyleneoxymethylimino, urea, guanidino, riboacetal, and amide. Not surprisingly, all oligonucleotide analogs of this type investigated were found to be completely resistant to degradation by nucleases. However, many of the analogs show poor water solubility and low hydrolytic stability. In addition, a major obstacle in the investigation of antisense properties of dephospho analogs is the laborious synthesis procedures required to make the monomer building blocks, combined with oligomer synthesis, which is not straightforward and often not amenable to automated solid-phase synthesis. The complete replacement of the phosphodiester linkage results in the introduction of local perturbations in the conformation of the duplexes formed by dephospho analogs with complementary DNA/RNA sequences. Summed over the entire length of the duplex, these perturbations can result in disruption of the hydrogen bonding and base stacking interactions required to hold the duplex together. For many of the dephospho analogs investigated, a reduced binding affinity is indeed observed. Despite this, some analogs, such as MMI and methylene carboxamide, show an increased binding affinity compared to unmodified oligonucleotides. This is probably due to a combination of factors, including reduced charge repulsion and flexibility in the linkage.

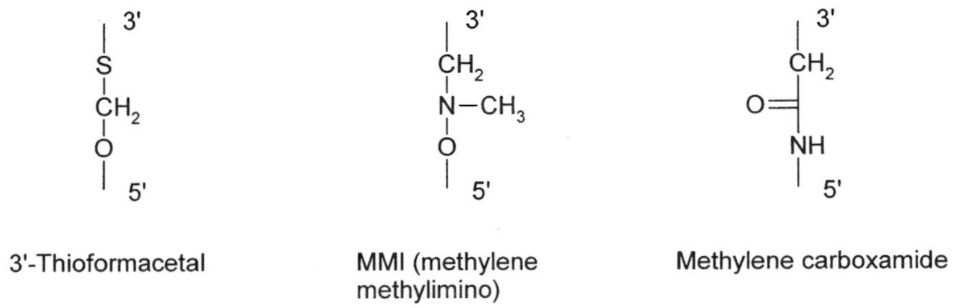

FIGURE 5 Examples of "dephospho" oligonucleotides.

V. REPLACEMENT OF THE INTERNUCLEOSIDE LINKAGE AND THE SUGAR

A. Polyamide Nucleic Acids

Peptide nucleic acids (PNA) are noncharged oligonucleotide analogs in which the entire sugar phosphate backbone is replaced by an *N*-aminoethylglycine-based polyamide structure (Fig. 6). They bind with higher affinity to complementary nucleic acids than their natural counterparts following Watson–Crick base pairing rules. However, in contrast to natural DNA, PNA binds in antiparallel and parallel orientation to complementary DNA and RNA, whereby the N terminus is equivalent to the 5′ end of nucleic acids. In case of the more stable antiparallel PNA · RNA duplex, the melting temperature is increased by approximately 1.5 K per base. Importantly, the discrimination of base mismatches has been reported to be better for PNA as compared to DNA. Not unexpectedly, PNA is extremely stable during incubation in serum, as it is neither recognized as substrate by nucleases nor by peptidases. PNA cannot stimulate RNase H cleavage. PNA directed to the coding part of the target mRNA was found to be less effective as

an antisense agent than phosphodiester and phosphorothioate oligonucleotides. However, if PNA is targeted to the 5′-nontranslated region, it can outperform the corresponding phosphodiester oligonucleotides in antisense inhibition studies. DNA/PNA chimeras with more than four nucleotides are able to stimulate the cleavage of RNA by RNase H on formation of a chimera–RNA duplex. The binding affinity of PNA/DNA chimeras to complementary DNA and RNA depends on the PNA:DNA ratio in the chimeras and increases with increasing PNA length. In contrast to pure PNA, 5′-DNA–PNA chimeras bind exclusively in the antiparallel orientation to DNA and RNA under physiological conditions. A further advantage of chimeras is their better solubility and higher cellular uptake relative to pure PNA.

The uptake of PNA can be substantially improved by coupling to carrier molecules. Thus, fusion of a 21-mer PNA to transporter peptides, such as transportan or pAntennapedia(43-58), facilitates efficient uptake of the conjugate by Bowes cells. Intrathecal administration of a PNA–pAntennapedia(43-58) conjugate, complementary to galanin receptor type 1 mRNA, resulted in decreased galanin receptor expression *in vivo*. Furthermore, fusion of a nuclear localization signal (NLS) to PNA can mediate translocation of a

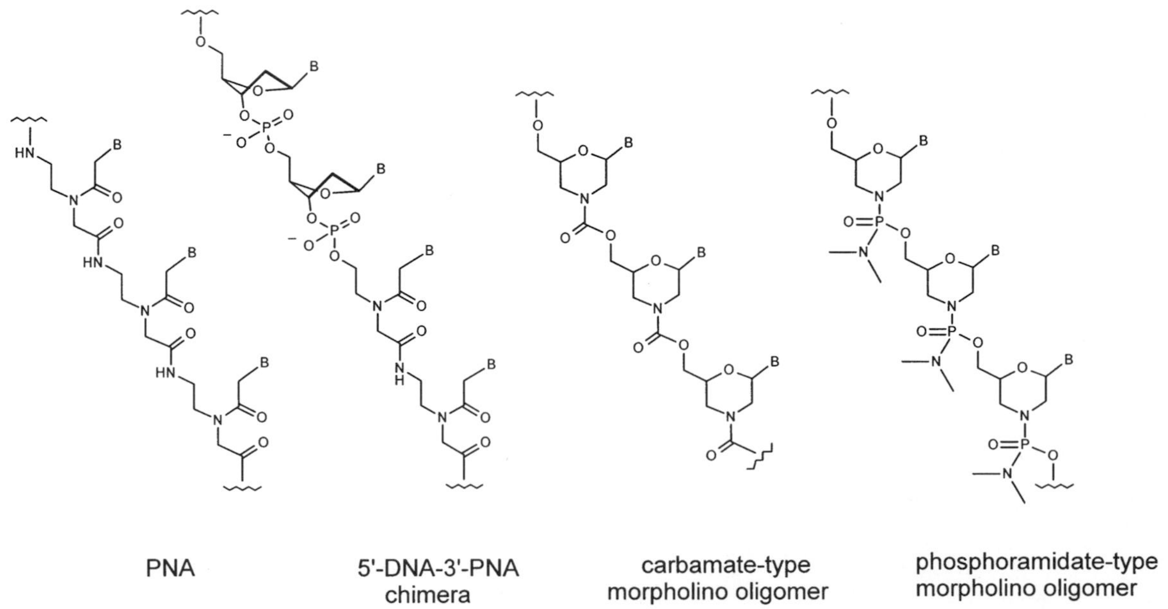

PNA   5′-DNA-3′-PNA   carbamate-type   phosphoramidate-type
                        chimera   morpholino oligomer   morpholino oligomer

FIGURE 6   Chemical structure of PNA and morpholino oligomers.

PNA–NLS conjugate to the nucleus. Specific uptake of PNA to cells expressing insulin-like growth factor 1 receptor (IGF1R) has been reported previously by conjugating PNA to a D-amino acid analog of IGF1. Surprisingly, intraperitoneal injection of a nonconjugated ("naked") PNA directed against the coding region of rat neurotensin (NT) receptor mRNA specifically downregulated NTR with a concomitant depression of behavioral and physiological responses to NT, suggesting that PNA administered ip could cross the blood–brain barrier.

B. Morpholino-Type Oligomers

Essentially two types of oligonucleotides are known in which the deoxyribose moiety is replaced by a morpholino moiety (Fig. 6). Morpholino units are connected by a carbamate bridge or, as a more recent modification, by a phosphoramidate bridge. Morpholino building blocks are readily obtained from ribonucleosides in a three-step reaction. Carbamate-type morpholino oligomers bind well to DNA, but binding to RNA is rather poor. In addition, they suffer from low solubility in water. These problems have been overcome with phosphoramidate-bridged morpholino oligomers. They bind to RNA with a higher affinity than natural oligodeoxynucleotides, they are highly resistant to nucleolytic degradation, and they are surprisingly soluble in water. Their mechanism of action is through steric blocking only, as they do not activate RNase H. Biological efficacy using this type of modified antisense oligonucleotides has been shown in numerous *in vitro* experiments using cell-free and culture cell systems. Results suggest that morpholino oligomers directed against cytokine targets can also function in animals.

VI. SUGAR-MODIFIED OLIGONUCLEOTIDES

A. 2′-Modified Oligonucleotides

Because RNA · RNA duplexes are generally more stable than DNA · RNA duplexes, the primary purpose for introducing 2′ modifications into oligonucleotides has been to enhance the binding affinity to target RNA by forcing the antisense oligomer into an "A" form geometry (by forcing the ribofuranosyl moiety into the 3′-endo conformation) and to increase nuclease resistance at the same time. This type of modification can be subdivided in 2′-O-alkyl RNA and other modifications at the 2′ position, such as 2′-fluoro or 2′-amino-substituted oligonucleotides (Fig. 7). 2′ Modifications have also been used in combination with modifications of the phosphate bridge, namely phosphorothioates or methylphosphonates.

The 2′-O-methylether of RNA is a naturally occurring modification found in selected positions in tRNAs, rRNAs, and snRNAs. The stability of heteroduplexes with RNA depends on the nature of the 2′ substituent, in particular on its electronegativity and the bulkyness of the O-alkyl group. 2′-Fluoro-modified oligonucleotides exhibit the highest increase in binding affinity, which for 2′-O-alkyl substituents decreases in the order 2′-O-(2-methoxyethyl)>2′-O-methyl>2′-O-allyl>2′-OH>2′-O-butyl>2′-O-dimethylallyl. In contrast, the 2′ amino modification

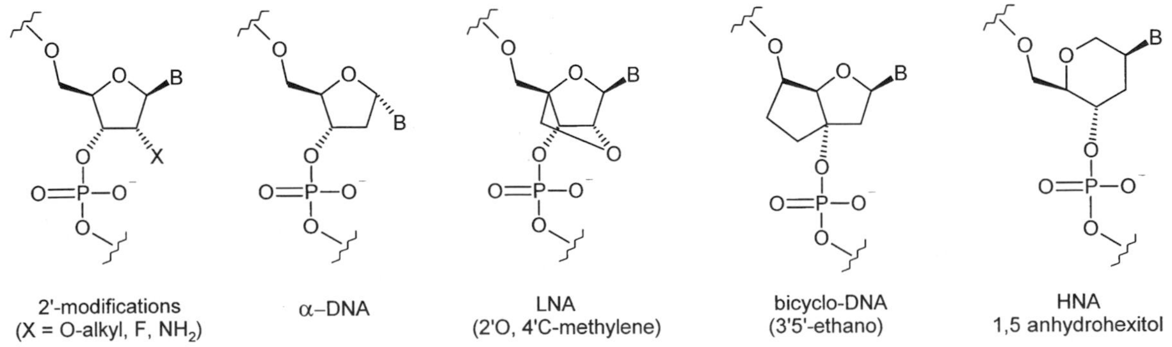

| 2′-modifications (X = O-alkyl, F, NH$_2$) | α–DNA | LNA (2′O, 4′C-methylene) | bicyclo-DNA (3′5′-ethano) | HNA 1,5 anhydrohexitol |

FIGURE 7 Examples of sugar modifications.

destabilizes the duplex with RNA, presumably due to electrostatic interactions between the 2′ amino group and the negatively charged phosphodiester function.

Surprisingly, the nuclease resistance was not increased over parent DNA with uniformly modified 2′-fluoro-oligonucleotides. It seems that the greater the bulk emanating from the 2′ position, the greater the gain in nuclease resistance (2′-O-methyl<2′-O-propyl·2′-O-pentyl). The 2′-O-(2-methoxyethyl) and 2′-O-(3-aminopropyl) derivatives are especially interesting because of both increased duplex stability and their superior nuclease resistance.

In all 2′ modifications, a uniform replacement throughout the oligonucleotide leads to the loss of RNase H activation, therefore these analogs have been used in chimeric oligonucleotides in combination with oligonucleotide portions that activate RNase H. Most interestingly, 2′-O-alkyl-modified antisense oligonucleotides have shown promising results in bioavailability studies after oral administration. 2′-O-alkyl modifications clearly play a big role in a newer generation of antisense oligonucleotides.

B. Conformationally Preorganized Nucleic Acids

Preorganization of the oligonucleotide in the A-form conformation (C-3′ endo) results in a lower entropy penalty upon duplex formation with target RNA. This led to the development of oligonucleotides with a conformationally restricted sugar phosphate backbone. Locked nucleic acid (LNA) is built up of monomers, where the 2′ oxygen is linked by a methylene bridge to the 4′ carbon forming a bicyclo[2.2.1]nucleoside, which are locked into a 3′-endo conformation (Fig. 7). LNA oligomers form complexes with complementary DNA or RNA with considerably higher affinity (+3 to +8 K per modification in mixed sequences) compared to their parent compounds. A somewhat similar approach uses "bicyclo nucleic acids," built up from monomer units containing a bicyclic sugar moiety (3′S,5′R)-2′-deoxy-3′,5′-ethano-β-D-ribofuranose, which have a preference for the 2′-endo conformation, which results in more stable duplexes with target DNA than their natural congeners. Yet another class of conformationally restricted analogs of RNA are the 1,5-an-

hydro-2-deoxy-D-altritol oligonucleotides (HNA). The six-membered hexitol ring can be considered as a mimic of furanose frozen in the 2′-exo-3′-endo conformation, again resulting in high duplex stability with complementary DNA (1.3 K per modification) or RNA (3.0 K per modification). All these analogs, LNA, HNA, and bicyclo-DNA, are resistant to 3′-exonuclease degradation.

C. α-Anomeric Oligonucleotides

α-Anomeric oligonucleotides (α-anomeric glycosylic bond) exhibit excellent hybridization properties. In some cases, the melting temperature of a duplex with RNA is almost doubled compared to β-anomeric oligonucleotides. This effect can be explained by the fact that the hybridization of α-oligonucleotides and β-DNA results in a parallel arrangement of the strands, whereas the natural double helix consists of antiparallel strands. Despite excellent binding properties and high nuclease resistance, α-anomeric oligonucleotides are usually not very efficient in antisense experiments, especially if they are directed against the coding part of the target mRNA. Because they lack the ability to activate RNase H, their mechanism of action is through steric blockage, which becomes efficient if the α-anomeric oligonucleotide is directed against the 5′-nontranslated mRNA region.

VII. MODIFICATION OF NUCLEOBASES

The chemical modification of heterocyclic nucleobases (Fig. 8) allows the modulation of binding affinity and molecular recognition properties, hence sequence specificity. For pyrimidines bases, the substitution of C5 with propynyl or hexynyl significantly enhances sequence specificity and binding affinity in the order of 1.5 K per modification. This can be explained by increased stacking interactions. Incorporation of 5-(1-propargylamino)-substituted pyrimidines into oligonucleotides enhances duplex stability even more as a result of the shielding of the negative charge/charge interactions in the duplex. Short oligonucleotides containing phenoxazine-type bases were found to penetrate cellular membranes. In-

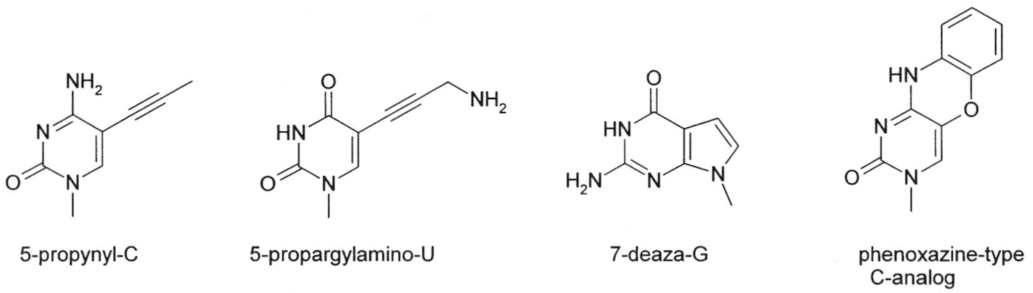

5-propynyl-C   5-propargylamino-U   7-deaza-G   phenoxazine-type C-analog

FIGURE 8 Examples of modifications of heterocyclic nucleobases.

terestingly, the ability to activate RNase H is retained in C5-alkynyl or phenoxazine-like cytosine-modified oligonucleotides. Duplex stabilizing effects have also been observed with the 7-propynyl-7-deaza purine modification. The use of 7-deaza modification in guanine is interesting for an additional reason: it retains Watson–Crick base pairing but prevents Hoogsteen base pairing and therefore prevents tetrad formation in GGGG motifs which may cause secondary structure formation and nonantisense effects. Imidazole-4-carboxamide can serve as a general base analog that may be introduced in place of all four natural bases without significant loss in duplex stability.

VIII. OLIGONUCLEOTIDE CONJUGATES

One of the simplest and most convenient methods to modify the properties of antisense oligonucleotides is the covalent attachment of nonnucleosidic molecules to 3′ or 5′ ends of the oligomers. Depending on the choice of conjugate and its point of attachment, it is possible to influence the stability, transport, cellular uptake, and hybridization properties of the oligonucleotide. In general, conjugates confer extra nuclease stability on the conjugate by hindering exonuclease digestion. In this context, 3′-end conjugates are especially desirable, as 3′-exonucleases predominate in human serum.

The attachment of conjugate molecules to the 5′ end of oligonucleotides is usually carried out in one of two ways: the reaction of a phosphoramidite or H-phosphonate derivative of the conjugate with the 5′ terminus of the oligomer during solid-phase synthesis

or the reaction of suitably activated conjugate molecules, such as active esters or iodo-acetamides, with 5′-amino- or mercapto-derivatized oligonucleotides in solution. A broad range of suitable derivatives of conjugate molecules, such as fluorescein, biotin, cholesterol, and dinitrophenyl, are commercially available for 5′ conjugation.

The most convenient method for the attachment of conjugates to the 3′ end of an oligonucleotide is to carry out solid-phase synthesis of the oligonucleotide on a solid support suitably derivatized with the conjugate molecule. Alternatively, the conjugation reaction can be carried out postsynthetically in solution, analogously to the method described earlier for 5′ conjugation.

A great deal of work in the area of oligonucleotide conjugates has been devoted to improving the cellular uptake of oligonucleotides. In this context, a wide variety of lipophilic molecules have been used as conjugates. For example, it has been demonstrated that attachment of cholesterol to oligonucleotides increases their cell association and uptake. In addition, the nuclear localization of cholesteryl oligonucleotides is increased compared to unconjugated oligonucleotides of the same sequence. Vitamin E and polyalkyl chains of various lengths have also been attached to oligonucleotides at both 3′ and 5′ ends, and in many cases, higher cellular association and uptake have been reported for these conjugates. It should be mentioned, however, that highly lipophilic moieties, such as cholesterol, can also interact strongly with cellular membranes, which often leads to complications in the interpretation of results from antisense experiments utilizing lipophilic oligonucleotide conjugates.

Intercalating agents, such as acridines, have been conjugated to oligonucleotides to enhance their duplex stability on binding to their target sequence, as well as cross-linking reagents, such as (2-chloroethyl)-amino groups and psoralen, which bind permanently to the target sequence. Nonspecific nucleic acid-cleaving molecules can be rendered sequence specific by covalently attaching them to oligonucleotides. Duplex formation of the oligonucleotide conjugate with its target sequence results in cleavage of the target adjacent to the site of hybridization. Most of these artificial endonucleases are metal complexes, such as texaphyrin/Europium, o-phenanthroline/Cu, EDTA/Fe, bleomycin/Fe, and bipyridinyl/Cu. This class of oligonucleotide conjugates is useful as a tool for probing oligonucleotide interactions *in vitro*.

More recently, oligonucleotides and PNA, conjugated to nuclear localization peptide sequences, have been synthesized, with the aim of influencing cellular uptake and intracellular distribution of oligonucleotides.

IX. DESIGN CONSIDERATIONS FOR ANTISENSE OLIGONUCLEOTIDES

The correct design of antisense oligonucleotides raises questions such as what is the optimal length of antisense oligonucleotides to achieve high inhibition of protein synthesis? What is the best chemistry to be used for the oligonucleotides in antisense experiments? Which chemical modifications can improve the cellular uptake of oligonucleotides by living cells? Are oligonucleotide derivatives that induce RNase H cleavage of the target mRNA after binding to RNA preferred over those derivatives that cannot stimulate RNase H? Unfortunately, there is no general answer to these questions, as many of these factors depend on each other and also on the biological assay system in which they are used. However, the following section discusses the different design considerations that may help in appropriately designing the antisense oligonucleotides for specific needs.

A. Oligonucleotide Length

The optimal length of an antisense oligomer depends on its chemical structure, which determines its bind-

ing affinity, but also on statistical considerations, as well as on the purpose of the experiment. A 17-mer base sequence appears statistically only once in the whole human genome. In the case of all-phosphorothioate oligonucleotides, even longer oligomers may be preferred to increase binding affinity, leading to stronger inhibition of protein biosynthesis. However, the longer the phosphorothioate, the higher the probability of undesired nonantisense effects. In the case of all-phosphorothioates, oligomers of 15 to 20 bases in length appear to work in many experiments. Under circumstances where point mutations (e.g., wild type vs mutant) must be discriminated, shorter oligomers will be more specific antisense agents. In general, the shorter the antisense oligonucleotide, the larger the difference in binding affinity for a single base mismatch. Especially for high-affinity oligomers, such as PNA or LNA, the optimal length may well be in the range of 12 to 14 bases. Considering that not all genes are expressed at the same time and that not all regions on the mRNA are really accessible due to its secondary structure, this length may provide both high specificity regarding base mismatches and sufficient selectivity regarding statistical limitations.

B. Critical Sequence Motifs

Phosphorothioate oligonucleotides containing CpG motifs have been found to have immunostimulatory activity by inducing certain cytokines. While this phenomenon can potentially be exploited for cancer therapy, it may not be desirable for other indications. In animal experiments, especially in rodents, the nonantisense effects caused by the CpG motif may lead to misinterpretation of the results. However, immune stimulation could be markedly decreased with oligonucleotides containing 5-methyl cytosine and further decreased by 2'-modification. Oligonucleotides containing four or more consecutive G nucleotides can form tetrameric structures, called G tetrads. These G tetrads were reported to cause nonantisense effects in cell-based assay systems by interacting with various proteins. Finally, certain sequence motifs can lead to secondary structures, which can obscure antisense activity by unintended binding of the oligonucleotide to proteins. While CpG and G tetrad effects can be suppressed by appropriate chemical modification, secondary structure folds can be circumvented only by selecting different target sequences.

C. Influence of Chemical Modification on the Mechanism of Action

1. Induction of RNase H

RNase H is an ubiquitous cellular ribonuclease that recognizes a DNA · RNA duplex and degrades the RNA strand of this duplex. Most modifications of the DNA part (oligodeoxynucleotide) influence the competency for RNase H stimulation. Backbone chemistries known today to support RNase H cleavage include phosphodiesters, phosphorothioates, phosphorodithioates, and boranophosphates. Although uniformly N3′ → P5′ phosphoramidate-modified oligonucleotide analogs do not support RNase H cleavage, the duplex formed by the anionic alternating N3′ → P5′ phosphoramidate-phosphodiester oligothymidylate and poly(A) was a good substrate for RNase H. Sugar chemistries known to support RNase H cleavage are natural β-D-deoxyribose, β-D-arabinose, and 2′-fluoro-β-D-arabinose.

2. Steric Blocking

RNase H-incompetent oligonucleotide analogs, such as methylphosphonates, PNA, morpholino oligomers, and 2′-O-alkyl oligoribonucleotides, are thought to work by a steric blocking mechanism, also referred to as an "occupancy only" mediated mechanism. In a pharmacological sense, the RNAse H-incompetent oligonucleotide analog binds as a competitive antagonist to the target RNA (receptor), thereby preventing the binding of natural effector molecules. When the RNase H-incompetent oligomer is targeted downstream of the AUG translational start signal, it is usually a poor antisense inhibitor of translation. However, RNase H-independent antisense oligomers can efficiently inhibit translation through a steric blocking mechanism when targeted against sequences in the mRNA region between the 5′ cap and the AUG start site. By directing oligonucleotide derivatives, which do not induce RNA cleavage, to regions of the pre-mRNA involved in the splicing, it is possible to correct aberrant splicing for certain human diseases. In order to allow inhibition of splicing of the pre-mRNA by antisense oligonucleotides, RNase H-incompetent oligomers, such as uniformly 2′-O-methyl-modified oligomers or PNA, must be used. Consequently, the chemical structure of an antisense oligonucleotide and the selection of its target sequence have to be coordinated to obtain optimal inhibition results.

3. Induction of RNase L

Another possibility for sequence-specific cleavage of RNA makes use of the ability of 2′5′-linked oligoadenylates, covalently bound to antisense oligonucleotides, to stimulate cellular ribonuclease L. However, in early studies, the antisense oligonucleotide part of these chimeras was modified as a phosphodiester or phosphorothioate oligodeoxynucleotide, which would also stimulate RNase H. Therefore, chimeric molecules composed of 2′-O-methylribonucleotides or PNA and 2′5′-tetraadenylate were synthesized that induce RNase L, but not RNase H.

D. Chimeric Oligonucleotide Analogs

At present, oligonucleotides with a uniformly phosphorothioate-modified backbone (all-phosphorothioates) are the best investigated and most widely used type of antisense agents, and most oligonucleotides in clinical trials are all-phosphorothioates. The side effects observed for all-phosphorothioates can be ascribed primarily to three different causes. First, they have a tendency for nonantisense effects, which are mainly due to undesired binding to proteins. Second, the activation of RNase H by partial oligonucleotide/RNA duplices of only five to seven nucleotides in length can cause nonspecific degradation of mRNA under certain conditions. Third, certain sequence motifs, such as CpG, are responsible for sequence-specific side effects, which can be potentiated by additional phosphorothioate modification. In principle, these limitations may at least be partly overcome by reducing the number of phosphorothioate linkages in the oligomers or by introducing secondary modifications. In case of the CpG motif, substitution of 2′-O-methylribonucleosides for CpG deoxynucleotides could minimize the undesired immunostimulatory effect of all-phosphorothioates.

After a number of different chemical structures introduced as uniform modification into oligonucleotides, it appears that none of the individual structures can fulfill the requirements of an optimal antisense agent. Therefore, various mixed backbone oligonucleotides, gap mers, or chimeric oligomers, in which the advantages of individual structural elements are combined, have been developed in recent years. The so-called gap mers consist of RNase H-incompetent 2′-O-methylribonucleotide wings, which enhance binding to RNA, while a window of six to eight deoxynucleotides limits recognition by RNase H cleavage to this part of the duplex. A typical mixed backbone oligonucleotide (MBO) consists of methylphosphonate and phosphorothioate backbone units, with the former providing excellent nuclease resistance and nonionic nature, while the phosphorothioate window allows activation of RNase H. The most important finding of recent antisense oligonucleotide research is, however, that MBOs or gap mers showed biological activity after oral administration to mice. An 18-mer phosphorothioate oligonucleotide, in which four deoxynucleotides at both 3′ and 5′ ends were substituted by 2′-O-methylribonucleotides, accumulated in tumor tissue after oral administration to mice and showed dose-dependent *in vivo* antitumor activity in SCID mice bearing xenografts of human cancers of the colon, breast, and lung after ip and oral administration (at 1 to 10 mg / kg).

Although PNA is extremely stable during incubation in serum and binds strongly to RNA, it does not stimulate RNase H in a duplex with RNA. In contrast, 5′-DNA–PNA (pseudo-3′) chimeras with more than four deoxynucleotides at the 5′ part of the oligomer can induce RNase H, show favorable solubility, and are completely resistant to 3′-exonucleases.

In minimally phosphorothioate modified oligonucleotides, the chemical modification is restricted to those parts of the oligomers critical to nuclease degradation. Unmodified oligodeoxynucleotides are degraded in serum by exo- and endonucleases, whereby the major degrading activity is a 3′-exonuclease. Therefore, capping of the 3′ end, or both 3′ and 5′ ends, by phosphorothioate linkages can significantly protect the oligonucleotide against 3′-exonuclease. However, these end-capped oligonucleotides are still subject to endonuclease degradation, thus limiting the successful use of this protection scheme. More promising is the "minimal protection" strategy, which is a combination of the end-capping technique and the protection

at internal pyrimidine residues, which are the major sites of endonuclease degradation. These minimally phosphorothioate-modified oligonucleotides turned out to be particularly useful, as they are sufficiently stable to exo- and endonucleases, while at the same time undesirable nonantisense effects are strongly suppressed. Furthermore, the minimal protection scheme can be easily combined with other secondary modifications, such as 2′-O-alkyl modification of ribose or C5-alkynyl modification of the pyrimidine bases, to enhance binding affinity and consequently the potency in antisense inhibition experiments.

See Also the Following Articles

ANTISENSE NUCLEIC ACIDS: CLINICAL APPLICATIONS • ANTISENSE: PROGRESS TOWARD GENE-DIRECTED CANCER THERAPY • RIBOZYMES AND THEIR APPLICATIONS

Bibliography

Agrawal, S. (1999). Importance of nucleotide sequence and chemical modifications of antisense oligonucleotides. *Biochim. Biophys. Acta* **1489**, 53–67.

Agrawal, S., and Zhao, Q. (1998). Mixed backbone oligonucleotides: Improvement in oligonucleotide-induced toxicity in vivo. *Antisense Nucleic Acid Drug Dev.* **8**, 135–139.

Cohen, J. S. (ed.) (1989). "Oligodeoxynucleotides: Antisense Inhibitors of Gene Expression." CRC Press, Boca Raton, FL.

Cook, P. D. (1998). Antisense medicinal chemistry. *Handb. Exp. Pharmacol.* **131**, 51–101.

Crooke, S. T. (1998). Basic principles of antisense therapeutics. *Handb. Exp. Pharmacol.* **131**, 1–50.

Freier, S. M., and Altmann, K.-H. (1997). The ups and downs of nucleic acid duplex stability: Structure-stability studies on chemically-modified DNA:RNA duplexes. *Nucleic Acids Res.* **25**, 4429–4443.

Herdewijn, P. (1999). Conformationally restricted carbohydrate-modified nucleic acids and antisense technology. *Biochim. Biophys. Acta* **1489**, 167–179.

Hyrup, B., and Nielsen, P. E. (1996). Peptide nucleic acids (PNA): Synthesis, properties and potential applications. *Bioorg. Med. Chem.* **4**, 5–23.

Iyer, R. P., Roland, A., Zhou, W., and Gosh, K. (1999). Modified oligonucleotides: Synthesis, properties and applications. *Curr. Opin. Mol. Ther.* **1**, 344–358.

Manoharan, M. (1999). 2′-Carbohydrate modifications in antisense oligonucleotide therapy: Importance of conformation, configuration and conjugation. *Biochim. Biophys. Acta* **1489**, 117–130.

Miller, P. S., and Ts'o, P. O. P. (1987). A new approach to

chemotherapy based on molecular biology and nucleic acid chemistry: Matagen (masking tape for gene expression). *Anti Cancer Drug Des.* **2,** 117–128.

Milligan, J. F., Jones, R. J., Froehler, B. C., and Matteucci, M. D. (1994). Development of antisense therapeutics: Implications for cancer gene therapy. *Ann. N. Y. Acad. Sci.*

Neckers, L., Whitesell, L., Rosolen, A., and Geselowitz, D. A. (1992). Antisense inhibition of oncogene expression. *Crit. Rev. Oncog.* **3,** 175–231.

Summerton, J. (1999). Morpholino antisense oligomers: The case for an RNase H-independent structural type. *Biochim. Biophys. Acta* **1489,** 141–158.

Taylor, J. K., and Dean, N. M. (1999). Regulation of pre-mRNA splicing by antisense oligonucleotides. *Curr. Opin. Drug Disc. Dev.* **2,** 147–151.

Uhlmann, E., and Peyman, A. (1990). Antisense oligonucleotides: A new therapeutic principle. *Chem. Rev.* **90,** 543–584.

Uhlmann, E., and Peyman, A. (1993). Oligonucleotide analogs containing dephospho-internucleoside linkages. *In* "Methods in Molecular Biology" S. Agrawal, (ed.), Vol. 20, pp. 355–389. Humana Press.

Uhlmann, E., Peyman, A., Breipohl, G., and Will, D. W. (1998). PNA: Synthetic polyamide nucleic acids with unusual binding properties. *Angew. Chem. Int. Ed.* **37,** 2796–2823.

Uhlmann, E. (2000). Recent advances in the medicinal chemistry of antisense oligonucleotides. *Curr. Opin. Drug. Disc. Dev.* **3.**

Verma, S., and Eckstein, F. (1998). Modified oligonucleotides: Synthesis and strategy for users. *Annu. Rev. Biochem* **67,** 99–134.

Wahlestedt, C., and Good, L. (1999). Antisense oligonucleotides: The way forward. *Curr. Opin. Drug Disc. Dev.* **2,** 142–146.

Wengel, J., Koshkin, A., Singh, S. K., Nielsen, P., Meldgaard, M., Rajwanshi, V. K., Kumar, R., Skouv, J., Nielsen, C. B., Jacobsen, J. P., Jacobsen, N., and Olsen, C. E. (1999). LNA (locked nucleic acid). *Nucleosides Nucleotides* **18,** 1365–1370.

Zamecnik, P. C., and Stephenson, M. L. (1978). Inhibition of Rous sarcoma virus replication and cell transformation by a specific oligodeoxynucleotide. *Proc. Natl. Acad. Sci. USA* **75,** 280–284.

Antisense Nucleic Acids: Clinical Applications

Georg Aue
Alan M. Gewirtz
University of Pennsylvania School of Medicine

GLOSSARY

antisense oligonucleotide Short sequences of nucleotides that are complementary to a sequence of targeted mRNA.
DNAzyme An RNA-cleaving DNA enzyme.
hairpin ribozyme Hairpin-shaped ribozyme.
hammerhead ribozyme Hammer-shaped ribozyme.
ribozyme RNA molecules with enzymatic strand-cleaving activity.

This article reviews the main approaches being used for clinically motivated gene squelching, discusses issues that remain to be solved before this approach can be widely applied, and, finally, reviews clinical trial data, which have already begun to accumulate.

I. INTRODUCTION

With their promise of high specificity and low toxicity, many believe that gene-targeted therapies will lead to a revolution in cancer therapeutics. Numerous gene therapy strategies are under development, one of which employs reverse complementary (antisense) nucleic acids to inhibit gene expression at the mRNA level. Simply stated, delivering an antisense nucleic acid into a cell where the gene of interest is expressed should lead to hybridization between the antisense sequence and the mRNA of the targeted gene. Stable mRNA–antisense duplexes cannot be translated and, depending on the chemical composition of the antisense molecule, can lead to the destruction of the mRNA by binding of endogenous nucleases, such as RNase H, or by intrinsic enzymatic activity engineered into the sequence. Although conceptually elegant, the utility of this approach for treating human malignancies remains unproven.

II. ANTISENSE STRATEGIES

A. Antisense Oligonucleotides (AS-ON)

AS-ONs are short sequences of nucleotides that are complementary to a sequence of targeted mRNA. Traditionally, this gene inhibition strategy has been designated "antisense" because of its reliance on the formation of reverse complementary (antisense) Watson–Crick base pairs between the targeted construct and the mRNA whose function is to be disrupted. The oligonucleotide strategy relies on either introducing the reverse complementary nucleic acid sequence to the target cell or by expressing the reverse complementary sequence in the target cell. Either DNA or RNA can be the reverse complement. Expressed nucleotides are made by one of the expression vectors used for gene therapy, such as an adenoviral, retroviral, or plasmid vector. This process can occur at any point between the conclusion of transcription and initiation of translation, or even possibly during translation. There are several possible mechanisms, including disruption of splicing, transport, or translation of the transcripts. Binding subsequently results in double helix formation. When hybridization between the target mRNA and the antisense oligonucleotide occurs, a duplex is created. This duplex prevents the ribosomal complex from completing the process of translation. Eventually it means that the appropriate tRNA cannot be assembled and the encoded peptide is not produced. Although theoretically appealing, the antisense approach is presently encumbered by a number of issues of efficacy and safety. Antisense oligonucleotides or modified antisense oligonucleotides are used for *in vivo* antisense applications because they have shown increased stability and nuclease resistance. This results in a longer serum half-life and allows the AS-ON to have more ample time to reach and interact with its target mRNA. Many oligonucleotides support the binding of RNase H at sites of RNA–DNA duplex formation. RNase H, a ubiquitous nuclear enzyme, is thought to be critical for antisense effectiveness because it functions as an endonuclease that recognizes and cleaves the RNA in the duplex. Studies seem to demonstrate that RNase H-dependent antisense effects are a nuclear event prior splicing, whereas RNase H-dependent oligonucleotides may affect splicing in transcript processing or may suppress gene expression after splicing has taken place. There is further evidence that in the absence of RNase H activity, antisense effects may be the result of interference with a certain type of translational initiation complex formation.

B. Ribozymes

Ribozymes are RNA molecules with enzymatic strand-cleaving activity. Their clinical potential is theoretically huge because of their ability to either cleave deleterious RNAs or repair mutant cellular RNAs. They form base pair-specific complexes with their target RNA molecule and catalyze the subsequent hydrolysis of the normally unreactive phosphodiester bonds that link the nucleotides in RNA. This results in strand cleavage of the target RNA, rendering it useless as a template for protein translation. Ribozymes can subsequently go on to ligate a new sequence of RNA to one of the cleavage products. Naturally occurring ribozymes have been used both to downregulate and to repair pathologic genes targeting mRNA. In comparison to RNase H-mediated antisense oligonucleotide degradation of transcripts, which relies on trimolecular kinetics, ribozymes should in theory increase transcript turnover through bimolecular kinetics. Ribozymes are RNase H independent, and the 2' modification improves stability and does not reduce the antisense effect. In comparison to AS-ONs, ribozymes can be expressed from a vector, which favors continuous production of these molecules intracellularly. Current gene therapy applications employ variations on naturally occurring ribozymes, but *in vitro* selection has provided new RNA and DNA catalysts, and research on trans-splicing and RNase P has suggested ways to harness the endogenous ribozymes of the cell for therapeutic purposes. It is thought that ribozymes perform effectively as enzymes. They are required not only to bind to substrate RNA, but also to dissociate from the cleaage product so that additional substrates can bind. Divalent metal ions play a crucial role in catalysis by ribozymes. There are reports that ribozymes require

Mg^{2+} to fold into their native structures. The hammerhead ribozyme and the hairpin ribozyme have drawn much research interest due to their rapid kinetics and size.

C. Hammerhead Ribozymes

Hammerhead ribozymes consist of a conserved catalytic core. They have the ability to cleave substrate RNA at NUH triplets 3′ to the H. Basically, N represents any nucleotide, U is uracil, and H represents any nucleotide but guanidine, although studies have shown that RNA may be less selective. The ribozyme will hybridize specifically to the RNA of interest by creating complementary sequences in the arms to sequences flanking the cleavage site. Subsequent cleavage will be directed at that targeted position. Critically important to hammerhead ribozymes are divalent metal ions such as magnesium. It is thought that the ions participate in the RNA unfolding and in the cleavage step itself. However, the Mg^{2+} requirement for *in vivo* studies usually exceed normal cell content by 5- to 10-fold. Therefore, there is some doubt regarding the application of hammerhead ribozymes to *in vivo* conditions.

D. Hairpin Ribozymes

Hairpin ribozymes basically consist of two domains connected by a hinge section (Fig. 1). One of the domains binds the substrate RNA to create two helical regions separated by a single-stranded loop. Cleavage occurs

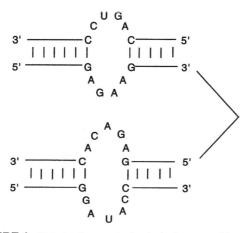

FIGURE 1 Hairpin ribozyme in the docked position: The two loop regions bind with each other in order to cleave the substrate RNA. Arrow indicates position of cleavage. Adapted from [3].

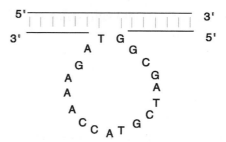

FIGURE 2 DNAzyme. Adapted from [4].

within the single-stranded area of the substrate RNA. The second domain is structured similarly, although the helices are formed by the ribozyme itself. The single-stranded region is the most important sequence for cleavage activity, whereas the helical portions can be almost any sequence as long as they form a double helix. The hinge acts like a joint mechanism and allows the two domains to be flexible to one another in space. It also allows the two domains to dock in an antiparallel orientation required for cleavagecatalysis.

E. DNAzymes

DNAzymes are essentially RNA-cleaving DNA enzymes. The structure of a DNAzyme consists of a catalytic domain of 15 deoxynucleotides and two substrate recognition domains of 8 nucleotides each (Fig. 2). The substrate recognition domains contain the necessary nucleotide sequence for specific binding to the RNA substrate. By composing the appropriate recognition domain sequences, it is possible to create DNAzymes that are able to cleave any RNA that contains a purine–pyrimidine junction. DNAzymes have two advantages over ribozymes: stability secondary to containing DNA instead of RNA and an inexpensive cost of production. However, DNAzymes must be proven to be able to achieve stable, efficient intracellular concentrations without toxicity and to perform targeted RNA cleavage. They must also have the ability to target the cell and cellular compartment of interest, as well as the ability to hybridize with the mRNA target *in vivo*.

III. ANTISENSE TARGETS

There are several main areas of interest in which antisense strategies are being investigated. Many of these strategies have important implications with respect to hematological disorders. Currently, application of the antisense approach to oncogenes is of intense interest. Various fusion genes associated with hematological malignancies have been studied. One of the best studied is the bcr/abl fusion mRNA from the Philadelphia chromosome [t(9:22) of chronic myelogenous leukaemia]. Anti-bcr/abl ribozymes in cell lines have been observed to produce effects such as decreases in bcr/abl mRNA and protein, kinase activity, and cell proliferation. Antisense research applied to oncogenes such as C-myb were carried out and led to clinical trials. The bcl 2 antisense oligonucleotide has drawn much attention. Involved in apoptosis, the bcl 2 protein and other cleavage substrates seem to mark one of the final steps of the apoptosis cascade. There is potential for application of antisense therapeutics in overcoming drug resistance. Several groups have investigated the resistance of tumor cells to chemotherapeutic drugs, a major limitation in cancer treatment. While many tumours are intrinsically resistant, others acquire resistance and eventually become increasingly unresponsive, not only to the initial drug, but also to other drugs to which the tumor has never been exposed. There is a paucity of information explaining this phenomenon; however, one interesting observation has been the increased expression of P-glycoprotein from the multidrug-resistant (or MDR 1) gene. Diseases that are results of viral infection provide other suitable targets for antisense methodology. The viral RNA sequences are unique to the infected cells and this provides an ideal target. Several viruses have been studied, mainly with hairpin ribozymes and hammerhead ribozymes, but also with oligonucleotides. Currently, HIV draws the most attention as a potential antisense target. Sickle cell disease is the most common heritable hematological disease. It was demonstrated that the region in the β-globin mRNA containing the sickle cell anemia mutation can be replaced with a γ-globin encoding sequence by the use of a trans-splicing group 1 ribozyme.

IV. PROBLEM SOLVING BEFORE CREATING ANTISENSE DRUGS

Although the antisense strategy is theoretically appealing, there are as yet several unresolved issues of efficacy and safety. For one, a variety of repair and editing enzymes, such as RNA unwindase and helicase, as well as the ribosomal complex itself, are able to unwind the RNA/DNA complex. Moreover, there remains difficulty in directing oligonucleotides within the body. Two additional problems include the large doses required for a therapeutic response, as well as the need for parenteral administration. Therefore, considerations, including mRNA site selection, drug delivery, and intracellular localization of the antisense agent, are important for the future development of an antisense drug.

In living cells, mRNA is usually folded to keep the transcript in a low-energy conformation. Therefore, most of the mRNA sequence is not accessible for hybridization and for potential mRNA targeting. A system for ribozyme targeting has been established to locate the accessibility of sequences within the transcript. Another approach to this problem is the utilization of a "molecular beacon." In this approach, molecules loaded with oligonucleotides are stem–loop shaped. The loop is the antisense to the targeted transcript. The second problem to overcome is the appropriate delivery of AS-ODN and ribozymes. The cellular uptake of naked oligonucleotides is poor and usually requires a vehicle for efficient delivery. A concept for delivery vehicles has been developed. Basically, through electrostatic interactions, a complex between negatively charged oligonucleotide phosphate groups and positively charged delivery vehicles is formed. Delivery vehicles such as cationic liposomes, fusogenic peptides, cationic porphyrins, and artificial virosomes have been tested. However, none of the delivery vehicles have been shown to be efficient in animal studies.

The mRNA can exist in cellular compartments such as the cytoplasm, nucleus, or nucleolus. To date it remains unclear where the AS-ON should target the mRNA. It also remains unclear in what cellular compartment the most antisense effect can be found. However, the location site might also depend on the type of AS-ON and its degradation. It appears that AS-ONs are inefficient when targets are located in the endosomes.

Although issues concerning the targets mentioned earlier could be addressed, problems remain with the antisense drug design itself. The chirality of the modified oligonucleotide and the formation of g quartets are some of the problems on which research studies are currently being performed.

V. CLINICAL TRIALS

Several oligonucleotide clinical trials have been published (Table I). This section discusses these trials.

In 1996, Bishop tested an antisense oligonucleotide against the phosphoprotein P53. Sixteen patients with either refractory acute myelogenous leukemia or advanced myelodysplastic syndrome participated in this phase 1 trial. None of the patients achieved complete remission. Apparently, toxicity was not directly related to the antisense drug.

In another study, Cunningham and colleagues utilized an ON for c-raf. Raf proteins play a central role in the mitogen-activated protein kinase signaling pathway and hence are involved in oncogenic transformation and tumor cell proliferation. ISIS 5132 is a 20 base antisense phosphorothioate oligodeoxyribonucleotide that specifically downregulates c-raf expression. Altogether 34 patients with a variety of solid tumors were treated. Two patients had prolonged stabilization of their disease, and one patient with ovarian carcinoma had a significant response with a 97% reduction in CA-125 levels. ISIS 5132 demonstrated antitumor activity at the doses tested. Side effects were minimal and could not be specifically related to ISIS 5132, according to the authors.

Advani and colleagues performed a phase 1 trial using an antisense oligonucleotide targeting protein kinase C α (ISIS 3521). It is believed that overexpression of protein kinase C α, a cytoplasmatic serine/threonine kinase involved in signal transduction, may promote the development of tumors. In this trial, ISIS 3521 was administered by continuous infusion. Out of 11 patients with progressive cancer who were treated, only one had stable disease for more than 3 months. Side effects included fever, chills, and hemorrhage, as well as flu-like symptoms.

The antisense oligonucleotide targeting protein kinase A (GEM231) was studied by Chen and co-workers in 1999. In this phase 1 trial studying a variety of refractory tumors, only 1 out of 13 patients with colon cancer had a slight decrease in a previously rising CEA level after 8 weeks of treatment. Overall the antisense drug was well tolerated: fever and flu-like symp-

toms occurred, as well as a prolonged partial thromboplastin time (PTT) and temporary liver enzyme elevation in 1 patient.

De Smet and colleagues presented a trial using Fomivirsen, a 21 nucleotide phosphorothioate oligonucleotide that is able to target the major immediate region (IE2) of cytomegaly virus (CMV). When injected into the human eye, it was assumed that Fomivirsen would be capable of inhibiting CMV from promoting CMV retinitis. In a clinical trial of patients with newly diagnosed CMV retinitis, time to progression was significantly delayed to 71 days in those who received Fomivirsen. De Smet and co-workers concluded that the time to progression was comparable with DNA polymerase inhibitors, such as IV gancyclovir or foscavir. Fomivirsen also delayed the progression of disease in patients who had failed other anti-CMV treatments. No systemic absorption of the drug could be detected. Reported adverse events were mild to moderate in intensity and either resolved spontaneously or were treatable with topical medications. Side effects included uveitis, vitritis, an increase in intraocular pressure, and cataracts. Locally administered Fomivirsen appears to effectively inhibit CMV retinitis using a mode of action complementary to existing DNA polymerase inhibitors.

In a patient dose-escalation protocol by Jansen, 14 patients with advanced malignant melanoma were given Augmerosen [BCL2 ASO (Augmerosen, Genasense, G3139)] either alone or plus standard dacarbazine treatment. Six patients had antitumor responses (one complete, two partial, three minor). Pharmacokinetic analysis demonstrated that steady-state plasma levels of G3139 are tolerable and maintained after repeated cycles.

Schreiber and co-workers tested the antisense oligonucleotide ISIS 2302 against the intercellular adhesion molecule 1 (ICAM 1) in patients with steroid refractory Crohn's disease. The trial did not prove clinical efficacy of ISIS 2302 based on the primary end point of the trial, i.e., no steroid treatment at week 14, and a Crohn's disease activity index less 150. However, positive trends were observed at the secondary end point at 26 weeks, although these data were not statistically significant. Overall, it was found that ISIS 2302 was safe. Side effects included injection site reaction, headache, pain, fever, rash, and flu-like symptoms. At this time of this publication, a

TABLE I

Antisense Oligonucleotide Trials

Target	Compound	Cancer	Additional chemo	No Pt phase	Toxicity	Year	Company	Reference	Response
P53		Yes		16	1 hematologic, fever, chills, hepatic, renal	1995	None	Bishop	No complete remission
Protein kinase A	GEM 231	Yes		13	1 fever, flu like symptoms	1999	Hybrion	Chen	1/13 tumor marker decrease
Protein kinase C	ISIS 3521	Yes		11	1 fever, myalgia, headache, thrombocytopenia	1999	ISIS	Advani	1/11 stable disease
RAS	ISIS 2503	Yes			1 fever, chills	1999	ISIS	Gordon	
C-RAF kinase	ISIS 5132	Yes		34	2 LFT, Hematologic toxicity, fever, nausea, weakness	1999	ISIS	Cunningham	6/34 stable disease
IE2	ISIS 2922 Fomivirsen	No/CMV		428	3 Locally applied: Uveitis, Inflammation, Cataract	1999	ISIS	De Smet	56% response
BCL2	G3139/Augmerosen	Yes	Dacarbacin	14	1 LFT, Hematologic toxicity, fever, nausea	2000	Genta	Jansen	6/14 regression or stable
ICAM 1	ISIS 2302	No/Crohn N		75	2 headache, pain, rash flu like symptom	2001	ISIS	Schreiber	Not significant

number of antisense trials in phase 1 and 2 have been reported. All of them so far have shown only a modest or no clinical efficacy. It does appear that antisense ONs have a lack of toxicity. If other problems, such as delivery, mRNA site selection, and localization, as well as drug design problems, can be resolved, the therapeutic potential for antisense drugs may one day be achieved. Despite these obstacles, optimism is high. Formiversen has been approved by the Food and Drug Administration for clinical use in cytomegaly retinitis. It is hoped that approval of additional compounds will be forthcoming in the near future.

See Also the Following Articles

Antisense: Medicinal Chemistry • Antisense: Progress Toward Gene-Directed Cancer Therapy • BCR-ABL • HIV • Multidrug Resistance • Myb • Ribozymes and Their Applications

Bibliography

Advani, R., Fisher, G. A., Grant, P., Yuen, A. R., Holmlund, J. T., Kwoh, T. J., and Dorr, A. (1999). A phase 1 trial of an antisense oligonucleotide targeted to protein kinase c alpha (ISIS 3521) delivered as a 24 hour continuous infusion (CI) *Proc. Am. Soc. Clin. Oncol.* **18,** A609.

Bishop, M. R., Iversen, P. L., Bayever, E., Sharp, G., Greiner, T., Copple, B. L., Ruddon, R., Zon, G., Spinolo, J., Arneson, M., Armitage, J. O., and Kessinger, A. (1996). Phase 1 trial of an antisense oligonucleotide OL (1)p53 in hematologic malignancies. *J. Clin. Oncol.* **14**(4), 1320–1326.

Chen, H., Ness, E., Marshall, J., Martin, R., Dvorchik, B., Rizvl, M., Marquis, J., Dahut, W., and Hawkins, M. (1999).

Phase 1 trial of a second generation oligonucleotide GEM231 targeted at type 1 protein kinase A in patients with refractory solid tumors. *Proc. Am. Soc. Clin. Oncol.* **18,** A610.

Cunningham, C. C., Holmlund, J. T., Schiller, J. H., Geary, R. S., Kwoh, T. J., Dorr, A., and Nemunaitis, J. (2000). *Clin. Cancer Res.* **6**(5), 1607–1610.

de Smet, M. D., Meenken, C. J., and van den Horn, G. J. (1999). *Ocul. Immunol. Inflamm.* **7**(3-4), 189–198.

Earnshaw, D. J., and Gait, M. J. (1997). Progress toward the structure and therapeutic use of the hairpin ribozyme. *Antisense Nucleic Acid Drug Dev.* **7,** 403–411.

Eckstein, F. (1996). The hammerhead ribozyme. *Biochem. Soc. Trans.* **24,** 601–604.

Gewirtz, A. M., Sokol, D. L., and Ratajczak, M. Z. (1998). Nucleic acid therapeutics: State of the art and future prospects. *Blood* **92,** 712–736.

Gordon, M., Sandler, A., Holmlund, J., Dorr, A., Battiato, L., Fife, K., Geary, R., Kwoh, T., and Sledge, G. (1999). A phase 1 trial of ISIS 2503, an antisense inhibitor of H ras, administered by a 24 hour weekly infusion to patients with advanced cancer. *Proc. Am. Soc. Clin. Oncol.* **18,** A604.

Jansen, B., Wacheck, V., Heere-Ress, E., Schlagbauer-Wadl, H., Hoeller, C., Lucas, T., Hoermann, M., Hollenstein, U., Wolff, K., and Pehamberger, H. (2000). *Lancet* **356**(9243), 1728–1733.

Kornblau, S. M., Konopleva, M., and Andreeff, M. (1999). Apoptosis regulating proteins as targets of therapy for hematological malignancies. *Exp. Opin. Invest. Drugs* **8**(12), 2027–2057.

Santoro, S. W., and Joyce, G. F. (1997). A general purpose RNA-cleaving DNA enzyme. *Proc. Natl. Acad. Sci. USA* **94,** 4262–4266.

Schreiber, S., Nikolaus, S., Malchow, H., Kruis, W., Lochs, H., Raedler, A., Hahn, E. G., Krummerl, T., and Steinmann, G. (2001). Absense of effecacy of subcutaneous antisense ICAM1 treatment of chronic active Crohn's disease. *Gastroenterology* **120,** 1339–1346.

Antisense: Progress toward Gene-Directed Cancer Therapy

Stanley T. Crooke

Isis Pharmaceuticals, Inc., Carlsbad, California

Antisense oligonucleotides are used to hybridize to a specific RNA molecule *in vivo* and thereby to inhibit its subsequent use; in most cases, the target RNA is a messenger RNA (mRNA), which cannot then be translated into a protein. Once the gene sequence of interest is known, an antisense oligonucleotide with the complementary sequence can be synthesized. Thus, antisense drugs represent the first class of drugs designed to work by binding to RNA. In fact, antisense technology has unfortunately been lumped together with gene therapy with which it has a few elements in common and should be considered a part of RNA-based drug discovery.

Selection of the sites in an RNA molecule at which optimal antisense activity may be induced is complex, dependent on the terminating mechanism and influenced by the chemical class of the oligonucleotide. Each RNA appears to display a unique pattern of sites of sensitivity. Within the phosphorothioate oligodeoxynucleotide class, studies have shown that antisense activity can vary from undetectable to 100% by shifting an oligonucleotide by just a few bases in the RNA target. Significant progress has been made in developing general rules that help define potentially optimal sites in RNA species, but to a large extent this must be determined empirically for each RNA target and every new chemical class of oligonucleotides.

I. THERAPEUTIC USES

Besides being useful for characterizing the roles of genes, antisense oligonucleotides have the potential for therapeutic use, to regulate the expression of certain genes, or to block an infection by a pathogenic bacterium or virus. The therapeutic use of oligonucleotides represents a new paradigm for drug discovery, as oligonucleotides have not been studied as potential drugs before and they are being used to intervene in processes that have not been considered as sites at which drugs might act. The affinity and the specificity of binding derive from the hybridization of two oligonucleotides and therefore are theoretically much greater than can be achieved with small molecules. Furthermore, the rational design of the nucleotide sequence of antisense oligonucleotide is much more straightforward than the design of small molecules interacting with proteins. Finally, it is possible to consider the design of antisense drugs to treat a very broad range of disorders, including those that are not amenable to other types of treatment.

The use of antisense oligonucleotides is still in its infancy, and the initial enthusiasm must be tempered by appropriate reservations concerning practical aspects. To be useful as a drug, an antisense oligonucleotide must be much more stable than ordinary nucleic acids, and it must be able to reach its desired site of action, the interior of a cell. Questions about the technology include: Can oligonucleotide analogs be created that have appropriate properties to be drugs?

Specifically, what are the pharmacokinetic, pharmacologic, and toxicologic properties of these compounds, and what are the scope and potential of the medicinal chemistry of oligonucleotides? Answers to most of these questions are now available for the phosphorothioate oligonucleotides and a growing number of analogs.

II. MECHANISMS OF ACTION

Figure 1 provides a summary of the mechanisms of action that have been reported for antisense drugs to date. It is helpful to divide the mechanisms into two classes: occupancy only and antisense-mediated cleavage. Antisense drugs may work by binding and obstructing an essential process (occupancy only) or by binding and inducing premature degradation of the target RNA.

Although there are examples of each potential mechanism identified in Fig. 1, RNase H has proven to be the most effective mechanism to date and is the mechanism about which the most is known. RNase H enzymes are a family of double strand RNA-binding

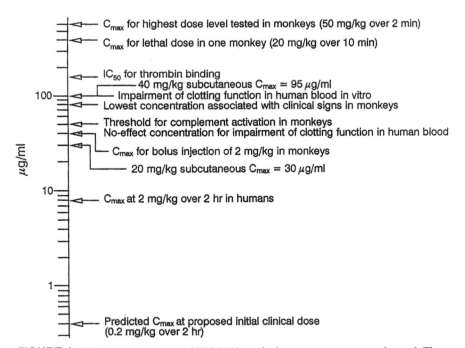

FIGURE 1 Plasma concentrations of ISIS 2302 at which various activities are observed. These concentrations are those of intact ISIS 23902 and were determined by extracting and analyzing plasma by capillary zone electrophoresis.

proteins that also bind to DNA–RNA duplexes and have the RNA in such duplexes. Thus, for any oligonucleotide analog that is DNA-like, these enzymes are involved in the activity of the drugs.

The other mechanisms described in Fig. 1 offer the potential for new chemical classes that take advantage of these mechanisms that to date are minimally studied. To be sure, numerous other mechanisms may be useful and are fruitful areas for future research.

III. PHOSPHOROTHIOATE OLIGODEOXYNUCLEOTIDES

To address the problem of stability, nonconventional oligonucleotides that are not susceptible to degradation or to hydrolysis by nucleases have been designed. Of the first generation of oligonucleotide analogs, the phosphorothioate class is best understood and has produced the broadest range of activities. Phosphorothioate oligonucleotides differ from normal in that one of the nonbridging oxygens in the phosphate group is replaced by a sulfur. The resulting compound is negatively charged, chiral at each phosphorothioate, and much more resistant to nucleases than a phosphodiester oligonucleotide.

A. Hybridization

The hybridization of phosphorothioate oligonucleotides to DNA and RNA has been thoroughly characterized. The melting temperature (T_m) of a phosphorothioate oligodeoxynucleotide bound to RNA is lower than for a corresponding phosphodiester oligodeoxynucleotide by approximately 0.5°C per nucleotide. Compared to RNA duplex formation, a phosphorothioate oligodeoxynucleotide has a T_m approximately 2.2°C lower per nucleotide. This means that to be effective *in vitro*, phosphorothioate oligodeoxynucleotides must be relatively long, typically at least 17 to 20 nucleotides, and invasion of double-stranded regions of the target RNA is difficult.

B. Interactions with Proteins

Phosphorothioate oligonucleotides bind to proteins. These interactions can be (i) nonspecific, (ii) sequence specific, or (iii) structure specific, each of which may have different characteristics and effects. Nonspecific binding to a wide variety of proteins has been demonstrated, most thoroughly with serum albumin. The affinity of such interactions is low; the dissociation constant (K_d) for albumin is approximately 200 μM, about the same as for its binding of aspirin or penicillin. Phosphorothioates also interact with nucleases and DNA polymerases; they are slowly metabolized by both endo- and exonucleases and are competitive inhibitors of these enzymes. When in an RNA–DNA duplex, phosphorothioates are substrates for ribonuclease H. At higher concentrations, phosphorothioates inhibit the enzyme, presumably by binding as a single strand. Again, the oligonucleotides appear to be competitive antagonists for the DNA–RNA substrate.

Phosphorothioates are competitive inhibitors of DNA polymerase α and β with respect to the DNA template and noncompetitive inhibitors of DNA polymerases γ and δ. They are also competitive inhibitors for the reverse transcriptase of HIV and inhibit its associated RNase H activity and human RNase H. Phosphorothioates inhibit various viral polymerases and also cause potent, nonsequence-specific inhibition of RNA splicing.

C. *In Vivo* Pharmacokinetics

Binding of phosphorothioate oligonucleotides to serum albumin and α$_2$-macroglobulin provides a repository for these drugs in the serum and prevents their rapid renal excretion. As serum protein binding is saturable, however, an intact oligomer may be found in urine with high doses, e.g., 15–20 mg/kg^{-1} administered intravenously to rats. Phosphorothioate oligonucleotides are rapidly and extensively absorbed after parenteral administration, as much as 70% within 4 h. Distribution of phosphorothioate oligonucleotides from blood after absorption or intravenous administration is extremely rapid, with distribution half-lives of less than 1 h. Clearance from the blood and plasma exhibits complex kinetics, with a terminal elimination half-life of 40 to 60 h in all species except humans, where it may be somewhat longer. Phosphorothioates distribute broadly to all peripheral tissues, although no evidence for significant penetration of the blood–brain barrier has been reported. Liver, kidney, bone marrow, skeletal muscle, and skin accumulate the highest amounts. Liver accumulates the drug most rapidly (20% of a dose within 1 to 2 h) and also eliminates it most rapidly (e.g., the terminal half-life is 62 and 156 h from liver and renal medulla, respectively). Within the kidney, oligonucleotides are probably filtered by the glomerulus and then reabsorbed by the proximal convoluted tubule epithelial cells, perhaps mediated by interactions with specific proteins in the brush border membranes. At relatively low doses, clearance of phosphorothioate oligonucleotides is due primarily to metabolism, mediated by exo- and endonucleases. Distribution within organs is complex. In the liver, the extent, kinetics, and effects of increasing doses on distribution to hepatocytes, Kupffer cells, and endothelial cells differ, although all three cell types take the drugs up.

D. Pharmacological Activities

Phosphorothioates have also been shown to have effects inconsistent with the antisense mechanism for which they were designed. Some of these effects are sequence or structure specific, whereas others are due to nonspecific interactions with proteins. These effects are particularly prominent in *in vitro* tests for antiviral activity, when high concentrations of cells, viruses, and oligonucleotides are often incubated together. The human immune deficiency virus (HIV) is particularly problematic, as many oligonucleotides bind to the gp120 protein. Moreover, uncertainty as to the mode of action of antisense oligonucleotides is certainly not limited to antiviral or just *in vitro* tests. These observations indicate that, before drawing conclusions, careful analysis of dose–response curves, direct analysis of target protein or RNA, and inclusion of appropriate controls are required. In addition to interactions with proteins, other factors can contribute to unexpected results, such as overrepresented sequences of RNA and unusual structures that may be adopted by oligonucleotides.

A relatively large number of reports of *in vivo* activities of phosphorothioate oligonucleotides have now appeared documenting activities after both local and systemic administration. However, for only a few of these reports have sufficient studies been performed to draw relatively firm conclusions concerning the mechanism of action by directly examining target RNA levels, target protein levels, and pharmacological effects, using a wide range of control oligonucleotides and examination of the effects on closely related isotypes. Thus, there is a growing body of evidence that phosphorothioate oligonucleotides can induce potent systemic and local effects *in vivo*, suggesting highly specific effects that are difficult to explain via any mechanism other than antisense.

E. Toxicological Properties

In rodents, the major adverse event is immune stimulation. In monkeys, sporadic reductions in blood pressure associated with bradycardia are often associated with activation of C-5 complement involving activation of the alternative complement pathway. All phosphorothioate oligonucleotides tested to date appear to induce these effects, although there may be slight variations in potency depending on their sequence and/or length. A second prominent toxicologic effect in the monkey is on blood clotting. The mechanisms responsible for these effects are probably very complex, but preliminary data suggest that direct interactions with thrombin may be at least partially responsible.

In humans, again the toxicological profile differs. When ISIS 2922 is administered intravitreally to patients with cytomegalovirus retinitis, the most common adverse event is anterior chamber inflammation, which is easily managed with steroids. A relatively rare and dose-related adverse event is morphological changes in the retina associated with loss in peripheral vision.

ISIS 2105, a 20-mer phosphorothioate designed to inhibit the replication of human papilloma viruses that cause genital warts, has been administered intradermally at doses as high as 3 mg/wart weekly for 3 weeks. Essentially, no toxicities have been observed. ISIS 2302 (an antisense inhibitor of ICAM) has been administered at doses of 2 mg/kg iv every other day for 1 month, with no significant adverse events, in normal volunteers and in more than 400 patients with various inflammatory diseases. Even higher doses of ISIS 3521 (PKCα inhibitor), ISIS 5132 (C-*raf* kinase inhibitor), and ISIS 2503 (Ha-*ras* inhibitor) have been administered to patients with a variety of malignancies without significant side effects.

F. Therapeutic Index

An attempt to put the toxicities and their dose–response relationships into a therapeutic context is shown in Fig. 2. This is particularly important because considerable confusion has arisen concerning the potential utility of phosphorothioate oligonucleotides for selected therapeutic purposes as a result of unsophisticated interpretation of toxicological data. As can be readily seen, the immune stimulation induced by these compounds appears to be particularly prominent in rodents and unlikely to be dose limiting in humans. Nor have hypotensive events in humans been observed to date; this toxicity appears to occur at lower doses in monkeys than in humans and certainly is not dose limiting in humans. On the basis of present experience, the dose-limiting toxicity in humans will likely result from blood clotting abnormalities, and this will be associated with peak plasma concentrations well in excess of 10 μg/ml. Thus, it would appear that phosphorothioate oligonucleotides have a therapeutic index that supports their evaluation for a number of therapeutic indications.

IV. CLINICAL ACTIVITIES

Significant therapeutic benefit has been reported in patients with cytomegalovirus retinitis treated with fomivirsen locally. Also, ISIS 2302 administered every other day for 1 month resulted in statistically significant improvement for 5 to 6 months in patients with steroid-dependent Crohn's disease in a randomized, double-blind, placebo-controlled trial. Additionally, ISIS 3521, an inhibitor of PKCα, has been reported to be active in patients with ovarian cancer, lymphomas, and non-small cell carcinoma of the lung. ISIS 5132 has been shown to reduce c-*raf* kinase levels in peripheral blood cells and displays suggestions of activity in patients with colon cancer. An inhibitor of BCL-2 has been reported to show activity in patients with non-Hodgkins lymphoma.

V. MEDICINAL CHEMISTRY OF OLIGONUCLEOTIDES

The core of any rational drug discovery program is medicinal chemistry. Although the synthesis of modified nucleic acids has been a subject of interest for some time (see DNA synthesis), the intense focus on

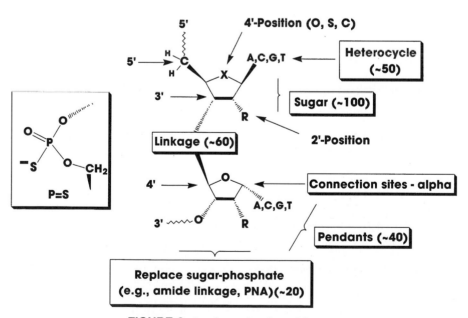

FIGURE 2 Isis oligonucleotide modifications.

the medicinal chemistry of oligonucleotides dates perhaps no more than the past five years. Modifications have been made to the base, sugar, and phosphate moieties of oligonucleotides (Fig. 2). The subjects of medicinal chemical programs include approaches to (i) create enhanced and more selective affinities for RNA or duplex structures, (ii) the ability to cleave nucleic acid targets, (iii) enhanced nuclease stability, (iv) cellular uptake and distribution, and (v) *in vivo* tissue distribution, metabolism, and clearance. Arguably, the most interesting modifications to date are those that alter the sugar moiety and the backbone. Modifications such as 2'-methoxyethoxy have been reported to enhance affinity for RNA, potency *in vivo*, provide a dramatic increase in stability, and reduce the potency for blood clotting and inflammatory effects. Also of interest are a number of modifications that replace the phosphate or the entire phosphate sugar backbone. Several novel chemical classes are being evaluated in animals and will shortly be studied in humans, so it seems likely that in the near future a variety of chemical classes with differing properties will be available.

See Also the Following Articles

ANTISENSE: MEDICINAL CHEMISTRY • ANTISENSE NUCLEIC ACIDS: CLINICAL APPLICATIONS • RIBOZYMES AND THEIR APPLICATIONS

Bibliography

Agrawal, S., Temsamani, J., and Tang, J. Y. (1991). Pharmacokinetics, biodistribution, and stability of oligodeoxynucleotide phosphorothioates in mice. *Proc. Natl. Acad. USA* **88,** 7595–7599.

Azad, R. F., Driver, V. B., Tanaka, K., Crooke, R. M., and Anderson, K. P. (1993). Antiviral activity of a phosphorothioate oligonucleotide complementary to RNA of the human cytomegalovirus major immediate-early region. *Antimicrob. Agents Chemother.* **37**(9), 1945–1954.

Barton, C. M., and Lemoine, N. R. (1995). Antisense oligonucleotides directed against p53 have antiproliferative effects unrelated to effects on p53 expression. *Br. J. Cancer* **71,** 429–437.

Bennett, C. F., and Crooke, S. T. (1996). Oligonucleotide-based inhibitors of cytokine expression and function. *In* "Ther. Modulation Cytokines" (B. B. Henderson and W. Mark, eds.), pp. 171–193. CRC Press, Boca Raton, FL.

Boyer, D. S., Lieberman, R. M., Antoszyk, A. A., Cantrill, H.,

Danis, R., Duker, J., Fish, R., Goldstein, D., Jaffe, G. J., Johnson, D. W., Kuppermann, B., Lalezari, J. P., Lambert, H. M., Mansour, S., Palestine, A. G., Park, S., Terry, B. G., Vrabec, T. R., and Muccioli, C. (1997). "Clinical Efficacy and Safety of Fomivirsen Sodium for the Treatment of CMV Retinitis Unresponsive to Other Antiviral Therapies." AAO Annual Meeting, San Francisco, CA.

Burgess, T. L., Fisher, E. F., Ross, S. L., Bready, J. V., Qian, Y., Bayewitch, L. A., Cohen, A. M., Herrera, C. J., Hu, S. F., Kramer, T. B., Lott, F. D., Martin, F. H., Pierce, G. F., Simonet, L., and Farrell, C. L. (1995). The antiproliferative activity of c-myb and c-myc antisense oligonucleotides in smooth muscle cells is caused by a nonantisense mechanism. *Proc. Natl. Acad. Sci. USA* **92,** 4051–4055.

Chen, H., Ness, E., Marshall, J., Martin, R., Dvorchik, B., Rizvi, N., Marquis, J., Dahut, W., and Hawkins, M. J. (1999). "Phase I Trial of a Second Generation Oligonucleotide (GEM 231) Targeted at Type I Protein Kinase a In Patients with Refractory Solid Tumors." Thirty-Fifth Annual Meeting of the American Society of Clinical Oncology, Atlanta, GA.

Chiang, M. Y., Chan, H., Zounes, M. A., Freier, S. M., Lima, W. F., and Bennett, C. F. (1991). Antisense oligonucleotides inhibit intercellular adhesion molecular 1 expression by two distinct mechanisms. *J. Biol. Chem.* **266**(27), 18162–18171.

Cornish, K. G., Iversen, P., Smith, L., Arneson, M., and Bayever, E. (1993). Cardiovascular effects of a phosphorothioate oligonucleotide to p53 in the conscious rhesus monkey. *Pharmacol. Comm.* **3,** 239–247.

Cossum, P. A., Sasmor, H., Dellinger, D., Truong, L., Cummins, L., Owens, S. R., Markham, P. M., Shea, J. P., and Crooke, S. (1993). Disposition of the 14C-labeled phosphorothioate oligonucleotide ISIS 2105 after intravenous administration to rats. *J. Pharmacol Exp. Ther.* **267**(3), 1181–1190.

Cossum, P. A., Truong, L., Owens, S. R., Markham, P. M., Shea, J. P., and Crooke, S. T. (1994). Pharmacokinetics of a 14C-labeled phosphorotioate oligonucleotide, ISIS 2105, after intradermal administration to rats. *J. Phamacol. Exp. Ther.* **269**(1), 89–94.

Crooke, S. T. (1992). Therapeutic applications of oligonucleotides. *Annu. Rev. Pharmacol. Toxicol.* **32,** 329–376.

Crooke, S. T. (1993). Progress toward oligonucleotide therapeutics: Pharmacodynamic properties. *FASEB J.* **7**(6), 533–539.

Crooke, S. T. (1995). "Therapeutic Applications of Oligonucleotides." R. G. Landes Company, Austin.

Crooke, S. T. (1996). Therapeutic applications of oligonucleotides in medicine. *Chem. Ind. (Lond.)* **3,** 90–93.

Crooke, S. T. (ed.) (1998). Antisense research and application. *In* "Handbook Experimental Pharmacology." Springer-Verlag, Berlin.

Crooke, S. T., Graham, M. J., Zuckerman, J. E., Brooks, D., Conklin, B. S., Cummins, L. L., Greig, M. J., Guinosso, C. J., Kornburst, D., Manoharan, M., Sasmor, H. M.,

Schleich, T., Tivel, K. L., Griffey, R. H., *et al.* (1996). Pharmacokinetic properties of several novel oligonucleotide analogs in mice. *J. Pharmacol. Exp. Ther.* **277**(2), 923–937.

Crooke, S. T., Grillone, L. R., Tendolkar, A., Garrett, A., Fratkin, M. J., Leeds, J., and Barr, W. H. (1994). A pharmacokinetic evaluation of ^{14}C-labeled afovirsen sodium in patients with genital warts. *Clin. Pharmacol. Ther.* **56**, 641–646.

Crooke, S. T., Lemonidis, K. M., Neilson, L., Griffey, R., Lesnik, E. A., and Monia, B. P. (1995). Kinetic characteristics of *Escherichia coli* RNase H1: Cleavage of various antisense oligonucleotide-RNA duplexes. *Biochem. J.* **312**(2), 599–608.

Crooke, S. T., and Mirabelli, C. K. (1993). "Antisense Research and Applications." CRC Press, Boca Raton, FL.

Dean, N. R., McKay, L., Miraglia, R., Howard, R., Cooper, J., Giddings, P., Nicklin, L., Meister, R., Ziel, S., *et al.* (1996). Inhibition of growth of human tumor cell lines in nude mice by an antisense oligonucleotide inhibitor of protein kinase C-.alpha. expression. *Cancer Res.* **56**(15), 3499–3507.

Dean, N. M., and McKay, R. (1994). Inhibition of protein kinase C-.alpha. expression in mice after systemic administration of phosphorothioate antisense oligodeoxynucleotides. *Proc. Natl. Acad. Sci. USA* **91**(24), 11762–11766.

Dorr, F. A., and Kisner, D. L. (1998). Antisense oligonucleotides to protein kinase C-a and C-raf kinase: Rationale and clinical experience in patients with solid tumors. "Antisense Research and Applications" (S. T. Crooke, ed.), Vol. 131, pp. 461–476. Springer-Verlag, Berlin Heidelberg.

Freier, S. M. (1993). Hybridization considerations affecting antisense drugs. *In* "Antisense Research and Applications" (S. T. Crooke and B. Lebleu, eds.), Vol. 67, pp. 67–82. CRC Press, Boca Raton, FL.

Galbraith, W. M., Hobson, W. C., Giclas, P. C., Schechter, P. J., and Agrawal, S. (1994). Complement activation and hemodynamic changes following intravenous administration of phosphorothioate oligonucleotides in the monkey. *Antisense Res. Dev.* **4**(3), 201–206.

Gao, W.-Y., Han, F.-S., Storm, C., Egan, W., and Cheng, Y.-C. (1992). Phosphorothioate oligonucleotides are inhibitors of human DNA polymerases and RNase H: Implications for antisense technology. *Mol. Pharmacol.* **41**, 223–229.

Gewirtz, A. M. (1998). Nucleic acid therapeutics for human leukemia: Development and early clinical experience with oligodeoxynucleotides directed a c-*myb*. *In* "Antisense Research and Application." (S. T. Crooke, ed.), Vol. 131, pp. 477–497. Springer-Verlag, Berlin.

Glover, J. M., Leeds, J. M., Mant, T. G. K., Amin, D., Kisner, D. L., Zuckerman, J. E., Geary, R. S., Levin, A. A., and Shanahan, W. R., Jr. (1997). Phase I safety and pharmacokinetic profile of an intercellular adhesion molecular-1 antisense oligodeoxynucleotide (ISIS 2302). *J. Pharmacol. Exp. Ther.* **282**(3), 1173–1180.

Graham, M. J., Crooke, S. T., Monteith, D. K., Cooper, S. R., Lemonidis, K. M., Stecker, K. K., Martin, M. J., and Crooke, R. M. (1998). In vivo distribution and metabolism of a phosphorothioate oligonucleotide within rat liver after intravenous administration. *J. Pharmacol. Exp. Ther.* **286**(1), 447–458.

Henry, S. P., Giclas, P. C., Leeds, J., Pangburn, M., Auletta, C., Levin, A. A., and Kornbrust, D. J. (1997). Activation of the alternative pathway of complement by a phosphorothioate oligonucleotide: Potential mechanism of action. *J. Pharmacol. Exp. Ther.* **281**, 810–816.

Henry, S. P., Grillone, L. R., Orr, J. L., Brunner, R. H., and Kornbrust, D. J. (1997). Comparison of the toxicity profiles of ISIS 1082 and ISIS 2105, phosphorothioate oligonucleotides, following subacute intradermal administration in Sprague-Dawley rats. *Toxicology* **116**(1-3), 77–88.

Henry, S. P., Novotny, W., Leeds, J., Auletta, C., and Kornbrust, D. J. (1997). Inhibition of coagulation by a phosphorothioate oligonucleotide. *Antisense Nucleic Acid Drug Dev.* **7**(5), 503–510.

Henry, S. P., Taylor, J., Midgley, L., Levin, A. A., and Kornbrust, D. J. (1997). Evaluation of the toxicity profile of ISIS 2302, a phosphorothioate oligonucleotide in a 4-week study in CD-1 mice. *Antisense Nucleic Acid Drug Dev.* **7**(5), 473–481.

Hertl, M., Neckers, L. M., and Katz, S. I. (1995). Inhibition of interferon-gamma-induced intercellular adhesion molecule-1 expression on human keratinocytes by phosphorothioate antisense oligodeoxynucleotides is the consequence of antisense-specific and antisense-non-specific effects. *J. Invest. Dermatol.* **104**, 813–818.

Hodges, D., and Crooke, S. T. (1995). Inhibition of splicing of wild-type and mutated luciferase-adenovirus pre-mRNAs by antisense oligonucleotides. *Mol. Pharmacol.* **48**(5), 905–918.

Hutcherson, S. L., Palestine, A. G., Cantrill, H. L., Lieberman, R. M., Holland, G. N., and Anderson, K. P. (1995). Antisense oligonucleotide safety and efficacy for CMV retinitis in AIDS patients. *35th ICAAC:* 204.

Iversen, P. (1991). In vivo studies with phosphorothioate oligonucleotides: pharmacokinetics prologue. *Anticancer Drug Des* **6**(6), 531–538.

Joos, R. W., and Hall, W. H. (1969). Determination of binding constants of serum albumin for penicillin. *J. Pharmacol. Exp. Ther.* **166**, 113.

Lima, W. F., Monia, B. P., Ecker, D. J., and Freier, S. M. (1992). Implication of RNA structure on antisense oligonucleotide hybridization kinetics. *Biochemistry* **31**(48), 12055–12061.

Majumdar, C., Stein, C. A., Cohen, J. S., Broder, S., and Wilson, S. H. (1989). Stepwise mechanism of HIV reverse transcriptase: Primer function of phosphorothioate oligodeoxynucleotide. *Biochemistry* **28**, 1340–1346.

Monia, B. P., Johnston, J. F., Ecker, D. J., Zounes, M. A., Lima, W. F., and Freier, S. M. (1992). Selective inhibition of mutant Ha-ras mRNA expression by antisense oligonucleotides. *J. Biol. Chem.* **267**(28), 19954–19962.

Monia, B. P., Johnston, J. F., Geiger, T., Muller, M., and Fabbro, D. (1995). Antitumor activity of a phosphorothioate oligodeoxynucleotide targeted against *C-raf* kinase. *Nature Med.* **2**(6), 668–675.

Monia, B. P., Johnston, J. F., Sasmor, H., and Cummins, L. L. (1996). Nuclease resistance and antisense activity of modified oligonucleotides targeted to Ha-ras. *J. Biol. Chem.* **271**(24), 14533–14540.

Monia, B. P., Lesnik, E. A., Gonzalez, C., Lima, W. F., McGee, D., Guinosso, C. J., Kawasaki, A. M., Cook, P. D., and Freier, S. M. (1993). Evaluation of 2′-modified oligonucleotides containing 2′-deoxy gaps as antisense inhibitors of gene expression. *J. Biol. Chem.* **268**(19), 14514–14522.

O'Dwyer, P. J., Stevenson, J. P., Gallagher, M., Cassella, A., Vasilevskaya, I., Monia, B. P., Holmlund, J., Dorr, A., and Yao, K. S. (1999). *C-raf*-1 depletion and tumor responses in patients treated with the c-*raf*-1 antisense oligodeoxynucleotide ISIS 5132 (CGP 69846)[1]. *Clin. Cancer Res.* **5**, 3977–3982.

Rappaport, J., Hanss, B., Kopp, J. B., Copeland, T. D., Bruggeman, L. A., Coffman, T. M., and Klotman, P. E. (1995). Transport of phosphorothioate oligonucleotides in kidney: Implications for molecular therapy. *Kidney Int.* **47**, 1462–1469.

Sanghvi, Y. S., and Cook, P. D. (1994). "Carbohydrate Modifications in Antisense Research." ACS Symposium Series No. 580. American Chemical Society, Washington, DC.

Srinivasan, S. K., Tewary, H. K., and Iversen, P. L. (1995). Characterization of binding sites, extent of binding, and drug interactions of oligonucleotides with albumin. *Antisense Res. Dev.* **5**(2), 131–139.

Stein, C. A., and Cheng, Y.-C. (1993). Antisense oligonucleotides as therapeutic agents: Is the bullet really magical? *Science* **261**, 1004–1012.

Vickers, T., Baker, B. F., Cook, P. D., Zounes, M., Buckheit, R. W., Jr., Germany, J., and Ecker, D. J. (1991). Inhibition of HIV-LTR gene expression by oligonucleotides targeted to the TAR element. *Nucleic Acids Res.* **19**(12), 3359–3368.

Wagner, R. W., Matteucci, M. D., Lewis, J. G., Gutierrez, A. J., Moulds, C., and Froehler, B. C. (1993). Antisense gene inhibition by oligonucleotides containing C-5 propyne pyrimidines. *Science* **260**(5113), 1510–1513.

Wu, H., Lima, W. F., and Crooke, S. T. (1999). Properties of cloned and expressed human RNase H1. *J. Biol. Chem.* **274**(40), 28270–28278.

Wyatt, J. R., Vickers, T. A., Roberson, J. L., Buckheit, R. W., Jr., Klimkait, T., DeBaets, E., Davis, P. W., Rayner, B., Imbach, J. L., and Ecker, D. J. (1994). Combinatorially selected guanosine-quartet structure is a potent inhibitor of human immunodeficiency virus envelope-mediated cell fusion. *Proc. Natl. Acad. Sci. USA* **91**(4), 1356–1360.

Yacyshyn, B. R., Bowen-Yacyshyn, M. B., Jewell, L., Tami, J. A., Bennett, C. F., Kisner, D. L., and Shanahan, W. R., Jr. (1998). A placebo-controlled trial of ICAM-1 antisense oligonucleotide in the treatment of Crohn's disease. *Gastroenterology* **114**(6), 1133–1142.

Anti-Vascular Endothelial Growth Factor-Based Angiostatics

Pär Gerwins
Lena Claesson-Welsh
Uppsala University

I. Introduction
II. Vascular Endothelial Growth Factor Antagonists
III. Receptor Antagonists
IV. Future Perspectives

GLOSSARY

antibodies Proteins in the blood that specifically bind and mediate an immune response to foreign proteins.

ATP-binding site The enzymatic activity of receptor tyrosine kinases (see later) requires ATP, which is bound to a specific lysine in the intracellular domain (the ATP-binding site). The enzymatic activity of receptor tyrosine kinases results in transfer of a phosphate group onto tyrosine residues in the receptor and cytoplasmic proteins.

growth factor A protein that is secreted from cells and stimulates this cell or other cell types to divide.

hypoxia Reduced oxygen tension, e.g., in growing tissues such as tumors.

receptor tyrosine kinase A cell surface-expressed protein that binds growth factors in a specific manner; binding results in activation of an intrinsic enzymatic activity: tyrosine kinase activity.

vascular endothelial growth factor A group of related growth factors important for endothelial cells.

Physiological processes such as embryonic development, wound healing, and menstruation are known to require the formation of new blood vessels, angiogenesis, to meet increased needs for oxygen and nutrients. Pathological processes, such as cancer growth and chronic inflammatory diseases, also depend on angiogenesis. A number of different growth factors are implicated in angiogenesis and one of these, vascular endothelial growth factor (VEGF), is the focus of attention due to its critical and specific role in angiogenesis. A number of approaches have been taken to inhibit the function of VEGF in order to inhibit angiogenesis and thereby halt the progress of diseases such as cancer.

I. INTRODUCTION

Vascular endothelial growth factor designates a still expanding family of growth factors. Currently known VEGF family members are denoted VEGF-A, placenta growth factor (PlGF), VEGF-B, -C, -D, and -E. VEGF-A (formerly denoted VEGF) occurs in several different isoforms, composed of 121, 165, 189, and 206 amino acid residues in humans. A number of features distinguish VEGF-A from other VEGF family members. Thus, expression levels of VEGF-A are markedly upregulated by reduced oxygen tension (hypoxia). VEGF-A induces increased permeability of vessels leading to edema. Furthermore, inactivation of one VEGF-A allele, of the existing two, leads to embryonic death halfway through the pregnancy due to lack of endothelial cells. Clearly, VEGF-A is criti-

cal for both establishment of the vascular system during development and angiogenesis.

VEGF-A binds to two distinct, but structurally related, cell surface receptors denoted VEGFR-1 (Flt-1) and VEGFR-2 (KDR/Flk-1). These are receptor tyrosine kinases, which are expressed on endothelial cells and a few other cell types. The function of VEGFR-1 is disputed. The intracellular part of VEGFR-1 contains a tyrosine kinase domain, the primary structure of which concurs with those of functional tyrosine kinases; still, it is very difficult to detect the expected activation of VEGFR-1 on VEGF-A binding. Inactivation of the VEGFR-1 gene leads to disorganization of vessels in the mutant embryos. This appears to be due to an increased number of endothelial cells, which fail to form functional vessels. Based on these features, VEGFR-1 has been suggested to have a negative regulatory function. VEGFR-2, however, is critical for the differentiation of endothelial cell precursors (angioblasts) into endothelial cells; inactivation of the VEGFR-2 gene results in embryonic death with

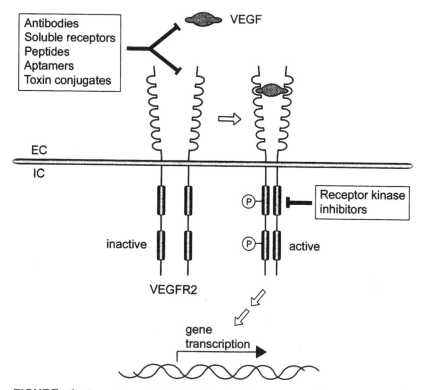

FIGURE 1 Strategies to inhibit VEGF-induced angiogenesis. Angiogenesis can be halted by preventing VEGF from binding to its receptors or by inhibiting the catalytic activity of the VEGF receptor.

features very similar to those observed in mice lacking expression of VEGF-A. VEGFR-1 expression is upregulated by hypoxia, and the VEGFR-1 promoter contains binding elements for the hypoxia-inducible transcription factor HIF-1. Such elements are lacking in the VEGFR-2 promoter, but VEGFR-2 appears to be upregulated during hypoxia through other mechanisms and there are increased levels of VEGFR-2 on proliferating endothelial cells.

The critical role of angiogenesis in the progression of human tumor diseases is now widely accepted. Impressive efforts aimed at suppressing angiogenesis in these tumor diseases have, in many cases, focused on the VEGF family of ligands and receptors, particularly VEGF-A and VEGFR-2. In principle, anti-VEGF-based angiostatics may be based on any of a number of different steps in the signaling cascade from the growth factor to the receptor, as outlined later. Figure 1 summarizes the different types of strategies that have been used to block the effects of VEGF-A/VEGFR-2 in tumor progression. It is noteworthy that tumor models may be dependent on only VEGF or a combination of different growth factors. A number of cancers (colon, esophagus, melanoma, renal, and nonsmall cell lung cancer) have been shown to depend on VEGF for their progression and metastasis and thus represent excellent target diseases for anti-VEGF therapy.

II. VASCULAR ENDOTHELIAL GROWTH FACTOR (VEGF) ANTAGONISTS

A. Neutralizing VEGF Antibodies

Therapy based on neutralizing VEGF-A antibodies has the advantage that the target protein is easily accessible, as compared with proteins contained within cells. The mechanism of action of anti-VEGF-A antibodies appear to be neutralization of VEGF-A followed by decreased vascularization of the tumors and consequent programmed cell death (apoptosis) of the tumor cells. Reduced vascular permeability as a consequence of VEGF-A neutralization is likely to also be valuable in the treatment. A number of different anti-VEGF-A antibodies with effects on expansion of a spectrum of tumor models have been described. Napoleone Ferrara and co-workers at Genentech iso-

lated a neutralizing antibody denoted A4.6.1. mAb 4.6.1 has been shown to efficiently suppress the progression of a number of human tumors, such as rhabdomyosarcoma (A673), glioblastoma multiforme (G55), leiomyosarcoma (SK-LMS-1), and prostate carcinoma (DU 145) inoculated in immunosuppressed mice. The tumor-arresting effect of 4.6.1 and other neutralizing VEGF antibodies is dependent on sustained treatment. Treatment with mAb 4.6.1 of E106 glioma-carrying mice affected vascularization of tumors regrowing after termination of the treatment; such tumors had fewer but larger vessels.

Hideo Suzuki and co-workers at Toagosei Co. have described another neutralizing anti-VEGF antibody denoted MV833, which was raised against a fusion protein encompassing the shortest form of VEGF-A, the $VEGF_{121}$ isoform. MV833 has been shown to suppress the growth of human gastric carcinoma (MT2) and other colon and gastric cancer tumors in mice. In these treatments, the effect of the neutralizing antibody appears not to be correlated with the levels of VEGF produced by the tumors. This is in contrast to other reports, such as that by Luo and colleagues, who examined the effects of a commercially available anti-VEGF antibody (AF-493-NA) on the growth of MM2 breast carcinoma and OG/Gardner lymphoma 6C3HED, which are two well-defined ascites tumors known to express moderate and low levels of VEGF, respectively. Whereas MM2 tumors were adversely affected by the anti-VEGF treatment, there was no effect on the growth of lymphomas, indicating that factors other than VEGF in the latter tumor type may stimulate angiogenesis. The characteristics of tumor growth may also be essential for the outcome of the anti-VEGF antibody treatment. Thus, the ovarian carcinoma SKOV-3 was injected subcutaneously or intraperitoneally, followed by treatment with the anti-VEGF A4.6.1 antibody by intraperitoneal injections. The subcutaneous tumors were inhibited by anti-VEGFA4.6.1 treatment, whereas the intraperitoneal tumors were resistant. The fact that the production of malignant ascites was decreased in anti-VEGF-treated animals carrying the intraperitoneal tumors indicated that the treatment as such was efficient, but that the growth of intraperitoneal SKOV-3 tumors in thin sheets over a large surface area could allow neoangiogenesis- and VEGF-independent growth of these tumors. It is also possible that growth factors other than VEGF, produced locally in the peritoneum, could compensate for VEGF.

The exact epitope that is recognized by neutralizing anti-VEGF antibodies probably differs, perhaps in a critical manner. A neutralizing antibody should, by definition, block the function of the growth factor by blocking its binding to the receptor. The receptor-binding part of VEGF has been mapped to the first 100 amino acid residues of the growth factor. It has been shown that antibodies raised against this amino-terminal domain of the VEGF molecule have better properties than antibodies raised against the entire VEGF protein in terms of homing of the antibody to the tumor vasculature and delayed clearing from the tumor tissue. Apart from the humanized version of the A4.6.1 antibody, epitopes of the different neutralizing anti-VEGF antibodies described in the literature have, in general, not been well defined. The humanized antigen-binding Fab fragment (Fab-12) derived from A4.6.1 has been cocrystallized with a fragment of VEGF (amino acid residues 8–109). The residues in VEGF critical for antibody binding turned out to be concentrated on one VEGF segment and distinct from those important for high-affinity binding to VEGFR-2, which are more generally distributed.

The humanized anti-VEGF antibody from Genentech has been analyzed for the effective dose range. The antibody is now in clinical trials. Side effects may include bleeding, e.g., from preexisting metastatic lesions.

B. Other VEGF-Neutralizing Agents; RNA "Aptamers," Peptides

Neutralization of VEGF function has also been achieved using synthetic oligonucleotides, so-called "aptamers", which are designed to specifically bind target proteins, such as growth factors, with high affinity. Ruckman and colleagues described an aptamer, which binds specifically to exon 7 in VEGF-A_{165}. This exon is not included in VEGF-A_{121}. The VEGF-A aptamer bound with high affinity to VEGF-A_{165}, but not to VEGF-A_{121} and prevented binding of ^{125}I-VEGF-A to VEGFR-1 and -2 *in vitro* and VEGF-A_{165}-induced vascular permeability *in vivo*. The retention and/or stability of the aptamer in plasma was increased considerably by attachment of a lipid group.

Highly specific VEGF-A-blocking peptides that are of lower molecular weights than other described VEGF antagonists have been identified in systematic approaches. Fairbrother and co-workers used multicopy display of random peptides in f1 filamentous phage particles to identify sequences that blocked the interaction of VEGF-A with its receptors. It is interesting that although no selection was applied, the identified peptides bound in an overlapping manner to the VEGFR-2 binding site on VEGF-A, whereas attempts to identify short peptides that block VEGF-A function have yielded sequences corresponding to the VEGF-A-binding sequence in VEGFR-2, again at micromolar concentrations.

C. Antagonistic Effects of VEGF–Toxin Conjugates

The concept that molecules, such as antibodies, could be carriers of toxins or drugs that would be presented specifically to the cell type reactive with this particular molecule has also been exploited to inhibit the function of VEGF. VEGF$_{165}$ or VEGF$_{121}$ fused with diphtheria toxin translocation and enzymatic domains is highly toxic to proliferating endothelial cells but not to other cell types and inhibits tumor growth of different types, such as Kaposi's sarcoma and ovarial cancer, causing hemorrhagic necrosis of tumor tissue, without affecting the vascularization of normal tissues.

III. RECEPTOR ANTAGONISTS

Antagonists directed toward VEGF receptors may have certain advantages over antagonists directed toward the growth factor, such as those outlined earlier. One argument supporting such a statement is that VEGF-A production is upregulated under hypoxic conditions and may accumulate in a sequestered manner, which makes it difficult to neutralize. Moreover, antagonists directed against VEGFR-2 will neutralize the action of all VEGF ligands that bind to this receptor, whereas antagonists raised against VEGF family members will be specific toward each individual ligand. This section summarizes different approaches that have been taken to generate VEGF receptor antagonists.

A. Dominant-Negative VEGF Receptors

VEGF receptor-1 exists as two forms; one is the classical transmembrane protein with the extracellular VEGF-binding domain, the transmembrane domain, and the intracellular tyrosine kinase domain. The second form is soluble and contains the six amino-terminal immunoglobulin-like folds of the extracellular domain of the receptor and is created by alternative splicing. Soluble VEGFR-1 is able to homodimerize with full-length cell surface expressed VEGFR-1 as well as VEGFR-2. Soluble VEGFR-1 is produced by the human placenta and becomes released in the maternal circulation. There is increased expression of soluble VEGFR-1 in preeclampsia. Soluble VEGFR-1 is also expressed by human endometrium, detectable in both epithelial and stromal cell fractions. Interestingly, the expression level of soluble VEGFR-1 is modulated during the menstrual cycle, with a threefold increased expression during the late proliferative stage. To examine the effect of soluble VEGFR-1 on tumor angiogenesis, Goldman and colleagues expressed soluble VEGFR-1 in HT-1080 human fibrosarcoma cells, which were injected subcutaneously into nude mice. The growth of the resulting tumor was initially reduced but accelerated at later stages, perhaps due to reduced expression of soluble VEGFR-1.

Although not occurring naturally, recombinant soluble VEGFR-2 has been tested for antitumor effects. In analogy with other engineered or naturally occurring truncated growth factor receptors, the affinity of VEGF-A binding to soluble VEGFR-2 is reduced as compared with the full-length VEGFR-2. A 250-fold excess of the soluble receptor over VEGF is required to block endothelial cell function *in vitro*. *In vivo*, expression of a dominant-negative VEGFR-2, lacking most of the intracellular domain, blocks the growth of glioblastoma as well as other model tumors.

B. Receptor Antibodies

A number of reports detail the properties of antibodies raised against the extracellular domain of VEGFR-2. Witte and colleagues raised a rat monoclonal antibody against the extracellular domain of mouse VEGFR-2 (denoted DC101), which neutralized the effects of VEGF. This antibody was shown to block tumor angiogenesis and thereby growth of murine Lewis lung, 4T1 mammary, and B16 melanoma tumors, as well as human epidermoid, glioblastoma, pancreatic, and renal tumor xenografts. Inhibition ranged from 70 to 92% and no side effects were noted. Interestingly, FGF-2-induced angiogenesis in implanted Matrigel plugs was inhibited by the anti-VEGFR-2 antibody, possibly indicating that FGF-2 may modulate the expression of VEGFR-2. Subsequently, antibodies reactive with human VEGFR-2 were isolated using a single-chain (sc) antibody phage display library. One scFv denoted p1C11 was isolated, which inhibited VEGF-A-induced VEGFR-2 activation and endothelial cell proliferation. The p1C11 bound to VEGFR-2 with an affinity equal to or higher than that of VEGF-A. Furthermore, the k_{off} rate for p1C11 was found to be very slow, indicating that the antibody remained tightly bound to the receptor for extended periods of time, thereby most likely increasing the efficiency of the treatment.

C. Receptor Kinase Inhibitors

The development of highly specific ATP analogs that bind to and block the ATP-binding site in receptor tyrosine kinases is the basis for efforts to develop VEGF receptor inhibitors as therapeutic tools in angiogenesis-related diseases. A number of compounds with distinct chemistry have been developed. The Sugen Company has focused on a series of 3-substituted indolin-2-ones. One compound, denoted SU5416, showed efficient blocking of VEGFR-2 activation. There was also some effect on the activation of another growth factor receptor, that for platelet-derived growth factor (denoted PDGFR), but no effect on the epidermal growth factor receptor, the insulin receptor, or FGF receptor. Growth of a number of model tumors, including melanoma, epidermoid carcinoma, lung carcinoma, glioma, prostatic carcinoma, and fibrosarcoma, was inhibited from 44 to 85% by daily intraperitoneal SU5416 treatment without any signs of toxicity. Interestingly, wound healing was not affected by treatment with the drug. Further development has resulted in the presentation of another ATP-blocking compound denoted SU6668, which blocks FGF, PDGF, and VEGF receptors. Oral or intraperitoneal administration of SU6668 had a striking effect on tumor growth and caused regression of established tumors at higher doses. The profound effect of SU6668 could be dependent on that several growth factor receptors are inhibited, each known to contribute to the angiogenic process. The efficiencies of SU5416 and SU6668 have been compared; the most profound difference between the two appeared to be the higher levels of endothelial and tumor cell apoptosis in animals treated with SU6668. However, although the growth of the primary tumor was inhibited, the growth of metastases was not affected. SU6668 is now in clinical phase II trials.

In a parallel effort to develop high-efficiency VEGF receptor inhibitors, Hennequin and co-workers presented the synthesis of substituted 4-anilinoquinazolines that were active *in vitro* and *in vivo*. The classical route of administration of VEGF angiostatics is by subcutaneous injection, which requires patients to be admitted to the clinic. It is therefore noteworthy that one of the 4-anilinoquinazolines, denoted ZD4190, could be administered orally, leading to efficient arrest of the growth of a number of human xenografted tumors in nude mice (breast, lung, prostate, and ovarian). Another novel VEGF receptor inhibitor, PTK 787 (4-anilino phtalazine), inhibits growth of VEGF-producing primary tumors, such as ovarian and renal cancer.

IV. FUTURE PERSPECTIVES

VEGF and VEGF receptors have been implicated in stimulating angiogenesis in a number of human solid tumors (bladder, breast, colon, gastrointestinal, glioma, renal, melanoma, and neuroblastoma). Strategies to block VEGF- or VEGF receptor-dependent angiogenesis in these diseases have been transferred from the laboratory to the clinic with an impressive pace. It is likely that future treatment of cancer will be combinatorial, i.e., not relying on any one single approach, but to a number of approaches aimed both at the tumor and at the vascular bed. The exact design of this treatment could be dependent on the type of tumor and the stage of disease. At this point, the prospects for VEGF angiostatics to be an efficient additional treatment strategy that could be added to conventional therapies for human tumor diseases look very promising. However, a number of issues still remain to be explored. One such issue is that of genetic drifting, i.e., does blockade of VEGF function promote the production, by the tumor cells, of another angiogenesis stimulator, such as FGF? This could be a particular problem for patients with slow-growing tumors. Furthermore, will treatment with VEGF angiostatics result in complete regression of tumors or will there be dormant metastases? Long-term treatment with VEGF angiostatics to keep these dormant tumors suppressed may pose problems with side effects not noticed this far. In this respect, it is noteworthy that the expression of VEGF receptor-1 and -2 is not, in contrast to general dogma, entirely restricted to the vascular endothelium. In order to further refine cancer treatment, it is important to continue exploring issues concerning specificity and efficiency.

Acknowledgments

Lena Claesson-Welsh is supported by the Swedish Cancer Foundation, the Novo Nordisk Foundation, and the Goran Gustafsson Foundation. Pär Gerwins is supported by King Gustaf the V:s 80-years Foundation, the Swedish Foundation for Strategic Research, the Harald and Greta Jeanssons Foundation, the Åke Wiberg Foundation, and Magnus Bergvalls Foundation.

See Also the Following Articles

ANTIBODY-TOXIN AND GROWTH FACTOR-TOXIN FUSION PROTEINS • ANGIOGENESIS AND NATURAL ANGIOSTATIC AGENTS • HEMATOPOIETIC GROWTH FACTORS • INTEGRIN-TARGETED ANGIOSTATICS

Bibliography

Dvorak, H. F. (2000). VPF/VEGF and the angiogenic response. *Semin. Perinatol.* **24,** 75–78.

Fairbrother, W. J., Christinger, H. W., Cochran, A. G., Fuh, G., Keenan, C. J., Quan, C., Shriver, S. K., Tom, J. Y., Wells, J. A., and Cunningham, B. C. (1998). Novel peptides selected to bind vascular endothelial growth factor target the receptor-binding site. *Biochemistry* **37,** 17754–17764.

Goldman, C. K., Kendall, R. L., Cabrera, G., Soroceanu, L., Heike, Y., Gillespie, G. Y., Siegal, G. P., Mao, X., Bett, A. J., Huckle, W. R., Thomas, K. A., and Curiel, D. T. (1998). Paracrine expression of a native soluble vascular endothelial growth factor receptor inhibits tumor growth, metastasis, and mortality rate. *Proc. Natl. Acad. Sci. USA* **95,** 8795–8800.

Hennequin, L. F., Thomas, A. P., Johnstone, C., Stokes, E. S., Ple, P. A., Lohmann, J. J., Ogilvie, D. J., Dukes, M., Wedge, S. R., Curwen, J. O., Kendrew, J., and Lambert-van der Brempt, C. (1999). Design and structure-activity relationship of a new class of potent VEGF receptor tyrosine kinase inhibitors. *J. Med. Chem.* **42,** 5369–5389.

Jayasena, S. D. (1999). Aptamers: An emerging class of molecules that rival antibodies in diagnostics. *Clin. Chem.* **45,** 1628–1650.

Kendall, R. L., and Thomas, K. A. (1993). Inhibition of vascular endothelial growth factor activity by an endogenously encoded soluble receptor. *Proc. Natl. Acad. Sci. USA* **90,** 10705–10709.

Laird, A. D., Vajkoczy, P., Shawver, L. K., Thurnher, A., Liang, C., Mohammadi, M., Schlessinger, J., Ullrich, A., Hubbard, S. R., Blake, R. A., Fong, T. A., Strawn, L. M., Sun, L., Tang, C., Hawtin, R., Tang, F., Shenoy, N., Hirth, K. P., McMahon, G., and Cherrington (2000). SU6668 is a potent antiangiogenic and antitumor agent that induces regression of established tumors. *Cancer Res.* **60,** 4152–4160.

Levitzki, A. (1999). Protein tyrosine kinase inhibitors as novel therapeutic agents. *Pharmacol. Ther.* **82,** 231–239.

Luo, J. C., Toyoda, M., and Shibuya, M. (1998). Differential inhibition of fluid accumulation and tumor growth in two mouse ascites tumors by an antivascular endothelial growth factor/permeability factor neutralizing antibody. *Cancer Res.* **58,** 2594–2600.

Mesiano, S., Ferrara, N., and Jaffe, R. B. (1998). Role of vascular endothelial growth factor in ovarian cancer: Inhibition of ascites formation by immunoneutralization. *Am. J. Pathol.* **153,** 1249–1256.

Millauer, B., Longhi, M. P., Plate, K. H., Shawver, L. K., Risau, W., Ullrich, A., and Strawn, L. M. (1996). Dominant-negative inhibition of Flk-1 suppresses the growth of many tumor types in vivo. *Cancer Res.* **56,** 1615–1620.

Rowe, D. H., Huang, J., Kayton, M. L., Thompson, R., Troxel, A., O'Toole, K. M., Yamashiro, D., Stolar, C. J., and Kandel, J. J. (2000). Anti-VEGF antibody suppresses primary tumor growth and metastasis in an experimental model of Wilm's tumor. *J. Pediatr. Surg.* **35,** 30–32; discussion 32–33.

Ruckman, J., Green, L. S., Beeson, J., Waugh, S., Gillette, W. L., Henninger, D. D., Claesson-Welsh, L., and Janjic, N. (1998). 2'-Fluoropyrimidine RNA-based aptamers to the 165-amino acid form of vascular endothelial growth factor (VEGF 165): Inhibition of receptor binding and VEGF-induced vascular permeability through interactions requiring the exon 7-encoded domain. *J. Biol. Chem.* **273,** 20556–20567.

Shibuya, M., Ito, N., and Claesson-Welsh, L. (1999). Structure and function of vascular endothelial growth factor receptor-1 and -2. *Curr. Top. Microbiol. Immunol.* **237,** 59–83.

Sun, L., Tran, N., Tang, F., App, H., Hirth, P., McMahon, G., and Tang, C. (1998). Synthesis and biological evaluations of 3-substituted indolin-2-ones: A novel class of tyrosine kinase inhibitors that exhibit selectivity toward particular receptor tyrosine kinases. *J. Med. Chem.* **41,** 2588–2603.

vanderSpek, J. C., and Murphy, J. R. (2000). Fusion protein toxins based on diphtheria toxin: Selective targeting of growth factor receptors of eukaryotic cells. *Methods Enzymol.* **327,** 239–249.

Witte, L., Hicklin, D. J., Zhu, Z., Pytowski, B., Kontanides, H., Rockwell, P., and Bohlen, P. (1998). Monoclonal antibodies targeting the VEGF receptor-2 (Flk1/KDR) as an antiangiogenic therapeutic strategy. *Cancer Metastasis Rev.* **17,** 155–161.

Xu, L., Yoneda, J., Herrera, C., Wood, J., Killion, J. J., and Fidler, I. J. (2000). Inhibition of malignant ascites and growth of human ovarian carcinoma by oral administration of a potent inhibitor of the vascular endothelial growth factor receptor tyrosine kinases. *Int. J. Oncol.* **16,** 445–454.

Zhu, Z., and Witte, L. (1999). Inhibition of tumor growth and metastasis by targeting tumor-associated angiogenesis with antagonists to the receptors of vascular endothelial growth factor. *Invest. New Drugs* **17,** 195–212.

APC (Adenomatous Polyposis Coli) Tumor Suppressor

Kathleen Heppner Goss
Joanna Groden
Howard Hughes Medical Institute and
University of Cincinnati College of Medicine

GLOSSARY

apoptosis Process by which cells undergo programmed cell death and which is characterized morphologically by membrane blebbing, nuclear condensation, and DNA fragmentation.

attenuated adenomatous polyposis coli A subtype of FAP characterized by fewer adenomas and a later age of onset associated with germline mutations of the 5' and 3' end of the APC gene.

β-catenin Multifunctional protein that is negatively regulated by APC and that controls the Wnt signaling pathway by associating with and activating the transcription of target genes by Tcf transcription factors.

differentiation Acquisition of a specified and specialized cell fate from a multipotent stem cell.

familial adenomatous polyposis coli (FAP) A rare, inherited colorectal cancer predisposition syndrome caused by germline mutation of the APC gene that is characterized by numerous adenomatous polyps carpeting the colonic mucosa.

loss of heterozygosity Loss or inactivation of the normal copy of a tumor suppressor gene or locus during tumor formation or progression.

methylation The most common epigenetic modification of DNA in human cancer, often resulting in the transcriptional silencing of tumor suppressor genes.

sporadic cancer Tumors that arise in the general population usually late in life and are the result of somatic gene mutations.

Tcf A family of architectural transcription factors that mediate Wnt signal transduction through association with β-catenin and binding to specific DNA recognition sequences.

Wnt signaling pathway An evolutionarily conserved signal transduction cascade that results in transcriptional activation of specific target genes important for developmental processes and cancer.

A decade ago, the first tumor suppressor gene associated with an inherited colorectal cancer predisposition was identified. The *APC* gene, germline mutations in which are found in persons with familial adenomatous polyposis coli (FAP), was mapped by linkage analysis of affected kindreds and isolated by positional cloning efforts. Importantly, the *APC* gene is mutated in more than 80% of sporadic colorectal cancers, suggesting that its alteration plays a critical role in the majority of tumors of the colorectal epithelium. Although the normal function of the *APC* gene product is not entirely understood, experiments indicate that it is involved in several key cellular processes, including proliferation, maintenance of chromosomal stability, differentiation, cell migration, and apoptosis.

I. INTRODUCTION

Some of the fundamental proteins involved in suppressing tumor development and progression were first identified as genes mutated in rare, inherited cancer predisposition syndromes. Similar to retinoblastoma and the *RB* gene, FAP and the *APC* gene are a good example of such an approach: mapping and isolating the gene mutated in the familial cancer syndrome, determining its incidence of mutation in sporadic cancer, identifying the normal function of the gene product, creating genetically engineered animal models to test therapeutic approaches, and, finally, establishing clinical approaches for chemoprevention and treatment of both familial and sporadic cancer.

The genetics of FAP and its similarity to the inheritance pattern of other tumor predisposition syndromes led to the designation of *APC* as a classical tumor suppressor gene. This designation has been supported by mutational inactivation of both copies of *APC* in familial and sporadic colorectal tumors and by its ability to inhibit tumor cell growth in culture. Functionally, APC is involved in diverse physiologi-

cal processes from cell growth to apoptosis in a number of cell types and organisms. More specifically, APC modulates the Wnt signal transduction cascade by regulating cellular levels of β-catenin and associates with additional proteins such as EB1 and DLG. Mutation of the *Apc* gene in mice has created the most commonly used and best-characterized mouse model of gastrointestinal tumor formation known as the *Apc*^{Min} mouse. Gene therapy and other therapeutic strategies are currently underway to exploit these animal and cell culture models of APC-mediated tumorigenesis.

II. FAMILIAL ADENOMATOUS POLYPOSIS COLI

Familial adenomatous polyposis coli is an inherited syndrome in which hundreds to thousands of colorectal adenomas carpet the colon of affected persons at a very young age, often in their teens, at a frequency of approximately 1 in 10,000. If untreated, colorectal cancer is unavoidable by the third or fourth decade of life. Although the large intestine is clearly the major organ affected, additional manifestations of FAP are common and include tumors of the central nervous system (CNS), stomach, upper gastrointestinal tract, pancreas and thyroid, osteomas, desmoids, dental abnormalities, epidermal cysts, and congenital hypertrophy of the retinal pigmented epithelium (CHRPE). The significant likelihood that at least one or more adenomas will become invasive dictates the recommended treatment for this disease, which is prophylactic resection of the colon in early adulthood.

FAP was first described in the medical literature in the 1920s and clearly demonstrated an autosomal dominant pattern of inheritance. The gene responsible for FAP, designated *APC*, was identified and cloned by linkage analysis of FAP families and conventional positional cloning strategies in 1991. The *APC* gene, which localizes to a 100-kb locus on chromosome 5q, is composed of 21 exons. Exon 15 is by far the largest exon, contains 75% of the 8535 bp of coding sequence, and is the target of most FAP germline mutations, as well as somatic mutations in sporadic tumors. In addition to the conventional form of APC encoded by exons 1–15, the *APC* gene includes alternatively expressed exons (.3, BS, .1, .2, 1, 9, and 10A) that contribute to alternate protein isoforms.

APC is a classical tumor suppressor gene that follows the "two-hit" model of gene inactivation: persons with FAP inherit one mutant copy in their germline and develop tumors from cells in which a second somatic mutation in the normal allele is acquired. The overwhelming majority of APC mutations, both germline and somatic, cause a premature stop codon in the open reading frame and result in a carboxy-terminally truncated gene product. To date, more than 1400 somatic and germline mutations in the APC gene have been described that span the entire coding sequence. Two of the most common germline mutations are 5-bp deletions in short, direct repeats at nucleotides 3927 and 3183 (codons 1309 and 1061) and comprise 18 and 12% of all germline APC mutations, respectively. In addition, some APC polymorphisms may be associated with an increased cancer risk and can segregate within specific populations. For example, a polymorphism at nucleotide 3920 is found in 6% of the Ashkenazi Jewish population and in 28% of Ashkenazi Jewish colon cancer patients with a family history of colon cancer. Although this T→A transversion does not create a stop codon directly, it generates a hypermutable polyadenine tract, prone to slippage during DNA replication, that increases the frequency of somatic mutation in this region of the APC gene. It is also likely there is some interdependence of the "two hits" that are acquired in APC. Individuals with germline mutations near codon 1300 tend to show allelic loss as the second or somatic mutational event, whereas FAP patients with other germline mutations most often acquire a second, truncating mutation in middle third of the coding sequence. This suggests that loss of function of one APC allele may apply selective pressure for cells to acquire a second mutant allele of APC.

There are genotype–phenotype correlations in FAP, as the clinical presentation of FAP is often associated with a specific APC mutation. For example, the "profuse" phenotype (more than 5000 adenomas) is associated with mutations between bases 3747 and 3990 (codons 1249 to 1330), whereas mutations 5′ or 3′ to this region are correlated with a "sparse" phenotype (fewer than 1000 adenomas). Mutations at the very 5′ and 3′ ends of the gene result in attenuated adenomatous polyposis coli (AAPC). AAPC is characterized clinically by often less than 100 adenomas developing later in life than FAP, although affected individuals still carry a significantly increased risk of colon cancer in comparison to the general population. Mutational and functional analyses suggest that AAPC alleles encode protein with residual function. Extracolonic disease is also associated with APC mutation position; CHRPE correlates with mutations 3′ of exon 9A, and desmoids are associated with mutations between bases 4335 and 4734 (codons 1445 to 1578).

III. ADENOMATOUS POLYPOSIS COLI AND SPORADIC CANCER

Colorectal cancer is one of the most common cancers in the developed world, accounting for over 135,000 new cases and 57,000 deaths in the United States this year. Unlike many tumor types, colorectal cancer progression from normal epithelium to malignancy is well defined histologically. Even before the APC gene was identified, chromosome 5q, where APC is localized, was implicated as a target for loss of heterozygosity (LOH) in studies of colon tumors of different stages in progression in the general population. Somatic APC mutations occur frequently and early in sporadic colorectal cancer. APC mutations are common in at least 50% of colorectal adenomas and approximately 80% of colorectal adenocarcinomas. In fact, APC inactivation is the earliest known genetic change in colorectal cancer progression and has been identified in the smallest detectable adenomas and aberrant crypt foci.

Somatic mutations in APC are similar to germline mutations in FAP in that they are often frameshifts, insertions, or deletions generating downstream stop codons. A well-defined region, the "mutation cluster region" (MCR), exists within the 5′ end of exon 15, between nucleotides 3000 and 4800 (codons 1000 to 1600). The MCR is the target for approximately 60% of somatic mutations identified, although it accounts for less than 20% of the coding sequence. The consequence of chain-terminating mutations in the MCR is a truncated APC protein unable to associate with and downregulate β-catenin (see later). Although there may be some selection for the mechanism of somatic mutation, it appears that inactivation of the normal copy of *APC* is the rate-limiting step in tumorigenesis. This property has earned *APC* the name of the "gatekeeper" of the colorectal epithelium, as its mutation early in tumor progression affects a number of cellular processes, which in turn facilitate the loss of growth control and accumulation of additional mutations.

Colorectal adenomas and adenocarcinomas are not the only tumor types associated with somatic mutation in the *APC* gene, although the frequency of mutation in colorectal tumors is very high compared to other tissues. APC mutations have been identified in other cancers of the gastrointestinal tract, including pancreas, stomach, and esophagus. In addition, a subset of sporadic breast cancers carry truncating mutations of *APC*, which is consistent with findings that a germline mutation of *Apc* in mice predisposes to mammary adenocarcinomas. Some specific subtypes of tumors from lung and the CNS also have mutations in *APC*, although at a relatively low frequency. Still other tumor types demonstrate a loss of chromosome 5q, although specific mutations in *APC* have not been confirmed.

Finally, an epigenetic mechanism of *APC* inactivation—silencing of the *APC* promoter region by DNA hypermethylation—has been demonstrated in some tumor types. Hypermethylation of normally unmethylated CpG islands in the promoters of some tumor suppressor genes, such as the cell cycle kinase inhibitor *p16* and the DNA mismatch repair gene *MLH1*, is associated with loss of expression of the gene products in sporadic cancers. In many cases, such silencing is effectively equivalent to inactivating mutation. Hypermethylation of the *APC* promoter has been described in up to 18% of sporadic colorectal adenomas and carcinomas, as well as a percentage of primary tumors and/or cell lines from the stomach, pancreas, liver, esophagus, bladder, kidney, lung, and breast.

IV. CELLULAR FUNCTIONS OF ADENOMATOUS POLYPOSIS COLI

APC is a very large, approximately 310-kDa protein with several putative functions in cell cycle control, differentiation, migration, apoptosis, and the maintenance of chromosomal stability. These processes are crucial in maintaining tissue homeostasis or in the maintenance of the proper number and orientation of cells. Identification of proteins that directly interact with APC has contributed greatly to the understanding of the mechanism by which APC mediates tumor suppression in the normal colorectal epithelium. The ultimate goal is to design better therapeutic and chemopreventive agents for colorectal cancer by dissecting the molecular pathways involving the APC protein.

A. Wnt Signal Transduction

Within the central third of the APC protein, there are three 15 amino acid and seven 20 amino acid repeats that are involved in regulating the Wnt signaling pathway (Fig. 1). The 15 amino acid repeats bind to the multifunctional β-catenin protein, whereas the 20 amino acid repeats mediate its downregulation. The association of β-catenin with APC facilitates phosphorylation of β-catenin by the serine-threonine kinase GSK3β. Also present in this APC/GSK3β/β-catenin complex are members of the axin family of proteins, including axin, axel, and conductin. Finally, a component of the E3 ubiquitin ligase, β-Trip, facilitates ubiquitin-mediated degradation of phosphorylated β-catenin at the proteasome complex. The p53-inducible protein Siah-1 has been implicated in mediating β-catenin degradation via a mechanism independent of GSK3β phosphorylation and β-TrCP through binding to the carboxy terminus of APC. It is clear that β-catenin degradation has many levels of regulation and represents an essential function of APC as a tumor suppressor.

When APC is mutated, β-catenin accumulates in the cytoplasm and is free to associate with members of the Tcf family of transcription factors. The β-catenin/Tcf complex in then transported into the cell nucleus by recognition of the nuclear localization signal in Tcf by a nuclear import receptor. β-Catenin also can be transported into the nucleus independent of Tcf. Nevertheless, β-catenin/Tcf complexes recognize and specifically bind Tcf consensus binding sites (5'-A/T A/T CAAAG-3') in the promoters of target genes. Tcf transcription factors are architectural in that Tcf binding bends but does not transactivate

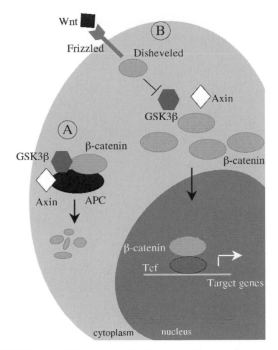

FIGURE 1 APC regulates the Wnt signaling transduction pathway. (A) Cytosolic levels of β-catenin are controlled by the formation of a complex that contains APC, β-catenin, GSK3β, and axin family members. As a result of phosphorylation by the GSK3β kinase, β-catenin is rapidly downregulated by ubiquitin-mediated degradation at the proteasome. (B) When APC is mutated, APC cannot bind and degrade β-catenin, resulting in β-catenin accumulation and association with members of the Tcf family of transcription factors. β-Catenin/Tcf complexes then modulate the transcription of target genes containing Tcf recognition sequences in their promoters. Similar to APC inactivation, the binding of some Wnt proteins to their receptors, frizzleds, inactivates the GSK3β kinase through the dishevelled proteins to generate a cytosolic pool of β-catenin. Although not shown, activation of the pathway is also achieved in cancer through inactivating *axin* mutations and activating *β-catenin* mutations in the GSK3β phosphorylation sites that render it nondegradable.

DNA directly. Therefore, the β-catenin/Tcf association alters the local promoter environment to change gene transcription profiles.

What are the transcriptional target genes affected by β-catenin/Tcf complexes and how do the targets affect tumor suppression by APC? To date, only a handful of gene targets have been described, each activated by β-catenin/Tcf binding. These genes include the cell cycle regulators *c-myc* and *cyclin D1*, the matrix-degrading metalloproteinase *matrilysin*, the hormone *gastrin*, and *PPARdelta*, which is involved in prostaglandin metabolism pathways. Expression of the

AP-1 transcription factors *c-jun* and *fra-1*, as well as the urokinase-type plasminogen activator receptor, is also upregulated by β-catenin/Tcf signaling and is associated with many types of cancer. Further studies are necessary to demonstrate that transcriptional changes in these and other genes are relevant to early tumor progression. In embryonic development, the Wnt signaling pathway is well conserved among species and is much better characterized. It is possible that some of the same transcriptional targets are important in tumor formation and development, considering that the two processes are strikingly similar in many ways. In addition, the balance of Tcf and β-catenin available for DNA binding is likely to determine the resulting transcriptional profiles. In the absence of β-catenin, for example, Tcf binding represses transcription through association with corepressors such as CBP and groucho. This observation implies that the Wnt pathway has complex levels of regulation, such that small changes in the local environment may have large effects on the transcription of critical growth regulatory genes.

Although many of the genes regulated by β-catenin/Tcf-mediated transcription are still unknown, the importance of this pathway in cancer is clear. With respect to APC, the MCR localizes to the region of the APC gene that encodes the 20 amino acid repeats that bind and downregulate β-catenin. Mutations in *β-catenin* itself, which keep the protein from being phosphorylated and degraded, are present in approximately 50% of colorectal tumors that do not contain APC mutations. The *Wnt* family includes oncogenes that, when overexpressed in tumors, result in GSK3β inhibition and accumulation of cytosolic β-catenin. Finally, mutations in *axin* have been described in hepatocellular carcinomas, and presumably would have an identical consequence. That at least four players in the Wnt signaling pathway are mutated in cancer underscores its importance in tumor development. This is not to say, however, that the only function of APC is to regulate β-catenin. Additional functions of APC other than in Wnt signaling are implied by experiments in more manipulable systems. The *Drosophila* APC homologue, for example, is not required for signaling through the β-catenin homologue, Armadillo, and in *Xenopus*, APC activity is positively associated with β-catenin signaling rather than negatively associated.

B. Cell Cycle Control

Like other tumor suppressors, including Rb and p53, APC regulates progression through the cell cycle. It became evident that APC had an effect on cellular proliferation when, in early experiments, normal *APC* was introduced into human colon adenocarcinoma cell lines with varied success. In many transfected cell lines, population doubling time, the ability to form colonies in soft agar, tumorigenicity in mice, and morphological characteristics were significantly changed upon addition of *APC*, and stable transfectants were impossible to propagate in other lines. Overexpression of *APC* in fibroblast and colon cancer cell lines inhibits progression from the G_1 to S phase of the cell cycle. This is a critical transition period in the cell cycle when cells are preparing for DNA replication. The cell cycle block by APC can be overridden by overexpressing specific components of the Rb pathway, including cyclin D1/CDK4, E1a, and E2F. Maintenance of the G_1/S checkpoint by APC is mediated through, at least in part, its ability to regulate β-catenin-mediated transactivation of targets such as *c-myc* and *cyclin D1*. Additional APC protein partners are probably also involved in controlling the G_1/S-phase transition. DLG, a PDZ domain-containing human homologue of the *Drosophila* discs large tumor suppressor, associates with the carboxy-terminal VTSV residues of APC; its overexpression alone is sufficient to inhibit S-phase entry. In addition, the ability of APC to block fully S-phase entry requires an intact DLG-binding domain. These data indicate two ways that APC controls entry into S phase: a β-catenin-dependent activation of transcription of cell cycle genes and a DLG-dependent signal transduction pathway.

APC is likely to be important at the G_2/M-phase cell cycle checkpoint in addition to the G_1/S-phase transition. During mitosis, APC accumulates at the kinetochore of chromosomes, a structure that links chromosomes to the mitotic spindle apparatus, along with members of the Bub family of checkpoint kinases. APC is a phosphorylation target of the M-phase kinase, p34^{cdc2}. Because this transition is the critical cell cycle checkpoint to ensure proper chromosome segregation and cytokenesis, this function of APC may be directly related to its role in maintaining chromosomal integrity and preventing mitotic errors (see later).

C. Maintenance of Chromosomal Stability

APC is thought to be important during mitosis because of its localization to the kinetochore and its modification by phosphorylation specifically at this time. In addition, its association with microtubules and microtubule-binding proteins is most likely important during mitotic checkpoints. The carboxy-terminal end of APC, particularly residues 2200–2400, is enriched in basic amino acids that enable binding to microtubules. This region is sufficient for microtubule colocalization when overexpressed in colon cancer cell lines and microtubule polymerization *in vitro*. APC also associates indirectly with microtubules through EB1, a member of the EB/RP family of tubulin-binding proteins. EB1 was identified as a protein partner of APC through a yeast two-hybrid library screen using the last 700 amino acids of APC. Given that a *S. cerevisiae* homologue of EB1 is required for a microtubule-dependent cytokinesis checkpoint, it is possible that APC and EB1 govern mitotic spindle integrity and/or proper chromosome segregation. APC/EB1 complexes are cell cycle regulated and may also be regulated by phosphorylation during the M phase, perhaps by the cell cycle-dependent kinase p34^{cdc2}. RP1, another member of the EB/RP protein family, also binds the carboxy terminus of APC, indicating that APC/microtubule complexes may contain several proteins. Further support for a role for APC in M phase comes from mouse cells with mutated *Apc* that display chromosome abnormalities and spindles with an abundance of microtubules that do not connect to the kinetochore properly. Because truncation of the last 250 amino acids of APC is associated with this phenotype, it is likely that the interaction of APC with microtubules, EB1, and/or M-phase kinases is involved in maintaining chromosomal integrity.

D. Migration

The identification of β-catenin, a component of the adherens junction, and plakoglobin, localized to the desmosome, as protein partners of APC suggested that APC may be important in cell migration and adhesion. In many ways, characterization of β-catenin function in the Wnt signaling pathway has overshadowed this function of APC, although several lines of evidence support the role of APC in epithelial cell motility and cell–cell contact.

Endogenous and exogenous full-length APC localize to the leading edges of migrating cells. This subcellular localization is dependent on the integrity of the microtubules, suggesting that APC may be involved in cell motility or adhesion through its association with the microtubule network at its carboxy terminus. *In vivo* evidence also supports a role for APC in migration. Migration of intestinal epithelial cells along the crypt–villus axis is altered in mice with either one mutant allele of *Apc* or overexpression of full-length APC; this phenotype is mediated by β-catenin dysregulation. In addition, mice homozygous for an *Apc* mutation die very early during embryonic development (during gastrulation), further suggesting that APC is required for cell migration and/or proliferation. It is possible that the *APC* mutation contributes to tumorigenesis by disrupting the integrity of the cadherin–catenin adhesion complexes in colorectal epithelial cells and altering cell–cell and cell–matrix adhesion. Because some target genes of Wnt signaling include *E-cadherin* and matrix-remodeling enzymes involved in cell motility, it is possible that APC affects migration through β-catenin and targets of transcription by β-catenin/Tcf. Studies suggest that APC may affect cell morphology and migration through association with Asef, a Rac-specific guanine nucleotide exchange factor, via the amino-terminal armadillo repeats of APC.

E. Differentiation

The pattern of APC expression along the colonic crypt and the fact that APC expression can inhibit cell proliferation suggest that APC may affect the differentiation of specific cell lineages. *In vivo*, the APC protein is found in epithelial cells in the lumenal half of the colonic crypt. This region of the crypt contains terminally differentiated, nondividing columnar epithelial cells, mucin-producing goblet cells, and neuroendocrine cells that are all derived from multipotent, proliferating stem cells at the base of the crypts. Alternatively expressed APC isoforms that contain any of the 5' exons (.3, BS, .2, or .1 but not exon 1) are detectable only in postmitotic, differentiated tissues and in early stages of differentiation in cell culture models. Furthermore, in neurons, APC expression is necessary for the initiation of the differentiated phenotype, but is not required for the maintenance of differentiation. It is also possible that some of the genes involved in cellular differentiation may be gene targets of the Wnt signaling pathway, as mice lacking a specific Tcf family member have a dramatic defect in intestinal stem cell proliferation.

F. Apoptosis

APC expression is restricted to the lumenal half of the nonproliferative, differentiated zone of intestinal epithelial cells. This region of the colonic crypt corresponds to the site of cell shedding during programmed cell death or apoptosis. Proper cell shedding is as important in maintaining homeostasis of the colonic epithelium as proliferation; its dysregulation can lead to tumor formation even if the cell cycle is properly controlled. To test whether APC is involved in regulating apoptosis, *APC* was inducibly expressed in one colorectal cancer cell line and demonstrated a 10-fold increase in the percentage of cells undergoing programmed cell death. In *Drosophila*, a null germline mutation of *apc* results in the apoptosis of retinal neurons and retinal degeneration, phenotypes that could be rescued by the concomitant inactivation of *Armadillo*/β-*catenin* or *Tcf*. Although the molecular basis of the effect of APC on apoptosis is not known, it is likely that at least some mechanisms are β-catenin dependent. In fact, overexpression of other components of the Wnt signaling pathway, such as dishevelled, is sufficient to induce apoptosis in an APC-dependent way. Finally, an amino-terminal fragment of APC is detectable in cells undergoing apoptosis that is the result of cleavage by the caspase family of apoptosis-specific proteases. It is possible that this proteolytic product of APC is functionally significant in apoptotic pathways.

V. ANIMAL MODELS AND THERAPEUTIC IMPLICATIONS

To understand APC functions and to test therapeutic approaches *in vivo*, several mouse models of intestinal polyposis have been developed by genetic manipulation of the *Apc* gene. Chemical mutagenesis and gene targeting by homologous recombination strategies have established mice predisposed to spontaneous intestinal adenomas at a young age and with complete penetrance. A handful of drugs have shown significant benefits with respect to tumor burden and life span using these models. For example, administration of nonsteroidal anti-inflammatory drugs to Apc^{Min} mice that carry a germline-truncating Apc mutation results in a dramatic reduction in adenoma formation. These data are supported by epidemiological evidence indicating a chemopreventive role for these drugs in patients with sporadic colorectal tumors and FAP. Consistently, tumor formation is suppressed in another Apc mutant mouse, $Apc^{\Delta716}$, in which a target of this family of drugs, cyclooxygenase-2 (COX-2), is ablated genetically or blocked with a specific inhibitor. Because COX-2 is overexpressed in mouse and human intestinal adenomas, it is an attractive target for abrogating tumorigenesis caused by APC mutation. Additional therapeutic agents that are effective in inhibiting tumor formation in mouse models of FAP include inhibitors of matrix metalloproteinases and DNA methyltransferase. Many of these and other related agents are being used currently as standard cancer therapy or in clinical trials.

One especially attractive therapeutic approach is to replace the mutant APC gene in tumors and the germline with a normal copy of APC using gene therapy strategies. Stable transfection of normal APC into colon cancer cell lines has been attempted with inconsistent success presumably because of the large size and growth-suppressive activity of APC. Approaches such as adenoviral infection or protein transduction may be alternative strategies. With respect to *in vivo* therapy, introduction and maintained expression of human APC into the colon of Apc^{Min} mice have been achieved using cationic liposomes. Further analysis is required to determine whether the expression of normal APC in this context can prevent tumor formation.

VI. CONCLUSION

APC mutation is an early and common event in sporadic colorectal tumor formation and is present in the germline of patients with an inherited predisposition to colorectal cancer known as familial adenomatous

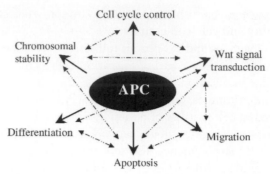

FIGURE 2 The APC tumor suppressor is implicated in diverse cellular processes, including cell cycle control (proliferation), Wnt signal transduction, cell migration, apoptosis, differentiation, and chromosomal stability. Many of the roles for APC in these processes overlap and are likely to be mediated, in part, by the ability of APC to regulate Wnt signaling through β-catenin downregulation. All of these functions contribute to the ability of APC to suppress tumor formation.

polyposis coli. Within the colorectal epithelium and perhaps other cell types, the APC tumor suppressor participates in numerous cellular functions, from proliferation to apoptosis and migration to proliferation (Fig. 2). Some of these APC functions are clearly attributable to its ability to regulate β-catenin levels and modulate the Wnt signal transduction pathway. The molecular basis of other APC functions involves association with additional protein partners, including EB1 and DLG, and cellular machinery, such as the microtubule network. Accordingly, additional investigation into the biology, biochemistry, and genetics of APC will no doubt result in the design of therapeutic and even chemopreventive strategies for inherited and sporadic colorectal cancer patients.

See Also the Following Articles

CELL CYCLE CONTROL • COLORECTAL CANCER: MOLECULAR AND CELLULAR ABNORMALITIES • DIFFERENTIATION AND CANCER: BASIC RESEARCH • TUMOR SUPPRESSOR GENES: SPECIFIC CLASSES • WNT SIGNALING

Bibliography

Fearnhead, N. S., Britton, M. P., and Bodmer, W. F. (2001). The ABC of APC. *Hum. Mol. Genet.* **10,** 721–733.

Fodde, R., Kuipers, J., Rosenberg, C., Smits, R. Kielman, M., Gaspar, C., van Es, J. H., Breukel, C., Wiegant, J., Giles, R. H., and Clevers, H. (2001). Mutations in the APC tumour suppressor gene cause chromosomal instability. *Nature Cell Biol.* **3,** 433–438.

Groden, J., Joslyn, G., Samowitz, W., Jones, D., Bhattacharyya, N., Spirio, L., Thliveris, A., Robertson, M., Egan, S., Meuth, M., and White, R. (1995). Response of colon cancer cell lines to the introduction of *APC*, a colon-specific tumor suppressor gene. *Cancer Res.* **55,** 1531–1539.

Groden, J., Thliveris, A., Samowitz, W., Carlson, M., Gelbert, L., Albertsen, H., Joslyn, G., Stevens, J., Spirio, L., Robertson, M., Sargeant, L., Krapcho, K., Wolff, E., Burt, R., Hughes, J. P., Warrington, J., McPherson, J., Wasmuth, J, Le Palier, D., Abderrahim, H., Cohen, D., Leppert, M., and White, R. (1991). Identification and characterization of the familial adenomatous polyposis coli gene. *Cell* **66,** 589–600.

Kawasaki, Y., Senda, T., Ishidate, T., Koyama, R., Morishita, T., Iwayama, Y., Higuchi, O., and Akiyama, T. (2000). Asef, a link between the tumor suppressor APC and G-protein signaling. *Science* 289, 1194–1197.

Kinzler, K. W., and Vogelstein, B. (1996). Lessons from hereditary colorectal cancer. *Cell* **87,** 159–170.

Liu, J., Stevens, J., Rote, C. A., Yost, H. J., Hu, Y., Neufeld, K. L., White, R. L., and Matsunami, N. (2001). Siah-1 mediates a novel beta-catenin degradation pathway linking p53 to the adenomatous polyposis coli protein. *Mol. Cell* **7,** 927–936.

Morin, P. J., Vogelstein, B., and Kinzler, K. W. (1996). Apoptosis and APC in colorectal tumorigenesis. *Proc. Natl. Acad. Sci. USA* **93,** 7950–7954.

Näthke, I. S., Adams, C. L., Polakis, P., Sellin, J. H., and Nelson, W. J. (1996). The adenomatous polyposis coli tumor suppressor protein localizes to plasma membrane sites involved in active cell migration. *J Cell Biol.* **134,** 165–179.

Spirio, L. N., Samowitz, W., Robertson, J., Robertson, M., Burt, R. W., Leppert, M., and White, R. (1998). Alleles of *APC* modulate the frequency and classes of mutations that lead to colon polyps. *Nature Genet.* **20,** 385–388.

Su, L. K., Burrell, M., Hill, D. E., Gyuris, J., Brent, R., Wiltshire, R., Trent, J., Vogelstein, B., and Kinzler, K. W. (1995). APC binds to the novel protein EB1. *Cancer Res.* **55,** 2972–2977.

Su, L. K., Vogelstein, B., and Kinzler, K. W. (1993). Association of the APC tumor suppressor protein with catenins. *Science* **262,** 1734–1737.

Taipale, J., and Beachy, P. A. (2001). The Hedgehog and Wnt signalling pathways in cancer. *Nature* **411,** 349–354.

Tetsu, O., and McCormick, F. (1999). Beta-catenin regulates expression of cyclin D1 in colon carcinoma cells. *Nature* **398,** 422–426.

Trzepacz, C., Lowy, A. M., Kordich, J. J., and Groden, J. (1997). Phosphorylation of the tumor suppressor adenomatous polyposis coli (APC) by the cyclin-dependent kinase p34. *J. Biol. Chem.* **272,** 21681–21684.

Ataxia Telangiectasia Syndrome

France Carrier
University of Maryland

Albert J. Fornace Jr.
National Cancer Institute, Bethesda, Maryland

GLOSSARY

ataxia The loss of muscular coordination.
autosomal Any chromosome except X and Y.
homozygote An individual carrying two of the same allele (one from each parent) in a particular loci.
linear energy transfer (LET) The energy absorbed by the medium through which an ionizing particle is traveling per unit length of the track of the particle, usually expressed in keV/μ.
recessive The allele phenotype that is obscured in a heterozygote individual by the dominant allele.
telangiectasia The dilatation of peripheral blood vessels.
tumor suppressor A gene product preventing the transformation of normal cells to tumor cells.

A taxia telangiectasia (AT) is an autosomal recessive disease with humoral and cellular immunologic defects. It is a unique combination of progressive neurological disease, immune dysfunction, and cancer predisposition in addition to a developmental disorder that manifests early in childhood. AT patients and cells derived from these patients are hypersensitive to ionizing radiation (IR) and certain radiometric chemicals. Doses of radiation commonly used in radiotherapy can cause fatal radiation burns in AT patients. The AT phenotypes manifest only in the homozygote population, but apparently normal adults, carrier of one mutated allele (heterozygote), may also be predisposed to certain types of cancer.

I. CLINICAL ASPECTS

A. Clinical Symptoms

Two symptoms, cerebellar ataxia and oculocutaneous telangiectasia, are considered the minimal criteria for a positive diagnosis of the ataxia telangiectasia disease. The earliest ataxic trait noted by parents is often difficulty in walking as early as the first year of life, but ataxia of the head and trunk may be present in early infancy; the ataxia, due to primary neuronal degeneration, progresses steadily and typically results in the patient's confinement to a wheelchair by early adolescence. Telangiectasia in or around the eyes usually develops between 3 and 6 years of age and later spreads in a symmetrical pattern to the eyelids, face, ears, and neck, and in particular sunlight-exposed and friction areas of the skin (Fig. 1). Abnormal differentiation of several tissues such as the liver and thymus results in a variety of anomalies including immune dysfunction. Although no specific hepatic lesions have been found in AT patients, their abnormal liver development might contribute to the high level of serum α-fetoprotein observed in almost all of them. In normal children under 1 year of age the levels of α-fetoprotein are higher than in older children but in AT patients the opposite, i.e., higher levels in older children, is found. The function of this protein still remains unknown; however, its glycosylation pattern indicates a hepatic origin. AT patients are also often affected by diverse developmental disorders such as gonadal abnormalities and short stature.

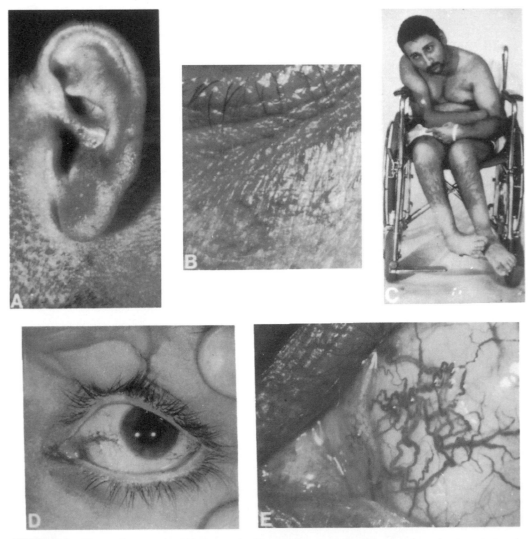

FIGURE 1 Ataxia telangiectasia. (A) Pinna of a 22-year-old patient showing many fine telangiectasia vessels. (B) Telangiectasia of the malar area and lower lid in another patient. (C) The 22-year-old patient, who is unable to walk unaided. (D) His eye shows interpalpebral telangiectasia. The tortuous vessels do not invade the cornea. (E) Interpalpebral telangiectasia. Reproduced from K. H. Kraemer (1977). Progressive degenerative diseases associated with defective DNA repair: Xeroderma pigmentosum and ataxia telangiectasia. *In* "Cellular Senescence and Somatic Cell Genetic: DNA Repair Process" (W. W. Nichols and D. G. Murphy, eds.). Symposia Specialists Inc., Miami, FL.

B. Cancer

The risk of developing malignancy in AT patients is about 1200-fold greater than that of an age-matched control population. The incidence of new cancer from age 10 on is estimated to be 1 in 10 patients each year. The vast majority, more than 85%, of the AT malignancies are acute lymphocytic lymphoma or leukemia. Other cancer predispositions have also been noticed in at least 38% of the patients; carcinomas of the breast, stomach, liver, pancreas, ovary, oral cavity, and salivary gland have been reported. Early studies have suggested an increased cancer predisposition in AT heterozygotes. The cancer most often associated with single gene carriers of this disease is breast cancer. However, the question of breast cancer predisposition in AT heterozygotes is still highly debated, mainly due to the fact that breast cancer families do not demonstrate linkage to the AT locus. The penetrance of AT mutations and the type of mutations may be at the basis of this debate. The risk of AT heterozygotes to develop breast cancer has been calculated at 11% by age 50 and at 30% by age 70. Since heterozygote cells in culture also show some sensitivity to radiation, it is possible that doses of radiation too small to produce any cancer risk in noncarriers induce cancer in heterozygotes. Cancer treatment in AT patients should be guided by their sensitivity to radiation and specific drugs to obtain successful results such as those with reduced doses of radiation in AT children.

C. Genetics and Frequency

Ataxia telangiectasia is a rare disease with a birth frequency anywhere between 1 in 80,000 to 1 in 300,000. The gene frequency of the AT allele has been estimated at 0.007 based on the assumption that AT is due to a mutation in both alleles of the AT gene. People that are heterozygote for the AT gene have been estimated at 1.4% of the U.S. white population. The genetics of this disease is fairly homogenous; linkage studies of 176 families from various parts of the world localize the major AT locus to the region between S1819(A4) and S1818(A2) at chromosome 11q22.3 in all but 7 families. In addition to the United States, cases of ataxia telangiectasia have been reported throughout Europe, Japan, China, Africa, the Middle East, India, and South and Central America. The frequency of the disease in the U.S. black population is similar to the proportion of black individuals in the general population, but the cancer rates in black AT patients in the United States are considerably higher than those in white patients. The differences between the two ethnic groups might reflect differences between the AT alleles or other genetic or environmental factors.

D. Tissue Radiosensitization

A universal characteristic of all AT patients is their hypersensitivity to radiation. The marked hypersensitivity is seen in both patients and cells derived from their normal tissue. Sensitivity of AT fibroblasts to ionizing radiation was first investigated in the mid-1970s due to reported fatal radiation burns in AT patients receiving radiotherapy for malignancies. Other severe reactions caused by the administration of standard radiotherapy to AT patients include ulcerative dermatitis, severe esophagitis, dysphagia, and deep tissue necrosis. It is estimated that the 1- to 9-mGy dose of radiation received in a diagnostic exposure is sufficient to increase considerably the risk of breast cancer in AT heterozygote women while a dose of 100–200 mGy is required to see a similar effect in normal individuals.

II. CELLULAR ASPECTS

A. Cellular Radiosensitization

The basis for AT cells radiosensitivity is still not completely understood but may be due to a slower rate of repair of DNA double strand breaks or to the continued existence of residual breaks (see repair parameters below). The radiosensitivity is exhibited by both a loss of colony formation ability and a higher frequency of chromosomal damage within individual cells. Although several abnormalities have been reported in cells from obligate AT heterozygotes, no clear effect on the capacity to stop DNA synthesis following irradiation (radiation-resistant DNA synthesis) has been demonstrated so far. Some studies indicate that radiosensitivity levels measured in AT heterozygotes by cell survival, chromosome aberrations, production of micronuclei, or flow cytometry are intermediate in between that of controls and AT homozygotes. However, others have pointed out that when larger scale blind evaluations were performed, sufficient overlap between heterozygotes and normal cells was obtained so that no assays could really distinguish between the two groups. Radiation sensitivity is defined by the steepness of a slope obtained from a survival curve when cells are exposed to graded doses of IR. The slope is proportional to $1/D_0$, where D_0 is the dose required to reduce cell survival to 37%. Normal human fibroblasts have typical D_0 values ranging from 1.2 to 1.4 Gy. AT cells, on the other hand, have D_0 values around 0.7 Gy. At 10% survival (D_{10}), AT cells are about twice as sensitive as normal cells. AT cells are also hypersensitive to certain radiometric chemicals (Table I), inhibitors of DNA topoisomerases, and restriction endonucleases. Some variability exists between the different AT cell lines, but AT cells in general are sensitive to compounds that induce DNA strand breaks most probably via free radical attack. The hypersensitivity of AT cells to the X-ray type of DNA-damaging agent is specific since AT cells are not hypersensitive to 254 nm UV radiation.

However, damage from densely ionizing radiation [α-particles, high linear energy transfer (LET)], which causes more extensive local damage to DNA, is less effective on AT cells, relative to normal, than damage from sparsely ionizing radiation (X-rays, low LET).

B. Neurodegeneration

Based on the various neuropathological anomalies, AT can be classified as a primary neuronal degeneration. Primary neuronal degeneration is a progressive disease characterized by the premature death of neurons in the absence of pathological evidence of a specific cause. The neurological abnormalities in AT include progressive cerebellar ataxia, dysarthric speech, movements of the extremities, peculiar eye movements called oculomotor dyspraxia, hyporeflexia or areflexia, and apparent arrest of cognitive development. At the autopsy, a marked atrophy of the cerebellar cortex primarily due

TABLE I
Cytotoxicity in Ataxia Telangiectasia (Homozygous)

Agent	Common effects	AT3B1	AT5B1	AT8B1	AT17IJE-F	AT19IJE-F	AT21IJE-F	AT22IJE-F
H_2O_2	Base damage / DNA single breaks				+	+	+	+
Ara-C	DNA polymerase inhibitor			+				
Nicotinamide	Inhibitor PARP			−				
Bleomycin	DNA strand breaks	+	+	+				
Hypoxia				+				
UV (254 nm)	Pyrimidine dimer			−				
MMS	Alkylating agent	−	+					
Actinomycin D	RNA synthesis inhibitor / Intercalating agent			+				
Streptonigrin	DNA strand breaks	+	+	+	+	+	+	+
Neocarzinostatin	DNA strand breaks			+				
Adriamycin	Intercalating agent			+	+	+	+	+
Paraquat	Herbicide			−	−	−	−	−
Saframycin A	Antitumor			−	−	−	−	−
Ellipticine	Intercalating agent			−	−	−	−	−
Chloroacetaldehyde	Cross-linking agent			−				
PMA	Tumor promoter					+		+
N-Ethyl-N-nitrosourea	Alkylating agent			+				
N-Hydroxy-AAF	DNA adducts			−				
4-Nitroquinoline-1-oxide	DNA adducts	−						

Note. Partial list of the cytotoxocity effects of different agents on AT homozygous lines. Because of the space constraint, references for each AT strain are not quoted; however, original references can be found in M. C. Paterson and P. J. Smith (1979). *Annu. Rev. Genet.* **13**, 291–318. Abbreviations: MMS, methyl methanesulfonate; PMA, phorbol myristate-acetate; PARP, poly-ADP-ribose polymerase; N-hydroxy-AAF, N-hydroxyacetylaminofluorene; (+), increase lethality compared to normal cells; (−), same lethality as normal cells.

to degeneration of the Purkinje and granular cells and, to a lesser extent, of basket cells is also observed. Eventually, the posterior and lateral columns of the spinal cord degenerate and the anterior horn cells are lost. The neuronal degeneration in the cervical area might contribute to the mental retardation observed in about 30% of all AT patients. The mental development may become arrested at a mental age of about 10 or 11 years. Radiosensitivity of AT cell lines is considerably greater than that of cell lines from other neurodegenerative diseases such as Huntington and Alzheimer diseases. This is even more clearly illustrated with cells from AT heterozygotes that have no clinical evidence of neurological abnormalities but are more radiosensitive than cells from patients with other radiosensitive diseases demonstrating significant neuronal degeneration.

C. Cell Cycle

Exposure of normal mammalian cells to DNA-damaging agents, particularly IR, results in transient inhibition or delay of their progression through the cell cycle at a number of different checkpoints, including G_1, S, and G_2. It is thought that these delays allow cells time to repair their DNA and avoid the passage of defective genetic information to the next generation. The importance of these checkpoints for the maintenance of cellular integrity is obvious in that the G_1/S checkpoint precedes DNA replication and that the G_2/M checkpoint precedes the segregation of chromosomes. It is now well established that a wild-type phenotype for the tumor suppressor p53 is necessary to observe a normal G_1 delay following IR. The involvement of p53 in such a critical point in the life of a cell is another indication of the importance of these delays since p53 mutations are found in the majority of human cancer cells. Anomalies in the progression of the AT cells through the cell cycle following exposure to IR have been described in virtually all of these cell cycle checkpoints. The abnormalities have been observed in several AT complementation groups and seem therefore to be universal in AT. In this respect, AT cells are somewhat like caffeine-treated cells which at high doses block multiple checkpoints. The first observation of a defect in the AT cell cycle checkpoints described their inability to stop DNA synthesis following irradiation and most likely referred to the S phase checkpoint since the DNA synthesis was measured 40 min after irradiation. The ra-

dioresistance to DNA synthesis allows the AT cells to proceed through S phase unchecked which results in a reduced mitotic delay and various cellular aberrations. However, increasing evidence suggests that the inability to stop the DNA synthesis cannot be responsible for the hypersensitivity as it was first thought. The two phenomenon, radioresistant DNA synthesis and sensitivity to cell killing, are dissociated in cell hybrids between AT lines and a normal line. In AT heterozygote, neither the radioresistant DNA synthesis nor the shortened mitotic delay is observed. Unlike the arrest in G_1 after IR, the IR-induced S phase arrest seems to be independent of p53. The correlation between p53 and a normal G_1 arrest is also reflected in the increased levels of the p53 protein. In AT homozygous, the G_1 delay and the normal increased p53 levels are not observed following a 1-hr exposure to 2 Gy of IR. The abnormal G_2 block in AT cells following ionizing radiation is more complex since although cells already in G_2 fail to arrest at the G_2-M checkpoint, cells irradiated in the G_1/S phase arrest when they reach G_2. This observation may reflect differences in the type of DNA damage that is produced in G_2 versus G_1. Furthermore, there may be distinct protein complexes (defective in AT) involved in processing and/or repair of one type of DNA lesion versus another. A correlation has been suggested between the number of cells arrested in G_2 and radiosensitivity, but in AT it seems that the number of cells arrested in G_2 correlates with an adverse prognostic indicator. The isolation of the AT gene has allowed a better understanding of the molecular basis of the defective checkpoints. This is described in more detail below (Section III).

D. Cytogenetics

Two types of basal (uninduced) cytogenetic abnormalities are seen in cells from AT patients: (i) an excess of "spontaneous" chromosome breaks (e.g., gaps, fragments) and rearrangements distributed randomly among the chromosomes, and (ii) clonal abnormalities usually involving chromosome 7 or 14. The incidence of these spontaneous changes varies among different patients and also within the same patient as a function of donor age and cell types, i.e., fibroblasts versus lymphoblast. The chromosomal translocations and inversions almost exclusively involve these six breakpoints: three T-cell receptor complexes, 7q35, 7q14, and

14q11, and three B-cell receptor complexes, 22q12, 14q32, and 2p12. All these sites are sites of gene rearrangements, implicating perhaps a common recombinase. These specific translocations are also observed in normal lymphocytes but at a lower frequency. Chromosomal aberrations also occur in fibroblasts but they are nonspecific and almost never involve the six sites mentioned earlier. The AT gene(s) site, 11q23, is never compromised in the chromosomal breakpoints, suggesting that this type of aberration is a consequence rather than a cause of the AT phenotype. Abnormalities in chromosome 14 are also associated with Burkitt lymphoma, Hodgkins disease, and various leukemia, indicating that this chromosome may contain a locus predisposing to lymphoproliferative malignancies. The proximity of the chromosomes 7 and 14 to some immunoglobin genes might be an indication that cytogenetic anomalies play a role in the immunodeficiency observed in AT. The type of aberrations produced in AT lines by radiation differs from that in control lines. In the mitosis following irradiation in the G_0 early G_1 stage of the cell cycle, AT cells show both chromosome and chromatid aberrations while only chromosomal aberrations are observed in normal lines. The reason for this particular response is still unclear, but it implies that some single-strand breaks persist for excessive periods in AT.

E. Immunodeficiency

The most consistent abnormality of the AT immune system is that invariably the thymus fails to develop normally, resembling an embryonic stage of development, and sometimes is even totally absent. Defects in both cellular or humoral immune system can occur. Severe recurrent lung infections are often the major cause of death in the affected patients. Humoral immunodeficiencies are found in most patients: 80% have IgG_2 deficiency, 60% have IgA deficiency, and approximately 50% have IgE deficiency. Despite the frequency of these humoral immunodeficiencies, deficiencies of IgM, IgG_1, and IgG_3 are uncommon. As mentioned earlier, the majority of the AT cancers are acute lymphocytic lymphoma or leukemia, but it is interesting that acute or chronic myeloid leukemia are completely absent. The combined immunodeficiency in AT patients is reminiscent of the phenotypes found in a mutant mouse model named severe combined immunodeficient mutation (scid). Cells from these mice are deficient in a recom-

bination process utilized in both DNA double-strand break repair and lymphoid variable (diversity)-joining [V(D)J] recombination. The resulting phenotype is therefore manifested in both cellular hypersensitivity to ionizing radiation and a lack of B- and T-cell immunity. The DNA-dependent kinase p350, recently identified as a strong candidate for the murine scid defect, is, however, normal in SV40-transformed AT cells (GM 5849). This indicates that even though AT and the scid mice share similar phenotypes, the affected mechanisms that regulate them are most likely different.

F. Repair Parameters

To this day, we still do not know whether the postulated accumulation of DNA damage in AT cells is due to primary defects in the DNA repair process, to a defect in some other system leading to secondary failure of DNA repair, to an abnormal signaling pathway, or to excessive damage to DNA. However, the increased sensitivity of AT to ionizing radiation derives most likely from an inability to recover from DNA breakage in the normal manner. Subtle defects in the ability to process DNA breaks such as accuracy of strand rejoining and persisting residual breaks may affect the ability to recover from DNA breakage. There are several conflicting reports in the literature concerning the capacity of AT cells to repair their damaged DNA. This confusion may have resulted from the differences in the sensitivity of the various techniques used. For example, cytogenetic experiments utilizing comparison of the breakage and rejoining of prematurely condensed chromosomes (pcc) indicated that after a dose of 6.0 Gy, both AT and normal cells had the same initial frequency of breaks and the same rate for rejoining of the breaks, but the fraction of breaks that did not rejoin was five to six times greater in the AT cells. It should be noted that the frequency of such events is orders of magnitude less than IR-induced DNA strand breaks. Fornace and Little, and subsequently others, using filter elution assays from the early 1980s, found no convincing differences between AT and normal lines in the ability to repair DNA strand breaks. Another technique, the pulse field gel electrophoresis, which detects double-stranded breaks in genomic DNA after low doses of γ-irradiation, indicated that the residual amount of unrepaired double-strand breaks in normal cells was 1.4% while it was 5.2 and 2.1% in AT cells and AT heterozygotes, respectively. There is also evidence of mis-rejoining of double-strand breaks in damaged plasmids. Interestingly, the cellular aberrations found in the next mitosis following the treatment of AT cells in G_1 with IR or electroporated restriction enzymes commonly involve only one chromatid. This suggests that AT cells have a defect in the repair of doublestrand breaks. However, the levels or activity of repair enzymes such as 5,6-dihydroxydihydrothymine, apurinic-site specific endonuclease, and ADP-ribose transferase are normal in AT. It seems therefore that a search for a specific DNA repair defect might not be the most likely way to find an explanation for the AT phenotype. Thus, it has been suggested that AT main defects might reside in the signaling of DNA repair. In that regard, phosphorylation of several key regulators of DNA repair has been described in an AT dependent manner (see Section III).

III. MOLECULAR ASPECTS

A. The AT Gene

Cloning of the AT gene opened the door to numerous molecular studies that had been awaited for quite some times. Several aspects of the AT field benefited from the identification of the AT gene, but one of the greatest advantages was probably that the long and tedious efforts required for the identification of different complementation groups could finally come to an end. Like other rare disease such as xeroderma pigmentosum, it was thought that the numerous AT phenotypes were caused by several genes. However, since roughly 97% of tested AT families link to chromosome 11, the possibility remained that a common multimeric molecule, with different subunits of the molecule being affected in different patients, leads to the indistinguishable AT phenotype between the complementation groups A, C, D, and E. Early linkage analysis clearly localized the AT gene from the complementation group A to a 3 cM region of chromosome 11q22-23. Subsequently, a more precise analysis involving 176 AT families localized the AT gene(s) within a 500-kb interval flanked by S1819 and S1818. This localization favored either a cluster of AT genes on chromosome 11 or intragenic defects in a single gene. There are several functional genes that have already been mapped to chromosome 11q22-23;

many of these genes have remained together for over 80 million years of evolution. There is also a number of diseases associated with this region, one of which, tuberous sclerosis, confers radiation hypersensitivity.

Data obtained from linkage analysis provided an alternative, positional cloning to the complementation group approach. Long-range cloning of the AT locus was performed by constructing a contig of yeast artificial chromosome (YAC) clones across the AT interval. Ultimately, a 5.9 kb cDNA clone obtained from a fibroblast cDNA library was isolated. The full sequence of this clone contained 5921 base pairs that include an open reading frame (ORF) of 5124 nucleotides. Northern blot analysis revealed a major transcript of approximately 13 kb in all tissues and cell types examined, and Southern blot analysis indicated considerable evolutionary conservation. The molecular cloning of a cDNA contig spanning the complete ORF predicts a product of 3056 amino acids. The carboxy terminal region of this protein shows considerable similarity to several yeast, *Drosophila,* and mammalian phosphatidylinositol-3' (PI-3) kinases that are involved in mitogenic signal transduction, meiotic recombination, cell cycle control, or DNA damage detection. The pleiotropic nature of the AT phenotype is therefore well served by this protein. This gene product, named ATM (AT mutated), is a serine/threonine protein kinase sharing the substrate recognition motif Ser/Thr-Gln-Glu of the phosphatidylinositol 3-kinase-like (PIKK) family of protein kinases. There is no evidence of alternative transcripts in the ORF, but complex alternative splicing in the 5' and 3' untranslated region has been observed. Posttranscriptional regulation of the transcript is therefore likely. A variety of cDNA expression vectors introduced into AT cells has been shown to complement the radiosensitivity phenotype. The ATM protein is predominantly found in the nucleus of proliferating cells but has also been observed in the cytoplasmic fraction of differentiated cells such as cerebellar neurons. ATM probably interacts with other proteins to facilitate its entry into the nucleus since there are no obvious nuclear localization signals in ATM primary sequence. ATM could thus possibly play different roles depending on its presence or absence in a given cellular compartment. ATM kinase activity is rapidly enhanced following treatment with agents that cause DNA double strand breaks (DSB) but is insensitive to other types of DNA damaging agents such as UV radiation and alkylating agents. Several laboratories using slightly different strategies have developed *ATM* knockout mice. All animals exhibit most of the noncentral nervous system features such as growth retardation, mild neurological dysfunction, male and female infertility, immunodeficiency, radiosensitivity, and predilection for thymic lymphoma. However, none of the animals reproduced the neurodegeneration changes observed in AT patients, even though one laboratory showed evidence of neuron degeneration in the cerebellar cortex of 2-month-old *ATM* $-/-$ mice. Mutations of the *ATM* gene, mainly characterized by premature truncation of the protein product, have been found in patients from all complementation groups. This indicates that *ATM* is probably the sole gene responsible for the AT disorder. Thus, the earlier complementation studies are not consistent with the current understanding of the genetic nature of this disease. Most AT patients are compound heterozygotes and have two different *ATM* mutations. At least 250 mutations have been described so far; a current list of *ATM* mutation can be found on the internet (http://www.vmresearch.org/atm.htm).

B. The ATM Substrates

Given that the ATM kinase is activated by agents that cause DSB, it is not surprising to find that most ATM substrates are involved in (1) cell cycle checkpoint, (2) stress response, or (3) DSB repair, all aspects of the cellular response to genotoxic stress.

1. Cell Cycle Checkpoint

Key regulators of all phases of the cell cycle have been identified as ATM substrates. The tumor suppressor p53 was the first cell cycle regulator identified and is among the best characterized substrates. In normal human hematopoietic and other cells, increases in the levels of the tumor suppressor p53 correlate with a transient G_1 arrest after irradiation. Cells that are mutant for p53 show no G_1 arrest but retain the G_2 arrest found typically after irradiation. In AT cells, the G_1 arrest and the p53 response is delayed. The suboptimal p53 activation is also reflected in the lower induction levels of the proteins Gadd45, MDM2, and p21$^{\text{WAF1/CIP1}}$, which are encoded by three p53 downstream effector genes. Moreover, the DNA-binding activity of p53 is also abnormal following IR in AT, and

failure to inhibit cyclin/cdk complexes by IR, an activity associated with p21$^{\text{WAF1/CIP1}}$ induction, has also been reported. However, the defective p53 activation might be specific to IR since induction of p53 by other DNA damaging agents appeared relatively normal in AT. Disruption of p53 function in normal fibroblasts (Fig. 2) results in increased spontaneous recombination rates and loss of the p53-dependent G_1/S cell cycle checkpoint. These two phenomena, also present in AT, indicate that an abnormal p53 response might contribute to the AT phenotype. In addition to these effects, a role for p53 in the mediation of the molecular abnormalities in AT has been demonstrated by insertion of mutant p53 protein, or viral protein known to degrade p53, in AT fibroblasts. Disruption of functional p53 in AT (Fig. 2), results in increased resistance to streptonigrin and IR mediated by a suppression of the apoptotic response. ATM regulates p53 control on the G_1 checkpoint by at least three different mechanisms. First, ATM phosphorylates p53 directly on Ser15 and increases its transcriptional activity. Second, ATM activates the checkpoint kinase 2 (chk2) by phosphorylating it on Thr68, which allows it to phosphorylate p53 on Ser20 and increases p53 stability by interfering with binding to the mouse double minutes 2 (MDM2) protein. MDM2 is the main mediator of the

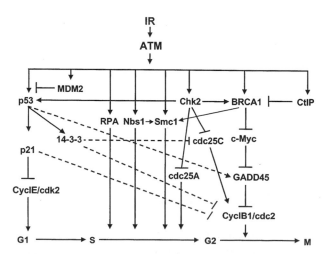

FIGURE 2   Ionizing radiation pathway. The AT gene product normally plays a role in the activation of several cellular responses following ionizing radiation. ATM activates key regulators of every phase of the cell cycle. Positive regulations are indicated by arrows while negative regulations are indicated by blunt arrows. Dashed lines indicate G_2 regulation mediated by p53 when cells enter G_2 with damaged DNA or are arrested in S phase (see details in the text).

proteoasome-mediated degradation of p53, where it functions as the E3 ligase in p53 ubiquitination process. The third mechanism used by ATM to regulate p53 action in G_1 is to phosphorylate MDM2 directly on Ser395, which prevents p53 export to the nucleus, a necessary step in p53 degradation.

Activation of chk2 by ATM provides also a mechanism for ATM's control of the G_2/M checkpoint. The activated chk2 can phosphorylate and inactivate the cdc25C phosphatase. This phosphatase is responsible for dephosphorylation and activation of cdc2, the kinase controlling entry into mitosis. ATM can also regulate the G_2/M checkpoint through the breast cancer susceptibility gene 1 (BRCA1). Similar to p53 regulation, ATM regulation of BRCA1 also involves three mechanisms. First, ATM phosphorylates BRCA1 directly on Ser1423 and Ser1525, chk2 in response to ATM phophorylates BRCA1 on another serine, Ser988, and, finally, ATM phosphorylates and inactivates CtIP, a negative regulator of BRCA1. The precise mechanism by which BRCA1 regulates the G_2/M checkpoint is not completely understood, but recent findings indicate a role as co-repressor. BRCA1 does not physically interact with DNA but rather associates with the proto-oncogene c-Myc and represses its transactivation. Among the different genes regulated by c-Myc is the growth arrest and DNA damage inducible gene GADD45. The expression of GADD45 can be repressed by c-Myc through a C/EBP element within the GADD45 promoter. Gadd45 binds to cdc2 and disrupts the cyclinB1/cdc2 complex, which results in the inhibition of the kinase activity and prevents cell cycle progression beyond G_2. By phosphorylating BRCA1, ATM may thus control the G_2/M checkpoint by allowing BRCA1 to relieve the transcriptional repression imposed by c-Myc on the GADD45 promoter. ATM can also control G_2 arrest through p53 when cells enter G_2 with damaged DNA or are arrested in S phase. Under these conditions, p53 inhibits cdc2 simultaneously by three transcriptional targets, GADD45, p21, and 14-3-3 sigma. The p21 protein may contribute to G_2 arrest by several mechanisms including direct binding to CyclinB1/cdc2 and inhibition of CAK, the kinase phosphorylating cdc2. The 14-3-3 protein is a direct substrate of p53 and binds to CyclinB1/cdc2 as well as Cdc25 and sequesters them in the cytoplasm.

The role of ATM in the regulation of the S-phase checkpoint is complex and involves the phosphoryla-

tion of several key regulators. Hyperphosphorylation of the replication protein A (RPA) following IR is reduced and delayed in AT cells. RPA is a three-subunit protein complex involved in the initiation and elongation stages of DNA replication and in repair. It seems that in AT cells, the underphosphorylation of RPA subunit, p34, is not due to the absence of RPA kinases but rather to a slower phosphorylation rate. This delay might be mediated by another kinase sharing similar substrate specificity such as DNA-PK or the ATM-related kinase ATR. On the other hand, the delay might be caused by reduced accessibility of RPA to repair sites. This might imply that there is a defect in AT chromatin structure. The evidences supporting this possibility are discussed below (repair parameters). Whether phosphorylation of RPA by ATM in response to IR is required for the S phase checkpoint is still not clear since overexpression of the ATM kinase domain is sufficient to restore the radioresistant DNA synthesis (RDS) defect without correcting the RPA phosphorylation status. Another important substrate of ATM for the S-phase checkpoint is the Nbs1 protein also known as nibrin or p95. Nbs1 is part of a large nuclease complex also containing Mre11 and Rad50 that is involved in repair of DSB generated at stalled replication forks. The nbs1 gene is mutated in the Nijmegen breakage syndrome (NBS), a syndrome sharing a variety of phenotypic abnormalities with ATM. Nbs1 is phosphorylated on Ser278, Ser343, Ser397, and Ser615 by ATM. Mutation of either Ser278 or Ser343 is sufficient to abrogate an S-phase checkpoint induced by IR. ATM binds directly to Nbs1; this interaction is enhanced upon DNA damage but ATM phosphorylation of Nbs1 does not affect Nbs1 binding to Mre11. However, ATM, the NBS proteins, and BRCA1 are part of a super complex named BASC (BRCA1-associated genome surveillance complex) that is thought to function as a sensor for DNA damage. It remains to be determined whether phosphorylation of Nbs1 by ATM affects the function of this large complex. One possible mechanism would be for ATM to help recruit the different members of the BASC complex as it helps recruit Nbs1, Mre11, and Rad50 to sites of DBS following IR. Another important ATM substrate for the S-phase checkpoint is the structural maintenance of chromosomes protein Smc1. ATM phosphorylates Smc1 on Ser957 and Ser966 in vivo and in vitro following IR. Optimal phosphorylation of Smc1 by ATM requires Nbs1 and BRCA1, but the reasons for this requirement are not clearly understood yet. It is possible that Nbs1 and BRAC1 are used as scaffold proteins to enhance ATM activity on Smc1. Mutations of the Smc1 protein at the ATM phosphorylation sites are sufficient to abrogate the IR-induced S-phase cell cycle checkpoint. As mentioned above, phosphorylation of chk2 by ATM provides a mechanism for ATM to control both G_1 and G_2 checkpoint. Phosphorylation of chk2 by ATM can also control the S-phase checkpoint through phosphorylation of the cdc25A phosphatase. Chk2 phosphosrylates cdc25A on Ser123 in response to IR in an ATM dependent manner. Phosphorylation of cdc25A triggers its degradation, which prevents dephosphorylation of cdk2 and arrest the cells in S phase.

2. Stress Response

Another class of substrates that are phosphorylated by ATM includes several important stress responsive proteins. ATM phosphorylates the non-receptor nuclear tyrosine kinase c-Abl on Ser465 in response to IR. This phosphorylation activates c-Abl which then phosphorylates its substrates such as the C-terminal repeated domain (CTD) of RNA polymerase II and the Jun N-terminal kinase (JNK), among others. JNK is a member of a subgroup of stress activated kinases known as the MAPKs that are activated by several cellular stresses including DNA damage. JNK stimulates the transcriptional activity of the AP-1 transcription factors such as c-*jun*. In AT cells, activation of the JNK pathway by IR is defective, but activation by UV radiation and protein synthesis inhibitors is intact. The inhibitor proteins known as IκB are also phosphorylated by ATM. IκB interacts with the transcription factor NFκB and prevent it from translocating to the nucleus by masking NFκB nuclear localization domain. Phosphorylation of IκB leads to its degradation and release of the NFκB to the nucleus where it can transactivate its downstream effector genes. NFκB is involved in the regulation of immunoglobulin genes and is a member of a gene family involved in lymphomagenesis. Moreover, NFκB is constitutively expressed at high levels in neurons, suggesting a possible link to central nervous symptoms in AT. Even though a functional ATM is required for IκB degradation, the pathway that leads to this degradation has not been elucidated yet but is likely to involve IKK, the kinase responsible for IκB phosphorylation.

3. DSB Repair

In addition to the Nbs1 protein, ATM also participates in the activation of other important proteins involved in DSB repair. The RAD51 protein is an indirect substrate of ATM; it is phosphorylated by c-Abl in an ATM dependent manner following IR exposure. Phosphorylation of RAD51 increases the interaction of RAD51 with RAD52, a complex mediating homologous recombinational repair.

C. Defect in Recombination and Chromatin Modification

A defect(s) in some form of DNA recombination in AT has been suggested based on the presence of spontaneously occurring chromosome translocations involving breakpoints in T-cell receptor (TCR) genes. Interestingly, the 70-fold increased frequency of TCR hybrid genes in AT lymphocytes does not affect the productivity nor the structure of the recombined TCR. This suggested that unlike the case with scid mice, the recombination process in AT cells is qualitatively normal. Using recombination vectors it has been shown that spontaneous intrachromosomal recombination rates are 30 to 200 times higher in AT fibroblasts line compared to normal cells, whereas extrachromosomal recombination frequencies are near normal. This indicates that the abnormality is specific to the AT chromosomal integrity and is not related to viral or plasmid DNA. The hyperrecombination rate is also particular to the AT phenotype and is not a consequence of defective DNA repair since cells from xeroderma pigmentosum patients, which are defective in excision repair, do not show abnormal recombination rates. The increased recombination rate is therefore an integral component of the AT phenotype and might contribute to genetic instability and an increased risk of cancer.

The defects in recombination may be linked to an ATM direct interaction with DNA and chromatin. ATM binds to meiotic chromosomes and is part of the recombination nodules, the structures thought to mediate chromatid exchanges. Fragmentation of meiotic chromosomes occurs at these sites in ATM deficient mice and may explain the infertility of these animals. A defective chromatin structure in AT has been suggested as a possible reason for the higher rate of conversion of

DNA double-strand breaks into chromosomes breaks. This was suggested based on apparent alterations of nucleosomal periodicity near the telomere chromatin. Moreover, a defective chromatin structure was also postulated to explain the inability of AT cells to stop DNA synthesis following exposure to IR. It is presumed that the defective chromatin structure could reduce accessibility of RPA to repair sites. The fact that in ATM deficient mice RPA remains attached to the ends of abnormal chromosomes fragments formed at the sites of the recombination nodules supports this possibility. There are several lines of evidence indicating that ATM could modulate the chromatin structure. First, transient dephosphorylation of histone H1, but not histone H3, following IR is ATM-dependent. Dephosphorylation of histone H1 is believed to increase chromatin decondensation. The exact pathways leading to H1 dephosphorylation have not been elucidated yet. Second, ATM rapidly interacts with the histone deacetylase HDAC1, both *in vivo* and *in vitro*. The amount of HDAC1 activity associated with ATM increases after IR. Histones deacetylation also decreases chromatin decondensation, which in turn is associated with increased radiosensitivity. A third line of evidence comes from ATM capacity to phosphorylate the histone H2A variant H2AX in response to DSB. Phosphorylation of H2AX at Ser139 is rapid (within 1–3 min) and specific to the sites of DNA damage. In yeast, H2AX phosphorylation causes chromatin decondensation, while in mammals it mediates the recruitment of repair or damage signaling factors such as BRCA1, Nbs1, RAD50, and RAD51 to the sites of DNA damage. H2AX phosphorylation following IR is severely compromised in *ATM* −/− cells but phosphorylation of H2AX can be restored by ectopic expression of ATM in these cells.

D. Abnormal Apoptosis

The control of the cell number in each lineage is determined by a balance between cell proliferation and cell death. The process regulating cell proliferation is highly regulated with numerous checks and balances. The regulation of cell death is now appearing to be as complex as cell proliferation. Differentiated cells have the ability to carry out their own death through the activation of an internal suicide program called apoptosis. The apoptotic process is usually turned on to eliminate cells that have developed improperly, have been produced in excess, or have sustained irreparable damage to their DNA. Apoptotic cell death is different from necrotic cell death which is a pathological form of death resulting from acute cellular injury. The difference between these two forms of death can be observed morphologically. Cells dying from necrosis will swell rapidly and lyse which will result in the leakage of cytoplasmic contents and the induction of an inflammatory response. An apoptotic cell undergoes a controlled autodigestion with the maintenance of the plasma membrane integrity and therefore no inflammatory response. In mouse, ATM is essential for IR-induced apoptosis in the developing nervous system. ATM-mediated apoptosis in the nervous system also required p53 and the pro-apoptotic effector Bax. The apoptotic response in ATM null mice is defective but the precise role of ATM in apoptosis is still debated. The conflicting results often reported in the literature may be associated with the cell types, the different apoptotic stimuli, or even the cellular states (proliferative vs quiescent) of the cells used by the investigators. Interestingly, AT fibroblasts are unusually sensitive to drugs that also produce internucleosomal DNA cleavage, characteristic of apoptosis. Widespread apoptosis was detectable in four A-T fibroblast lines, AT22IJE, AT4BVI, AT5BIVA, and AT2SFSV, representing complementation groups A, C, and D, but not in two control lines. Apoptosis began 24 hr after exposure to X rays or streptonigrin (radiomimetic agent) and peaked 72 to 96 hr following treatment. No apoptotic differences were detected between AT and control fibroblasts following exposure to 30 J/m^2 of UV irradiation. Streptonigrin also induced widespread apoptotis in A-T lymphoblasts but not in control lymphoblasts. The interval between exposure of cells to apoptotic agents and the induction of apoptosis can be short, being detected in some instances as soon as 4 hr after exposure. The significant delay in AT to trigger the apoptosis machinery might be due to a defect in the same pathway responsible for the loss of G$_1$ delay since p53 is required for radiation-induced apoptosis. Recent evidence, however, suggests that c-Abl may rather link ATM to p73, a member of the growing p53-like family that is not induced by DNA damage but plays a role in damage-induced apoptosis. In response to ATM phosphorylation, c-Abl phosphorylates and activates p73. As mentioned above, one of the AT gene domains shares homology with PI-3 kinase. PI-3 kinase is required for the prevention of apoptosis in rat pheochromocytoma cells by nerve growth factor. This facet of the AT gene might correlate with the increased nerve cell death in AT and the increased apoptosis in cultured AT cells exposed to DNA-damaging agents.

IV. FUTURE DIRECTIONS

Since the cloning of the ATM gene, tremendous efforts have been directed at delineating ATM functions in cell cycle regulation, sensing of DNA damage, and initiation of DNA repair mechanisms. The predominantly nuclear localization of the protein is in good agreement with these important cellular functions. However, it is now becoming evident that ATM probably plays other important roles in cellular homeostasis that may be mediated by the small pool of cytoplasmic protein. For example, ATM could react with ROS (reactive oxygen species) in the cytosol and affect the redox state of a cell. Several lines of evidence are supporting a role for ATM in the oxidative stress response. For instance, increased levels of ROS have been detected in the cerebellum of ATM deficient mice. The absence of ATM may thus result in oxidative damage and cause the degeneration of cerebellar neurons. The variety of symptoms and cellular AT phenotypes indicate that certain AT substrates are likely to be involved in mechanisms other than the ones related to the DNA damage response. Substrates found in the cytosol, such as the translational regulatory protein 4E-BP-1, are good examples of this possibility. ATM phosphorylates this regulatory protein in response to insulin stimulation. There is also evidence that ATM may be linked to growth factor mediated pathways such as the insulin-like growth factor-1 receptor (IGF-1R). Transcriptional expression of IGF-1R appears to be ATM-dependent. The identification of the different proteins interacting with ATM as well as the ATM domains involved in these interactions will allow the development of drugs that can specifically target a given pathway and will eventually lead to efficient treatments for this devastating disease. Future treatments will also probably include different genetic approaches such as anti-sense ATM to sensitize radioresistant tumors to radiation. The most challenging symptom that remains to be alleviated is the progressive neurodegeneration. Targeting ATM or smaller part of the gene to the Purkinje cells will be a difficult challenge but the use of ATM −/− mice models will surely help direct these efforts. Identification of the AT gene is a major breakthrough; the discovery of this pleiotropic gene will provide tools to better understand several fundamental cellular mechanisms that have implications far beyond the AT syndrome.

See Also the Following Articles

CELL CYCLE CHECKPOINTS • EWING'S SARCOMA (EWING'S FAMILY TUMORS) • IMMUNE DEFICIENCY: OPPORTUNISTIC TUMORS • LI-FRAUMENI SYNDROME • MOLECULAR ASPECTS OF RADIATION BIOLOGY • PEDIATRIC CANCERS, MOLECULAR FEATURES • RECOMBINATION • TELOMERES AND TELOMERASE

Bibliography

Carrier, F., and Fornace, A. J., Jr. (1996). Ataxia-telangiectasia syndrome. In "Encyclopedia of Cancer" (J. R. Bertino, ed.), Vol. 1, pp. 100–111. Academic Press, San Diego.

Falck, J., Mailand, N., Syljuasen, R. G., Bartek, J., and Lukas, J. (2001). The ATM-Chk2-Cdcc25A checkpoint pathway guards against radioresistant DNA synthesis. *Nature* **410**, 842–847.

Kim, S.-T., Xu, B., and Kastan, M. B. (2002). Involvement of the cohesin protein, Smc1 in Atm-dependent and independent responses to DNA damage. *Gene Devel.* **16**, 560–570.

Lavin, M. F. (1999). ATM: the product of the gene mutated in ataxia telangiectasia. *Intl. J. Biochem. Cell. Biol.* **31**, 735–740.

Meyn, M. S. (1999). Ataxia-telangiectasia, cancer and the pathobiology of the ATM gene. *Clin. Genet.* **55**, 289–304.

Mullan, P. B., Quinn, J. E., Gilmore, P. M., McWilliams, S., Andrews, H., Gervin, C., McCabe, N., McKenna, S., White, P., Song, Y.-H., Maheswaran, S., Liu, E., Haber, D. A., Johnston, P. G., and Harkin, D. P. (2001). BRCA1 and GADD45 mediated G2/M cell cycle arrest in response to antimicrotubule agents. *Oncogene* **20**, 6123–6131.

Rotman, G., and Shiloh, Y. (1999). ATM: A mediator of multiple responses to genotoxic stress. *Oncogene* **18**, 6135–6143.

Shiloh, Y. (2001). ATM (ataxia telangiectasia mutated): expanding roles in the DNA damage response and cellular homeostasis. *Biochem. Soc. Trans.* **29**, 661–666.

Shiloh, Y. (2001). ATM and ATR: networking cellular responses to DNA damage. *Curr. Opin. Genet. Devel.* **11**, 71–77.

Taylor, W. R., and Stark, G. R. (2001). Regulation of the G2/M transition by p53. *Oncogene* **20**, 1803–1815.

Autocrine and Paracrine Growth Mechanisms in Cancer Progression and Metastasis

Garth L. Nicolson

The Institute for Molecular Medicine, Huntington Beach, California

GLOSSARY

autocrine growth factors Growth factors that are made by and that act on the same cell.

metastasis The spread of tumor cells via the lymph, blood, or body cavities to near or distant sites where new secondary tumors are formed.

paracrine growth factors Growth factors that are made and secreted by one cell and that act on adjacent cells in a tissue or organ.

tumor diversification Generation of heterogeneous subpopulations of tumor cells with differing phenotypes.

tumor instability Changes in tumor cell properties caused by irreversible modifications in the coding sequences of genes and by quantitative changes in gene expression.

tumor progression Sequential changes in tumorigenic and malignant properties of tumors that occur with time *in vivo*. The changes generally tend toward more malignant, dangerous states.

O ne of the most important characteristics of cancer cells is their ability to grow in unusual locations, especially at metastatic sites. The successful proliferation of cancer cells is due to their responses to local (paracrine) growth factors and inhibitors and their production and responses to their own (autocrine) growth factors. As tumors grow and evolve (tumor progression), they undergo changes in their growth and other properties. For example, when tumor cells invade and spread to other sites at the early stages of malignant tumor progression, there is a tendency for many common cancers to metastasize and grow preferentially at particular sites, suggesting that unique tissue paracrine growth mechanisms may dominate the growth signals processed by metastatic cells. At somewhat later stages of tumor progression, where widespread dissemination to various tissues and organs occurs, autocrine growth mechanisms may dominate. The progression of malignant cells to completely autonomous growth states can occur, and at this stage of tumor progression cell proliferation may be independent of growth factors or inhibitors.

I. INTRODUCTION

Most patients succumb to their metastatic disease, not their primary tumors; therefore, controlling the spread and growth of malignant cells at metastatic sites is an important challenge. Malignant tumors are characterized by differences in various properties, and those that are functionally involved in invasion and metastasis are among the most important properties of cancer cells that determine their survival and growth at secondary sites.

In addition to their invasive and metastatic properties, highly malignant cells are characterized by progressive changes in their genomes, particularly in genes that regulate and encode products important in certain phenotypic properties. Highly malignant cells are not particularly stable and they continually drift in their phenotypic properties. In some cases, such phenotypic drift in cancer cell properties is virtually undetectable, but in other cases it can be dramatic and result in obvious tumor cell heterogeneity. Advanced primary tumors that have not yet metastasized and cancers that have metastasized are made up of very dynamic, unstable cellular assemblages. The individual cancer cells that are unstable do not always undergo phenotypic drift. In some cases they interact with other tumor and normal cells that can stabilize the cell population as a whole and reduce the tendency for individual cells to diversify and become more variable in a variety of properties.

If malignant cells break loose from their primary site as individual cells or small groups of cells, some of these cells can diversify further and become even more heterogeneous in their properties. As stated earlier, this can occur because individual cells are modulated in their phenotypic properties by interactions with other cells. Once removed from these interactions, cancer cells undergo phenotypic diversification. Therefore, the invasion of individual cells away from the initial tumor site and into new tissue compartments can lead to cancer cells with differing properties from the primary tumors from which they were derived. However, most cellular properties do not change detectably as tumor cells in advanced primary tumors metastasize to distant sites. This may be due to the fact that advanced primary tumors have already undergone significant diversification and change.

Tumor cells progress to the malignant state and eventually the metastatic state in a process that is thought to occur by a stepwise series of genetic and epigenetic (nongenetic) changes. These changes occur apparently randomly, and accumulating enough changes necessary for a cancer cell to become highly metastatic can take years. Such metastatic cells were previously thought to be very rare cells that occasionally arose within the primary tumor, and it was thought that only these rare phenotypically stable cells were the cells capable of metastasizing. Although tumor progression can result in stepwise nonreversible changes and acquisition of a number of phenotypic properties that are important in the process of metastasis, it is now thought that tumor progression to the metastatic phenotype depends less on the selection of rare, stable metastatic cells than on the inherent instabilities of the tumor cells that comprise the primary neoplasm. This notion was advanced by Victor Ling, Ann Chambers, Richard Hill, and their colleagues at the Ontario Cancer Institute. They envisaged that malignant tumor cells are constantly undergoing rapid dynamic phenotypic changes in a process they called dynamic heterogeneity. Independently from the group in Canada, my colleagues and I at the University of Texas M. D. Anderson Cancer Center studied this phenomenon and termed it phenotypic drift. In either scheme individual cancer cells are thought to be changing constantly from the metastatic to nonmetastatic phenotype and back to the metastatic phenotype. When the rate of change favors the appearance of metastatic cells, a tumor progresses to a more malignant phenotype capable of metastasizing.

Tumor phenotypic instability is probably due, in part, to essentially irreversible qualitative changes in gene structure (gene mutations, deletions, transpositions, amplifications, etc.) that can result in altered gene products and to dynamic quantitative changes in gene expression. The quantitative changes in gene expression result in transient changes in the amounts of various gene products in individual cancer cells. The net result is cellular variability within a primary tumor and eventually transient or, in some cases, even permanent acquisition of the metastatic phenotype by individual malignant cells. It is probably these unstable, highly malignant cells that ultimately give rise to tumor colonies at other sites. This could explain the problem in determining the particular molecular characteristics of metastatic cells. If metastatic cells possess unstable properties important in malignancy, these would be expected to be difficult to identify.

In contrast to the various unstable properties of metastatic cells, the proliferative properties required for survival and growth of metastatic cells at secondary sites must remain relatively stable if metastases grow to detectable sizes. Without stable tumor cell growth, only micrometastases would be present, and these would not be expected to kill the host. Thus an understanding of the process of malignant cell growth and its interference at metastatic sites may be important in the development of new therapies for restraining the growth of established metastases.

II. CANCER PROGRESSION AND PARACRINE GROWTH OF METASTATIC CELLS

As cancer progresses and individual cancer cells eventually acquire more malignant phenotypes, under the proper circumstances, they can invade and metastasize to near and distant sites. For many cancers this process is not random and cannot be explained by the anatomic site of the cancer or mechanical properties of cancer cells. Many cancers metastasize to sites unexpected on the basis of their circulatory or lymphatic connections or on their ability to mechanically lodge in the first lymph node or capillary bed encountered by cancer cells released from the primary cancer site. For example, the metastasis of cutaneous malignant melanoma to the brain but ocular malignant melanoma to the liver, prostate carcinoma to the bone, or colon carcinoma to the liver are examples of nonrandom metastatic spread. In addition, during tumor progression the evolving malignant cells can change in their tissue-metastatic properties. This observation has been made for a number of different histologic classes of cancer.

At the initial stages of metastasis, many possess a tendency to metastasize to particular sites. This so-called organ specificity or organ preference of metastasis occurs at early stages of metastatic progression, but at later stages of progression where metastasis is widespread and many secondary sites are involved, more organs and tissues are colonized by metastatic cells. Strictly speaking, the site specificity of cancer metastasis is usually only a *preference* for colonizing certain sites; it is not entirely a site-specific process, except for very few cancers. Nonetheless, it is an important phenomenon that appears to be based on the unique properties of the cancer cells as well as the host microenvironments. This notion was first advanced over 100 years ago by Stephen Paget, who was treating breast cancer patients in London. Paget advanced the "seed" and "soil" hypothesis that individual cancer cells or seeds can only grow in suitable soil. In terms of their growth properties, neoplastic cells that progress to the metastatic phenotype and colonize distant sites should be less dependent on their usual growth signals and more growth responsive to growth signals at their new metastatic sites.

The increased responsiveness of some cancer cells to paracrine growth factors or decreased responsiveness to paracrine growth inhibitors expressed differentially at particular metastatic sites could explain why certain cancers show a preference for metastatic growth at certain sites. This could also explain the finding of increased numbers or affinities of particular growth factor receptors and enhanced responses to certain growth factors. Overexpression of specific growth factor receptors correlates with progression and metastasis of certain cancers. For example, the epidermal growth factor (EGF) receptor is often associated with poor prognosis or enhanced metastasis in breast, lung, and bladder cancers and melanomas. In some cases, overexpression of an oncogene, such as c-erbB-2/neu-encoded putative growth factor receptor, is associated with poor prognosis of breast and ovarian carcinomas. Other examples of alterations exist in growth factor receptors, but in general, those growth factor receptors that are probably important in metastasis are usually the ones that change in their expression in highly metastatic cancers.

The overexpression of growth factor receptors has been accomplished experimentally by gene transfer techniques, and the biological properties of the recipient cells can be tested in suitable animal hosts. For example, in my department at the University of Texas M. D. Anderson Cancer Center, Dihua Yu, Mienchie Hung, and I found that the transfer of a mutated c-erbB-2/neu oncogene into benign cells resulted in conversion to the metastatic phenotype. Although the changes in metastatic properties and enhanced growth potential of the growth factor receptor gene-transferred cells can be explained by oncogene transfer, this experimental result is not always found. Changes in the metastatic properties of c-erbB-2/neu gene-transferred cells occurred concomitant with changes in several metastasis-associated properties, including increased adhesion to microvessel endothelial cells, particularly endothelial cells derived from the target organs for metastasis, increased invasiveness of extracellular matrix and reconstituted basement membrane matrix, increased cell motility in response to organ-derived chemotactic factors that stimulate directed tumor cell invasion, and increased responses to organ-derived paracrine growth factors. In these experiments we found that the oncogene-mediated conversion of benign tumor cells to metastatic cells was accompanied by changes in growth factor receptor expression and growth factor responses as well as by changes in the expression of other gene products involved in various steps of the metastatic process.

To test the hypothesis that organ growth properties are important in organ preference of metastasis, we found that the organ preference of metastatic cell growth, at least at the initial stages of metastatic progression, was related to the differential responses of metastatic cells to paracrine growth factors and inhibitors secreted by the target organ tissues. Therefore, differentially expressed paracrine growth factors and inhibitors in different organs and tissues probably determine, to some degree, the growth potentials of cancer cells at metastatic sites. Thus cancers, at least at their initial stages, should be dependent on paracrine growth factors released from surrounding normal cells. After progression to the metastatic phenotype, growth factor responses are often changed, and they should be more compatible with the responses to cytokines expressed at secondary metastatic sites.

Tumor models have been used to demonstrate that the organ preference of metastasis is related to enhanced growth responses mediated by cytokines, growth factors, and inhibitors released at secondary organ sites. Using lung- and ovary-colonizing murine melanoma sublines and liver- and lung-metastasizing large cell lymphoma cell lines, we demonstrated that tumor cell growth in serum-limited culture medium was differentially stimulated by soluble factors released from different organ tissues. In these examples, lung- and liver-metastatic tumor cells were growth stimulated better by factors released from lung and liver tissue, respectively. In contrast, other tissue-conditioned media inhibited or had no effect on tumor cell growth.

Tissue-derived growth-promoting substances have been identified and partially purified from the culture medium conditioned by certain organ tissues. For example, we purified to homogeneity a lung-derived metastatic cell growth factor from lung-conditioned medium, and from its amino acid sequence we were able to identify the growth factor as a transferrin. Transferrins are iron-transferring ferroproteins that are required for cell growth. Some years ago Pedro Cuatrecasas found that transferrins are more than iron transport proteins and that they have mitogenic properties beyond their nutrient transport. The tissue-derived transferrins that we isolated are probably used as paracrine growth stimulators in several tissues. The transferrin isolated from lung tissue-conditioned medium was the first tumor cell growth factor purified to homogeneity on the basis of its ability to differentially stimulate the growth of highly metastatic cells. We examined a number of different tumor metastatic systems and found that several other metastatic cell lines were more responsive to transferrin. To demonstrate that a transferrin-like activity in tissue-conditioned medium is responsible, in part, for the stimulation of metastatic cell growth, transferrin-like molecules were removed from tissue-conditioned medium. After the removal of transferrin molecules, most of the growth properties of the organ tissue-conditioned medium were lost.

Other organ compartments are also important sites of metastatic involvement and apparently have their own set of important cytokines. For example, bone is an important metastatic site for prostate cancer, and transferrin was found to be a major growth factor for bone-metastasizing prostatic carcinoma cells. How are transferrins used as specific organ cytokines if they are found at several organ sites? The answer may be that the relative concentrations of the transferrins and other cytokines in different tissues are different. Using a series of melanoma cell lines of differing metastatic potentials to sites such as brain, we found that brain- and lung-colonizing melanoma lines responded best to the lowest concentrations of transferrins and expressed the highest numbers of transferrin receptors. Transferrin receptor numbers were highest in brain metastatic lines and decreased in the following order: high brain-metastasizing ability > high lung-metastasizing ability > intermediate lung-metastasizing ability > poor metastatic capability. Thus, a hierarchy of transferrin expression exists in different organs and may be important in determining metastatic cell growth. Cancer cells with greater numbers of transferrin receptors (or different affinities) may be more successful at growing at sites that express low concentrations of transferrin molecules.

Brain is an example of an organ that is not particularly susceptible to metastatic colonization. Brain metastases are rarely produced by cancers, but in some malignancies, such as melanoma and breast cancer, brain metastases are quite commonly found. For malignant cells to metastasize to brain, it may be advantageous for them to express high numbers of particular growth factor receptors, such as transferrin receptors, and respond to low concentrations of growth factors, such as the transferrins. Further support for the evolution of enhanced transferrin re-sponsiveness and the metastasis of various tumor cells comes from the selection of high transferrin receptor-expressing variants from poorly metastatic cells. The high transferrin receptor-expressing cells displayed increased spontaneous metastatic properties and grew faster compared to low transferrin receptor-expressing cells. Brain-metastasizing cancer cells appear to also respond to other paracrine growth factors at secondary sites, and it is likely that paracrine sources of transferrin provide only one of several growth factors important in determining the organ preference of metastatic cell growth. Differences in the concentrations of various cytokines, growth factors, and inhibitors may be important in providing the correct environment for metastatic cell growth.

The normal functions of paracrine growth factors are not known, but they might be involved in controlling cell growth and local tissue regeneration during wounding and inflammation. Metastases often occur at the sites of trauma or tissue damage. Thus the normal role of the paracrine growth factors and growth inhibitors is probably in organ repair.

Another source of organ-derived growth-promoting molecules are extracellular matrix, tissue stroma, and basement membranes. Extracellular matrix and basement membranes contain tightly bound growth factors that can be released by tumor cell degradative enzymes and stimulate tumor cell growth. Extracellular matrix molecules themselves may modulate tumor cell growth and the state of tumor cell differentiation. For example, the maintenance of normal breast cells is dependent on lactogenic hormones and extracellular matrix, and matrix molecules can regulate gene expression and growth of particular normal cells. Metastatic cells often show differential growth responses to extracellular matrix molecules. Using extracellular matrix obtained from several organs, Lola Reid and collaborators at the Albert Einstein Medical Center found that metastatic mammary carcinoma and hepatoma cells were differentially stimulated to grow at low cell densities by organ matrix isolated from the target organs for metastasis formation. However, they did not find the same pattern of growth stimulation if metastatic cells were plated at high cell densities on the various extracellular matrices, suggesting that extracellular matrix growth stimulatory molecules are more important at the early stages of cancer cell growth, such as in micrometastases, rather than at the later stages of cell growth at high cell densities, such as would be expected in gross clinically detectable metastases. Thus the unique growth microenvironments for cancer cells in various organs and tissues are probably determined collectively by tumor cell responses to cell-bound, matrix-bound, and soluble paracrine factors.

III. PARACRINE GROWTH INHIBITORS OF METASTATIC CELLS

Cancer cells also receive and process paracrine negative growth signals. Only a few organ-derived paracrine growth inhibitory molecules have been identified. In most cases these have turned out to be well-known cytokines, such as the transforming growth factor-β (TGF-β) family. Certain organ cells can release potent growth inhibitors that prevent the growth of malignant cells, and these factors could be important in determining metastatic cell growth at particular sites. For example, kidney cell-conditioned medium is particularly inhibitory for many cancer cells, and most cancers and metastatic model systems fail to metastasize to the kidney. The most potent growth inhibitor released by kidney tissue has been identified as TGF-β1. TGF-β1 can inhibit the growth of several highly metastatic cell lines. Not all metastatic cells are growth inhibited by TGF-β, but this family of cytokines is very important in cancer metastasis. An interesting finding is the growth stimulation of metastatic cells by TGF-β and the inhibition of growth of tumor cells from primary sites, but this does not appear to be a general phenomenon.

The growth responses of malignant cells can change during progression to more malignant phenotypes. For example, the growth responses of early lateral growth phase human melanoma cells and more advanced vertical growth phase melanoma cells have been studied by Robert Kerbel and Meenhard Herlyn. Only the vertical growth phase melanomas are dangerous, and patients with these lesions are at risk to develop metastases. Studies on the responses of melanoma cells to positive and negative growth cytokines indicated that the more progressed melanoma cells lose responsiveness to negative growth inhibitors.

The molecule responsible for differentially inhibiting the growth of early lateral growth phase melanoma cells was purified and shown to be interleukin-6 (IL-6), a well-known hemopoietic cytokine. This cytokine is produced by a variety of tissues, among them keratinocytes, endothelial cells, fibroblasts, macrophages, and monocytes. The inhibitory responses to recombinant IL-6 were not duplicated with more advanced vertical growth phase melanoma cells. It was subsequently established that the more highly progressed metastatic cells uniformly lost responsiveness to a variety of growth inhibitors. Loss of paracrine inhibitor responses could be as important to the formation of metastasis as changes in paracrine growth factor responsiveness.

IV. SOURCES OF PARACRINE GROWTH FACTORS AND INHIBITORS

The sources of paracrine growth factors and inhibitors in various organ tissues are largely undetermined. Parenchymal cells, fibroblasts, endothelial cells, mast cells, and macrophages, among other cell types, and factors from acellular sources, including interstitial extracellular matrix and basement membranes, could collectively provide various growth factors and inhibitors. Some of the growth factors expressed by parenchymal cells are released as soluble molecules, whereas some are not released and require cell–cell or cell–matrix contact. When lung- and liver-colonizing malignant melanoma cells were cocultured with normal hepatocytes, Max Burger and colleagues found that only liver-colonizing melanoma cells were growth stimulated. The stimulation required cell-to-cell contact with the hepatocytes and was not duplicated with liver tissue-conditioned medium. Thus in some metastatic systems, organ parenchymal cells are important sources of tumor cell growth stimulation.

Microvascular endothelial cells are important in metastatic cell growth. Using lung- and liver-colonizing large cell lymphoma cells, we showed that conditioned medium from organ-derived microvessel endothelial cells could substitute for organ tissue-conditioned medium in tumor cell proliferation assays. Interestingly, liver-colonizing large cell lymphoma cells responded best to conditioned medium from liver sinusoidal endothelial cells, whereas lung-colonizing lymphoma cells responded best to conditioned medium from lung microvessel endothelial cells. Removal of transferrin from the lung endothelial cell-conditioned medium resulted in a reduction of mitogenic activity, but some activity remained that was not associated with transferrin. Endothelial cells can respond, in turn, to growth and motility factors, called angiogenesis factors, released by malignant cells. A reciprocal relationship may exist between tumor cells and specific organ-derived normal cells (Fig. 1). This relationship extends to other cell types as well as to extracellular matrix. Thus malignant cells can stimulate as well as be stimulated by normal host cells.

Fibroblasts isolated from different tissues have been used to differentially stimulate the growth of cancer cells. Using lateral and vertical growth phase melanoma cells, the growth responses of these cells to fibroblasts from various tissue sources have been tested in cocultures. Fibroblasts isolated from dermal tissue generally inhibited the growth of early lateral growth phase human melanoma cells but had stimulatory or little effect on more advanced vertical growth phase melanoma cells. In this case, the inhibitory molecule

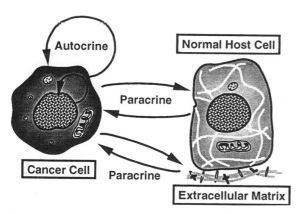

FIGURE 1 Reciprocal interactions between malignant cells and their cellular microenvironments. Cancer cells release paracrine factors that can affect host cells, such as parenchymal cells, endothelial cells, fibroblasts, mast cells, granulocytes, macrophages, and tissue extracellular matrix. In turn, the host cells and matrix can release paracrine factors that stimulate or inhibit tumor cell proliferation. Tumor cells can also synthesize autocrine factors that can act inside the cell (private or intracellular) or outside the cell (public or extracellular).

responsible was identified as IL-6 released by dermal fibroblasts. We also found that metastatic and non-metastatic mammary carcinoma cells responded differentially to tissue-derived fibroblast-conditioned medium, and this was related to the organ preference of metastasis. The highest growth stimulation was from fibroblasts isolated from lung and mammary gland, targets for metastatic cell growth in this system. The fibroblast-derived growth factor was not related to transferrin because we demonstrated that the organ-derived fibroblasts did not synthesize detectable amounts of transferrin. Peter Jones has examined the growth properties of bladder carcinomas of different grade and invasive properties. Using bladder carcinomas of differing grade, differentiation, and invasive properties, only the poorly differentiated high-grade, invasive bladder carcinoma cells were growth stimulated by bladder-derived fibroblasts. When prostate carcinoma cells were cocultured with fibroblasts from different tissue sources, an interesting relationship was found. Similar to the reciprocal relationship between cancer cells and endothelial cells, bidirectional stimulation of growth was seen by Lelung Chung when conditioned medium from prostate carcinoma cells was tested with conditioned medium from bone fibroblasts. Because bone is a common site of prostate metastases, this suggested that prostate carcinoma cells stimulate and are stimulated by target bone fibroblasts. This reciprocal or bilateral relationship between metastatic cells and host cells in the target site for metastasis appears to be an important feature of metastatic cell colonization (Fig. 2).

Mast cells are another source of mitogens and motility factors for metastatic cells. Similar to the process of inflammation, mast cells are attracted to tumor sites by the release of mast cell mediators. Mast cells often associate at the periphery of tumors and can release tumor cell mitogens and motility factors that can differentially affect the growth and motility of malignant cells. With Mustafa Dabbous we found that only highly metastatic mammary cells attracted large numbers of mast cells into the tumor periphery. Mast cells isolated from the tumor periphery were found to release factors that differentially stimulated the growth of the highly metastatic but not poorly metastatic cells. A function for the mast cell mitogens was shown *in vivo* by administering drugs that are

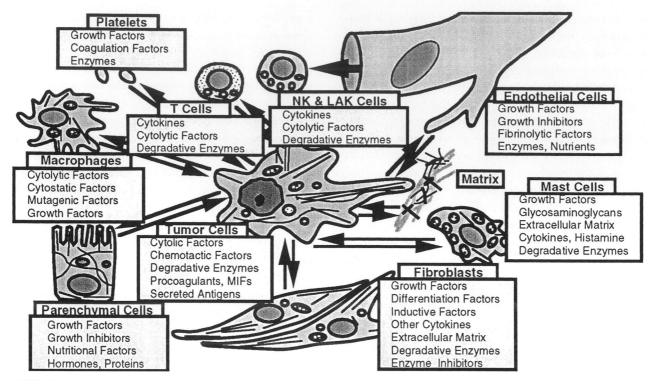

FIGURE 2   Tumor microenvironment and the role of paracrine cytokines in regulating tumor cell growth, differentiation, and malignant properties. Reciprocal or bidirectional interactions between various cells in the tumor microenvironment are important in the establishment of the tumor microenvironment.

mast cell stabilizers to animals receiving metastatic cell implants. Mast cell stabilizers prevented the release of mast cell contents and reduced the growth and metastases of the highly metastatic cells growing at their normal organ sites.

V. AUTOCRINE GROWTH MECHANISMS IN CANCER METASTASIS

Cancer cells have the capacity to synthesize and release multiple growth factors that can act on the tumor cells themselves in tumor cell autocrine loop mechanisms. This can occur either by extracellular release of the growth factor and its binding to an appropriate extracellular receptor on the same cell (public or extracellular autocrine mechanism) or by ligand–receptor interaction inside the cell (private or intracellular autocrine mechanism, Fig. 1). When highly malignant and metastatic cells are examined for the synthesis of autocrine growth factors, they are commonly found to make and use a variety of growth factors. Interestingly, these are often the same growth factors that normally stimulate the growth of normal cells from which the tumor cells were derived.

Autocrine growth factors play an important role in neoplastic transformation, but their role in cancer metastasis is somewhat less clear. Studies on tumor cells derived from primary and metastatic sites or sequential selection of malignant or metastatic variants have yielded important but inconclusive data on the role of autocrine growth factors in metastasis. As tumors progress to more malignant or metastatic phenotypes, they generally become less dependent on serum-derived growth factors for their growth and they begin to produce polypeptide growth factors, suggesting that autocrine growth mechanisms may be involved in metastasis formation. There are, however, examples where the autocrine production of a growth factor by malignant cells did not correlate with tumor progression or stage. For example, the production and secretion of melanoma growth-stimulating activity by melanoma cells and bombesin-like (gastrin-releasing peptide) activity by small cell lung carcinoma cells were not related to tumor stage or tumor progression. The usual result is a loss of growth factor responsiveness with tumor progression to the metastatic phenotype. For example, Meenhard Herlyn and collaborators found that cell lines established from dysplastic nevi had similar growth factor requirements to normal melanocytes, whereas malignant melanoma cell lines had reduced requirements for a variety of growth factors. Only cell lines established from melanoma metastases could be quickly adapted to *in vitro* growth in serum-free medium. When they sequentially selected human melanoma cell lines that were established from a primary melanoma lesion for their ability to invade a reconstituted basement membrane, they showed that only the most invasive tumor cell variants were spontaneously metastatic in nude mice and that these same cell lines were less serum dependent for growth in tissue culture. Selection for growth in serum-free medium resulted in increases in invasive and metastatic properties, but the selected melanoma cell lines were unstable and in the absence of continued selective pressure reverted back to the phenotype of the parental cell line. The relative instability of metastasis-associated properties was mentioned earlier, and transient changes in gene expression are expected when a strong selective pressure is removed from a population of inherently unstable malignant cells.

The release of autocrine cytokines can also produce effects on neighboring cancer cells. The release of a cytokine from one tumor cell and its effect on neighboring cells is a form of paracrine signaling among tumor cell populations that may be important in modifying the properties of the tumor. In a few cases, the clonal effects of tumor cells on surrounding tumor cells have been examined and found to affect tumor cell properties, especially malignant cell properties. When we examined the interclonal interactions of a series of melanoma cell lines, we found that the expression and the display of a cell surface glycoprotein that later was identified as a growth factor receptor were affected by clonal cell interactions along with metastatic properties. Here the interclonal tumor cell interactions stabilized the phenotypic properties of the malignant cells, but when the malignant cells were grown separately, they quickly lost their metastatic and organ growth properties. Thus tumor cell–cell and host cell–tumor cell interactions are important in the metastasis and growth of malignant cells.

In some tumor systems, both paracrine and autocrine signals are important in metastasis. For example, hepatocyte growth factor, which is also known as scatter factor (HGF/SF), plays autocrine and paracine roles in both cell motility and growth. The HGF/SF receptor at the cell surface is encoded by the oncogene *met* or its normal cell counterpart, c-*met*. HGF/SF has been shown to be synthesized by a number of mesenchymal cell types, and it can act as a paracrine stimulator of metastasis at specific organ sites, such as liver and lung. Certain melanoma cells selected for liver-specific metastasis overexpress the HGF/SF receptor, and exposure of these cells to HGF augments cell motility and invasive behavior. Upregulation of c-*met* in these cells and its HGF/SF receptor by various methods increases liver colonization ability but does not change the organ metastatic specificities of these cells. Treatment of certain mammary adenocarcinoma cells with HGF stimulates their ability to metastasize to lung.

VI. GENE TRANSFER AND METASTATIC CELL GROWTH PROPERTIES

Transfer of a growth factor gene or a growth factor receptor gene into suitable untransformed recipient cells can result in these cells acquiring malignant growth characteristics. For example, we found that transfection of the transferrin receptor gene resulted in an increased ability to grow in serum-free medium with transferrin as the sole supplement along with acquisition of the metastatic phenotype. In other experiments, transfer of the oncogene c-*sis* that encodes the platelet-derived growth factor (PDGF) receptor, c-*erb*B-1 that encodes the EGF receptor, or c-*erb*B-2/*neu* that encodes a growth factor-related receptor by use of viruses increases the growth potential of the gene-transferred cells, resulting in oncogenic transformation. In some cases, however, the transfer of a growth factor gene does not result in neoplastic transformation unless the encoded growth factor is synthesized in a form that can be cell secreted and bind to a cell surface receptor. For example, Michael Klagsbrun found that the addition of basic fibroblast growth factor (bFGF) by itself or transfer of the bFGF gene alone was not transforming to recipient cells. However, when the bFGF gene was fused to a secretion signal sequence to facilitate bFGF secretion, only the chimeric signal peptide–bFGF gene was transforming. In this example, the appropriate location of the growth factor was important to its ability to signal growth. In addition to tumor cell growth, FGFs are also important in endothelial cell proliferation and angiogenesis.

Using gene transfer techniques to stimulate cells to secrete growth factors and become transformed in the process assumes that the technique itself does not cause other changes in the recipient cell. This turns out to be important because highly malignant cells are also unstable, and the gene transfer techniques can destabilize cells in a process that leads to cellular instability, diversification, and cellular heterogeneity. Controversy exists as to whether additional genomic changes are required for the transformation of cells that have received growth factor genes. An example of this is the use of transforming sequence containing a gene for one of the PDGF polypeptide chains. The PDGF molecule is made up of two polypeptide (A and B) chains. Only the B chain gene was found to have a transforming sequence in at least two retroviruses, a class of transforming virus that has a propensity to pick up critical host gene sequences that can transform normal cells to neoplastic cells. The PDGF receptor homologue that constitutes the c-sis retroviral gene is oncogenic, suggesting the importance of growth factor genes and their receptors in neoplastic transformation. Although overexpression of the c-sis oncogene can result in neoplastic transformation, the addition of excess PDGF to untransformed cells does not reproduce this phenomenon. This apparent paradox can be explained by considering that the increased rate of cell proliferation caused by PDGF probably results in expansion of a subpopulation of preneoplastic cells that are potential targets for oncogenic transformation. Alternatively, the insertion of the growth factor gene itself causes mutation of cellular genes or other changes that are necessary for neoplastic transformation.

Gene transfer techniques have been used to test for the involvement of autocrine growth mechanisms in metastasis formation. Transfection of human breast cancer cells with the HGF/SF gene establishes an autocrine loop, and these cells demonstrate a greater propensity to metastasize to the lung. Cotransfection of murine 3T3 cells with genes encoding HGF/SF and its receptor results in cells that acquire the metastatic phenotype, especially lung-metastatic ability. Arnold Greenberg and collaborators used a transforming chimeric bFGF gene construct to transfect untransformed but highly unstable preneoplastic cells. The signal peptide–bFGF chimeric gene-transfected cells formed experimental metastases, whereas the bFGF gene-transfected cells without the signal peptide did not. In addition to experiments where untransformed cells were converted to malignancy by transfer of a gene encoding a growth factor that the recipient cells can respond to, cells have been transfected with growth factor genes encoding factors that they normally cannot respond to. For example, untransformed NIH-3T3 cells are not normally responsive to colony-stimulating factor-1 (CSF-1) because they lack the CSF-1 receptor. Using v-fms-transfected cells (v-fms is an oncogene encoding a CSF-1-like receptor), Greenberg and collaborators found that an addition of exogenous CSF-1 stimulated cell growth. In vivo the v-fms-transformed cells formed experimental metastases, whereas the untransformed cells did not. The addition of exogenous CSF-1 to v-fms-transformed cells before injection into animals resulted in greater numbers of experimental metastases in mice. However, if v-fms-transformed cells were allowed to grow under culture conditions where autocrine growth factor-conditioning could occur, and then the cells were treated with CSF-1, the opposite effect was obtained and the v-fms-transformed cells formed fewer metastases. This inhibitory effect was probably due to downregulation of the CSF-1 receptors on the v-fms-transfected cells by excess exogenous CSF-1. The differing effects of growth factors on the transfected NIH-3T3 cells were explained as being due to receptor occupancy and growth factor saturation effects. Although the levels of secreted autocrine growth factors, their receptors, and receptor occupancy were not determined, the saturation of growth factor receptors by exogenous growth factors could cause effects other than growth stimulation, such as growth inhibition or differentiation. Different concentrations of certain growth factors can have opposite effects on the same cell system. Often low concentrations of cytokines and growth factors can be stimulatory, whereas high concentrations of the same factor can be inhibitory. In addition, as discussed earlier, the transfer of genes into unstable cells can result in cellular diversification and heterogeneity.

Another example of loss of responsiveness with tumor progression is the loss of hormone responses with progression of breast cancer. Loss in estrogen dependency of MCF-7 breast cancer cells after transfection with the v-H-*ras* oncogene has been seen by Marc Lippman and collaborators. In contrast to parental MCF-7 cells, *ras*-transfected MCF-7 cells were tumorigenic in the absence of infused estrogens, and the transfected cells secreted TGF-α, TGF-β, and insulin-like growth factor-I, without a change in their cell surface growth factor receptor densities. Because advanced breast cancers often become refractory to estrogens and other hormones, this suggests that as malignant cells become more advanced, they become less dependent on systemic hormones and they possibly secrete higher amounts of autocrine growth factors. In support of this notion is the loss of hormone responsiveness of breast cancers as they progress *in vivo*. Breast cancers that are initially responsive to 17β-estradiol lose their hormone responsiveness as they progress to more malignant and aggressive, hormone-independent phenotypes. They can also increase their synthesis and secretion of autocrine growth factors. These findings are consistent with a generalized loss of growth factor regulation and an increase in autocrine growth mechanisms with progression to more malignant cellular phenotypes.

VII. NEW APPROACHES TO CANCER THERAPY

The information on growth requirements, expression of growth factor receptors, and growth inhibitor receptors by malignant cells should be useful in developing new therapeutic approaches to limiting the growth of metastatic cancers. Specific approaches used to limit the proliferation of tumor cells include the administration of growth inhibitors or analogs of growth factors or the use of antibodies against growth factor receptors to deliver toxins to highly metastatic

cells. For example, John Mulshine and collaborators found that a bombesin/gastrin-releasing peptide is a commonly found autocrine growth factor made by small cell lung cancer cells, and bombesin analogs have been used to inhibit the growth of the lung carcinoma cells *in vitro* in clonogenic growth assays and *in vivo* in xenographs in nude mice. Alternatively, to inhibit autocrine/paracrine growth pathways, antibodies have been administered that bind to the growth factors and remove or prevent them from interacting with tumor cells. For example, bombesin/gastrin-releasing peptides can be eliminated by administering monoclonal antibodies against these factors. A phase I clinical trial using a monoclonal antibody against a bombesin/gastrin-releasing peptide indicated that the effects of the bombesin/gastrin-releasing peptide can be partially blocked without apparent toxicity.

The employment of antibodies against growth factor receptors has been effective in preventing tumor growth. John Mendelson and collaborators and Ralph Reisfeld independently were among the first to use monoclonal antibodies against the EGF receptor to inhibit the growth of human tumors in nude mice. One of the monoclonal antibodies that Mendelson and colleagues used was also found to activate macrophage- and complement-dependent lysis of cancer cells *in vitro*, suggesting that the effects of growth factor receptor antibodies on the growth of tumor cells *in vivo* could be due, in part, to blocking host responses against the tumor. The formation of metastases from implants of human melanoma cells in severely immunodeficient mice has been blocked with a monoclonal antibody against the EGF receptor. When the antibody Fc or tail portion was removed, the tailless monoclonal antibody did not inhibit metastasis, suggesting that the Fc or tail portion of the antibody contributed to the anti-metastatic effect, possibly by an antibody-dependent host cell effector mechanism.

Various investigators have coupled the antibodies to toxins or toxin subunits to increase the effectiveness of antigrowth factor receptor monoclonal antibodies in suppressing the growth and metastasis of human tumors. Using extremely toxic molecules covalently bound to the targeting monoclonal antibody, specific killing of malignant cells has been achieved. The chimeric toxin–antibody molecules can produce antitumor effects without apparent side effects and suppression of white blood cells, even though these normal cells also express the growth factor receptors. Although it remains to be demonstrated that every last malignant cell can be killed with such toxin–antibody conjugates, the use of potent toxin conjugates to specifically kill metastatic cells at secondary sites may be an achievable goal that is well within our technical ability.

VIII. GROWTH RESPONSES OF METASTATIC CELLS AND MALIGNANT PROGRESSION

During the progression of malignant tumors there is often a tendency for the most malignant cells in a tumor cell population to lose expression of growth factor or inhibitor receptors and lose responsiveness to particular growth factors or inhibitors. The loss of these responses in highly metastatic cancer cells and the ability of such cancers to colonize and grow at distinct secondary sites may be explainable by considering each stage of cancer progression. At the early stages of metastasis, many cancers show restricted or-

gan preference of metastatis, whereas at the final stages near host death, these same cancers often colonize multiple organ and tissues sites. The explanation for this is that cancers progress from mainly paracrine growth stimulatory and inhibitory mechanisms at the initial stages of metastatic progression to mainly autocrine stimulatory mechanisms at the final terminal stages (Fig. 3). As discussed earlier, highly advanced cancers can secrete a variety of growth factors that could serve as autocrine sources of growth stimulation independent of their microenvironments. This could explain the loss of organ preference of metastasis seen at the later stages of cancer progression, whereas at earlier stages of cancer progression fewer organs are usually involved. Eventually metastatic progression continues and alterations in tumor cells may produce what has been termed an acrine (lack of regulation) state where malignant cells have lost their usual growth factor and inhibitor responses and are refractory to growth regulation by cytokines and growth factors and inhibitors. Because acrine malignant cells are not expected to respond to endogenous or exogenous growth factors or inhibitors, they should be the ultimate autonomous cells.

The concept that growth stimulatory and inhibitory

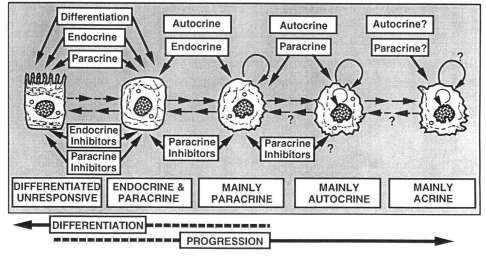

FIGURE 3 Progression of malignant cancer cells results in alterations in their responsiveness to host-derived growth stimulatory and inhibitory molecules and synthesis of autocrine growth factors. Tumor cell differentiation is shown as a possible process to the left and tumor cell progression to the right. Tumor progression can result initially in an increase in paracrine growth factor responses, as in the case of organ preference of metastatic colonization. As tumor progression continues, however, loss of paracrine growth factor and growth inhibitor responsiveness occurs and increases in autocrine growth factor production occur with more widespread tissue metastatic colonization. Eventually, tumor progression can result in a complete loss of growth factor/inhibitor responses (acrine state) and metastatic colonization of virtually any tissue can occur.

responses are altered during cancer progression has important significance for the development of new therapies for metastatic cancers. If highly progressed metastatic cells are more refractory to growth regulation, then it is unlikely that therapeutic intervention using analogs of growth inhibitors, monoclonal antibodies against growth factors or their receptors, or other means of suppressing growth-stimulating molecules or enhancing growth-inhibitory molecules will be useful in highly advanced cancers. Because these highly progressed cancers are often unstable and produce cell progeny that are unstable and undergo rapid changes in their gene expression programs, it is unlikely that therapies based on growth properties of malignant cells will succeed at the terminal stages of cancer progression. Their use must be at the earliest stages of cancer progression and metastasis, where malignant cells are still responsive to growth signals.

See Also the Following Articles

HEMATOPOIETIC GROWTH FACTORS • MOLECULAR MECHANISMS OF CANCER INVASION • TUMOR CELL MOTILITY AND INVASION

Bibliography

Aaronson, S. A. (1991). Growth factors and cancer. *Science* **254,** 1146–1153.

Cavanaugh, P. G., Jia, L.-B., Zou, Y. Y., and Nicolson, G. L. (1999). Transferrin receptor overexpression enhances transferrin responsiveness and the metastatic growth of a rat mammary adenocarcinoma line. *Breast Cancer Res. Treat.* **56,** 203–217.

Nicolson, G. L. (1987). Tumor cell instability, diversification, and progression to the metastatic phenotype: From oncogene to oncofetal expression. *Cancer Res.* **47,** 1473–1487.

Nicolson, G. L. (1991). Gene expression and tumor progression to the metastatic phenotype. *Bioessays* **13,** 337–342.

Nicolson, G. L. (1988). Cancer metastasis: Tumor cell and host organ properties important in colonization of specific secondary sites. *Biochim. Biophys. Acta* **948,** 175–224.

Nicolson, G. L. (1991). Molecular mechanisms of cancer metastasis: Tumor and host properties and the role of oncogenes and suppressor genes. *Curr. Opin. Oncol.* **3,** 75–92.

Nicolson, G. L. (1993). Cancer progression and growth: Relationship of paracrine and autocrine growth mechanisms to organ preference of metastasis. *Exp. Cell Res.* **204,** 171–180.

Nicolson, G. L. (1993). Paracrine and autocrine growth mechanisms in tumor metastasis to specific sites with particular emphasis on brain and lung metastasis. *Cancer Metast. Rev.* **12,** 325–343.

Nicolson, G. L., Menter, D., Herrmann, J., Cavanaugh, P., Jia, L.-B., Hamada, J., Yun, Z., and Marchetti, D. (1994). Tumor metastasis to brain: Role of endothelial cells, neurotrophins and paracrine growth factors. *Crit. Rev. Oncogen,* **5,** 451–471.

Rodeck, U., and Herlyn, M. (1991). Growth factors in melanoma. *Cancer Metast. Rev.* **10,** 89–101.

Vande Woude, G. F., Jeffers, M., Cortner, J., Alvord, G., Tsarfaty, I., and Resau, J. (1997). Met-HGF/SF: Tumorigenesis, invasion and metastasis. *Ciba Found. Symp.* **212,** 119–130.

Volpe, J. P. (1988). Genetic instability of cancer: Why a metastatic tumor is unstable and a benign tumor is stable. *Cancer Genet. Cytogenet.* **34,** 125–134.

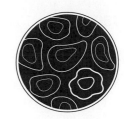

Bcl-2 Family Proteins and the Dysregulation of Programmed Cell Death

John C. Reed
The Burnham Institute

GLOSSARY

apoptosis A cell death process involving characteristic morphological changes, including nuclear fragmentation and chromatin condensation; plasma membrane blebbing and cytoplasmic vacuolarization; and cell shrinkage, culminating in cell disintegration into small fragments ("apoptotic bodies"). Apoptosis occurs in many types of cells during the process of programmed cell death and is also induced by a wide variety of stimuli, including chemotherapeutic drugs and radiation.

***bcl-2;* Bcl-2** Acronyms for the B-cell lymphoma/leukemia-2 gene or the protein encoded by this gene, respectively. As implied by its name, *bcl-2* was first discovered because of its activation in many B-cell lymphomas.

Bcl-2 antagonist-X (Bax) A proapoptotic protein that heterodimerizes with Bcl-2 and several other antiapoptotic members of the Bcl-2 family.

permeability transition pore A multi-protein complex that controls permeability of the inner mitochondrial membrane. Components include the adenine nucleotide translocator in the inner membrane and the voltage-dependent anion channel in the outer membrane.

programmed cell death   A physiological cell death process that removes extraneous cells formed during fetal development and removes older cells to make room for newer ones in adult tissues as part of normal tissue homeostasis.

t(14;18)   A chromosomal translocation seen frequently in malignant B-cell lymphomas that involves fusion of a portion of the long arm of 18 where the *bcl-2* gene resides with the immunoglobulin heavy chain locus on the long arm of chromosome 14.

Bcl-2 family proteins play a central role in the regulation of apoptosis. The Bcl-2 family is composed of at least 24 members in humans and includes both cell death suppressors, such as the founding family member Bcl-2, and death inducers, such as Bax. Abnormalities in the expression of the Bcl-2 family protein occur commonly in cancers and contribute to a state of apoptosis resistance, with important consequences for a variety of aspects of tumor biology, including chemo- and radioresistance. Developing knowledge about the biochemical mechanisms of Bcl-2 family protein is beginning to suggest strategies for restoring apoptosis sensitivity in tumors.

I. PROGRAMMED CELL DEATH: ROLE IN TISSUE KINETICS AND NEOPLASTIC DISEASES

Although originally described in the context of fetal development, programmed cell death (PCD) is a normal physiological mechanism that plays an essential role in normal tissue homeostasis in adults. In any tissue with self-renewal capacity where new cells are produced through cell division, there must exist an opposing mechanism for the removal of cells at a commensurate rate if overall cell numbers are to be held constant. That mechanism is PCD, also referred to often as "physiological cell death" or "apoptosis." Enormous amounts of cell death occur in all of us; in fact, some estimates suggest that in the course of a typical year, each of us will produce and then in parallel eradicate through cell death a mass of cells equivalent to our entire body weight. To put the issue into

perspective, for example, adults typically produce 50–70 billion cells each day, necessitating a means for eradication of cells at an equivalent rate. Consequently, the average life span of some types of leukocytes is on the order of only hours to days. Similarly, keratinocytes in the skin turnover approximately every 2 weeks and intestinal epithelial cells about every 6 to 8 days. This constant cycle of cell birth followed by cell death creates a flux of cells through all tissues with regenerative capacity and provides a mechanism for rapidly responding to situations where there may arise a temporary need for greater cell numbers, such as during infections when a demand for an increased number of neutrophils and lymphocytes might occur.

Unfortunately, this normal physiological process of PCD can become dysregulated, leading to disease. Excessive cell death occurring via the apoptotic mechanism is currently believed, for example, to contribute to the depletion of cells in neurodegenerative diseases, heart failure, and AIDS. Conversely, defects in PCD mechanisms that lead to insufficient cell death impart a selective survival advantage on cells and thus can contribute to the origins of cancer. In this regard, at least two mechanisms exist through which cells may accumulate in the body: (1) increased rates of cell division and (2) decreased rates of cell death. To the extent that cell turnover is important in maintaining normal numbers of a particular cell type within a tissue, dysregulation of cell death mechanisms can be just as important to the neoplastic process as alterations in cell cycle regulation. A cell clone therefore that acquires the ability to survive for long periods of time but that proliferates at normal rates will nevertheless enjoy a selective growth advantage relative to its normal counterparts and undergo clonal expansion *in vivo*.

Of course, combinations of genetic alterations leading to both accelerated rates of cell growth and diminished rates of cell death within the same neoplastic cell clone can and often do occur during tumor progression, but some malignancies probably arise primarily through alterations in either cell division or cell death mechanisms. Indolent B-cell neoplasms such as follicular non-Hodgkin's lymphoma and B-cell chronic lymphocytic leukemia (CLL) are good examples of malignancies that occur primarily because of dysregulation of cell death mechanisms. These neoplastic diseases also serve to introduce the subject of this article, as the founding member of the Bcl-2 family of apoptosis-regulating genes was discovered due to its important involvement in indolent B-cell malignancies.

Normally, the average life span of B lymphocytes is approximately 5 to 7 days. In follicular B-cell lymphomas and B-CLLs, however, neoplastic cells survive for very long periods of time *in vivo*. Most of the malignant B cells are in the G_0/G_1 phase of the cell cycle, indicating that they are not proliferating at increased rates, consistent with the primary defect being in cell death as opposed to cell replication mechanisms. The natural history of these neoplastic disorders is also consistent with this hypothesis in that the malignant cells accumulate gradually in the patient. Median survivals with one or two drug therapies are often in the range of 5 to 8 years, as opposed to aggressive high-grade B-cell lymphomas where 1 to 2 years is more typical for many patients, despite use of combination chemotherapy. Although typically running an indolent course, however, the unrelenting neoplastic cell expansion that occurs in follicular B-cell lymphomas and B-CLL nevertheless eventually crowds out normal marrow elements and disrupts normal immune cell responses, ultimately leading to lethal complications that result in death in the majority of patients. In part, the low growth fraction of these B-cell disorders may also account for the current incurability of follicular lymphomas and B-CLLs, as most anticancer therapeutics are predicated upon the assumption that the malignant cells replicate faster than normal cells. Similar scenarios have been revealed for many types of more common cancers, including many adenocarcinomas of the prostate, breast, and colon—to name a few.

In addition to the role that defective PCD plays in cell accumulation, apoptosis resistance also plays prominent roles in a number of cellular behaviors of relevance to tumor formation and progression. For example, defects in apoptosis can render tumor cells resistant to eradication by immune cells. Apoptosis dysregulation also overcomes the cell death that would normally result from miscues in cell cycle control and genome mismanagement. Most anticancer drugs and radiotherapy rely on apoptotic machinery, and thus defects in cell death mechanisms can render tumor cells relatively more resistant to these cancer therapies. Apoptosis dysregulation also contributes to tumor metastasis, allowing epithelial cells to survive in a suspended state without attachment to extracellular matrix proteins and promoting intravascular survival of tumor cells lodged in distal capillary beds. Thus, proper control of apoptosis is critical for avoiding malignancy and for counteracting tumor progression.

II. Bcl-2 FAMILY PROTEINS

Bcl-2 family proteins play a central role in the regulation of apoptosis. The relative ratios of anti- and proapoptotic Bcl-2 family proteins dictate the ultimate sensitivity or resistance of cells to various apoptotic stimuli, including growth factor/neurotrophin deprivation, hypoxia, radiation, anticancer drugs, oxidants, and Ca^{2+} overload. Not surprisingly, then, alterations in the amounts of these proteins have been associated with a variety of pathological conditions, characterized by either too much (cell loss) or too little (cell accumulation) cell death, including cancer, autoimmune disorders such as lupus (where a failure to eradicate autoreactive lymphocytes occurs), immunodeficiency associated with HIV infection, and ischemia–reperfusion injury during stroke and myocardial infarction, among others. In humans, 24 members of the Bcl-2 gene family have been described, many of them expressed in tissue-specific manners or fulfilling cell-specific roles in death regulation *in vivo*.

The founding member of the Bcl-2 family of apoptosis-regulating proteins is B-cell lymphoma/leukemia-2 (Bcl-2), which gets its name because of its involvement in B-cell lymphomas and leukemias. The protein encoded by the *BCL-2* gene is an inhibitor of PCD, blocking cell death induced by a wide variety of physiological and experimental stimuli. The *BCL-2* gene was first discovered by virtue of its involvement in the t(14;18) chromosomal translocations that occur in >85% of follicular non-Hodgkin's lymphomas in Western countries and which fuse the *BCL-2* gene on chromosome 18 with the immunoglobulin heavy chain (IgH) locus on chromosome 14. Before the *BCL-2* gene was molecularly cloned, it was hypothesized that a cellular oncogene would be found on chromosome 18 at the breakpoints of t(14;18) translocations by analogy to the t(8;14) translocations of Burkitt lymphomas, which had been previously shown to bring the *c-MYC* gene at 8q24 into juxtaposition with the IgH locus at 14q32. These t(8;14) translocations generally did not directly alter the coding regions of the *c-MYC* gene but did place *c-MYC* into a *cis* configuration with powerful transcriptional enhancer elements located within the IgH locus, thus deregulating the expression of this protooncogene. Because B-cell neoplasms were known to frequently contain either t(11;14) or t(14;18) translocations involving the IgH locus at 14q32, it was theorized that additional cellular protooncogenes resided on chromosomes 11 and 18, and these loci were termed, *BCL-1* and *BCL-2*, respectively, by Croce and colleagues.

Since the discovery of Bcl-2, multiple members of this family of apoptosis regulators have been revealed in humans and other animal species, including mammals, birds, amphibians, and other vertebrates, as well as nematodes, insects, marine sponges, and other invertebrates. Bcl-2 homologues are also found in several animal viruses, including BHRF-1 the Epstein–Barr Virus (EBV), which transforms B lymphocytes, ORF16 in Herpes Virus Saimiri, Kbcl-2 in Kaposi sarcoma-associated virus human herpes virus-8 (HHV8), a member of the herpes virus family implicated in endothelial cell malignancy, the African swine fever virus gene 5HL, and the adenovirus E1b-19kD protein, which serves as a functional homologue of Bcl-2, although sharing little amino acid sequence identity with it.

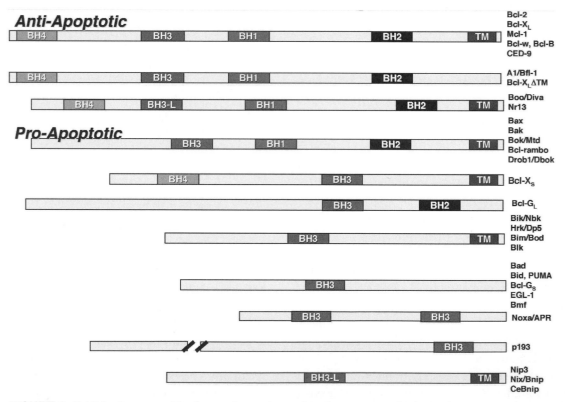

FIGURE 1 Bcl-2 family proteins. The diagram depicts the topological organization of Bcl-2 family proteins, with respect to the presence of BH domains and TM domains. The proteins are grouped into antiapoptotic (top) and proapoptotic (bottom), with multidomain proapoptotic and BH3-only proteins included. Most proteins depicted represent human or mouse family members, but a few examples of Bcl-2 homologues from lower organisms are also included, such as Ced-9 and Egl-1 of *C. elegans* and DBok of *Drosophila*. Viral homologues are not included.

Cellular Bcl-2 family proteins include at least four subgroups that can be distinguished based on differences in their structures and mechanisms of regulating cell death, as discussed later. In this regard, up to four conserved domains have been identified in Bcl-2 family proteins based on amino acid sequence alignments, referred to as Bcl-2 homology (BH) domains, BH1, BH2, BH3, and BH4 (Fig. 1). Mutagenesis studies suggest that all four of these domains are important for the antiapoptotic function of Bcl-2. Also, all cellular antiapoptotic Bcl-2 family proteins contain all four of these domains. However, many Bcl-2 family proteins possess only a subset of the BH domains, including a diverse group of proapoptotic proteins, which contain only the BH3 domain (so-called, "BH3-only proteins). The viral homologues of Bcl-2 may represent a fifth group, as some share very limited amino acid sequence identity with cellular Bcl-2 family members and at least some (e.g., E1b-19kD of adenovirus) may function through different mechanisms than antiapoptotic counterparts encoded in cellular genomes.

III. Bcl-2 FAMILY PROTEINS CONTROL AN EVOLUTIONARILY CONSERVED PATHWAY FOR CELL DEATH

A variety of experimental observations have pointed to Bcl-2 as a critical regulator of an evolutionarily conserved cell survival mechanism. Hints of the importance of Bcl-2, for example, have come from the finding that Bcl-2 homologues can be found within the genomes of some viruses. Given the sparse economy of viral genomes, the observation that several Herpes family viruses, for example, have bothered to include a Bcl-2 homologue speaks to the potential importance of Bcl-2 as a regulator of cell survival. In addition to molecular virology, genetic studies in lower organisms, specifically the nematode *Caenorhabditis elegans*, have revealed a homologous gene, *ced-9*. Hyperfunction of *ced-9* prevents all programmed cell deaths that normally occur in the worm during development. Without *ced-9*, worm embryos undergo massive apoptotic cell death early in development. Thus, in the worm, the Ced-9 protein appears to function as a master switch that determines the life and death fate of cells. Furthermore, human Bcl-2 can rescue Ced-9-deficient embryos, demonstrating that these genes are functional homologues and suggesting that the cell death pathway controlled by Bcl-2 is evolutionarily conserved. The human Bcl-2 protein is also active when expressed in Sf9 insect cells, where it has been shown to delay apoptosis induced by baculovirus infection, again arguing that the pathway regulated by Bcl-2 is well conserved through evolution. Finally, in this regard, the human Bcl-2 protein has also been shown to function in yeast, *Saccharomyces cerevisiae*, where it can promote the growth of mutant strains of yeast that have defects in antioxidant pathways under conditions of aerobic metabolism and can also neutralize toxicity of the Bcl-2 antagonist Bax, which is discussed in detail later.

Studies of Bcl-2 function using gene transfer approaches in mammalian cells have demonstrated that overproduction of this oncoprotein can render cells relatively more resistant to induction of apoptosis by a wide variety of stimuli. Among the experimental situations in which Bcl-2 has been shown to provide protection from cell death are (1) growth factor deprivation from hematopoietic, lymphoid, and fibroblastic cells; (2) neurotrophic factor withdrawal from neurons; (3) UV and γ radiation; (4) heat shock; (5) some types of cytotoxic lymphokines (tumor necrosis factor-α); (6) calcium ionophores; (7) some types of viruses; (8) excitotoxic neurotransmitters such as L-glutamate; (9) agents that induce free-radical production; and (10) essentially all anticancer chemotherapeutic drugs. This broad range of stimuli, with their numerous biochemical mechanisms of action in cells, argues that Bcl-2 functions at a distal point in a pathway leading to cell death. Thus, despite the various upstream "signals" that are generated by these stimuli, eventually they must utilize the same final common pathway to kill cells, as Bcl-2 can provide protection from all of them. Nearly all of the cell death-inducing stimuli mentioned earlier have been shown to trigger apoptotic, as opposed to necrotic, cell death. However, Bcl-2 can also protect cells from necrosis in some circumstance, especially when mitochondria are involved in the underlying pathology. Thus, the forms of cell death that Bcl-2 can obviate are not necessarily limited to those that resemble apoptosis or various other manifestations of physiological cell death and can include necrosis in at least some circumstances.

IV. LOCATIONS OF Bcl-2 FAMILY PROTEINS

Many Bcl-2 family proteins contain a hydrophobic stretch of amino acids near their carboxyl terminus, which allows them to insert posttranslationally into intracellular membranes (Fig. 1). Among the more prominent membrane locations of these proteins are mitochondria. Indeed, many of the functions of Bcl-2 family proteins center on mitochondria and the roles that these organelles play in cell life and death. Moreover, some Bcl-2 family proteins that are extramitochondrial can be triggered to translocate to and interact with these organelles. For example, the BH3-only protein Bim is sequestered in a complex with the dynein light chain on microtubules, but can be released in response to specific stimuli, translocating to the surface of mitochondria. Similarly, the proapoptotic protein Bid lies latent in the cytosol until it becomes cleaved by a protease, thus removing an N-terminal autoinhibitory domain. Cleaved Bid then undergoes myristylation and targets to mitochondrial membranes. These and other examples not cited here teach us that interaction with mitochondrial membranes represents an important aspect of the function of Bcl-2 family proteins.

It should be noted, however, that significant portions of the total pool of Bcl-2 within cells, as well as many other Bcl-2 family members, are integrated into the membranes of the endoplasmic reticulum (ER) and nuclear envelope. In fact, at least one of the viral antiapoptotic proteins, E1b-19K of adenovirus, is found exclusively in the nuclear envelope. While less is understood about the roles of Bcl-2 family proteins at these extramitochondrial locations, hints of activities related to transport of either ions or proteins between cytosol and either ER or nucleus have surfaced in the course of experimentation. Taken together, therefore, it seems that the actions of Bcl-2 in cells are not relegated solely to protecting mitochondria during cellular confrontation with apoptosis-inducing insults and stimuli. Although mitochondria are clearly a major site of action of Bcl-2 family proteins, some studies provide evidence that under specific circumstances they may regulate cell life and death events by acting at other locations. Deciphering the mechanisms involved seems likely to generate important insight into the full repertoire of mechanisms of Bcl-2 family proteins in the future.

V. INTERACTIONS AMONG Bcl-2 FAMILY PROTEINS: A NETWORK OF HOMO- AND HETERODIMERS

Probably all Bcl-2 family proteins are capable of interacting with at least one, if not several, other family members. Nearly all Bcl-2 family proteins contain a dimerization domain called BH3, representing a ~16 amino acid amphipathic α helix that inserts into a hydrophobic crevice on the surface of selected other members of the family. A complex network of homo- and heterodimers thus has been demonstrated among Bcl-2 family proteins, the functional significance of which remains elusive in many instances. Bcl-2, for example, readily forms homodimers, but whether this is fundamental to its antiapoptotic function is controversial. The proapoptotic proteins Bax and Bak can homodimerize and seem even to multimerize within membranes, which correlates with their proapoptotic activity, as discussed later. However, here too, a direct cause-and-effect relation between homodimerization/multimerization is lacking at present.

BH3-only proteins may be the most straightforward in terms of understanding the functional significance of their interactions with other Bcl-2 family members. Although all BH3-only proteins identified to date induce apoptosis, overall, they generally lack an intrinsic activity as promoters of cell death and instead rely exclusively on their BH3 domain for interacting with other Bcl-2 family members. BH3-only proteins bind in a BH3-dependent manner to either anti- or proapoptotic members of the family, which typically contain several of the BH domain (so-called "multidomain" proteins). In binding these multidomain members of the family, BH3-only proteins either inhibit or activate the multidomain proteins. For example, several BH3-only proteins, including

Bcl-X$_S$, BAD, Bik, Bim, Hrk, Puma, Noxa, Bcl-G$_S$, and Bmf, interact with anti-apoptotic Bcl-2 family members but not proapoptotic members, apparently functioning as transdominant inhibitors of apoptosis suppressors such as Bcl-2 and Bcl-X$_L$. Conversely, the Bid protein can interact with its BH3 domain with either antiapoptotic or proapoptotic multidomain family members. Interactions with apoptotic proteins such as Bcl-2 and Bcl-X$_L$ result in suppression of their cell survival effects. In contrast, interactions of Bid with killer proteins such as Bax and Bak seem to activate these proteins, arousing them from a resting state.

Based on these differences in structure and function, it has been proposed that four subgroups of Bcl-2 family proteins can be envisioned, including (i) multidomain apoptosis suppressors (group I) such as Bcl-2 and Bcl-X$_L$; (ii) multidomain killers (group II) such as Bax, Bak, and Bok; (iii) BH3-only antagonists of Bcl-2, Bcl-X$_L$, and other group I proteins (Group III) such as BAD, Bik, Bim, and Bcl-G; and (iv) BH3-only agonists of Bax, Bak, and other group II multidomain proapoptotic proteins (group IV) such as Bid. However, additional subgroups of Bcl-2 family proteins may eventually emerge as our understanding of the mechanisms of these proteins improves. For example, while details remain sketchy, Nip3 and Nix proteins may rely more on their transmembrane (TM) domain than their BH3 domain for promoting apoptosis. Also emerging are descriptions of unorthodox BH3-only proteins, where a BH3 domain or its functional equivalent is embedded within proteins that serve other functions. Examples of such unorthodox BH3-only proteins include the transcription factor TR3, a member of the steroid/retinoid family that can be triggered to translocate from the nucleus to mitochondria, interacting with Bcl-2 and Bcl-X$_L$, and inducing apoptosis. RAD9 and 2′-5′-oligoadenylate synthetase probably represent additional examples of proapoptotic proteins that carry cryptic BH3-like domains and which can be enticed to exploit those BH3-like domains under certain specified conditions, thereby linking diverse cellular pathways to the core apoptosis machinery of cells (Fig. 2).

The viral homologues of Bcl-2 may constitute a fifth group (group V) (not shown). Where tested, all of these genes so far have been found to suppress apoptosis, and it is speculated that they may serve to

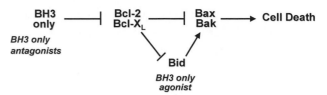

FIGURE 2 Linking signal transduction and cell stress to activation of BH3-only proteins. Examples of some BH3-only proteins are provided. In response to specific signals or environmental circumstances, expression of BH3-only proteins is induced at the transcriptional level (Noxa; Puma; Hrk) or through alternative splicing (Bcl-Xs; Bcl-Gs), or the proteins (already present) can become activated from a latent or sequestered state (Bad; Bim; Bmf; Bid).

keep host cells alive during viral replication. Many of these viral Bcl-2 family proteins share very limited sequence identity with their cellular counterparts. Furthermore, at least some of them may function in ways at least partly different from antiapoptotic Bcl-2 family members encoded in cellular genomes.

VI. STRUCTURES OF Bcl-2 FAMILY PROTEINS

A milestone in our understanding of Bcl-2 family protein function was achieved when the three-dimensional structure of a Bcl-2 family protein, Bcl-X$_L$, was determined for the first time, revealing striking structural similarity with the pore-forming domains of the bacterial toxins, such as diphtheria toxin (DT) and the colicins. Since then, three-dimensional structures have been obtained for Bcl-2 and for the proapoptotic family members Bax and Bid. The structures of these Bcl-2 family proteins and the pore-forming domains of DT and colicins consist entirely of α helices connected by variable length loops. Each structure contains a pair of core hydrophobic helices that are long enough to penetrate the lipid bilayer and which are shielded from the aqueous environment by a surrounding shell of amphipathic (one side hydrophilic and the other hydrophobic) α helices that orient their hydrophobic surfaces toward the central core helices and their hydrophilic surfaces outward.

Studies of the bacterial toxins suggest that under appropriate conditions, the central hydrophobic helices efficiently insert through the lipid bilayer as one step in the process of pore formation. True to their structural similarity with these bacterial toxins, recombinant Bcl-2, Bcl-X_L, Bax, and Bid proteins can form pores in synthetic membranes, including liposomes and planar bilayers, either forming discrete ion-conducting channels with various conductance states or making large pores in membranes.

It should be noted that with the exception of Bid, BH3 domain proteins are not predicted to share similar protein folds with the multidomain members of the Bcl-2 family. Thus, the view has emerged that multidomain members of the Bcl-2 family may possess an intrinsic function as channels or pore-forming molecules, whereas most BH3-only proteins lack an intrinsic function and operate as transregulators.

Because both antiapoptotic (Bcl-2; Bcl-X_L) and proapoptotic (Bax; Bid) proteins are capable of forming channels in membranes, it remains unclear at present how this pore-forming activity relates to the bioactivities of these proteins. Probably the most popular hypothesis is that proapoptotic multidomain proteins such as Bax and Bak form large channels in mitochondrial membranes that cause release of apoptosis-inducing proteins normally sequestered in these organelles. In this case, antiapoptotic family members are envisioned primarily as antagonists, which somehow impair multimerization of Bax and Bak in membranes, thus precluding pore formation. Consistent with this model, it has been demonstrated that cells from mice in which both *bax* and *bak* genes have been ablated cannot be rescued by overexpression of Bcl-2 or Bcl-X_L, suggesting that these antiapoptotic proteins are lacking in function in contexts where they have no killer proteins to oppose (Fig. 3).

However, this model fails to take into account some hints that even Bcl-2 may possess an intrinsic function as a suppressor of cell death. For example, ectopic expression of Bcl-2 in yeast suppresses cell death induced by oxidative damage and heat shock, and yet these simple eukaryotes possess no Bax homologues. Thus, alternative models in which channel-like attributes might be operative must be entertained. One idea is that proteins such as Bcl-2 (death blocker) and Bax (death promoter) transport the same molecules but in opposite directions across biological membranes. Alternatively, it could be that both Bcl-2 and

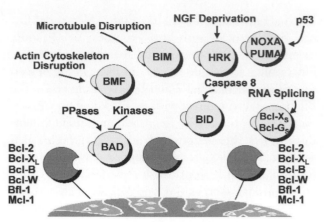

FIGURE 3 Proposed model for physical and functional interactions among Bcl-2 family proteins. A speculative model that attempts to relate interactions among Bcl-2 family proteins to their function as regulators of apoptosis is presented. Bax/Bax (or Bak/Bak) homodimers are proposed to trigger or be required for a cell death pathway. Bcl-2 and other survival proteins such as Bcl-X_L can interact with and oppose the cytotoxic actions of Bax (Bak) and promote cell survival. BH3-only proteins antagonize the function of Bcl-2 (Bcl-X_L) by forming heterodimers with it, thus preventing Bcl-2 (Bcl-X_L) from interacting physically or functionally with Bax (Bak). The Bid protein can bind both multidomain antiapoptotic (Bcl-2; Bcl-X_L) and multidomain proapoptotic (Bax; Bak) proteins. Bcl-2/Bcl-X_L and Bid mutually neutralize each other, whereas Bid activates Bax/Bak.

Bax have similar transport functions, possibly allowing transport of deleterious molecules that induce cell death. In this case, it might be speculated that heterodimerization of Bcl-2 and Bax plugs the pores so that the critical issue is not whether Bcl-2 or Bax is present individually but rather the ratio of these proteins. This model would be consistent with data suggesting that the excessive amounts of Bcl-2 can paradoxically promote cell death rather than block it in some circumstances and with the finding that Bax and Bak can unexpectedly exhibit cytoprotective rather than cytotoxic functions in some cellular contexts. Finally, it is entirely possible that heterodimerization of death blockers such as Bcl-2 and death promoters such as Bax creates chimeric channels with transport or regulatory properties are different from either Bcl-2 or Bax channels alone.

In addition, many other issues remain unresolved about the Bcl-2 and Bax protein channels, such as the diameter of the channels and how many Bcl-2, Bcl-X_L, or Bax proteins it takes to create an aqueous channel in membranes. In the case of DT, the channels are evidently large enough to transport a protein, as the primary function of DT is thought to be for allowing transport of the ADP-ribosylation factor subunit of the toxin from lysosomes and endosomes into the cytosol. In contrast, bacterial colicins transport ions. Thus, transport of ions or proteins could fit with some of the phenotypes ascribed to Bcl-2 family proteins, such as volume control of mitochondria (e.g., organelle swelling and rupture), release of apoptogenic proteins from mitochondria (see later), and effects on Ca^{2+} transport and intracellular pH regulation.

VII. MITOCHONDRIA AND APOPTOSIS REGULATION BY Bcl-2 FAMILY PROTEINS

Mitochondria play a central role in apoptosis regulation. Although mitochondria-independent pathways for apoptosis also exist, these organelles have been linked to cell death associated with a broad array of stimuli, insults, stresses, and environmental conditions. Bcl-2 family proteins have been implicated in the regulation of two important aspects of mitochondria pathophysiology: (a) mitochondrial permeability transition (PT) pore opening and (b) release of apoptogenic proteins from mitochondria into the cytosol. During apoptosis induced by myriad insults and stimuli, the electrochemical gradient ($\Delta\Psi$) across the inner mitochondrial membrane becomes dissipated. This loss of $\Delta\Psi$ has been attributed to the opening of a large conductance inner membrane channel commonly referred to as the mitochondrial PT pore. Although the structure and biochemical composition of the PT pore remain poorly defined, its constituents are thought to include both inner membrane proteins, such as the adenine nucleotide translocator (ANT), and outer membranes proteins, such as porin (voltage-dependent anion channel), which operate in concert, presumably at inner and outer membrane contact sites, to create a channel with a ~1.5-kDa diameter. The opening of this nonselective channel in the inner membrane allows for an equilibration of ions within the matrix and intermembrane space of mitochondria, thus dissipating the electro-chemical gradient, uncoupling the respiratory chain, and leading to organellar swelling (volume dysregulation). Other constituents of the PT pore complex include the peripheral benzodiazapine receptor (PBR), an outer membrane protein that binds protoporphyrin IX with nanomolar affinity and which also is regulated by some types of small molecule drugs, including benzodiazepines.

Several potentially lethal events follow from mitochondrial PT pore opening. For example, electrons that normally would find their way through the respiratory chain to molecular oxygen are instead shunted into free radical production. Mitochondrial ATP production also grinds to a halt, but presumably adequate intracellular stores typically persist, as ATP depletion is not a general feature of apoptosis and indeed would preclude it usually. The volume dysregulation that occurs upon PT pore opening leads to entry of water into the protein-rich matrix of mitochondria, causing the matrix space to expand. Because the inner membrane with its folded cristae possesses a larger surface area than the outer membrane, this matrix volume expansion can eventually cause the outer membrane to rupture, releasing proteins located within the intermembrane space into the cytosol. In this regard, several proteins have been described that can trigger or contribute to apoptosis when released from mitochondria into the cytosol. These proteins include cytochrome c, Smac (Diablo), Omi (HTRAZ), endonuclease G (EndoG), and apoptosis-inducing factor (AIF) (Fig. 4).

A. Cytochrome c

Cytochrome c plays a critical role in linking mitochondrial damage to activation of a family of intracellular proteins responsible for apoptosis—the caspases. Caspases are a family of intracellular cysteine proteinases that cleave their target substrates at aspartic acid residues within specific sequence contexts. Caspase activation represents a sine qua non of apoptosis. These proteins are not degradative proteases, but rather clip specific substrates within cells. It is the specific proteolytic events executed by caspases that account directly or indirectly for most of the morphological and biochemical characteristics of the apoptotic cell.

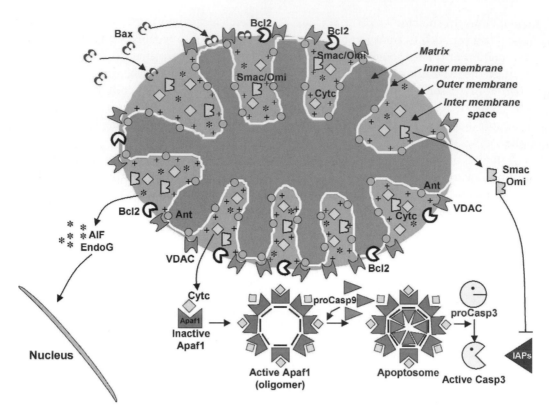

FIGURE 4 Bcl-2 family proteins, guardians of mitochondria. The mitochondria-dependent pathway for apoptosis is governed by Bcl-2 family proteins. Both proapoptotic and antiapoptotic Bcl-2 family proteins exist, and many of these proteins physically bind each other, forming a complex network of homo- and heterodimers. Mitochondria are well know for their life-sustaining production of ATP, but these organelles can also function as engines for cell death due to the release cytochrome *c* (activator of Apaf1/caspases), Smac and Omi (IAP inhibitors), AIF (endonuclease activator), EndoG (endonuclease), and other apoptosis-relevant proteins that they normally sequester. Probably the chief function of Bcl-2 family proteins is to regulate the release of cytochrome *c* and other apoptogenic proteins from mitochondria. The release of sequestered proteins is induced by proapoptotic Bcl-2 family proteins and is suppressed by antiapoptotic family members. Some of these proteins operate as pore formers or ion channels, probably explaining their effects on mitochondrial membrane permeability.

Caspases lie in a latent state as inactive zymogens (proenzymes) in essentially all animal cells, becoming activated under conditions that culminate in apoptosis. This activation typically involves cleavage of the caspase zymogen at aspartyl residues, either by itself or by other caspase molecules. Eleven caspases have been identified in the human genome, some of which play roles as initiators of apoptosis pathways and others which function downstream in a proteolytic cascade as effectors of apoptosis.

When mitochondria are involved in the apoptotic mechanism, cytochrome *c* represents the critical link that communicates changes in mitochondrial permeability with activation of cytosolic procaspases. Cytochrome *c* activates caspases through its effects on a protein called apoptosis protease-activating factor-1 (Apaf-1). Apaf-1 lies in a latent state in the cytosol of cells. Upon binding cytochrome *c*, however, Apaf-1 oligomerizes and then binds the pro-form of a specific caspase, procaspase-9, presumably because of cytochrome *c*-induced conformational changes in the Apaf-1 protein. This results in proteolytic activation of procaspase-9, possibly through a trans-processing mechanism facilitated by the binding of the multiple procaspase-9 molecules to the Apaf-1/cytochrome *c* complex (the so-called "induced proximity" mechanism). The redox state of cytochrome *c* is apparently unimportant for its function as a coactivator of caspases. However, methylated cytochrome *c* from yeast is inactive, implying a need for specific structural features of animal cytochrome *c* that allow binding to and activation of Apaf-1. Heme binding is also critical, as apocytochrome *c* does not trigger caspase activation.

The beauty of this system is that apocytochrome *c* can be produced in the cytosol by translation from a nuclear-encoded gene and then transported into mitochondria for heme attachment, without killing the cell. Because cytochrome *c* is essential for execution of oxidative phosphorylation, cells cannot discard this molecule and still produce ATP through aerobic respiration. This dependence on cytochrome *c* for respiration, therefore, presumably ensures that nearly all cells retain the cytochrome *c*-based mechanism for apoptosis, perhaps explaining in part why all animal cells seem to be capable of undergoing apoptosis if stimulated appropriately or hit hard enough.

Studies with cells that have been genetically engineered to be deficient in cytochrome *c*, Apaf1, or procaspase-9 (through homologous gene recombination; "knockouts") have provided unequivocal evidence that these proteins are essential for linking mitochondria to caspase activation and thus to the apoptosis program. However, even cells lacking cytochrome *c*, Apaf1, or procaspase-9 can be triggered to activate caspases and undergo apoptosis through alternative mitochondria-independent pathways. Furthermore, cells deficient in cytochrome *c*, Apaf1, and procaspase-deficient cells can also be killed through nonapoptotic mechanisms involving mitochondrial participation, without a necessity for involving caspase family proteinases.

B. Smac and Omi (HtrA2)

In cells, caspases are kept in check by a family of antiapoptotic proteins called inhibitors of apoptosis proteins (IAPs). Several of the IAPs bind and directly inhibit caspases, serving as intracellular proteinase inhibitors. Humans contain at least eight IAP family genes, some of which are inappropriately overexpressed in cancers.

Smac (Diablo) and Omi (HtrA2) are inhibitors of the IAPs. These proteins are encoded in the nuclear genome, produced in the cytosol, and then imported into mitochondria in association with proteolytic removal of their N-terminal leader peptides. The excision of the leader peptide from Smac and Omi creates a new N terminus, which begins with alanine and bears four amino acids that dock into a pocket on the surface of the BIR domains of certain IAPs. Smac and Omi, thus, compete with active caspases for binding to IAPs. The result is Smac and Omi dislodge caspases from the grip of IAPs, freeing these proteinases to induce apoptosis.

The normal mitochondrial function of Smac is unknown. Omi (HtrA2), in contrast, is a serine proteinase, which presumably functions in the processing of intramitochondrial proteins.

C. Endonuclease G

Another protein released during apoptosis is EndoG. This endonuclease is highly conserved and appears to be released from mitochondria during apoptosis in vertebrate (mammals) and invertebrate (*C. elegans*) species, where it contributes to digestion of the nuclear genome. Although genomic digestion is not absolutely critical for programmed cell death, it does play a role in the disposal of corpses.

D. Apoptosis-Inducing Factor

The AIF protein is a 50-kDa flavoprotein and putative activator of cellular endonucleases. Analogous to cytochrome *c*, AIF is encoded in the nuclear genome and transported through the cytosol as an inactive precursor, which gains competency as a promoter of cell death upon proteolytic removal of its N-terminal mitochondria-targeting leader peptide and conjugation to flavonucleotides. When added to exogenous nuclei or microinjected into cells, AIF induces cleavage of genomic DNA at ~50-kbp intervals and causes chromatin condensation typical of early stages of apoptosis. Embryos devoid of AIF fail to undergo cavitation, implying a requirement of this protein for cell death at a very early stage in formation of the preimplantation embryo. However, AIF-deficient cells appear to be unimpaired in their ability to undergo apoptosis in response to a wide variety of exogenous stimuli, including many that invoke the mitochondrial pathway.

E. Bcl-2 Family Proteins and Regulation of Mitochondria-Dependent Steps in Apoptosis Programs

Where do Bcl-2 and its homologues fit into this story of mitochondrial PT pore opening and release of apoptogenic proteins? Overexpression of Bcl-2 or similar antiapoptotic members of the Bcl-2 family such as Bcl-X$_L$ confers protection upon mitochondria, making it more difficult for many stimuli to induce PT pore opening and to trigger release of cytochrome c and other mitochondrial proteins. Conversely, overexpression of the proapoptotic protein Bax or similar proapoptotic family members induces loss of $\Delta\Psi$ and release of cytochrome c. The mechanisms by which Bcl-2 prevents and Bax promotes these destructive changes in mitochondria, however, are far from clear.

It has been hypothesized that Bcl-2 family proteins directly participate in regulation of the PT pore. In support of this idea are experiments in which attempts were made to purify the multiprotein PT pore complex from mitochondria and reconstitute it in synthetic liposomes, demonstrating copurification of Bax. Moreover, the partially purified PT pore complex retains many of its expected functional characteristics when reconstituted in liposomes, including suppression of pore opening by recombinant Bcl-2 protein but not by mutants of Bcl-2 that fail to suppress apoptosis in intact cells. Functional interactions of Bcl-2 family proteins with the adenine nucleotide translocator (ANT) in membranes have also been reported in experiments where ion conductances by ANT have been measured in the presence and absence of added recombinant Bcl-2 (Bcl-X$_L$) or Bax (Bak). Similarly, Bcl-2 and Bcl-X$_L$ have been claimed to compete with Bax and Bak for binding to VDAC, the porin-like channel protein of the outer membrane. Moreover, it has been claimed that Bax and Bak collaborate with VDAC in producing channels of sufficient size to permit escape of cytochrome c.

Even if Bcl-2 family proteins do interact with components of the PT pore complex in mitochondrial membranes, the question that remains to be answered is how do proteins ranging in mass from cytochrome c (~15 kDa) to Smac (dimer of ~100 kDa mass) transit from their normal place of residence in the space between the inner and the outer mitochondrial membranes across the outer membrane to enter the cytosol? Two competing models have been advanced involving either swelling-dependent or -independent mechanisms. The most popular swelling-dependent mechanism envisions Bcl-2 family proteins as regulators directly or indirectly of the ANT in the inner membrane. In this scenario, opening of the ANT causes an immediate dissipation of $\Delta\Psi$, followed by volume dysregulation, osmotic swelling of mitochondria, and secondary release of apoptogenic proteins as a result of rupture of the outer membrane. A variation on this model has also been proposed envisioning that mitochondrial volume dysregulation with matrix swelling and outer membrane rupture can occur independent of PT pore opening, perhaps as a result of changes in the function of some of the various ion transporters found in the inner membrane. The competing model for explaining how proteins are released from mitochondria hypothesizes that pores are created *de novo* in the outer membrane, allowing escape of some proteins (such as cytochrome c), while leaving the permeability of the inner membrane intact. Both models are supported by abundant data, which has not helped to resolve the issue. An added complication is the observation that certain caspases can induce PT pore opening when applied to isolated mitochondria *in vitro* and caspase inhibitory drugs can often delay $\Delta\Psi$ dissipation in intact cells stimulated to undergo apoptosis. Thus, sorting out events that are causative from those that are a downstream effect of caspase activation can be problematic.

Thus, a central question of apoptosis research is which comes first: (a) dissipation of $\Delta\Psi$ due to PT pore opening, followed by cytochrome c release due to organellar swelling and rupture, or (b) release of cytochrome c, resulting in failed electron transport from complex III to IV and a subsequent decline in $\Delta\Psi$? Comparisons of the time-courses of cytochrome c release and mitochondrial $\Delta\Psi$ loss in cells undergoing apoptosis caused by growth factor deprivation or cytotoxic anticancer drugs have provided evidence that cytochrome c release often precedes $\Delta\Psi$ loss in most types of cells. In this scenario, it has been argued that only a portion of the total available cytochrome c need be released into the cytosol to result in caspase activation, and thus sufficient cytochrome c remains bound to the external surface of the inner membrane (associated with cytochrome c oxidase) to sustain electron transport and $\Delta\Psi$. However, time-lapse video microscopy suggests that cytochrome c release is an "all-or-none" phenomenon, rather than a problem of slow leakage.

Clearly, much remains to be learned about the relative importance of the PT pore in apoptosis induced by various stimuli and the relation of PT pore regulation to the functions of Bcl-2 family proteins. Importantly, more than one mechanism for the release of proteins from mitochondria is probably possible, perhaps accounting for some of the discrepancies found in the literature. Thus, selective permeabilization of the outer membrane resulting in protein release without $\Delta\Psi$ dissipation is almost certainly involved in apoptosis induction by many physiologically relevant stimuli (such as growth factor deprivation), whereas PT pore opening can be triggered by oxidative injury or calcium overload (e.g., ischemia reperfusion injury), causing an immediate loss of $\Delta\Psi$ and secondary organellar rupture due to osmotic swelling. Curiously, Bcl-2 family proteins seem to regulate both pathways, suggesting diversity in their mechanisms.

VIII. Bcl-2-BINDING PROTEINS: CLUES TO ADDITIONAL FUNCTIONS

Further clues to the mechanism of action of Bcl-2 and its homologous proteins have come from the discovery of other Bcl-2-interacting proteins that do not share amino acid sequence homology with Bcl-2. To date, Bcl-2 or its antiapoptotic homologues have been reported to bind a plethora of additional proteins, including (a) p23-R-Ras, a member of the Ras family of low molecular weight GTPases; (b) p72-Raf-1, a serine/threonine-specific protein kinase; (c) BAG-1 (Bcl-2-associated AthanoGene-1) and BAG3, proteins that interact with and regulate Hsp70 family molecular chaperones; (d) p53BP2, a p53-binding protein; (e) Pr-1, a prion protein; (f) Smn1, a protein implicated in the regulation of RNA splicing and causally linked to spinal muscular atrophy; (g) TCTP, a Ca^{2+}-binding protein of uncertain function; (h) Bap31, a resident ER protein that binds caspase-8; (i) BAR, an integral membrane protein found in membranes of mitochondria and ER that also binds

Caspase-8; (j) BI-1, a multipass transmembrane protein implicated in apoptosis suppression; (k) calcineurin, a Ca^{2+}/calmodulin-dependent protein phosphatase; (l) Flip (MRIT), an antagonist of caspases-8 and -10; (m) the Caspase-activator Apaf1, (n) Aven, an Apaf1-binding protein; and (o) other proteins. Debate reins as to the relative importance of each of these interacting proteins for the antiapoptotic function of Bcl-2 and its relatives.

In mammalian systems, it may be that these alternative interaction partners play an ancillary role in cell death regulation, linking various signaling events to the core apoptosis machinery by modulating the functions of Bcl-2, Bcl-X_L, and their relatives. In contrast, a clear role for interactions with a nonhomologous protein in the mechanism of a Bcl-2 homologue has been demonstrated in the nematode *C. elegans*. In this invertebrate animal, the Bcl-2 homologue binds and suppresses Ced-4, an Apaf1-like caspase activator. In the worm, binding of Ced-9 to Ced-4 correlates tightly with the antiapoptotic function of this Bcl-2 homologue. It remains to be seen, however, whether a similar scenario exists in higher eukaryotes. Even in other invertebrates such as *Drosophila melanogaster*, the function of Bcl-2 family proteins as guardians of the mitochondria seems more akin to the mammalian system than to *C. elegans*.

IX. EFFECTS OF Bcl-2 ON CELL PROLIFERATION

Evidence that Bcl-2 and its antiapoptotic cousins Bcl-X_L and Bcl-W can delay cell cycle entry ($G_0 \rightarrow G_1$ transition) or slow $G_1 \rightarrow S$ phase progression has been obtained for several types of cells. The mechanism responsible for this putative link of antiapoptotic proteins to an antiproliferative pheonotype is unclear, but raises the possibility that one of the cytoprotective mechanisms of Bcl-2 may involve encouraging cells to remain quiescent and thus less vulnerable to a variety of cytotoxic insults that seem to preferentially affect dividing cells.

Candidate proteins that can potentially speed cell cycle rates and whose function may be inhibited by overexpression of Bcl-2 include the transcription factors NF-κB and NF-AT. Inhibition of entry into the nucleus and/or successful transactivation of target genes by NF-κB and NF-AT has been reported in Bcl-2 overexpressing cells. In the case of NF-AT, a transcription factor first identified because of its ability to stimulate the expression of lymphokine and lymphokine receptor genes in lymphocytes, it has been shown that dephosphorylation of NF-AT by calcineurin is required for NF-AT translocation from the cytosol into the nucleus. The ability of Bcl-2 to bind calcineurin, sequestering it at membranes where it cannot dephosphorylate NF-AT in the cytosol, may provide an explanation for at least one mechanism by which Bcl-2 contributes to cell cycle arrest. It should be noted, however, that the wild-type Bcl-2 protein does not cause a cell cycle delay in all types of cells and indeed has been shown to enhance rather than inhibit cell proliferation in some cellular contexts.

X. POSTTRANSLATIONAL MODIFICATIONS OF Bcl-2 FAMILY PROTEINS

Several Bcl-2 family proteins can be regulated by posttranslational modifications to the proteins. The best documented involve either phosphorylation or proteolytic cleavage.

A. Phosphorylation

Some of the antiapoptotic Bcl-2 family proteins, including Bcl-2 and Bcl-X_L, contain a long flexible loop region that is rich in proline residues and appears to suppress their prosurvival functions through uncertain mechanisms. The loop region of Bcl-2 undergoes phosphorylation at serine 70, serine 87, or other sites in response to specific stimuli. Phosphorylation at serine 70 by protein kinase C (PKC) has been reported to enhance the survival-promoting activity of Bcl-2. However, in most circumstances where phosphorylation of Bcl-2 occurs, a reduction of Bcl-2 activity has been suggested. Much attention has been given to the phosphorylation of Bcl-2 induced in response to microtubule-targeting drugs, such as paclitaxel, vincristine, and nocodazole. These phosphorylation events appear to suppress apoptosis suppression by Bcl-2, as evidenced by site-specific mutagenesis experiments in

which nonphosphorylatable mutants of Bcl-2 are more potent protectors against death induced by these agents. Although not uniformly seen in all studies, phosphorylation of Bcl-2 following exposure to microtubule-targeting drugs has been reported to impair heterodimerization with Bax. Phosphorylated Bcl-2 binds the peptidyl prolinyl isomerase (PPIase), Pin, a protein that interacts in a phosphorylation-dependent manner with Cdc2 substrates during mitosis. The significance of this interaction of phosphorylated Bcl-2 with Pin is unknown, but suggests the possibility that Pin induces changes in the conformation of Bcl-2 that impair its antiapoptotic function. The kinases responsible for phosphorylation of Bcl-2 following exposure to microtubule-targeting drugs are uncertain, but cases have been made for the involvement of various cyclin-dependent kinases, microtubule-associated kinases (MAPKs), and Jun N-terminal kinase (JNKs). It has also been suggested that phosphorylation of Bcl-2 may control ubiquitination and proteasome-dependent degradation of this protein in response to cytokine stimulation (TNFα). In this case, however, dephosphorylation rather than phosphorylation seems to correlate with degradation of Bcl-2. Interestingly, mutations have been identified in the loop region of Bcl-2 in lymphomas containing t(14;18) chromosomal translocations involving the *BCL-2* gene, sometimes occurring in association with transformation from low-grade follicular lymphoma to aggressive diffuse large cell non-Hodgkin's lymphoma.

The BH3-only protein, BAD, is tightly regulated by phosphorylation/dephosphorylation. Heterodimerization of BAD with Bcl-X_L is inhibited by phosphorylation, which can be induced by several kinases, including Akt (PKB), Raf1, Pak1, and Rsk. The inactivation of BAD by phosphorylation provides a mechanism for functionally linking a variety of growth factor receptors to the suppression of apoptosis. Excessive signaling by these growth factor receptors is common in cancer and may explain in part the apoptosis-resistant state of many tumors. Some phosphorylated forms of BAD bind 14-3-3, which helps sequester the protein in a form that precludes it from being readily dephosphorylated. Among the phosphatases that can reverse phosphorylation of BAD is calcineurin, which has been shown to cause BAD dephosphorylation in situations where Ca^{2+} influx occurs. Dephosphorylation of BAD correlates with translocation of the protein from cytosol to the surface of mitochondria, where BAD can be found in a complex with Bcl-2 or Bcl-X_L.

Although largely unexplored, it seems likely that additional examples of regulation of Bcl-2 family proteins by phosphorylation will emerge over time.

B. Proteolysis

Some Bcl-2 family members are cleaved by proteases, thus altering their activities in profound ways. For example, the loop regions of Bcl-2 and Bcl-X_L contain typical recognition sequences for effector caspases and are sites of cleavage *in vitro* and *in vivo*. Caspase-mediated cleavage of Bcl-2 and Bcl-X_L converts these cytoprotective molecules into killers, which probably operate as transdominant competitors with intact Bcl-2 and Bcl-X_L. Interestingly, at least one example of a mutation in the caspase cleavage site of Bcl-2 has been described in a cancer cell line.

The proapoptotic protein Bid is also a target of caspases. Specifically, Bid is cleaved by the initiator protease, caspase-8. Cleavage of Bid arouses this protein from a latent state, exposing an N-terminal segment that undergoes subsequent myristoylation and causing Bid to target mitochondrial membranes where it interacts via its BH3 domain with multidomain members of the family. Because caspase-8 becomes activated by several TNF family cytokine receptors, the Bid protein provides a mechanism for cross talk between the death receptor pathway for apoptosis and the mitochondrial pathway. Interestingly, many types of cells do not express Bid, suggesting that this cross talk pathway is available only in some circumstances.

The Bax protein can also become cleaved, probably by a calpain-like protease. It has been speculated that this cleavage of Bax activates this protein or enhances its proapoptotic function. Details, however, remain unavailable at present.

XI. DYSREGULATION OF *BCL-2* FAMILY GENES IN CANCERS

Multiple examples exist of dysregulation of the expression of *BCL-2* family genes in cancers. The *BCL-2* gene, for instance, is probably pathologically overexpressed in roughly half of all human cancers, including large proportions of adenocarcinomas of the breast, colon, stomach, and prostate; squamous cell carcinomas of the lung, head and neck, and skin; and small round cell tumors such as small cell lung cancer, neuroblastoma, and others. Although the mechanisms remain unclear, overexpression of Bcl-2 in solid tumors does not appear to be associated with structural alterations in the *BCL-2* gene, unlike the situation in lymphomas where t(14;18) translocations are commonly responsible. Amplification of the *BCL-2* gene has been reported in some lymphomas, suggesting another mechanism for dysregulation of this cell survival gene in tumors. Hypomethylation of the *BCL-2* gene promoter has also been described in CLL, in association with overproduction of Bcl-2 mRNA and protein. The roles of gene amplification, hypomethylation, and mutation in the pathological overexpression of *BCL-2* seen in many solid tumors remain largely unexplored to date. In addition to Bcl-2, overexpression of other antiapoptotic members of the family has been reported in specific types of cancer, including Bcl-X_L, Mcl-1, and Bcl-W.

In contrast to the common overexpression of the antiapoptotic protein such as Bcl-2 in cancer, reduced expression of proapoptotic proteins such as Bax can also be found in some types of malignancies. Moreover, frameshift mutations have been described in the *BAX* gene in hematopoietic and solid tumors in humans, resulting in a failure to produce the Bax protein. These mutations occur most commonly in a homopolymeric stretch of eight guanosine nucleotides and are typically associated with microsatellite instability. Data from tumor xenograph studies have also provided evidence that loss of *BAX* expression due to such frameshift mutations confers a selective growth advantage on tumor cells and thus supports data from *bax* knockout mice, which have suggested a tumor suppressor function for this proapoptotic gene. Examples of decreases in the expression of other proapoptotic Bcl-2 family members have also been revealed, such as the marked reduction of Bak seen in many colon cancers.

The relative contributions of transcriptional and posttranscriptional mechanisms to the dysregulation of *BCL-2* family genes in cancers are mostly unknown.

However, several transcription factors have been shown to regulate the expression of Bcl-2 family genes, including p53, NF-κB, RXR, RAR, PPARγ, estrogen receptor (ER), Stats, Sp1, Ets, and others. Furthermore, for some *BCL-2* family genes, this transcriptional regulation seems to be direct, involving physical interactions of these transcription factors with *cis*-acting elements in the promoter regions of the *BCL-2* family genes. For example, tumor suppressor p53 can bind and directly transactivate the promoters for human *BAX*, *PUMA*, and *NOXA*. This property of p53 thus provides a plausible link between DNA damage and apoptosis. Similarly, NF-κB family transcription factors probably directly induce the promoters of the antiapoptotic genes *BCL-X* and *BFL1*.

These links between transcription factors and expression of *BCL-2* family genes may have therapeutic implications in some instances. For example, the use of retinoids in the treatment of acute myelogenous leukemia (AML) may owe its success in part to the ability of retinoids to downregulate the expression of *BCL-2* and *BCL-X* in these leukemias. The same appears to be true of antiestrogens in breast cancer, where it has been shown that *BCL-2* is an estrogen-dependent gene. Thus, many opportunities exist for exploiting emerging knowledge about the regulation of *BCL-2* family genes by agents that modulate the activity of steroid/retinoid family transcription factors for the improved treatment of cancer.

XII. Bcl-2 REGULATES RESISTANCE TO CHEMOTHERAPY AND RADIATION

Although defects in the regulation of the physiological cell death pathway (such as overexpression of *BCL-2*) can clearly contribute to the origins of cancer by causing cells to live longer than they would normally be programmed to do, loss of cell death mechanisms can also figure prominently in the treatment of cancer. This is because nearly all drugs currently available for the treatment of malignancies ultimately kill cancer cells by activating endogenous cellular pathways for apoptosis. Thus, cancer cells that have dysregulation of these cell death pathways tend to respond more poorly to anticancer drugs. The same is also true for γ radiation.

Conclusive evidence has been provided indicating that increases in Bcl-2 protein levels render cancer cells more resistant to induction of cell death by a wide range of anticancer drugs. Included among these drugs are inhibitors of deoxynucleotide triphosphate synthesis and antimetabolites (methotrexate, thymidyl synthase inhibitors, cytosine arabinoside, fludarabine, 2 chloro-deoxyadenosine, 5-flurouracil), microtubule-targeting drugs (vincristine, vinblastine, paclitaxel), topoisomerase inhibitors (etoposide, camptothecin, mitoxantrone), DNA intercalators (adriamycin, daunomycin), glucocorticoids (dexamethasone), alkylating reagents (BCNU, nitrogen mustards, cyclophosphamide), and cisplatin. Moreover, using antisense approaches to achieve reductions in Bcl-2 protein levels, it has been possible to reverse chemoresistance in some circumstances. This observation has prompted attempts to apply synthetic nuclease-resistant antisense oligonucleotides targeted against *BCL-2* in clinical trials. Promising results have been obtained in phase I and II studies, and pivotal phase III trials for patients with myeloma, melanoma, and other forms of malignancy are presently underway. In most of the advanced clinical trials, as in prior animal models, *BCL-2* antisense is being used as a chemosensitizer, in conjunction with conventional cytotoxic anticancer drugs.

The drug resistance imparted to cancer cells by overproduction of the Bcl-2 protein is different from all other previously described forms of drug resistance. First, the spectrum of drugs to which Bcl-2 confers resistance is the broadest defined to date and presumably reflects the facts that (1) all of these drugs, as well as radiation, ultimately kill cancer cells by triggering endogenous cellular pathways for apoptotic cells death and (2) Bcl-2 regulates a distal step in this cell death pathway. Thus, despite the diversity of their biochemical mechanisms of action, all of these drugs have in common the ability to activate the programmed cell death pathway at some point that lies upstream of Bcl-2. Second, unlike some other previously defined mechanisms of drug resistance, Bcl-2 does not prevent entry of drugs into cells (contrast with *mdr-1* overexpression) nor does it alter the extent to which drugs induce damage to DNA or the rate at which cells repair damaged DNA. Rather, with Bcl-2 overproduction, drugs still enter cells and induce damage, but this damage is somehow ineffectively translated into signals for cell death. In fact, it has been shown that anticancer drugs can still induce cell cycle arrest when Bcl-2 is present at high levels, but the cells typically fail to die at higher frequencies compared to cells with low Bcl-2. Thus, Bcl-2 can convert anticancer drugs from cytotoxic to cytostatic. Furthermore, when drugs are removed from cultures, a scenario that is analogous to the cessation of drugs that occurs clinically between cycles of chemotherapy, BCL-2-expressing cells can often reinitiate cell growth far more frequently than their control counterparts, based on clonigenic cell assays. Presumably, therefore, because they do not die as easily when exposed to drugs, cells with elevated levels of Bcl-2 protein are able to survive through the period of drug treatment and then repair drug-induced damage and resume their proliferation when drugs are withdrawn. Taken together, these observations suggest that Bcl-2 and its related proteins define a new category of drug resistance genes, i.e., those that regulate the physiological cell death pathway.

XIII. UTILITY OF Bcl-2 FAMILY PROTEINS AND GENES AS PROGNOSTIC MARKERS IN CANCER

The t(14;18) translocation, which commonly activates the BCL-2 gene in non-Hodgkin's lymphomas, can serve as a tumor-specific marker for diagnosis as well as for monitoring of treatment of patients using various molecular techniques, including highly sensitive polymerase chain reaction (PCR) methods. Indeed, one of the first applications of PCR to human cancer involved detection of t(14;18) breakpoints in DNA isolated from patients with lymphoma. One of the applications where the use of PCR for monitoring the presence of residual tumor cells has had its greatest utility is in autologous bone marrow transplantation, both for determining the success of bone marrow-purging procedures (which are designed to eliminate malignant cells from the patient's harvested marrow specimen before transplantation) and for detecting malignant cells after transplanation in the peripheral blood. Data from several studies have suggested that prolonged disease-free survival correlates with the ability to purge the marrow to PCR negativity and with absence of PCR-detectable cells in the

peripheral blood when monitored at frequent intervals after transplantation. These promising data suggest the possibility of predicting relapse based on PCR status and making clinical decisions based on that information.

Immunohistochemical methods have also been employed for the detection of Bcl-2 in clinical samples. In patients with intermediate-grade non-Hodgkin's lymphomas, high levels of Bcl-2 protein, as assessed by immunostaining, are commonly associated with shorter relapse-free and overall survival, indicating that Bcl-2 represents an adverse prognostic marker, which confers independent prognostic information. However, positive correlations between Bcl-2 and worse prognosis have not been uniformly found, suggesting that additional factors are also important.

In addition to lymphomas, assessment of Bcl-2 status by immunostaining has shown promise of prognostic utility in patients with other types of malignancy. For instance, high levels of Bcl-2 immunostaining are commonly associated with an unfavorable clinical outcome in prostate cancer, where overexpression of Bcl-2 has been associated with a risk of progression to hormone refractory, metastatic disease. High levels of Bcl-2 protein, as determined by indirect immunofluorescence with flow cytometric analysis, have also been correlated with a poor response to therapy in patients with AML. However, Bcl-2 immunopositivity has been associated with better prognosis in at least one study of nonsmall cell lung cancer, particularly the squamous type. The treatment of these patients, however, was surgical, and thus findings are irrelevant to the issue of Bcl-2 and chemoresistance. Bcl-2 has also been consistently correlated with a better prognosis for women with early stage (I and II) carcinoma of the breast. It has been speculated that this association of Bcl-2 expression with a favorable outcome in breast cancer may be linked to the observation that BCL-2 is an estrogen-dependent gene in the mammary gland, and thus tumors that express BCL-2 are also highly likely to have functional estrogen receptors (ER). ER-positive breast cancer generally is less aggressive and potentially can be controlled using antiestrogens.

In addition to Bcl-2, suggestions of prognostic utility of other Bcl-2 family members have also begun to emerge. For example, loss of BAX expression was associated with poor responses to chemotherapy and shorter survival in a study of women with metastatic breast cancer (stage IV) treated with combination chemotherapy. Given their role in chemoresistance, radioresistance, and also metastasis, it seems likely that multiple examples will eventually appear in which tumor-specific changes in the expression of Bcl-2 family proteins correlate with the clinical outcome for patients with cancer.

XIV. THERAPEUTIC OPPORTUNITIES

Although our understanding of the mechanisms responsible for regulating expression and function of Bcl-2 family proteins remains far from complete, rapidly emerging data are beginning to suggest some novel approaches to the treatment of cancer. The therapeutic strategies that can be envisioned include traditional small molecule drugs, antisense oligonucleotides, and gene therapy. With respect to small molecule drugs, for example, proof-of-concept experiments using BH3 peptides suggest that molecules which mimic the BH3 domain can be used to induce apoptosis by binding to the same crevice on the surface of Bcl-2, Bcl-X$_L$, or similar antiapoptotic proteins, which is used for heterodimerization among Bcl-2 family proteins. Nonpeptidyl compounds that function as BH3 mimics have been described, laying a foundation for drug development. Alternatively, antisense approaches for interfering with the expression of antiapoptotic BCL-2 family genes can be envisioned, and indeed are already under evaluation in advanced clinical trials in humans using BCL-2 antisense phosphorothioate oligonucleotides. Conversely, restoring the expression of proapoptotic Bcl-2 family genes in tumors is a possibility for gene therapy approaches. Already, intratumoral injection of adenoviruses carrying p53 has advanced to clinical trials, suggesting the possibility of using proapoptotic Bcl-2 family genes in a similar manner to achieve locoregional control of resistant tumors. Finally, myriad opportunities exist for exploiting the transcriptional and signal transduction pathways that impinge on Bcl-2 family proteins and their genes for indirectly regulating the activity or expression of these important apoptosis regulators. Such applications could involve small molecule drugs that activate various retinoid/steroid family transcription factors or that inhibit protein kinases. With improved knowledge at the molecular and structural level of the mechanisms of action of Bcl-2 and related proteins and with increasing information about the mechanisms that regulate the expression of BCL-2 family genes in normalcy and neoplasia, it should eventually be possible to develop novel treatments for cancer that specifically seek to modulate the physiological cell death pathway, thereby encouraging cancer cells to commit suicide.

Acknowledgments

I thank the present and past members of our laboratory whose talents and untiring efforts resulted in many of the experimental observations discussed in this review. Thanks also go to R. Cornell and A. Sawyer for manuscript preparation and to the National Cancer Institute, the California Breast Cancer Research Program, the Department of Defense, and CaP-CURE for generous financial support.

See Also the Following Articles

Caspases in Programmed Cell Death • Cell Cycle Checkpoints • Chronic Lymphocytic Leukemia • DNA Damage, DNA Repair, and Mutagenesis • Epstein-Barr Virus • Lymphoma, Non-Hodgkin's • Pancreatic Cancer: Cellular and Molecular Mechanisms

Bibliography

Bredesen, D. E. (2000). Apoptosis: Overview and signal transduction pathways. *J. Neurotrauma* **17,** 801–810.

Chao, D. T., and Korsmeyer, S. J. (1998). Bcl-2 family: Regulators of cell death. *Annu. Rev. Immunol.* **16,** 395–419.

Croce, C. M., Erikson, J., Tsujimoto, Y., and Nowell, P. C. (1987). Molecular basis of human B- and T-cell neoplasia. *Adv. Viral Oncol.* **7,** 35.

Green, D., and Kroemer, G. (1998). The central executioners of apoptosis: Caspases or mitochondria? *Trends Cell Biol.* **8,** 267–271.

Green, D. R., and Reed, J. C. (1998). Mitochondria and apoptosis. *Science* **281,** 1309–1312.

Gross, A., McDonnell, J., and Korsmeyer, S. (1999). BCL-2 family members and the mitochondria in apoptosis. *Genes Dev.* **13,** 1899–1911.

Häcker, G., and Vaux, D. L. (1995). A sticky business. *Curr. Biol.* **5,** 622–624.

Huang, D. C., and Strasser, A. (2000). BH3-only proteins: Essential initiators of apoptotic cell death. *Cell* **103,** 839–842.

Kelekar, A., and Thompson, C. B. (1998). Bcl-2-family proteins: The role of the BH3 domain in apoptosis. *Trends Cell Biol.* **8,** 324–330.

Korsmeyer, S. J. (1992). Bcl-2 initiates a new category of oncogenes: Regulators of cell death. *Blood* **80,** 879.

Kroemer, G., and Reed, J.C. (2000). Mitochondrial control of cell death. *Nature Med.* **6,** 513–519.

Matsuyama, S., and Reed, J. C. (2000). Mitochondria-dependent apoptosis and cellular pH regulation. *Cell Death Differ* **7,** 1155–1165.

Minn, A., Swain, R., Ma, A., and Thompson, C. (1998). Recent progress on the regulation of apoptosis by Bcl-2 family members. *Adv. Immunol.* **70,** 245–279.

Pellegrini, M., and Strasser, A. (1999). A portrait of the bcl-2 protein family: Life, death, and the whole picture. *J. Clin. Immunol.* **19,** 365–377.

Reed, J. C. (1994). Bcl-2 and the regulation of programmed cell death. *J. Cell Biol.* **124,** 1.

Reed, J. C. (1997). Double identity for proteins of the Bcl-2 family. *Nature* **387,** 773–776.

Reed, J. (1998). Bcl-2 family proteins. *Oncogene* **17,** 3225–3236.

Reed, J. C. (2000). Mechanisms of apoptosis (Warner/Lambert Award). *Am. J. Pathol.* **157,** 1415–1430.

Rudin, C., and Thompson, C. (1997). Apoptosis and disease: Regulation and clinical relevance of programmed cell death. *Ann. Rev. Med.* **48,** 267–281.

Sachs, L., and Lotem, J. (1993). Control of programmed cell death in normal and leukemic cells: New implications for therapy. *Blood* **82,** 15.

Schendel, S., Montal, M., and Reed, J. C. (1998). Bcl-2 family proteins as ion-channels. *Cell Death Differ.* **5,** 372–380.

Thompson, C. B. (1995). Apoptosis in the pathogenesis and treatment of disease. *Science* **267,** 1456–1462.

Vander Heiden, M. G., and Thompson, C. B. (1999). Bcl-2 proteins: Regulators of apoptosis or of mitochondrial homeostasis? *Nature Cell Biol.* **1,** E209–E216.

Vaux, D. L. (1993). Toward an understanding of the molecular mechanisms of physiological cell death. *Proc. Natl. Acad. Sci. USA* **90,** 786.

Vaux, D. L., Haecker, G., and Strasser, A. (1994). An evolutionary perspective on apoptosis. *Cell* **76,** 777.

Vaux, D., and Korsmeyer, S. (1999). Cell death in development. *Cell* **96,** 245–254.

Vaux, D. L., and Strasser, A. (1996). The molecular biology of apoptosis. *Proc. Natl. Acad. Sci. USA* **93,** 2239–2244.

Williams, G. T. (1991). Programmed cell death: Apoptosis and oncogenesis. *Cell* **65,** 1097.

Williams, G. T., and Smith, C. A. (1993). Molecular regulation of apoptosis: Genetic controls on cell death. *Cell* **74,** 777.

Yang, E., and Korsmeyer, S. J. (1996). Molecular thanatopsis: A discourse on the Bcl2 family and cell death. *Blood* **88,** 386–401.

BCR/ABL

Anna Butturini
Children's Hospital Los Angeles, California

Ralph B. Arlinghaus
M.D. Anderson Cancer Center, Houston, Texas

Robert Peter Gale
Center for Advanced Studies in Leukemia, Los Angeles, California

GLOSSARY

Abelson proto-oncogene (ABL) A 230-kb, 11 exon proto-oncogene located at 9q34. It encodes p145^{ABL}, a protein with nonreceptor tyrosine kinase activity. ABL is responsible for the transforming activity of Abelson murine leukemia virus (*v-ABL*). In the t(9;22) translocation typical of chronic myelogenous leukemia (CML), the ABL breakpoint is in the first intron; sequences 3′ the breakpoint are juxtaposed to BCR to form BCR/ABL.

acute lymphoblastic leukemia (ALL) Leukemia characterized by bone marrow and blood replacement by immature lymphoid cells. Only a subset of ALL (15–35% in adults, 5–15% in children) has the t(9;22) translocation, usually as only chromosomal abnormality.

BCR/ABL The chimeric gene created by the t(9;22) translocation typical of CML, which juxtaposes BCR and ABL genes. Breakpoints in different regions of BCR gene result in fusion genes of different length and consequently in different BCR/ABL mRNAs and proteins. P210$^{BCR/ABL}$ is present in >95% of CML, P190$^{BCR/ABL}$ is present in 5–35% of acute lymphoblastic leukemia (ALL), and the less common P230$^{BCR/ABL}$ is present in a rare form of CML, chronic neutrophilic leukemia (CNL). All BCR-ABL proteins have tyrosine kinase activity.

Breakpoint cluster region (BCR) A 155-kb, 23 exon gene located at 22q11. It encodes p160^{BCR}, a protein with two serine-rich domains involved in binding to the ABL SH2, a GDP exchange domain called DBL homology domain, a pleckstrin homology (PH) domain, and a GAP domain. In the t(9;22) translocation typical of CML, BCR breakpoints are in the major (M-BCR), minor (m-BCR), or the less common u-BCR cluster regions; sequences 5′ the breakpoint are juxtaposed to ABL to form BCR/ABL.

chronic myelogenous leukemia Leukemia characterized by the presence of t(9;22) translocation in hematopoietic cells of myeloid and lymphoid lineage (suggesting an initial event in an early multipotent hematopoietic precursor). Clinically, CML has two phases: chronic and acute. The chronic phase is characterized by an increased number of mature granulocytes and myeloid precursors in blood. The acute phase is similar to acute leukemia. During the chronic phase, the t(9;22) translocation is the only chromosome abnormality detected in leukemia cells. In contrast, additional chromosome changes may develop in the acute phase.

P190$^{BCR/ABL}$ The 190-kDa protein with tyrosine kinase resulting from a break in BCR at the m-BCR region and its fusion to ABL. It is present in 2–20% of ALL and in rare CML. P190$^{BCR/ABL}$ may cause leukemia. Among BCR-ABL proteins, P190$^{BCR/ABL}$ has the greatest tyrosine kinase activity.

P210$^{BCR/ABL}$ The 210-kDa protein with tyrosine kinase resulting from a break in BCR at the M-BCR region and its fusion to ABL. It is typical of CML, but is also present in about 2–15% of ALL. P210$^{BCR/ABL}$ is the major factor in causing leukemia.

P230$^{BCR/ABL}$ The 230-kDa protein with tyrosine kinase resulting from a break in BCR at the u-BCR region (exon 19 or 20) and its fusion to ABL. It is present and may have a causal role in CNL (chronic neutrophilic leukemia, a variant of CML).

BCR/ABL is a fusion gene containing 3'ABL sequences juxtaposed to 5' BCR sequences. It usually results from the t(9;22)(q34;q11) translocation. In cells with this translocation, the derivative chromosome 22 is referred to as Philadelphia (*Ph^1*) chromosome.

I. INTRODUCTION

BCR/ABL is the molecular hallmark of chronic myelogenous leukemia. It is also present in about 20–50% of B-lineage acute lymphoblastic leukemia in adults, about 5–15% of B-lineage ALL in children, and 2–10% cases of acute myeloblastic leukemia (AML). The presence of the t(9;22) translocation in hematopoietic cells of multiple lineages *in vivo* and/or in colony assays suggests that the BCR/ABL fusion happens in multipotent hematopoietic precursors in CML and in at least a subset of ALL with either P190$^{BCR/ABL}$ or P210$^{BCR/ABL}$. The cause of breaks in BCR and ABL and following BCR/ABL fusion is uncertain. In early hematopoietic cells, regions containing BCR and ABL genes are adjacent during S phase; this may facilitate that process.

Studies of transgenic mice and in mice transplanted with BCR/ABL-transfected bone marrow cells indicate that BCR/ABL causes CML and ALL-like leukemia. The mechanism of leukemogenesis is still unknown, but it is likely related to the activated tyrosine kinase activity of BCR/ABL.

II. CHARACTERISTICS OF BCR/ABL

Different BCR/ABL genes result from the fusion of ABL to different parts of BCR. ABL breakpoints typically occur in the first 175-kb intron. Consequently, all BCR/ABL genes contain ABL exons 2 to 11 (a2 to a11). BCR breakpoints are also intronic but occur in different regions.

In most CML and in about 50% of adults with *Ph^1* positive ALL, BCR breakpoints are in a 5.8-kb region called the *major breakpoint region* (M-BCR), which spans between exons 12 to 16 (also called b1 to b5). The most common breakpoints are between exons 13 (or b2) and 14(or b3) and exons 14 and 15 (or b4). The sequences 5' to the BCR breakpoint are joined in frame to the truncated ABL so that either a b2a2 or a b3a2 junction is created and processed into two different 8.5-kb RNAs, with or without the exon 14 (or b3) sequences. In about 5–10% of CML with b3a2 junctions, both RNAs are present because of alternative splicing of exon 14 sequences. Both these RNAs are translated into a 210-kDa protein, P210$^{BCR/ABL}$.

In about 50% of *Ph^1* positive adult ALL, in most childhood *Ph^1* positive ALL, and in rare CML, BCR breakpoints are in the first intron, in a segment called the *minor breakpoint region* (m-BCR), between exon 1 (also called e1) and 2 (or e2). The first exon of BCR is joined to the truncated ABL in the e1a2 junction; this chimeric gene is transcribed into a 7-kb RNA and is translated into a 190-kDa protein, P190$^{BCR/ABL}$ (also called P185$^{BCR/ABL}$).

In about 5% of CML, a third breakpoint is located

further 3′ from M-BCR, between exons 19 (e19, also called c3) and 20 (e20 or c4), in a segment termed u-BCR. In the e19a2 junction, most of the BCR gene is fused to the truncated ABL; this chimeric gene is translated into a 230-kDa protein, P230$^{BCR/ABL}$.

III. BCR/ABL PROTEINS

A. Structure

BCR/ABL proteins contain BCR-encoded sequences at the N terminus and ABL-encoded sequences at the C terminus. As discussed, P190$^{BCR/ABL}$, P210$^{BCR/ABL}$, and P230$^{BCR/ABL}$ have the same ABL-encoded sequences, but different BCR-encoded sequences. Like the normal ABL product, P145^{ABL}, BCR/ABL proteins have a SH1 domain with tyrosine kinase activity, a phosphotyrosine-binding SH2 domain, a SH3 domain that binds proteins with proline-rich domains, and two more C-terminal domains— one DNA and the other F-actin binding. Also, both BCR/ABL and ABL have three nuclear localization sequences and a nuclear export sequence. The N terminus of BCR included in all BCR/ABL proteins has a coiled-coil motif (possibly responsible for the increased tyrosine kinase activity of BCR/ABL proteins; see later), a serine–threonine kinase activity, and tyrosine-phosphorylated residues that bind proteins with certain SH2 domains (like the GRB2 adapter protein; see later). P210$^{BCR/ABL}$ and the longer P230$^{BCR/ABL}$ also have a GDP–GTP exchange factor domain. All BCR/ABL proteins are autophosphory-lated on tyrosine residues, most within BCR exon 1 and ABL SH1 domains.

Fusion of ABL to BCR generates a tetrameric quaternary structure with greater tyrosine kinase activity than the normal ABL product (P190$^{BCR/ABL}$ the greatest) and the ability to interact with multiple adapter proteins, such as GRB2, CRK oncogene-like protein (CRKL), and CBL.

B. Function

The precise functions of BCR/ABL proteins in leukemia development are unclear. Different from normal ABL product, which moves from nucleus to cytoplasm, BCR/ABL proteins are cytoplasmic only. This is apparently due to reduced nuclear import. Tyrosine kinase activity may have a role in BCR/ABL localization; BCR/ABL proteins with reduced tyrosine kinase activity due to mutations or treatment with inhibitors can be imported in the nucleus. As has been suggested, the location of BCR/ABL might control BCR/ABL functions. Intranuclear BCR/ABL may have proapoptotic activity, as described for nuclear ABL. In contrast, cytoplasmatic BCR/ABL may prevent apoptosis (see later).

Cytoplasmatic BCR/ABL proteins may also complex with the normal BCR protein (that may act as inhibitor) and bind and/or phosphorylate other proteins (Table I). CRKL, an adapter protein, is considered the major substrate of BCR/ABL activity, but other adapter proteins, GRB2 and CBL, may also be affected. Directly or via activation of the RAS cascade, BCR/ABL-activated adapter proteins

TABLE I
Proteins Reported to Interact with BCR/ABL and Possible Implications

Protein	Function	Results of interaction with BCR/ABL
BCR	?	Inhibition of BCR/ABL activity
CRKL	Adaptor protein	Transduction of BCR/ABL signal
CBL	Adaptor protein	Transduction of BCR/ABL signal
SHC	Adaptor protein	Transduction of BCR/ABL signal
GRB2	Adaptor protein	Transduction of BCR/ABL signal
BAP-1	Phosphoserine binding adaptor protein	?
p62 Dok	Adaptor protein	Transduction of BCR/ABL signal
RIN1	Small G-protein (GTPase)	Transduction of BCR/ABL signal

influence the growth factor (GF) signaling pathway, mitogen-activated protein kinases (MAPKs), transcription factors, and adhesion proteins.

IV. BCR/ABL TRANSFORMATION

A. *In Vitro* and Animal Data

Like v-ABL, P190$^{BCR/ABL}$ and P210$^{BCR/ABL}$ transform murine and human fibroblasts and hematopoietic cells and cell lines *in vitro*. In these experiments, transformation is measured as the ability to generate foci in liquid culture and colonies in semisolid medium.

Animal studies suggest a definitive role of BCR/ABL proteins in leukemogenesis. Irradiated mice transplanted with bone marrow cells transfected with a construct carrying the P210$^{BCR/ABL}$ encoding gene develop a disease resembling chronic phase CML. Other animals develop acute leukemia. The type of leukemia correlates with the BCR/ABL construct and mouse strain. Improvements in technology allow development of a myeloid leukemia in virtually all mice in 3–6 weeks. Notably, when bone marrow from mice with CML-like disease is transplanted to irradiated secondary recipients, they develop acute leukemia, mimicking transformation from chronic to acute phase typical of CML in humans. The same results, including chronic and acute leukemia, are observed in animals transplanted with hematopoietic cells transfected with constructs encoding P190$^{BCR/ABL}$ and P230$^{BCR/ABL}$. The only difference is the timing to leukemia development. Animals receiving P190$^{BCR/ABL}$-transformed cells develop acute leukemia earlier than those receiving P210$^{BCR/ABL}$- and P230$^{BCR/ABL}$-transformed cells.

Additional data derive from transgenic animals. About one-half of P190$^{BCR/ABL}$ mice develop pre-B leukemia/lymphoma within 6 months. These cancers initially have a normal karyotype, but rapidly develop abnormal subclones. These animals express P190$^{BCR/ABL}$ in several tissues but they do not develop any nonhematopoietic tumors.

B. Pathogenesis

Cellular mechanisms of BCR/ABL transformation are also unclear. *In vitro* experiments show that the major requirements for transforming activity are functional tyrosine kinase activity and the presence of phosphorylated tyrosine residues at position 177 in BCR exon 1 (which affect binding to Grb2 adapter proteins) and position 1294 in the ABL SH1 domain. How this results in transformation is uncertain. Three major hypotheses have been formulated: defective adherence of immature hematopoietic cells, inhibition of apoptosis, and development of growth factor independence; these are not mutually exclusive.

Data about defective adherence derive from *in vitro* long-term hematopoietic culture studies in CML, indicating that *Ph*^{1} positive progenitor cells tend not to adhere to the stroma. Interestingly, cells transformed by BCR/ABL genes show increased integrin functions. The adhesion proprieties can be restored by antisense oligonucleotides against BCR/ABL, tyrosine kinase inhibitors, or interferon-α.

Data on inhibition of apoptosis and growth factor independence mostly derive from *in vitro* studies in growth factor-dependent murine and human cell lines, where transfection with the P210$^{BCR/ABL}$-encoding gene overcomes growth factor dependence for both survival and growth. The effect on survival is possibly due to the inhibition of apoptosis and depends on tyrosine kinase activity; the effect on growth may also depend on the autocrine secretion of cytokines or effects on intracellular growth factor signaling. In experiments using normal hematopoietic cells, P210$^{BCR/ABL}$ initially decreases, but does not eliminate the need for exogenous growth factor (such as in *in vitro* colony assays of human CML chronic-phase cells).

Another unanswered aspect of BCR/ABL-induced leukemogenesis is the relationship between BCR/ABL proteins and distinct types of leukemia (including the transition between chronic- and acute-phase CML). Several models are proposed. One is that the different BCR/ABL proteins have different transforming potentials, which determine the type of leukemia (i.e., P190$^{BCR/ABL}$ may have a stronger leukemogenic potential, therefore it can directly cause acute leukemia; P210$^{BCR/ABL}$ may only be able to initiate leukemia, but further genetic changes are needed). A second model is that the transforming potentials of BCR/ABL proteins are similar, but the type of leukemia relates to the type of cells where the transformation occurs (i.e., when the e1a2 junction event does take place in lymphoid precursors, it causes ALL, whereas when the same b2a2 junction occurs in multipotent precursors, CML is the result). Each model is both supported and contradicted by experimental and clinical data. How BCR/ABL predisposes to further genetic changes is also unclear. BCR/ABL may increase the risk of DNA damage by the formation of reactive oxygen species, by affecting cell cycle regulation, and/or by altering apoptosis signaling.

V. BCR/ABL TRANSCRIPTION

Data on transcriptional control of BCR/ABL are limited. In CML, transcription of BCR/ABL is controlled by a BCR promoter located in a 270-bp region 5′ of BCR. Little is known about BCR/ABL transcription and expression during hematopoietic differentiation in chronic-phase CML and in the subset of ALL with multilineage involvement. Some data suggest that P210$^{BCR/ABL}$ is not expressed in early hematopoietic precursors.

VI. CLINICAL IMPLICATIONS

A. Effect on Prognosis

BCR/ABL-positive leukemias have a poor response to cytotoxic therapy. Conventional chemotherapy is ineffective in CML and moderately effective in BCR/ABL-positive ALL. In children, the 5-year disease-free survival (DFS) rate is 5–20% in BCR/ABL-positive ALL versus 70–90% in BCR/ABL-negative ALL. The corresponding figures in adults are 0–10% and 40–60%.

Allogeneic bone marrow transplantation (BMT) is very effective in chronic-phase CML (possibly because of immune-mediated mechanisms, see later), but less effective in acute-phase CML or BCR/ABL-positive ALL. Why BCR/ABL-positive cells respond poorly to chemotherapy is unknown. Different causes, as chemoresistance or leukemia origin in a noncycling cell, have been postulated.

As discussed previously, there are different BCR/ABL proteins. Several studies tried to correlate the type of BCR/ABL proteins and disease features. In CML, P210$^{BCR/ABL}$ is almost universal; the type of transcript (b2a2 vs b3a2) does not affect the duration of the chronic phase. Persons with a b3a2 transcript might have a higher platelet count and those with the rare P190$^{BCR/ABL}$ may have monocytosis. Finally, P230$^{BCR/ABL}$ is associated with the neutrophilia/thrombocytosis variant of CML (also termed chronic neutrophilic leukemia) and possibly with a prolonged chronic phase.

In Ph^1 positive ALL, there are differences in age distribution of the BCR/ABL proteins. P210$^{BCR/ABL}$ is uncommon in children, whereas adults have the same probability of having either P190$^{BCR/ABL}$ or P210$^{BCR/ABL}$. In this setting, the type of protein does not affect outcome.

B. BCR/ABL as a Marker of Minimal Residual Leukemia

Polymerase chain reaction (PCR) is increasingly used to diagnose Ph^1 positive leukemias. Because breakpoints in ABL and BCR are intronic and may vary, the mRNA encompassing the BCR/ABL junction is copied and the product is amplified (RT-PCR). This technique allows the detection of one positive cell in 10^3–10^5 normal cells and is commonly used to monitor response to therapy in responding patients. Reliable semiquantitative RT-PCR procedures are now available, but their value remains to be demonstrated. Other techniques, such as *in situ* hybridization, are used less commonly for the same purpose. The ability of these techniques to predict relapse, and consequently their use in guiding therapies, is still controversial.

C. Immunity to BCR/ABL

The analysis of outcome after allogeneic BMT suggests that immune antileukemia mechanisms operate in CML. For example, graft-versus-host disease (GVHD) is associated with a decreased risk of relapse. Also, allogeneic T cells can induce remission in persons relapsing after BMT. The cellular bases of these antileukemia mechanisms (also called graft-versus-leukemia, GVL) are unknown. They may be in part cytokine mediated. Notably, therapy with interferon-α is effective in persons with chronic phase CML, causing a hematological response in >50% of the cases and complete disappearance of Ph^1 positive cells in about 5% of the cases. GVL may also be T cell mediated. Possible targets are BCR-ABL proteins. The hypothesis that cytoplasmatic BCR/ABL proteins may function as leukemia-specific antigens is based on the possibility of being processed and presented on the cell surface in the context of the HLA complex. *In vitro* and animal data sustain this hypothesis. Data in humans are still controversial. Clinical trials using BCR/ABL peptides for the immunization of patients with CML are in progress.

D. Anti-BCR/ABL Therapy

As discussed previously, BCR/ABL is central in leukemia development. Consequently, many attempts have been made to design therapeutic strategies based on inhibiting BCR/ABL protein synthesis or their functions. Few compounds were tested in clinical studies. Preliminary results are promising using an inhibitor of ABL protein kinase activity, STI570, in persons with CML and Ph^1 positive acute leukemia. Phase I studies indicated modest toxicity. In most persons with CML in the chronic phase, STI570 is followed by normalization of blood cellularity. In about 30% of these persons the number of bone marrow Ph^1 positive cells decreased dramatically. A longer follow-up is necessary to assess whether these changes translate in cure. In persons with CML in the chronic phase or in Ph^1 positive leukemia, a response also occurs, but it is often partial or transient; again, a longer follow-up is needed to determine whether a subset of persons may have long-term benefits from STI570. Many efforts are now dedicated to understanding the mechanisms of resistance to STI750 and how to improve its clinical efficacy, as well as to define its role in the treatment of leukemia.

See Also the Following Articles

Acute Lymphoblastic Leukemia • Acute Myelocytic Leukemia • Chronic Lymphocytic Leukemia • Chronic Myelogenous Leukemia: Etiology, Incidence, and Clinical Features • Chronic Myelogenous Leukemia: Prognosis and Current Status of Treatment • Graft versus Leukemias and Graft versus Tumor

Bibliography

Arlinghaus, R. (1998). The involvement of Bcr in leukemias with the Philadelphia chromosome. *Crit. Rev. Oncogen.* **9**, 1–18.

Butturini, A., and Gale, R. P. (1995). Chronic myelogenous leukemia as a model of cancer development. *Sem. Oncol.* **22**, 374–379.

Butturini, A., and Gale, R. P. (1995). Graft versus leukemia in man. *In* "Technical and Biological Components of Marrow Transplantation" (C. D. Buckner, ed.), pp. 299–314. Kluwer Academic Press, New York.

Druker, B. J., Sawyers, C. L., Kantarajian, H., Resta, D., Reese, S. F., Ford, J., Capdeville, R., and Talpaz, M. (2001). Activity of a specific inhibitor of the BCR-ABL tyrosine kinase in the blast crisis of chronic myelogenous leukemia on acute lymphoblastic leukemia with the Philadelphia chromosome. *N. Eng. J. Med.* **344**, 1038–1042.

Druker, B. J., Talpaz, M., Resta, D., Peng, B., Buchdunger, E., Ford, J., Lydon, N. B., Kantarajian, H., Resta, D., Capdeville, R., Ohno-Jones, S., and Sawyers, C. L. (2001). Clinical efficacy and safety of a specific inhibitor of the BCR-ABL tyrosine kinase in chronic myelogenous leukemia. *N. Eng. J. Med.* **344**, 1031–1037.

Faderl, S., Talpaz, M., Estrov, Z., O'Brien, S., Kurzrock, R., and Kantarjian, H. M. (1999). The biology of chronic myeloid leukemia. *N. Engl. J. Med.* **341**, 164–172.

Groffen, J., de Jong, R., Haataja, L., Kaartinen, V., and Heisterkamp, N. (1999). Phosphorylation substrates and altered signalling in leukemias caused by BCR/ABL. *Leukemia* **13**(Suppl. 1), 81–82.

Groffen, J., Voncken, J. W., van Schaick, H., and Heister-kamp, N. (1992). Animal model for chronic myeloid leukemia and acute lymphoblastic leukemia. *Leukemia* **6**(Suppl. 1), 44–46.

Li, S., Ilaria, R. L., Jr., Million, R. P., Daley, G. Q., and Van Etten, R. A. (1999). The P190, P210, and P230 forms of the BCR/ABL oncogene induce a similar chronic myeloid leukemia-like syndrome in mice but have different lymphoid leukemogenic activity. *J. Exp. Med.* **189**, 1399–1412.

Sawyers, C. L. (1999). Chronic myeloid leukemia. *N. Engl. J. Med.* **340**, 1330–1340.

ten Bosch, G. J., Kessler, J. H., Joosten, A. M., Bres-Vloemans, A. A., Geluk, A., Godthelp, B. C., van Bergen, J., Melief, C. J., and Leeksma, O. C. (1999). A BCR-ABL oncoprotein p210b2a2 fusion region sequence is recognized by HLA-DR2a restricted cytotoxic T lymphocytes and presented by HLA-DR matched cells transfected with an (b2a2) construct. *Blood* **94**, 1038–1045.

Vigneri, P., and Wang, J. Y. (2001). Induction of apoptosis in chronic myelogenous leukemia cells through nuclear entrapment of BCR/ABL tyrosine kinase. *Nature Med.* **7**, 228–234.

Yu, Y., Ma, G., Lu, D., Lin, F., Xu, H. J., Liu, J., and Arlinghaus, R. B. (1999). Bcr: A negative regulator of the Bcr-Abl oncoprotein. *Oncogene* **18**, 4416–4424.

Bladder Cancer: Assessment and Management

Mark D. Hurwitz

Brigham and Women's Hospital and Harvard Medical School

GLOSSARY

cystectomy Surgical removal of the urinary bladder.
detrusor The bladder muscle.
transurethral resection of bladder tumor Surgical excision performed for diagnosis and treatment of superficial bladder cancers or as part of coordinated therapy when combined with radiation and chemotherapy for bladder preservation in the treatment of muscle invasive disease.

Bladder cancer is relatively common with an estimated incidence worldwide of 250,000 cases per year. In 2000, approximately 53,000 cases were diagnosed in the United States, accounting for 6% of all cancers and 3% of cancer deaths. The male:female ratio in the United States approaches 3:1; for men, bladder cancer is the fourth most common diagnosed site of malignancy. The median age for diagnosis is 65 and presentation at less than 40 years of age is rare. In developed countries, approximately 92% of bladder cancers are transitional cell carcinomas, 6% squamous cell carcinomas, and the other 2% include adenocarcinomas, sarcomas, lymphomas, and other rare variants.

I. ANATOMY

A. Gross Anatomy

The urinary bladder is a readily expandable muscular organ composed principally of a smooth muscle called the detrussor. The bladder is tetrahedral when empty with four surfaces approximating an equilateral triangle with each side approximately 12 cm in length. When full, the bladder is ovoid in shape. Several regions are defined when referring to bladder anatomy. The base, or fundus, of the bladder is the posterior portion that faces inferiorly and posteriorly. The ureters enter the bladder obliquely through the base and posterolateral to the urethral orifice. Together, these three orifices define an area referred to as the trigone. Additional regions include the superior aspect of the bladder, termed the dome, the anterior aspect of the tetrahedron, the apex, and the inferior angle leading to the urethra, referred to as the bladder neck.

When empty, the bladder lies entirely with the pelvis but when fully expanded may reach superiorly to the umbilicus and lie directly beneath the anterior abdominal wall without interceding peritoneum. Superiorly, the bladder is draped by peritoneum. In males the peritoneum descends posteriorly over the bladder base to line the rectovesical pouch. The seminal vesicles rest against the base with the prostate positioned inferiorly directly under the bladder neck. In females the peritoneum reflects posteriorly onto the uterus without covering the base. The cervix and anterior wall of the vagina lie further inferior against the base.

Draining lymph nodes include all of the nodes within the true pelvis. Regional lymph nodes pertinent to staging and management include perivesical, hypogastric, obturator, internal and external iliac, presacral, and sacral lymph nodes.

B. Histological Anatomy

The bladder lining consists of three principal layers between the bladder lumen and the detrusor muscle or muscularis propria. A thin transitional epithelium lines the bladder lumen under which is a basement membrane overlying a loose connective tissue layer termed the lamina propria. A variably present and generally poorly defined layer of smooth muscle may be found within the lamina propria termed the muscularis mucosa. In pathologic evaluation it is important to distinguish between muscularis propria and muscularis mucosa in properly defining muscle invasive disease.

II. EPIDEMIOLOGY AND ETIOLOGY

In certain parts of the world, high rates of *Shistosoma haematobium* infection are associated with a high incidence of squamous cell carcinoma. For instance, in

Egypt, bladder cancer accounts for approximately 18% of all cancers, of which three-quarters are squamous cell carcinomas.

Smoking is the most important known risk factor for bladder cancer in both men and women. Approximately 50% of all bladder cancers in men and over a third in women are attributed to tobacco use. The relative risk for smokers of developing bladder cancer is estimated to be between 2.80 and 5.33 as compared to nonsmokers.

An association of aromatic amines with bladder cancer was first noted over a century ago. Several occupations have been linked to an increased risk of bladder cancer, including workers in the dye and rubber industries. In the United States, occupational exposure is linked to approximately 10–20% of all bladder cancers.

Notable among other etiologic factors is phanacetin, which is no longer available in most countries. Other analgesic agents, however, have not been associated with increased risk. Dietary habits may also be linked to bladder cancer, although results of epidemiological studies are not conclusive. In general, high-fat diets have been linked to increased risk, whereas vitamin A and carotene may decrease risk. Artificial sweeteners have not been convincingly linked to an increased risk of bladder cancer in humans.

Squamous cell carcinoma of the bladder is linked to chronic inflammation, leading first to squamous metaplasia. Carcinogenesis is thought to be induced by spontaneous genetic mistakes made during the regenerative and reparative processes. In countries where shistosomiasis is endemic, squamous cell carcinoma is the predominant pathologic variant of cancer of the bladder. Infection is associated with chronic inflammation of the bladder mucosa that results from the deposition of ova in the bladder wall by *S. haemotobium*. Chronic cystitis resulting from the long-term use of indwelling catheters, calculi, or bladder diverticulum is also linked to the development of squamous cell carcinoma.

In addition to environmental factors, there are well-established genetic factors associated with a predisposition to bladder cancer. The finding of high rates of transition cell carcinoma in various ethnic groups in association with other disease processes, such as with

Balkan nephropathy, provided the first suggestion of a genetic link to the development of bladder cancer. Several chromosomal aberrations have now been linked to bladder cancer. Most commonly noted is loss of all or part of chromosome 9 on which a tumor suppressor locus involved in bladder cancer has been mapped and designated DBC1. The level of risk this confers has yet to be determined. Selective loss of a region on 9q is associated with Ta disease, whereas loss of a region on 9p is associated with more aggressive T1 disease. Allelic loss of 11p and 17p, the site of p53, has been associated with high-grade tumors. Abnormalities of 1p, 1q, 3p, 4q, 6p, 6q, 11p, 13q, and 18q are also reported.

III. SCREENING AND DIAGNOSIS

A. Clinical Signs and Symptoms

The most common sign associated with bladder cancer is asymtomatic hematuria in 70–80% of patients. Approximately 20% of patients present with asymptomatic microscopic hematuria alone. Symptoms, when present, include dysuria, frequency, or urgency in 30–50% of patients.

B. Laboratory Analysis

1. Cytology

Urinary cytology should be performed for all patients with hematuria or those with urinary irritative symptoms in whom infection has been ruled out. Cytology alone cannot be used to rule out bladder cancer due to low sensitivity, particularly for low-grade lesions; however, a positive finding is predictive of the presence of a high-grade transitional cell tumor.

2. Tumor Markers

There is active interest in developing noninvasive tests to diagnose and monitor bladder cancer. No standard test yet exists, however, for screening due to limitations in regard to sensitivity and/or specificity, which clinically manifests as a high false-positive rate. Bladder tumor antigen (BTA) garnered much interest initially, but lacks a desirable degree of sensitivity to detect low-grade lesions and appears inferior to cytol-

ogy in detecting high-grade tumors. The presence of inflammatory conditions, common in the population most likely to be screened, limits the specificity of this test as well. Nuclear matrix protein 22 (NMP 22) has demonstrated an improved ability to detect low-grade lesions as compared with cytology or BTA; however, 30% of low-grade lesions are still not detected with this assay.

Additional markers, including fibrin-related assays, telomerase, and assays for hyaluronidase and hyaluronic acid, which are associated with angiogenesis, have been studied. While each of these markers shows promise in at least one regard as compared with other available tests, further assessment is necessary before any of these markers enter clinical practice.

3. Molecular Biology

Other biomarkers for bladder cancer have been studied, including p53, p27, p21, Ki-67, microvascular counts (factor VIII-related antigen), and DNA content/ploidy. A study by the National Cancer Institute Bladder Tumor Marker Network of 109 patients with primary transitional cell cancer (stages T2–T3, grade 2 or higher) found no correlation of the presence of lymph node metastases at cystectomy with Ki67, microvascular counts, or DNA content/ploidy with the finding of lymph node metastases at cystectomy in patients with muscle-invasive, grade ≥2 bladder cancer. A trend was noted for p53, however, and others have noted a positive correlation with survival for patients with T2 tumors that were p53 negative who underwent bladder preservation. While p53 has potential for clinical applicability in bladder cancer management, further investigation is warranted before such a practice can be standardized.

IV. EVALUATION AND STAGING

All patients should undergo a thorough history and physical examination, including rectal exam and pelvic exam in women. Laboratory studies include urinalysis, urine cytology, complete blood count, and serum chemistries, including liver function tests. Cystoscopic evaluation with bimanual examination under anesthesia is essential. An intravenous urogram is advised prior to cystoscopy to evaluate the upper tracts, as synchronous primaries elsewhere in the uro-genital tract are not uncommon and suspicious find-ings can be assessed at the time of cystoscopy. In ad-dition to biopsy, transurethral resection (TUR) can be performed as indicated at the time of cystectomy. Patients with muscle invasive disease should undergo metastatic work-up, including computed tomography or MRI of the pelvis, chest X ray, and bone scan.

The current 5th edition AJCC staging system, in-troduced in 1997, is provided in Fig. 1. In review of the literature, it is important to be aware of differ-ences between the current staging system and prior classifications. The American classification, com-monly known as the Marshall–Jewitt classification, was the first system employed in wide use (Fig. 2). The current AJCC system is largely a modification of this original staging system, which was developed based on clinicopathologic studies correlating the

Primary Tumor (T)

TX	Primary tumor cannot be assessed
T0	No evidence of primary tumor
Ta	Noninvasive papillary carcinoma
Tis	Carcinoma *in situ*: "flat tumor"
T1	Tumor invades subepithelial connective tissue
T2	Tumor invades muscle
T2a	Tumor invades superficial muscle (inner half)
T2b	Tumor invades deep muscle (outer half)
T3	Tumor invades perivesical tissue
T3a	microscopically
T3b	macroscopically (extravesical mass)
T4	Tumor invades any of the following: prostate, uterus, vagina, pelvic wall, abdominal wall
T4a	Tumor invades prostate, uterus, vagina
T4b	Tumor invades pelvic wall, abdominal wall

Regional Lymph Nodes (N)

Regional lymph nodes are those within the true pelvis; all others are distant lymph nodes.

NX	Regional lymph nodes cannot be assessed
N0	No regional lymph node metastasis
N1	Metastasis in a single lymph node, 2 cm or less in greatest dimension
N2	Metastasis in a single lymph node, more than 2 cm but not more than 5 cm in greatest dimension, or multiple lymph nodes, none more than 5 cm in greatest dimension
N3	Metastasis in a lymph node more than 5 cm in greatest dimension

Distant Metastasis (M)

MX	Distant metastasis cannot be assessed
M0	No distant metastasis
M1	Distant metastasis

Stage Grouping

0a	Ta	N0	M0
0is	Tis	N0	M0
I	T1	N0	M0
II	T2a	N0	M0
	T2b	N0	M0
III	T3a	N0	M0
	T3b	N0	M0
	T4a	N0	M0
IV	T4b	N0	M0
	Any T	N1	M0
	Any T	N2	M0
	Any T	N3	M0
	Any T	Any N	M1

FIGURE 1   The 5th edition (1997) AJCC staging criteria for bladder cancer.

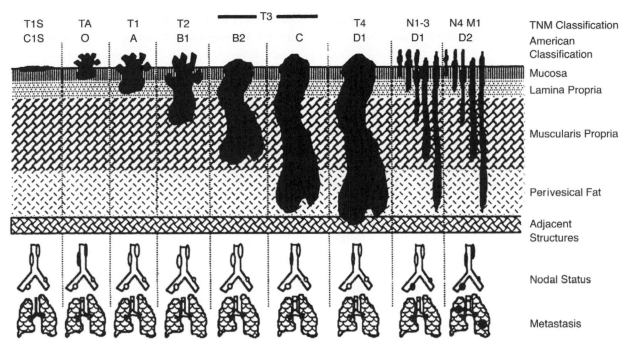

FIGURE 2 Diagrammatic comparison of the Marshall–Jewitt staging system with 4th edition (1992) AJCC staging criteria. Note the differences in the distinction of T2 vs T3 disease from 4th to 5th edition criteria.

depth of tumor penetration into and through the muscularis propria with risk of lymph node and distant metastases. The current AJCC staging criteria most notably differs from the Mashall–Jewitt and prior AJCC classifications in distinguishing T3 disease as requiring invasion of perivesical tissue as opposed to deep muscle invasion now classified as T2b.

V. NATURAL HISTORY

A. Superficial Bladder Cancer

The large majority of bladder cancers diagnosed are within the superficial category. Superficial bladder cancer includes stages Ta, T1, and Cis. This grouping includes a diverse spectrum of disease ranging from low-grade papillary (Ta) lesions with a very low risk of recurrence or progression and over 95% 5-year survival to high-grade carcinoma *in situ* (Cis) with high rates of recurrence and progression to invasive disease with significant mortality rates within 5 years. These differences in biologic behavior appear to reflect differing molecular routes to carcinogenesis.

Both stage and grade have significant prognostic value. Ta lesions are over twice as common as T1.

Both recurrence and especially progression are more common with T1 lesions. Muscle invasive subsequently develops in over a third of T1 patients but is uncommon for stage Ta tumors. Within the T1 category, muscularis mucosa invasion has been associated with an increased risk of recurrence and progression but cannot always be reliably identified. Grade is also clearly linked to prognosis with low-grade lesions, most commonly found with stage Ta associated with long-term survival in the range of 95%, whereas high-grade tumors, typically stage T1, confer a survival rate of 50% over 10 years. The presence of dysplasia elsewhere in the bladder and tumor size have been linked to progression, whereas the finding of multiple tumors confers a greater risk of recurrence but has not been clearly linked to an increased risk of progression.

B. Invasive Bladder Cancer

Invasive cancer equates with muscle invasion and at a minimum T2 disease. Muscle invasive disease also carries a high risk of distant disease. Death due to invasive disease is most commonly the result of the failure to control distant metastatic disease. Therefore, the treating physician must recognize both issues pertinent to local control as well as risk of distant metastases in considering appropriate treatment for muscle invasive disease.

VI. TREATMENT

A. Superficial Bladder Cancer

Grade 1 and 2 Ta lesions have a 50% probability of recurrence but low rates of progression. TUR alone is generally sufficient treatment for low-grade Ta lesions. Regular follow-up with urine cytology and cystoscopy is required, however, due to risk of recurrence. High grade Ta lesions are unusual and have a recurrence risk of 60% with an intermediate risk of progression. In addition to TUR, intravesical therapy with Bacillus Calmette Guerrin (BCG) or mitomycin should be considered and regular follow-up evaluation is required. Low-grade T1 lesions have similar risks of recurrence and progression and may be managed in the same manner as high-grade Ta lesions. T1, grade 3 tumors have a high risk of both recurrence and progression. Careful attention to the pathologic assessment of the TUR specimen must be made to ensure that there is adequate muscle tissue to rule out muscle invasive disease. Intravesical therapy should be administered to all patients followed by repeat TUR at 6–8 weeks. If negative, further intravesical therapy, most commonly BCG, is advised. If still positive, additional intravesical therapy followed by repeat TUR or cystectomy are standard options.

Carcinoma *in situ* has very high rates of both recurrence and progression, often in separate sites from the original tumor, following initial TUR. All patients require intravesicle therapy, most standardly BCG, followed by repeat cystoscopy. For patients with complete response, maintenance intravesical therapy for up to 3 years is generally advised. For patients with persistent or recurrent disease after at least two cycles of BCG, cystectomy warrants strong consideration.

B. Invasive Bladder Cancer

1. Cystectomy

Standard local treatment for nonmetastatic muscle invasive disease is radical cystectomy. Radical cystec-

tomy offers excellent local control, thus optimizing survival for patients without metastatic disease at the time of surgery. Also, as compared with bladder-sparing approaches, there is far more extensive clinical experience with cystectomy and unless there is a multidisciplinary team dedicated to alternative approaches, cystectomy should be considered the appropriate management option for muscle invasive disease. In men, this operation involves a cytoprostatectomy with removal of the bladder, prostate, seminal vesicles, proximal vas deferens, and at least a portion of the proximal urethra. In women, radical cystectomy classically involves removal of the bladder, urethra, anterior vaginal wall, uterus, fallopian tubes, and ovaries. Local control for stage T2 and T3a disease is excellent and generally exceeds 90%. Distant failure remains a significant problem, however, and remains the principal cause for mortality.

For patients with a tumor that has extended outside the bladder wall, including T3b, T4, or N1 disease, primary treatment is radical cystectomy, provided that resection is considered feasible. If the extent of tumor renders the patient inoperable, neoadjuvant chemotherapy or occasionally radiation therapy may be utilized. Following surgery, adjuvant chemotherapy is generally recommended for patients with T3b or T4 disease as well as any patient found to have nodal metastases due to the high risk of distant failure.

2. Urinary Diversion and Reconstruction

Options for urinary diversion have expanded over the past several decades with a concomitant favorable impact on quality of life. The first urinary diversion was performed in 1852 by John Simon by creating an artificial fistula between the ureters and the rectum in a patient with bladder extrophy. Subsequently, novel techniques, including cutaneous continent diversions and neobladder development, were first attempted. Limitations in surgical technique, sepsis, and renal dysfunction resulting from chronic reflux and infection limited the advancement of these innovative techniques until the second half of the 20th century.

The ileal conduit introduced in 1950 represented an advance over the previously widely used ureterosigmoidostomy. Although this approach does not offer continent diversion, it remains popular as it is relatively straightforward both from a surgical standpoint and in regard to long-term patient management. Shortly after the introduction of the ileal conduit, continent diversions were developed. Two popular techniques utilizing a catheterizable stoma to empty the reservoir are the Indiana and Kock pouches. Catheterization is performed periodically. The Indiana pouch utilizes an 8- to 10-cm segment of ileum for the afferent catheterizable limb with a 25- to 30-cm segment of detubularized cecum and ascending colon used for the reservoir to which the ureters are attached. The Koch pouch utilizes a 70- to 80-cm segment of ileum with the ends configured into afferent and efferent limbs and the middle segment is approximated into a urinary reservoir. Both procedures involve placement of a stoma, most commonly in the right lower quadrant of the abdomen, which requires periodic catheterization. Continence rates of over 95% are reported with both procedures.

Alternatively, an intestinal reservoir, commonly made from an ileal segment, may be anastomosed directly to the male urethra. Newer techniques are now available to allow for a similar approach in selected female patients for whom a segment of urethra may be spared. The external sphincter is used to achieve continence and voiding is accomplished with abdominal straining. Daytime and nighttime continence rates of over 90 and 75%, respectively, may be achieved with this approach.

3. Bladder Preservation

Selected patients with muscle invasive bladder cancer may have bladder preservation without a compromise in survival as compared with similarly staged patients undergoing cystectomy. In carefully selected patients, partial cystectomy may be an option but should not be considered standard therapy. Partial cystectomy is most commonly proposed for patients with isolated lesions of the dome of the bladder without associated Cis. A more widely applied approach involves TURB and chemoradiotherapy. An analysis of published data from three institutions and two prospective trials conducted by the Radiation Therapy Oncology Group of combined modality therapy for patients with muscle-invading bladder cancer using selective bladder preservation or cystectomy indicated that the overall 5-year survival rates were comparable to other series of im-

mediate cystectomy. The best results achieved with bladder preservation involve a combination of aggressive TURB, radiation, and chemotherapy.

Investigators at Massachusetts General Hospital were among the first to establish the feasibility of bladder preservation. Fifty-three consecutive patients with muscle-invading bladder cancer (stages T2 through T4, NXM0) were treated with transurethral surgery, followed by two cycles of MCV (methotrexate, cisplatin, and vinblastine), and then radiation (4000 cGy) with concurrent cisplatin administration. Patients who had complete responses received additional chemotherapy and radiotherapy (6480 cGy). With median follow-up of 48 months, 45% were alive and free of detectable tumor. In 58%, the bladder was free of invasive tumor and functioning well; of the 28 patients who had complete responses after initial treatment, 89% had functioning tumor-free bladders.

A subsequent phase III study of bladder preservation with or without neoadjuvant chemotherapy following TURB has revealed no advantage to the use of MCV before radiation with concurrent cisplatin. Overall survival was comparable to historical surgical series. The decreased toxicity resulting from exclusion of MCV may lead to bladder preservation in a greater number of patients.

While several studies now support the use of bladder preservation as a viable alternative in selected patients, radical cystectomy remains the "gold standard" approach to the treatment of muscle invasive disease, and bladder preservation should be undertaken by a multimodality team dedicated to such an approach. Proper patient selection is also of importance. The ideal candidate for bladder preservation is a patient with well or moderately differentiated T2 disease. Evidence of hydronephrosis is a contraindication to bladder preservation. In addition, patients undergoing bladder preservation should have a complete response on second-look cystoscopy following moderate-dose radiation (approximately 4000 cGy) and chemotherapy, as otherwise cystectomy should be considered. Close follow-up of patients undergoing bladder preservation is also required, as 20–30% will develop superficial recurrences amenable to TURBT with or without intravesical therapy. A smaller number of patients may experience an invasive recurrence.

Radiation therapy as single modality therapy is

indicated for patients medically unsuitable for cystectomy and chemotherapy. Local control rates of 25–45% have been obtained with total dose of approximately 6500cGy. Additional radiation techniques, including hyperfractionation or interstitial brachytherapy as advocated by several European institutions, may result in increased complete response and enhanced survival with acceptable toxicity.

C. Metastatic Disease

For most patients with metastatic disease, palliation is the primary goal. Chemotherapeutic regiments tailored to the extent of disease, patient's performance status, and comorbidities should be considered as front-line therapy. A report of a multi-institutional randomized study comparing gemcitobine and cisplatinum with M-VAC, a combination of methotrexate, vinblastine, adriamycin, and cisplatin considered as standard therapy, yielded comparable results, including response rate and overall survival. The gemcitabine/cisplatinum regiment was significantly less toxic, however, lending support to its use as standard therapy for patients with metastatic disease for whom multiagent chemotherapy is warranted. Patients most likely to benefit from such therapy are those considered good risk, which includes patients with high performance status and without visceral metastases.

While palliation is generally the goal in the setting of metastatic disease, long-term survival may be accomplished in certain good risk patients. For selected patients, multimodality therapy, including chemotherapy with partial or complete cystectomy, or aggressive radiation therapy may yield long-term survival. Patients must be carefully selected to ensure a reasonable expectation of benefit in the setting of increased treatment toxicity.

For patients with significant comorbidities or far advanced disease, effective palliation with the minimum amount of treatment is of primary importance. A short course of radiation therapy to a total dose in the range of 3000 cGy is generally very effective in palliating bleeding or pain due to either primary disease or bony metastases. A slightly longer course of radiation may be required to address urinary obstruction due to either primary disease or nodal metastases. Chemoradiosensitization with single agent cisplat-

inum or taxol may be considered in selected patients without a significant increase in morbidity. Alternatively, single agent chemotherapy alone may be considered, but response rates to single agents are generally low. Minimally invasive interventional options, including urinary stent placement, may also be used to address obstruction to preserve renal function. Occasional patients may benefit from toilet cystectomy with ileal conduit to address extensive local symptoms for which aggressive chemoradiotherapy may be contraindicated or attempted and found to be ineffective.

See Also the Following Articles

COLORECTAL CANCER: EPIDEMIOLOGY AND TREATMENT • ESOPHAGEAL CANCER • GASTRIC CANCER • KIDNEY, EPIDEMIOLOGY • LIVER CANCER • OVARIAN CANCER • PANCREATIC CANCER, CELLULAR AND MOLECULAR MECHANISMS • PROSTATE CANCER

Bibliography

Bricker, E. (1990). Bladder substitution after pelvic evisceration. *Surg. Clin. North Am.* **30,** 1511.

Esrig, D., Elmajian, D., Groshen, S., Freeman, J. A., Stein, J. P., Chen, S. C., Nichols, P. W., Skinner, D. G., Jones, P. A., and Cote, R. J. (1994). Accumulation of nuclear p53 and tumor progression in bladder cancer. *N. Engl. J. Med.* **331**(19), 1259.

Greenlee, R. T., Murray, T., Bolden, S., Wingo, P. A. (2000). Cancer Statistics, 2000. CA *Cancer J Clin.* **50**(1), 7.

Hautmann, R., Egghart, G., Frohnberg, D., *et al.* (1988). The ileal neobladder. *J. Urol.* **139,** 39.

Lianes, P., Charytonowicz, E., Cordon-Cardo, C., Fradet, Y., Grossman, H. B., Hemstreet, G. P., Waldman, F. M., Chew, K., Wheeless, L. L., and Faraggi, D. (1998). Biomarker study of primary nonmetastatic versus metastatic invasive bladder cancer: National Cancer Institute Bladder Tumor Marker Network. *Clin. Cancer Res.* **4**(5), 1267.

Olumi, A. F. (2000). A critical analysis of the use of p53 as a marker for management of bladder cancer. *Urol. Clin. North Am.* **27**(1), 75.

Pagano, F., Bassi, P., Galetti, T., *et al.* (1991). Results of contemporary radical cystectomy for invasive bladder cancer: A clinicopathological study with emphasis on the inadequacy of the tumor, nodes, and metastases classification. *J. Urol.* **145,** 45.

Sandberg, A. A., and Berger, C. S. (1994). Review of chromosome studies in urologic tumors. II. Cytogenetics and molecular genetics of bladder cancer. *J. Urol.* **151,** 545.

Scher, H., Bahnson, R., Cohen, S., Eisenberger, M., Herr, H., Kozlowski, J., Lange, P., Montie, J., Pollack, A., Raghaven, D., Richie, J., and Shipley, W. (1998). NCCN urothelial cancer practice guidelines: National Comprehensive Cancer Network. *Oncology* **12**(7A), 225.

Shipley, W. U., Winter, K. A., Kaufman, D. S., Lee, W. R., Heney, N. M., Tester, W. R., Donnelly, B. J., Venner, P. M., Perez, C. A., Murray, K. J., Doggett, R. S., and True, L. D. (1998). Phase III trial of neoadjuvant chemotherapy in patients with invasive bladder cancer treated with selective bladder preservation by combined radiation therapy and chemotherapy: Initial results of Radiation Therapy Oncology Group 89-03. *J. Clin. Oncol.* **16**(11), 3576.

von der Maase, H., Hansen, S. W., Roberts, J. T., Dogliotti, L., Oliver, T., Moore, M. J., Bodrogi, I., Albers, P., Knuth, A., Lippert, C. M., Kerbrat, P., Sanchez Rovira, P., Wersall, P., Cleall, S. P., Roychowdhury, D. F., Tomlin, I., Visseren-Grul, C. M., and Conte, P. F. (2000). Gemcitabine and cisplatin versus methotrexate, vinblastine, doxorubicin, and cisplatin in advanced or metastatic bladder cancer: Results of a large, randomized, multinational, multicenter, phase III study. *J. Clin. Oncol.* **18**(17), 3068.

Bladder Cancer: Epidemiology

Mimi C. Yu
Ronald K. Ross
University of Southern California/Norris Comprehensive Cancer Center

I. Introduction
II. Demographic Patterns
III. Genetic/Environmental Risk Factors

GLOSSARY

***N*-acetyltransferase** An enzyme system that is coded by two distinct genes, NAT1 and NAT2, in humans. NAT2 catalyzes the N-acetylation of arylamines in the liver, whereas NAT1 catalyzes the O-acetylation of arylamines in the bladder.

arylamines A class of chemicals with selective members linked either definitively or suggestively to human bladder cancer.

CYP1A2 An inducible enzyme that catalyzes the N-oxidation of arylamines in the liver.

glutathione *S*-transferase A family of enzymes that detoxify reactive chemical entities by promoting their conjugation to glutathione.

nitrosamines A class of chemicals capable of inducing bladder cancer in rodents.

Bladder cancer is the 11th most common cancer on a worldwide basis, accounting for 3–4% of all malignant tumors worldwide. About 220,000 new cases are diagnosed annually. Three-fourths of the patients are men, and a disproportional number of cases (two-thirds) occur in developed (as opposed to developing) countries.

I. INTRODUCTION

The two most established etiologic risk factors for bladder cancer are cigarette smoking and occupational exposure to selected arylamines. Smoking is believed to account for 50% of all cases diagnosed among men in the United States today. In the United States and most developed countries, the industrial use of established or suspected carcinogenic arylamines has been banned or under strict regulatory guidelines for decades. The extent of occupational exposure as a cause of bladder cancer in the United States today is unclear.

II. DEMOGRAPHIC PATTERNS

A. Histopathology

The uroepithelial lining of the human bladder can become transformed to tumor cells with markedly different histopathologies. Approximately 90% of tumors of the urinary bladder in the United States are of transitional cell type, 7% are squamous, 2% are glandular, and 1% are undifferentiated. In contrast, in Egypt and parts of the Middle East where infection with *Schistosoma haematobium* is endemic, squamous cell carcinomas of the bladder constitute 55–80% of all bladder cancer diagnoses.

Transitional cell carcinomas occur in at least three distinct morphological forms, which have different natural histories and prognoses. Almost 80% of transitional cell bladder cancers diagnosed in the Western world are papillary noninfiltrating tumors. Another 3–5% are nonpapillary and noninfiltrating (i.e., carcinoma *in situ*). The remaining transitional cell carcinomas invade into the underlying stroma of the bladder.

B. International Variation

Bladder cancer shows an almost 10-fold international variation in incidence. High-risk populations include non-Latino whites in the United States and most Western Europeans with age-standardized rates in men clustering around 25 per 100,000 population per year. Asians (including Chinese, Japanese, and Indians) are at low risk for this malignancy, with annual age-standardized rates in men around 3–6 per 100,000 population.

C. Sex, Age, and Race

In nearly all populations, men are 2.5 to 5.0 times more likely to develop bladder cancer than women. The incidence of bladder cancer rises monotonically with age. The disease is rare prior to age 35, and two-thirds of the cases occur in people aged 65 or older.

There is marked racial–ethnic variation in bladder cancer incidence. In the United States among all major racial–ethnic groups, non-Latino white men possess the highest incidence of bladder cancer. Their rate is twice those in Latino and African-American men and 2.5 times higher than those in Chinese- and Japanese-American men. A similar pattern is observed in women, although within race, the male rate is about 3–4 times higher than the female rate. Table I shows the age-adjusted incidence rates of bladder cancer in Los Angeles County, California, by major racial–ethnic groups during 1972–1995.

D. Time Trends

In the United States, the incidence of bladder cancer in both men and women increased steadily between 1950 and 1985 such that the 1985 rates are approximately 50% greater than in the 1950 rates. It appears that the bladder cancer rate in the United States peaked in the mid-1980s for both men and women regardless of race–ethnicity. In Los Angeles, there is clear indication of declining incidence among non-Latino white men and women since their peak rates in the mid-1980s. This secular trend is not apparent among other racial–ethnic groups of Los Angeles.

In contrast, mortality rates in both sexes have decreased steadily since 1950 such that the 1950 death

TABLE I

Age-Adjusted Incidence Rates of Bladder Cancer
(per 100,000 Person-Years) in Men and Women of
Los Angeles County, California, by Major
Racial–Ethnic Groups (1972–1995)[a]

Race–ethnicity	Male	Female	Male:female
Non-Latino white	24.5	6.2	4.0
African-American	13.1	5.0	2.6
Latino	12.1	3.4	3.6
Japanese	8.5	2.8	3.4
Chinese	9.5	2.6	3.3
Filipino	5.6	0.9	6.2
Korean	9.4	1.9	4.9
All race–ethnic groups	20.6	5.4	3.8

[a]Based on data from the Los Angeles County Cancer Surveillance Program/Surveillance Epidemiology and End Results (SEER) Cancer Registry; age adjustment according to the 1970 United States population.

rate is approximately 50% higher than the corresponding rate in the 1990s. The decline in mortality rates is consistent with the observed improvement in survival over the same time period.

III. GENETIC/ENVIRONMENTAL RISK FACTORS

A. Occupational Exposures

The first known cause of human bladder cancer was occupational exposure to a class of chemicals known as the arylamines, which include the now established bladder carcinogens 2-naphthylamine, 4-aminobiphenyl (4-ABP), and benzidine. A century ago there was already anecdotal evidence that these chemicals might be the cause of bladder cancer in exposed workers in the textile dye industry. In the 1950s, Case and colleagues provided definitive epidemiologic data showing a substantially elevated risk of bladder cancer in exposed workers in the textile dye and rubber tire industries. In the United States and most developed countries, the industrial use of 2-naphthylamine has been banned since the late 1950s, and the industrial use of other established or suspected carcinogenic arylamines is under strict regulatory guidelines.

Several other occupational groups have been consistently shown to exhibit an elevated risk of bladder cancer, including truck drivers, leather workers, painters, and aluminum smelters. Causes of the enhanced bladder cancer risk among these workers are not known.

B. Cigarette Smoking

The epidemiologic literature linking cigarette smoking to bladder cancer development is extensive, beginning with the original observations of Lillienfeld and colleagues in 1956. Generally speaking, cigarette smokers have a roughly twofold risk of bladder cancer relative to lifelong nonsmokers, and risk increases with an increasing number of cigarettes smoked on a regular basis. Risk among ex-smokers is lower than among current smokers for a given duration and dose of smoking, but like other smoking-related cancers, risk does not appear to ever return to the baseline risk of lifelong nonsmokers. A large-scale epidemiologic study in Los Angeles suggested that female smokers may experience a higher bladder cancer risk than male smokers with a comparable duration and dose of smoking habits; these first observations require confirmation. There is no evidence that the inhalation pattern and the type of cigarettes smoked (filtered versus nonfiltered, low versus higher tar) materially modify bladder cancer risk. Bladder cancer is only weakly linked to pipe and cigar smoking and not at all to the use of smokeless tobacco.

The precise mechanism by which cigarette smoking causes bladder cancer has not been established. Nonetheless, aromatic amines, including 2-naphthylamine and 4-ABP, are present in tobacco smoke in small quantities and are the leading candidates as the specific etiologic agents. Also, tobacco tars can induce bladder papillomas and carcinomas in mice.

Cigarette smoking is by far the most important contributor to bladder cancer development on a population basis, and 50% of all male bladder cancer cases in the United States can be attributed to this lifestyle factor. However, important differences in the worldwide demographic distribution of bladder cancer versus lung cancer whose major cause is also cigarette smoking suggest that one or several additional factors must play a role in modifying the risk of smoking-related bladder cancer. In addition, non-Latino white men of Los Angeles County share comparable smoking habits (both in terms of duration and amounts smoked per day) with their non-white (African-American and Asian-American) counterparts and yet exhibit an incidence of bladder cancer that is 2–2.5 times that of the latter groups. In New Zealand, Maori men have a 50% higher smoking rate but one-third the rate of bladder cancer relative to European men.

These seemingly disparate observations suggest one or a combination of the following possibilities. (1) Differences exist among populations in the metabolism of smoking-related carcinogens, and these differences substantially alter the risk of smoking-related bladder cancer. (2) Other exogenous agents (e.g., dietary factors) are important modifiers of susceptibility to smoking-induced bladder cancer. (3) Other, as yet unidentified, major causes of bladder cancer exist in the United States and elsewhere.

C. Alterations in Metabolism of Tobacco Carcinogens

The carcinogenic arylamines present in cigarette smoke (or in the workplace) require metabolic activation to transform into fully carcinogenic agents (Fig. 1). The first step in this process is N-oxidation, which is catalyzed by the hepatic cytochrome P4501A2 isoenzyme (CYP1A2). This enzyme system is inducible by a number of environmental factors, including cigarette smoking itself, so that there is considerable individual and population variability in the activity of this enzyme. Urine-based assays, which employ caffeine as the test compound, are available to assess N-oxidation phenotype. There is as yet no epidemiologic data directly showing the CYP1A2 phenotype as a risk factor for bladder cancer.

The metabolically active form of the arylamines (the hydroxylamines) are electrophilic and can form

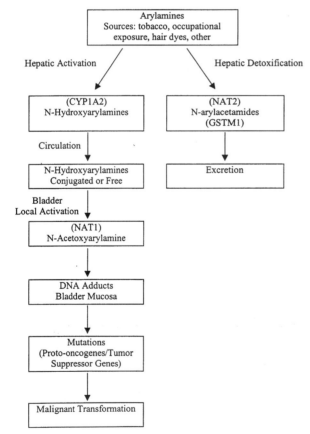

FIGURE 1 Overview of current understanding of arylamine-induced bladder cancer pathogenesis.

adducts with hemoglobin and/or circulate freely or as their glucuronide conjugates and be excreted through the kidney. These latter compounds are hydrolyzed in the acidic environment of the bladder lumen, and with or without further bioactivation by N-acetyltransferase 1 (NAT1, see later) to form a highly electrophilic N-acetoxy derivative, can covalently bind to urothelial DNA. Misrepair of the damage to DNA induced by these adducts can lead to mutations in proto-oncogenes and/or tumor suppressor genes, a critical step in the process of changing a normal cell to a malignant phenotype. An examination of ABP hemoglobin adducts versus DNA adducts in exfoliated urothelial cells of cigarette smokers and nonsmokers has shown a close correlation between levels of the two adducts, thus establishing the former as a valid biomarker for ABP exposure in human studies.

Alternatively, arylamines can be catalyzed by competing detoxification pathways. The best established of these enzymatic pathways is N-acetylation, which is regulated by N-acetyltransferase activity in the liver. N-Acetyltransferase in humans is coded by two distinct genes, NAT1 and NAT2. NAT2, a noninducible system, has long been known to exhibit polymorphism, and the NAT2 phenotype (rapid or slow acetylator) primarily reflects enzyme activity in the liver. A number of "mutant" alleles at the NAT2 locus have been identified, and it has been shown that individuals possessing any two of these mutant alleles display a slow acetylator phenotype (and, therefore, detoxify carcinogenic arylamines less efficiently). There are a number of assays for NAT2 phenotypic determination, including two urine-based tests, both of which employ caffeine as the test compound.

A number of case-control studies of bladder cancer have investigated the relationship between NAT2 phenotype and/or genotype and bladder cancer risk. Overall evidence suggests a relative risk for bladder cancer of about 1.3–1.5 in slow versus rapid acetylators; risks are higher when data are confined to subjects with a documented exposure to arylamines.

It was relatively recently that NAT1 was shown to be polymorphic, and at least two selective probes have been identified. Appreciable NAT1 but low NAT2 activities have been observed in bladder tissues or cells. Because O-acetylation of N-hydroxy arylamine in the bladder can lead to the highly electrophilic

N-acetoxy derivative that covalently binds to urothelial DNA, a rapid NAT1 genotype theoretically could be associated with an increased bladder cancer risk. Preliminary data show heightened susceptibility toward bladder cancer from cigarette smoking among carriers of the NAT1*10 allele, the putative high-activity allele, especially in the presence of the NAT2 slow acetylation genotype. These data await confirmation by larger studies. At present, no firm conclusion can be drawn regarding the effect of the NAT1 genotype on bladder cancer risk.

Glutathione S-transferase M1 (GSTM1) is part of a family of enzymes that detoxify reactive chemical entities by promoting their conjugation to glutathione. GSTM1 is polymorphic in humans; about half of the U.S. non-Latino white population lacks both copies of the gene and hence exhibits no GSTM1 enzymatic activity. Metabolites of several polycyclic aromatic hydrocarbons that are present in cigarette smoke are known substrates for GSTM1. Metabolites of other carcinogenic compounds in cigarette smoke, including arylamines and nitrosamines, are also potential substrates.

A number of case-control studies conducted in the United States and Western European populations have examined the possible protective role of GSTM1 in bladder cancer development. Most have reported a significant excess of GSTM1 null genotype/phenotype among bladder cancer cases relative to controls, with the larger studies consistently observing a relative risk for bladder cancer of about 1.5–1.7 in GSTM1 null individuals.

D. Dietary Factors

1. Artificial Sweeteners

In the 1970s, a number of laboratory experiments showed that saccharin, a combination of cyclamate and saccharin, and a cyclamate metabolite can each induce bladder tumors in rats when given in very high doses. Later studies showed that these compounds are also capable of promoting the effects of other animal carcinogens. These experimental observations raised concerns that human exposure to these chemicals, although at levels many folds lower than those administered to experimental animals, may lead to bladder cancer development. Numerous case-control and co-

hort investigations have addressed this possible diet–cancer association. The overall evidence does not support the use of artificial sweeteners as a risk factor for human bladder cancer.

2. Caffeine-Containing Beverages

Caffeine is a mutagen in some in vitro systems and can increase the transformation rate of cells treated with chemical carcinogens. Coffee consumption as a possible cause of bladder cancer has been a major focus of numerous case-control and cohort investigations. The totality of evidence does not support coffee drinking as a direct risk factor for bladder cancer. Other caffeine-containing beverages, including tea and cola, have been examined for their potential role in bladder cancer development. Again, data are largely negative.

3. Other Dietary Factors

It has been hypothesized that vitamin A and the vitamin A precursor β-carotene (or other carotenoids) may reduce the risk of epithelial cancers, including bladder cancer. In rodents, vitamin A analogs can prevent the induction of bladder cancer by chemical carcinogens, including N-nitrosamines. Results of epidemiologic studies to date have been inconclusive. Some studies have found an increased risk of bladder cancer among individuals with a low intake of vitamin A and β-carotene, whereas others have observed no such associations.

N-Nitrosamines are chemicals that can produce bladder cancer in rodents. Human exposure to nitrosamines or their precursors can be via tobacco smoke or ingestion of cured meat such as hot dogs and salami. Nitrosamines can be formed in vivo from ingested nitrates and secondary amines by nitrate-reducing bacteria in the human bladder, and vitamin C can block this in vivo nitrosamine formation. Results of epidemiologic studies to date on either dietary nitrosamines or vitamin C have been inconclusive.

E. Drinking Water Contaminants

1. Chloroform/Other Chlorination By-products

Chlorine has been the method of choice for water purification since the early 1900s and is currently added to approximately 75% of the drinking water supply in the United States. The presence of chlorine and organic contaminants in water can lead to the formation of halogenated organic compounds, such as chloroform and bromodichloromethane, which are rodent carcinogens. Due to a higher level of organic precursors in surface water that is also subjected to more intense chlorination, the content of such chlorination by-products is more than 60-fold higher in treated surface water relative to treated groundwater. Epidemiologic studies have been consistent in showing a modest increase in bladder cancer risk (40% increase in risk for the highest exposure category) in subjects with long-term exposure to chlorinated surface water relative to those with no exposure.

2. Inorganic Arsenic

Arsenic is a naturally occurring element whose inorganic form has been known for a long time to cause lung (via inhalation) and skin (via ingestion) cancers in humans. Much of the epidemiologic evidence definitively linking inorganic arsenic exposure to bladder cancer development was derived from studies conducted in a black foot disease-endemic area of Taiwan where the bladder cancer incidence is 5–30 times higher than the general population of Taiwan. Black foot disease is a peripheral vascular disorder that can result from chronic arsenic exposure, and Taiwan residents in affected areas are exposed to extraordinarily high levels via the drinking of artesian well water. There is no evidence that the relatively low level of arsenic in drinking water in the United States is associated with bladder cancer development.

F. Iatrogenic Factors

1. Analgesics

Phenacetin-based analgesics have been known for a long time to cause cancer of the renal pelvis, which are transitional cell carcinomas, in humans. Later experimental and epidemiologic data showed the compound to be carcinogenic to the bladder as well. Phenacetin has been banned from most Western countries, including the United States, since the late 1970s. Acetaminophen has served as the phenacetin

substitute in many analgesic brands after the ban, but is itself a major metabolite of phenacetin in humans. There is no evidence to date that acetaminophen use is associated with bladder cancer.

Nonsteroidal anti-inflammatory agents (NSAIDs), including aspirin, are recognized chemopreventive agents for colon cancer, presumably via their inhibitory actions on the expression of cyclooxygenase (COX) 2, an inducible enzyme that has been linked to many aspects of the multistep process of colon carcinogenesis. Experimental data also point to the involvement of COX-2 in bladder cancer development. A large-scale case-control study in Los Angeles reported a statistically significant reduced risk of bladder cancer among regular, long-term users of NSAIDs. These novel observations, which carry obvious public health significance, require confirmation.

2. Cyclophosphamide/Chlornaphazine

Cyclophosphamide and chlornaphazine are alkylating agents that have been used to treat malignant as well as nonmalignant diseases. Both agents are experimental tumorigens. Follow-up studies of patients treated with these two agents have definitively linked them to human bladder cancer development.

G. *Schistosoma haematobium*

Schistosomiasis is hyperendemic in Egypt and parts of the Middle East where bladder cancer is among the top three most frequently diagnosed cancers. The histological profile of the disease in these regions is distinct in that over two-thirds of the cases are squamous cell carcinomas (as compared to 5% in the United States). Cases are mainly diagnosed between ages 40 and 49 years, considerably younger than those occurring in schistosomiasis-free areas. Considerable experimental and epidemiologic data have established *S. haematobium* as a causal agent of human bladder cancer. The observation that levels of nitrate, nitrite, and *N*-nitrosamines are significantly higher in the urine of infected versus uninfected individuals raised the possibility that *N*-nitroso compounds (which, as noted earlier, are bladder carcinogens in rodents) may be involved in schistosomiasis-associated bladder cancer.

H. Hair Dyes

Hair dyes contain arylamines, and most oxidative-type (or permanent) hair dyes are mutagenic in the Ames assay. These observations became especially relevant when it was noted that individuals with occupational exposure to these chemicals (hairdressers, barbers, and beauticians) are at an elevated risk for bladder cancer. Results of several epidemiologic studies examining personal use of hair dyes irrespective of types of dyes (permanent, semipermanent, or temporary rinse) showed no material increase in bladder cancer risk among users. However, a study in Los Angeles, which examined personal hair dye use according to types of dyes, showed a statistically significant frequency- and duration-dependent increase in bladder cancer risk specifically with the use of permanent dyes. No increases in risk were noted among users of semipermanent dyes or temporary rinses. This novel observation requires confirmation.

See Also the Following Articles

Cancer Risk Reduction (Diet/Smoking Cessation/Lifestyle Changes) • Colorectal Cancer: Epidemiology and Treatment • Kidney, Epidemiology • Liver Cancer: Etiology and Prevention • Prostate Cancer • Tobacco Carcinogenesis

Bibliography

Badawi, A. F., Mostafa, M. H., Probert, A., and O'Connor, P. J. (1995). Role of schistosomiasis in human bladder cancer: Evidence of association, aetiological factors, and basic mechanisms of carcinogenesis. *Eur. J. Cancer Prev.* **4,** 45–59.

Castelao, J. E., Yuan, J.-M., Gago-Dominguez, M., Yu, M. C., and Ross, R. K. (2000). Nonsteroidal anti-inflammatory drugs and bladder cancer prevention. *Br. J. Cancer* **82,** 1364–1369.

Castelao, J. E., Yuan, J.-M., Skipper, P. L., Tannenbaum, S. R.,

Gago-Dominguez, M., Crowder, J. S., Ross, R. K., and Yu, M. C. (2001). Gender- and smoking-related bladder cancer risk. *J. Natl. Cancer Inst.* **93,** 538–545.

Chiou, H.-Y., Hsueh, Y.-M., Liaw, K.-F., *et al.* (1995). Incidence of internal cancers and ingested inorganic arsenic: A seven-year follow-up study in Taiwan. *Cancer Res.* **55,** 1296–1300.

Elcock, M., and Morgan, R. W. (1993). Update on artificial sweeteners and bladder cancer. *Regul. Toxicol. Pharmacol.* **17,** 35–43.

Gago-Dominguez, M., Castelao, J. E., Yuan, J.-M., Yu, M. C., and Ross, R. K. (2001). Use of permanent hair dyes and bladder-cancer risk. *Int. J. Cancer* **91,** 575–579.

Hein, D. W., Doll, M. A., Fretland, A. J., Leff, M. A., Webb, S. J., Xiao, G. H., Devanaboyina, U. S., Nangju, N. A., and Feng, Y. (2000). Molecular genetics and epidemiology of the NAT1 and NAT2 acetylation polymorphisms. *Cancer Epidemiol. Biomark. Prev.* **9,** 29–42.

Marcus, P. M., Vineis, P., and Rothman, N. (2000). NAT2 slow acetylation and bladder cancer risk: A meta-analysis of 22 case-control studies conducted in the general population. *Pharmacogenetics* **10,** 115–122.

Morris, R. D., Audet, A.-M., Angelillo, I. F., Chalmers, T. C., and Mosteller, F. (1992). Chlorination, chlorination by-products, and cancer: A meta-analysis. *Am. J. Public Health* **82,** 955–963.

Parkin, D. M., Whelan, S. L., Ferlay, J., Raymond, L., and Young, J. (1997). "Cancer Incidence in Five Continents," Vol. VII. IARC Scientific Publications No. 143, International Agency for Research on Cancer, Lyon.

Skipper, P. L., and Tannenbaum, S. R. (1994). Molecular dosimetry of aromatic amines in human populations. *Environ. Health Perspect.* **102**(Suppl. 6), 17–21.

Vineis, P., Malats, N., Lang, M., d'Errico, A., Caporaso, N., Cuzick, J., and Boffetta, P. (1999). "Metabolic Polymorphisms and Susceptibility to Cancer." IARC Scientific Publications No. 148, Lyon.

Viscoli, C. M., Lachs, M. S., and Horwitz, R. I. (1993). Bladder cancer and coffee drinking: A summary of case-control research. *Lancet* **341,** 1432–1437.

Yu, M. C., and Ross, R. K. (1998). Epidemiology of bladder cancer. *In* "Carcinoma of the Bladder: Innovations in Management" (Z. Petrovich, L. Baert, and L. W. Brady, eds), pp. 1–13. Springer-Verlag, Berlin.

Bleomycin

John S. Lazo
University of Pittsburgh

I. Chemistry
II. Mechanism of Action
III. Cellular Pharmacology
IV. Pharmacokinetics
V. Toxicity
VI. Resistance

GLOSSARY

ataxia telangiectasia A syndrome resulting from the loss of a DNA repair enzyme and characterized by immunodeficiency affecting both B- and T-type lymphocytes.

DNA repair Enzymatic correction by covalent modification of damaged DNA.

drug resistance The failure of a tumor to respond to an anticancer drug.

half-life Time required for a 50% decrease in blood levels of a drug.

pulmonary fibrosis A syndrome characterized by deposition of excessive extracellular matrix components, including collagen and fibronectin, which prevents proper gas exchange in the lungs.

Bleomycin was isolated as copper chelate in broths from a fungal strain of *Streptomyces verticillus* by Umezawa and colleagues. The first clinical trials were initiated in 1965 and since then bleomycin has emerged as a useful agent for the treatment of Hodgkin's disease, non-Hodgkin's lymphoma, testicular cancer, malignant pleural effusions, cancer of the cervix and penis, and head and neck cancer. With the exception of the treatment of pleural effusions, bleomycin is always used in combination with other chemotherapeutic agents. When used in combination with vinblastine sulfate and *cis*-diamminedichloroplatinum to treat patients with germinal neoplasms of the testis, it has produced high cure rates, and deletion of bleomycin from this regimen compromises therapeutic efficacy. There are several unique aspects of bleomycin, including (a) its chemical structure, which is a rather large, metal-binding, glycopeptide; (b) its unusual mechanism of action; and (c) its limited toxicity to normal hematopoietic tissue.

I. CHEMISTRY

The term bleomycin is used to describe what is actually a family of glycopeptides with a common bleomycinic acid core (Fig. 1). Individual bleomycins differ only in their terminal alkylamine moiety designated as R in Fig. 1. Clinically used bleomycin predominantly contains two bleomycins: A_2 and B_2. Many hundreds of bleomycin analogs have been either isolated or synthesized, but none has yet been found to have superior clinical activity.

The native compound isolated from *S. verticillus* is a blue-colored Cu(II)-coordinated complex with a 1:1 stoichiometry. Bleomycin can also complex *in vitro* with a number of endogenous and exogenous metals, including Cu(I), Fe(II), Fe(III), Co(II), Co(III), Zn(II), Mn(II), and Mn(III). The metal coordination chemistry of bleomycin has been the subject of considerable study with general agreement for a square-pyramidal complex. Undisputed participants are the N-1 of the pyrimidine, the N of the imidazole, and the secondary amine. The assignment of the remaining ligands is still debated. Clinical bleomycin is formulated metal free due to the phlebitis seen with the Cu(II)-chelated bleomycin used in early clinical trials. Umezawa posited the generally accepted theory that after injection the apobleomycin quickly complexes with Cu(II) in the blood and the Cu(II) is replaced by intracellular Fe(II) to form the pharmacologically competent species. Outstanding questions remain with this theory, however, including the identity of the intracellular reductant for Cu(II), the fate of the reduced Cu, the subcellular site where the putative Cu/Fe exchange occurs, and the source for the Fe. Because of these issues, some have suggested that there may be a possible biological role for Cu(I)bleomycin.

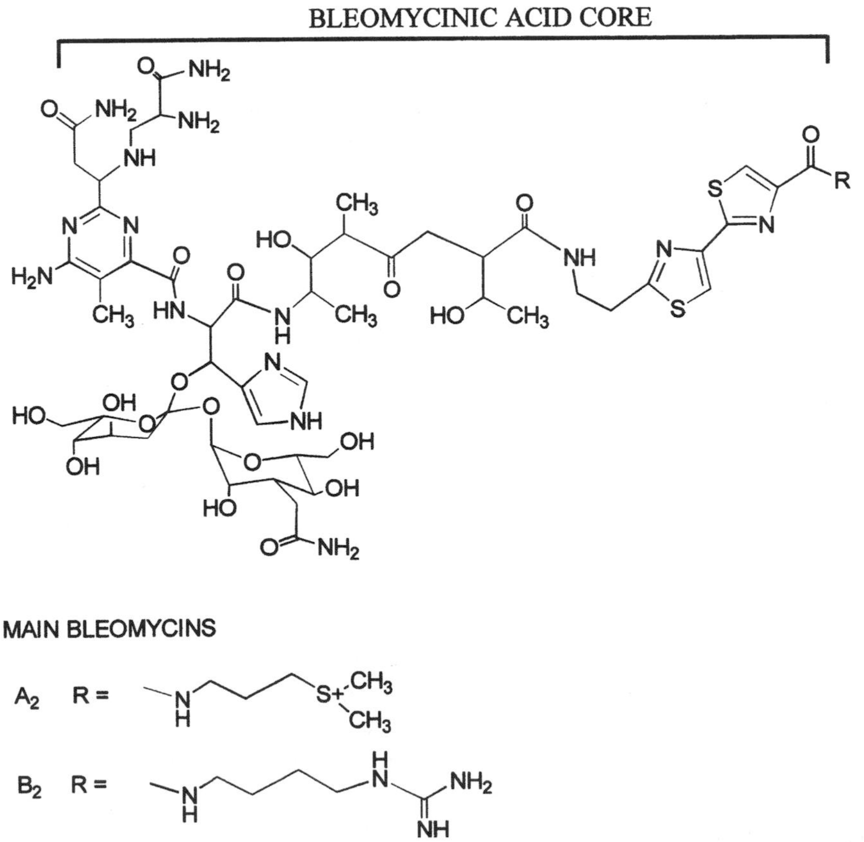

FIGURE 1 Chemical structure of the major components in clinically used bleomycin.

II. MECHANISM OF ACTION

Prescient studies by Umezawa and co-workers implicated DNA damage as causal for cellular toxicity. Single and double strand DNA damage is readily observed with isolated DNA and cultured cells incubated with pharmacologically relevant concentrations of bleomycin. Predictably, cells with DNA repair deficiencies are more sensitive to the toxic actions of bleomycin than wild-type cells. Electrostatic binding and partial intercalation of the drug into the minor groove place it in a position to cleave DNA preferentially at GpC and GpT sequences. The positively charged terminus of bleomycin also participates in DNA binding. Unlike most DNA-damaging agents, bleomycin attacks neither the phosphate linkages nor the nucleic bases. Rather, in its "activated" form, bleomycin abstracts a hydrogen from the C-4′ of a neighboring deoxyribose on DNA. The process of activation has been well studied *in vitro*; it first requires the binding of dioxygen to Fe(II)bleomycin. This "activated" form of bleomycin is then competent to initiate DNA degradation. During the DNA cleavage process, Fe(II)bleomycin functions catalytically as a ferrous oxidase with the oxidation of Fe(II) to Fe(III). The oxidized Fe(III) can be regenerated by a variety of endogenous reductants, including NADPH and cytochrome P450 reductase. If DNA is not present, the "activated" bleomycin can engage in suicide chemistry, in which a complex mixture of DNA cleavage-incompetent degradation products forms. When bleomycin is incubated in the presence of DNA, at least one toxic bleomycin degradation product has been observed that is not capable of attacking DNA, which challenges the notion that DNA is the sole target for bleomycin. Indeed, evidence exists for bleomycin-mediated damage to bacterial cell walls, small organic molecules, and all three major classes of RNA, although the relative contribution of this damage to tumor cell toxicity remains unknown.

At a macromolecular level, DNA cleavage is reflected in chromosomal gaps, deletions, and fragments found with cytogenetic studies of whole cells. Cultured cells seem to be most susceptible to bleomycin in the G_2 or mitotic phases of the cell cycle, which might reflect a more open chromatin structure with enhanced accessibility to the drug. Bleomycin readily causes both high molecular weight DNA fragments that are >500 kbp as well as smaller 180- to 200-bp fragments, which are associated with breaks at the linker regions between nucleosomes. Interestingly, these small fragments are similar in size to those formed during apoptosis in many cells. Both large and small fragments are the direct result of bleomycin-induced double strand DNA breaks, which occur at a 1:10 ratio with single strand DNA breaks. Unlike single strand DNA damage, which can be readily repaired, double strand damage is not thought to be repairable and is presumed lethal. The relatively high frequency of presumably lethal double strand DNA breaks seen with bleomycin is thought to result from the highly electronegative attributes of the products of DNA damage, namely 3′-phosphoglycolate and 5′-phosphate, found on the opposing strand, which could promote access of a second cleavage-competent bleomycin molecule. Product analysis after DNA cleavage consistently confirms a preferential release of thymidine or thymine-propenal, with lesser amounts of the other three bases or their propenal adducts. This inclination for thymine base attack probably reflects the aforementioned partial intercalation of bleomycin between base pairs in which at least one strand contains a GpT sequence.

II. CELLULAR PHARMACOLOGY

Because bleomycin is relatively large and positively charged, it is not rapidly or effectively internalized and large concentration gradients normally exist between the extracellular space and the cellular interior. Tumor cells appear to selectively retain bleomycin for unknown reasons, which has been the basis for the use of bleomycin with radionuclides for tumor imaging. The importance of the plasma membrane as a barrier is readily documented by permeablization studies in which intracellular bleomycin concentrations soars and toxicity is greatly enhanced. The mode of cellular entry has not been resolved. It may be mediated by adsorptive endocytosis or by binding to cell surface proteins that facilitate entry. Once internalized, bleomycin presumably translocates to the nucleus and interacts with DNA.

The only known metabolism of bleomycin in mammalian cells is mediated by a neutral cysteine protease called bleomycin hydrolase, which forms the non-toxic and DNA cleavage-incompetent deamido-bleomycin. Bleomycin hydrolase is a homohexameric enzyme comprising identical subunits of 455 amino acids that form a barrel-like structure with all of the active sites situated within the central channel in a manner resembling the organization of a 20S proteosome. Molecular, biochemical, and structural studies suggest that bleomycin hydrolase is a member of the papain superfamily of cysteine proteases, containing their signature cysteine, histidine, and arginine in the active site. Bleomycin hydrolase may have a biological role in processing the amyloid precursor protein associated with Alzheimer's disease and the production of major histocompatibility complex class I ligands. The human bleomycin hydrolase is located at 17q11.2 and has one polymorphic site encoding either a valine or an isoleucine in the carboxyl terminus. Mice made deficient in bleomycin hydrolase not only have abnormal skin, but also are much more sensitive to the toxic actions of bleomycin.

IV. PHARMACOKINETICS

Because of its size, charge, and peptide-like structure, bleomycin is not orally active and is administered by intravenous, intramuscular, or occasionally by subcutaneously or intracavitary routes (Table I). For historical reasons, it is formulated in units (U). A variety of microbiological, biochemical, chromatographic, and immunological methods have been developed to determine the pharmacokinetics of bleomycin. Bleomycin is primarily excreted in the urine (approximately 45–70% in the first day), and in patients with normal serum creatinine, a rapid, two-phase drug disappearance from plasma is seen. The half-lives of plasma loss are 24 min and 2–4 h for the initial and terminal phases (Table I). Peak plasma concentrations reach 1–10 mU/ml for normal intravenous bolus doses of 15 U/m². The mean half-life after intramusclar injection is approximately 2.5 h. As might be expected, abnormal renal function can have a dramatic effect on bleomycin pharmacokinetics. Thus, it is prudent to consider decreasing the dose of bleomycin if there is any sign of impaired renal function.

TABLE I

Key Pharmacologic and Pharmacokinetic Features of Bleomycin

Absorption	Intravenous, intramuscular, subcutaneous, intrapleural
Metabolism	Deamidation and inactivation by bleomycin hydrolase
Elimination	Renal: 45–70% in the first 24 h
Pharmacokinetics	$T_{1/2\alpha} = 24$ min $T_{1/2\beta} = 2$–4 h
Mechanism of action	Single and double strand DNA breaks
Major toxicity	Pulmonary interstitial infiltrates and fibrosis
	Dermal desquamation, especially of fingers and elbows
	Raynaud's phenomenon
	Hypersensitivity reactions

V. TOXICITY

Unlike most other antineoplastic agents, bleomycin is not generally associated with myelosuppression. The most prominent untoward effects of bleomycin are pulmonary and dermal toxicity. It has been hypothesized that sensitivity of the skin and lungs reflects low levels of the inactivating enzyme bleomycin hydrolase. Approximately half of the patients treated with once- or twice-daily doses of bleomycin develop erythema, induration, and hyperkeratosis. These changes occur predominantly on digits, hands, joints, and areas of previous irritation. Pulmonary toxicity is manifest as a subacute or chronic interstitial pneumonitis, with cough, dyspnea, and bibasilar pulmonary infiltrates on chest radiographs. This can lead to progressive interstitial fibrosis, hypoxia, and death, especially when patients receive total cumulative doses in excess of 450 U. Pulmonary function tests, particularly a rapid fall in carbon monoxide diffusing capacity, are of possible value in predicting a high risk of pulmonary toxicity in patients.

Bleomycin has emerged as a valuable experimental reagent to probe the molecular pathobiology of pulmonary fibrosis because of the reproducibility and rapidity in the generation of pulmonary fibrosis in animal models. Intratracheal instillation of a single small dose of bleomycin in mice or hamsters causes a robust lung fibrosis within several weeks. Bleomycin causes direct toxicity to alveolar endothelial and epithelial cells, inducing epithelial apoptosis, intraalveolar inflammation, cytokine release by alveolar macrophages, fibroblast proliferation, and collagen deposition. Such studies have revealed the prominent role of cytokines, including TGF-β, TNF-α, interleukin 1β, interleukins 2, 3, 4, 5, and 6, have in the fibrotic process.

VI. RESISTANCE

Bleomycin has a relatively limited antitumor profile in humans presumably because of the intrinsic resistance to the drug. Because bleomycin is almost always used in combination with other agents, most of our information about the mechanism of resistance has been generated with laboratory cells grown in culture; most of the focus has been on acquired rather than intrinsic resistance. It is generally assumed that information about acquired resistance will be useful in understanding intrinsic resistance. Mechanisms that have been observed for acquired resistance in tumor cells include decreased drug accumulation, increased drug inactivation, and increased DNA damage repair. In contrast to many other natural products, bleomycin is not affected by P-glycoprotein. The precise mechanism for the reduced drug content in resistant cells, however, is unknown. Increased drug inactivation can result from an increase in bleomycin hydrolase. Because Fe(III)bleomycin requires reduction to be reactivated, sulfhydryl groups on proteins and peptides are potential reactivators. Thus, tumor lines with elevated levels of glutathione are more sensitive to bleomycin. Decreases in either intracellular glutathione or proteins that are thiol rich, such as metallothionein, might be an alternative mechanism of resistance. Fibroblasts from patients with ataxia telangiectasia, which are deficient in DNA repair, are more sensitive to bleomycin compared to fibroblasts from normal patients. Studies from many laboratories indicate that cells can repair some of the bleomycin-induced DNA breaks using DNA polymerase β as well as other repair complexes. Nonetheless, only a few cell lines with acquired resistance to bleomycin have been found and these have modest alterations in their DNA repair capacity. Thus, the role of altered DNA repair in acquired bleomycin resistance has not been established.

Acknowledgments

The author is supported in part by the Fiske Drug Discovery Fund and grants from the National Cancer Institute (CA43917, CA52995, and CA78039).

See Also the Following Articles

AKYLATING AGENTS • CELLULAR RESPONSES TO DNA DAMAGE • HYPOXIA AND DRUG RESISTANCE • LYMPHOMA, HODGKIN'S DISEASE • LYMPHOMA, NON-HODGKIN'S

Bibliography

Burger, R. M. (1991). Cleavage of nucleic acids by bleomycin. *Chem. Rev.* **98,** 1153–1169.

Hecht, S. M. (1986). The chemistry of activated bleomycin. *Acc. Chem. Res.* **1986,** 383.

Joshua-Tor, L., Xu, H. E., Johnston, S. A., and Rees, D. C. (1995). Crystal structure of a conserved protease that binds DNA: The bleomycin hydrolase, Gal6. *Science* **269,** 945–950.

Lazo, J. S., Hoyt, D. G., Sebti, S. M., and Pitt, B. R. (1990). Bleomycin: A pharmacologic tool in the study of the pathogenesis of interstitial pulmonary fibrosis. *Pharmacol. Ther.* **47,** 347–348.

Lefterov, I. M., Koldamova, R. P., and Lazo, J. S. (2000). Human bleomycin hydrolase regulates the secretion of amyloid precursor protein. *FASEB J.* **14,** 1837–1847.

Levi, J. A., Raghavan, D, Harvey, V., Thompson, D., Sandeman, T., Gill, G., Stuart-Harris, R., Snyder, R., Byrne, N., and Herestes, Z. (1993). The importance of bleomycin in combination chemotherapy for good-prognosis germ cell carcinoma. *J. Clin. Oncol.* **11,** 1300–1305.

Montoya, S. E., Ferrell, S. E., and Lazo, J. S. (1997). Genomic structure and genetic mapping of the human neutral cysteine protease bleomycin hydrolase. *Cancer Res.* **1,** 413–418.

Rusnak, J. M., Calmels, T. P. G., Hoyt, D. G., Kondo, Y., Yalowich, J. C., and Lazo, J. S. (1996). Genesis of discrete higher order DNA fragments in apoptotic human prostate carcinoma cells. *Mol. Pharmacol.* **49,** 244–252.

Schwartz, D. R., Homanics, G. E., Hoyt, D. G., Klein, E., Abernethy, J., and Lazo, J. S. (1999). The neutral cysteine protease bleomycin hydrolase is essential for epidermal integrity and bleomycin resistance. *Proc. Natl. Acad. Sci. USA* **96**(8), 4680–4685.

Stoltze, L., Schirle, M., Schwartz, G., Schroter, C., Thompson, M. K., Hersh, L. B., Kalbacher, H., Stevanovic, S., Rammensee, H. G., and Schild, H. (2000). Two new proteases in the MHC class I processing pathway. *Nature Immunol.* **1,** 413–418.

Umezawa, H. (1983). Studies of microbial products in rising to the challenge of curing cancer. *Proc. R. Soc. Lond. B* **217,** 257–276.

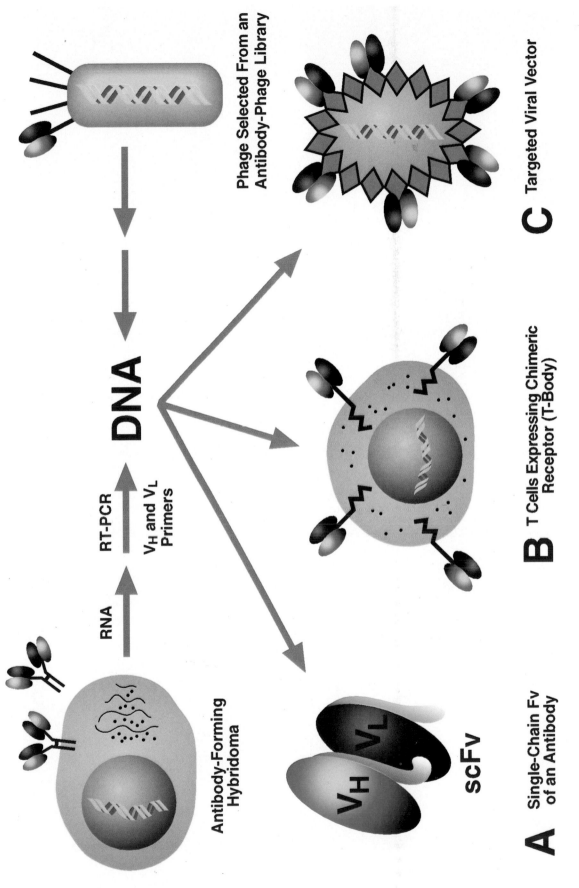

RNA

RT-PCR

V_H and V_L Primers

DNA

Antibody-Forming Hybridoma

Phage Selected From an Antibody-Phage Library

A Single-Chain Fv of an Antibody

scFv

V_H

V_L

B T Cells Expressing Chimeric Receptor (T-Body)

C Targeted Viral Vector

Sources of antibody-derived V region constructs and their use in gene therapy. Antibodies are selected by screening of monoclonal antibody-producing B cell hybridomas (top left) or by phage display technology (top right); the DNA encoding the variable regions is used in the configurations shown below. (A) Single chain Fv (scFv) consisting of the heavy chain and light chain variable regions (V_H and V_L) expressed in a single construct and connected by a peptide linker sequence. scFv may be expressed intracellularly in the cytoplasm or nucleus and used to modulate the expression or function of specific proteins to which they bind. (B) Single chain antibody constructs can be linked to a T-cell activation chain and transduced into patient-derived effector cells to produce "T bodies." The antibody-derived recognition element redirects the specificity of the cytotoxic effector cell to a tumor marker of choice. (C) Antibodies may also be used as recognition elements to control the specificity of the viral vectors used to deliver gene therapy. Such modified viral envelopes may have broadened specificity, enabling a virus that previously infected only rodent cells to now infect human cells, or they may be used to limit infection to a specific cell lineage or to cells expressing a tumor marker. See article ANTIBODIES IN THE GENE THERAPY OF CANCER.

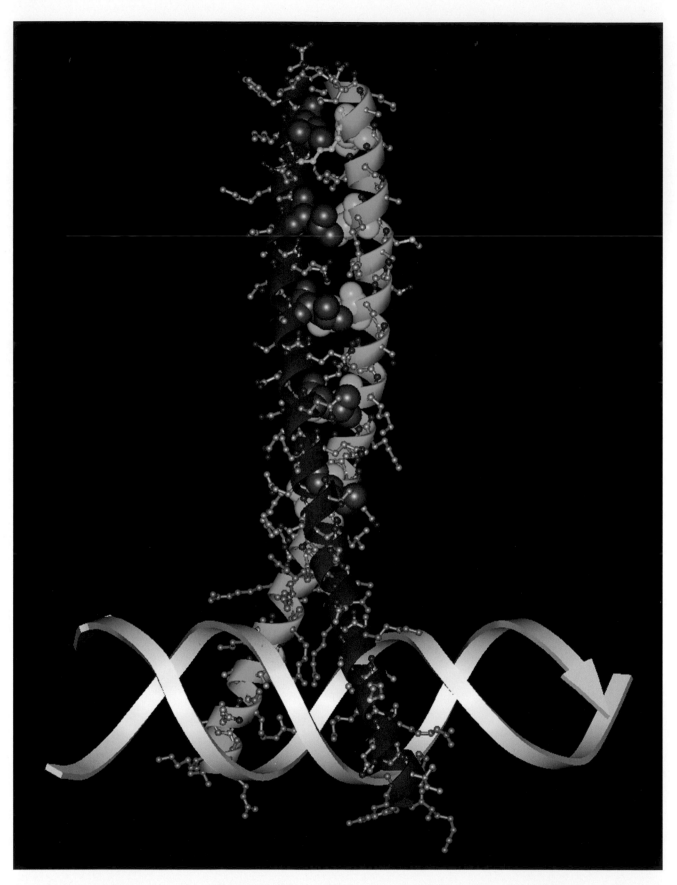

Crystal structure of Fos-Jun complex with DNA. A ribbon model represents the α helices of Fos (red) and Jun (green). The DNA helix is depicted in yellow. The leucines of the zipper are depicted in a space-filling model, whereas the other amino acid side chains are represented in a ball-and-stick model. The side chains of the basic amino acids in the DNA binding domain are colored blue. See article FOS ONCOGENE.

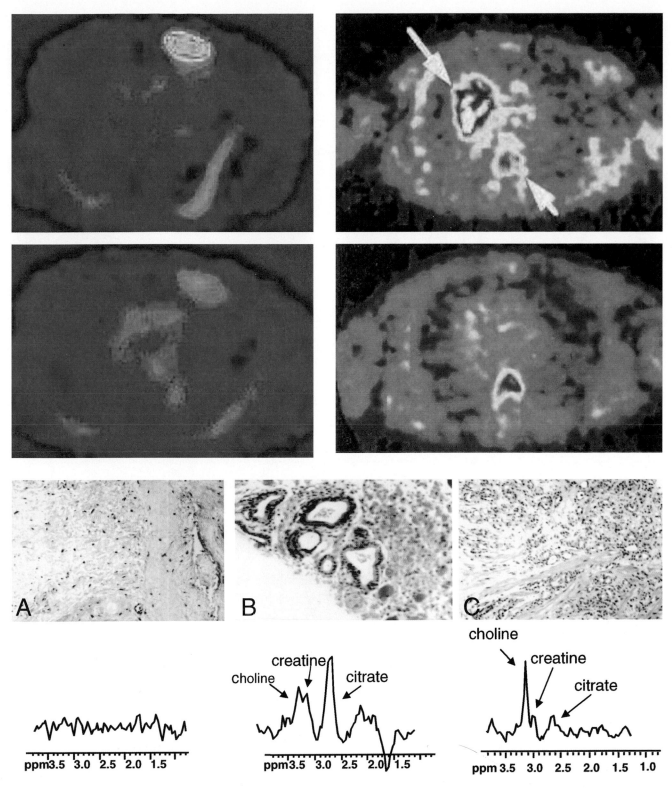

(Top) Left, patient with estrogen-receptor positive metastases of breast cancer in the pleural space. ^{18}F-Fluoroestradiol is the probe. Upper panel, PET image obtained prior to therapy, showing uptake by the tumor (oval at top of picture). Lower panel, same image slice after 7 days of tamoxifen therapy. Right, patient with primary lung cancer, evaluated with ^{11}C-dThd as the probe. Upper panel, PET image prior to therapy. Note extensive uptake of ^{11}C-dThd in both tumor (large arrow) and vertebral space (smaller arrow). Lower panel, patient is evaluated on day 6, after a dose of cisplatin on day 1 and etoposide on days 1–3. Tumor is still present anatomically, but has stopped taking up ^{11}C-dThd for DNA synthesis/cell proliferation. See article PET IMAGING AND CANCER. (Bottom) Differentiation of necrotic tissue, glandular BPH, and malignant tissue by 1-H MRS. (A) Representative spectrum of necrosis and corresponding histologic slide of necrotic biopsy tissue. (B) Representative spectrum of BPH and corresponding histologic slide of BPH biopsy tissue. (C) Representative spectrum of prostate cancer and corresponding histologic slide of malignant biopsy tissue. See article METABOLIC DIAGNOSIS OF PROSTATE CANCER BY MAGNETIC RESONANCE SPECTROSCOPY.

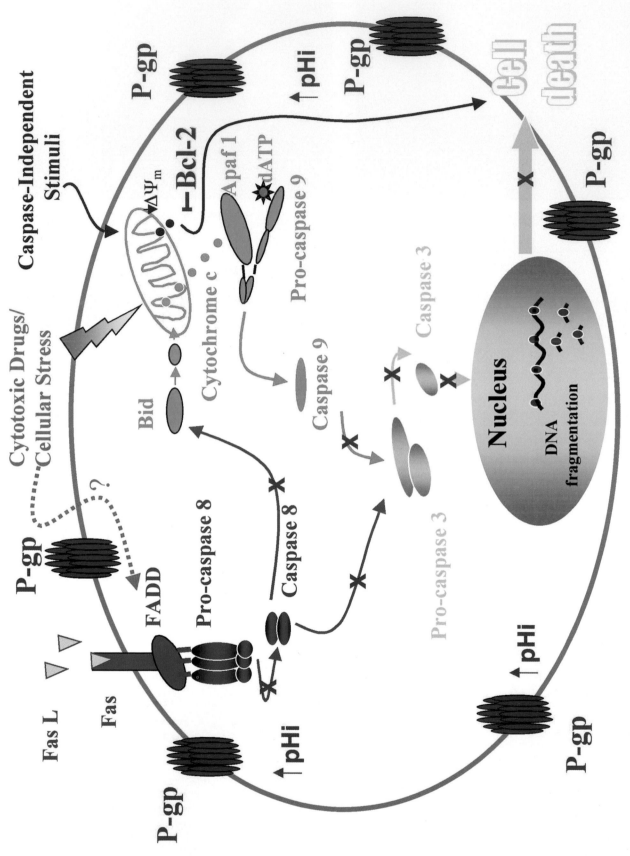

Regulation of apoptosis by P-gp. Expression of functional P-gp results in an increase in intracellular pH (pHi) and inhibition of caspase 8 and caspase 3 activation. The activation of caspases and the release of cytochrome c from the mitochondria may be optimal in an acidic cytosolic environment. It is therefore possible that both apoptosis pathways are affected by a P-gp-mediated increase in pHi as indicated by the red crosses. Expression of P-gp may also disrupt formation of the DISC (Fas receptor, FADD, and caspase 8) at the cell surface by an as yet unidentified mechanism. See article P-GLYCOPROTEIN AS A GENERAL ANTIAPOPTOTIC PROTEIN.

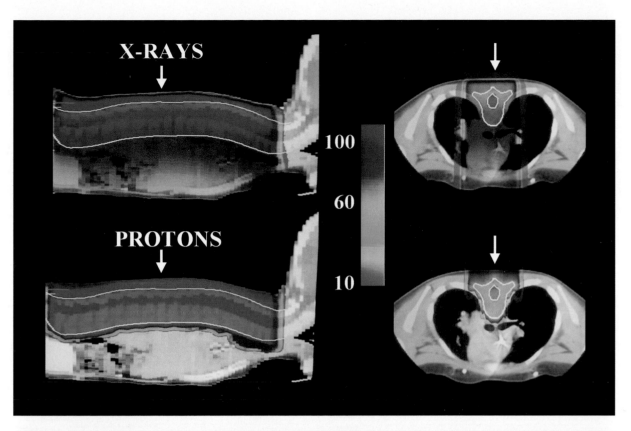

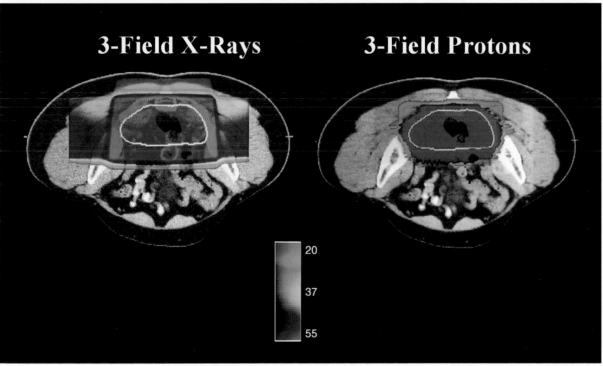

(Top) Comparison of photon and proton single posterior portals for spinal axis irradiation in the treatment of medulloblastoma. The photon plan results in irradiation of normal tissues and organs in the thorax, abdomen, and pelvis. For protons, there is no dose beyond the bony spine, which is uniformly irradiated to prevent irregular bone growth. The color scale is a percentage of prescription dose. (Bottom) A treatment plan comparison for rectal carcinoma using photons (left) and protons (right). Both plans use three treatment fields (posterior, right, and left laterals). The photon plan irradiates a larger volume of normal tissues/organs in the abdomen and pelvis. The color scale is total dose (Gray). See article PROTON BEAM RADIATION THERAPY.

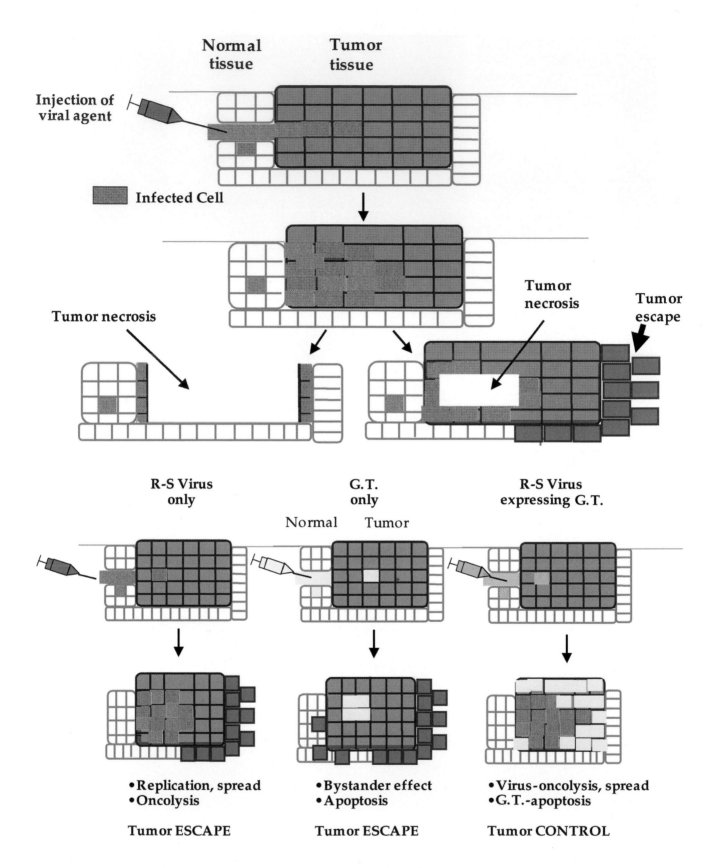

Schematic representation of tumor-selective viral replication and cell killing (top) and tumor-selective tissue necrosis (bottom). Top panel demonstrates that viral replication and spread within a tumor mass can lead to tumor eradication or, if viral killing and spread are not efficient enough, localized tumor necrosis with tumor escape at the margins. Bottom panel shows the potential advantages of combining replication-selective viruses (R-S Virus) and standard gene therapy (G.T.) to allow spread and bystander effect killing of tumor cells. See article REPLICATION-SPECIFIC VIRUSES FOR CANCER TREATMENT.

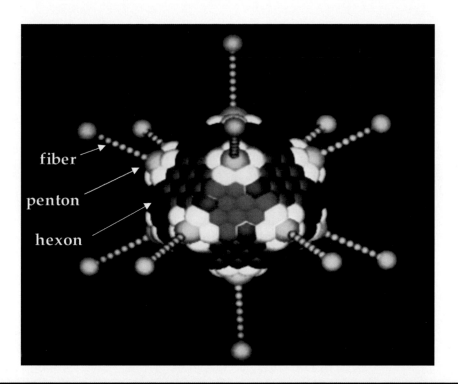

fiber

penton

hexon

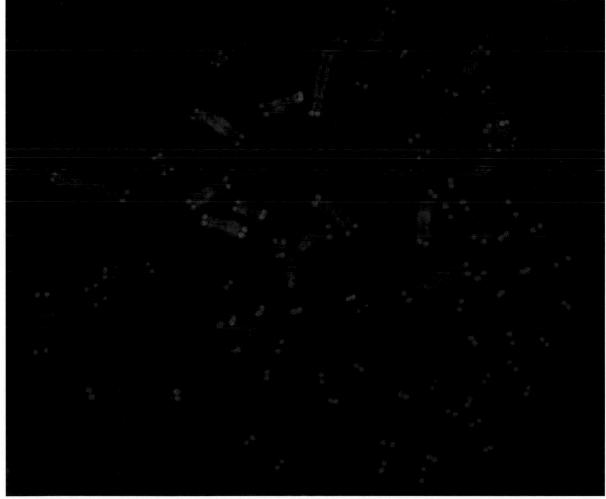

*(Top) Human adenovirus coat structure. See article REPLICATION-SPECIFIC VIRUSES FOR CANCER TREATMENT.
(Bottom) Human metaphase showing telomeres as detected by fluorescent in situ hybridization using a telomeric probe.
Telomeres are at the end of each chromosome and look like red colored caps. See article TELOMERES AND TELOM-
ERASE.*

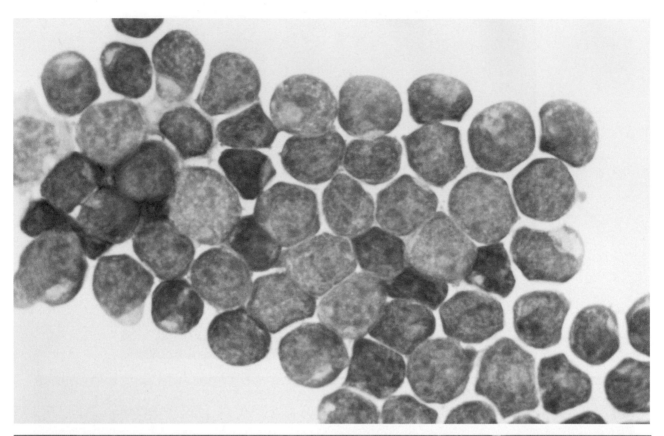

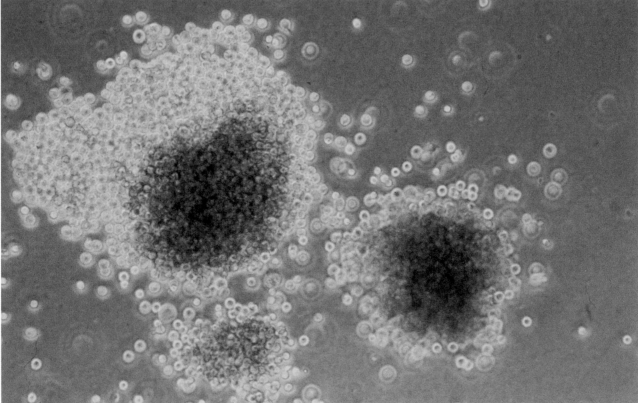

(Top) CD34⁺ selected HSC from a patient with multiple myeloma. CD34⁺ cells are heterogeneous with respect to proliferative capacity and lineage commitment. The totipotent stem cells comprise about 5% of the total and have the appearance of small lymphocytes. CD34⁺ cells that are committed to become myeloid or erythroid progenitors appear blastic. (Bottom) A myeloid colony is shown, a colony-forming unit granulocyte-macrophage (CFU-GM) having grown in semisolid medium innoculated with mobilized blood CD34⁺ cells. The CFU-GM represents the progeny of a single CD34⁺ cell committed to the myeloid lineage. See article STEM CELL TRANSPLANTATION.

Bone Tumors

Richard Gorlick
Paul A. Meyers
Memorial Sloan-Kettering Cancer Center

GLOSSARY

diaphyses The shafts of a long bone. The usual location for a Ewing's sarcoma to arise.

Huvos grade Grading system for the degree of necrosis observed in a definitive surgical specimen following induction chemotherapy. Grade IV indicates that no viable tumor cells are observed. Grade I indicates that the tumor is fully viable. Grades II and III are intermediate. The prognostic value of the Huvos grading has been reproduced in multiple osteosarcoma clinical trials.

induction chemotherapy Chemotherapy administered after the diagnosis is established and prior to definitive surgery. Analogous to other tumor systems, this is the period of chemotherapy that eliminates bulk disease rapidly. Following induction chemotherapy and definitive surgery, virtually all patients have no clinical evidence of disease. Induction chemotherapy has also been referred to as preoperative chemotherapy and neoadjuvant chemotherapy.

limb salvage surgery An *en bloc* resection of a tumor with wide margins, which preserves normal anatomy. The resected region is usually replaced by an autologous graft, allograft, or endoprosthesis.

metaphyses A conical section of bone between the shaft (diaphysis) and the end (epiphysis) of a long bone. The usual location for an osteosarcoma to arise.

Paget's disease A metabolic bone disorder characterized by excessive bone resorption and disorganized new bone formation. Osteosarcoma arises in adults in bones involved by Paget's disease.

staged thoracotomies In osteosarcoma, this refers to two sequential operations to resect pulmonary nodules from both lungs of patients with metastatic disease. When the lungs are deflated, a surgeon can palpate and resect nodules that are smaller than can be visualized on radiographic studies because the lesions are calcified. The lesions are described as feeling like grains of sand.

Malignant bone tumors are relatively uncommon, with approximately 2500 new cases diagnosed in the United States each year. The two most common malignant bone tumors are Ewing's sarcoma (including primitive neuroectodermal tumors of bone) and osteosarcoma, which primarily afflict children and adolescents. Fibrosarcoma, chondrosarcoma, and malignant fibrous histiocytoma, which can involve bone or soft tissue, occur later in life. A variety of benign bone tumors occur as well, including aneurysmal bone cysts, osteoblastoma, osteoid osteoma, osteochondroma, enchondroma, desmoplastic fibroma, giant cell tumors (can be malignant), and eosinophilic granuloma among other rare histologic variants. These lesions, although capable of local recurrence, rarely metastasize, thus the management is primarily surgical. Because a full discussion of each of these clinical entities is not possible, the remainder of this article focuses on comparing and contrasting features of the two most common malignant bone tumors: Ewing's sarcoma and osteosarcoma (Table I).

I. EPIDEMIOLOGY

Both Ewing's sarcoma and osteosarcoma have a peak incidence during the second decade of life and are rare before the age of 5. Ewing's sarcoma has a slightly younger age distribution, being the most common malignant bone tumor in children less than 10 despite a lower overall incidence. Ewing's sarcoma is rare over age 30, whereas osteosarcoma is seen in adults, particularly in bones with long-standing Paget's disease. Both tumors have a slight preponderance in males. As an unusual epidemiologic feature, Ewing's sarcoma has a very low incidence in blacks and Chinese as compared to whites. Osteosarcoma does not display a racial predilection.

II. PATHOGENESIS

We know limited amounts about the etiology of Ewing's sarcoma and osteosarcoma. Except for a potential association with skeletal (such as aneurysmal bone cyst) and genitourinary anomalies (such as hypospadias), there are no identified predisposing factors for Ewing's sarcoma. The peak age of incidence in Ewing's sarcoma and osteosarcoma coincides with a period of rapid bone growth in young people. Supporting a correlation between rapid bone growth and the evolution of osteosarcoma are several observations, including patients with osteosarcoma tend to be taller than their peers. At the same time, these tumors frequently arise in patients both before and after the adolescent growth spurt. Radiation exposure is a well-documented etiologic factor for osteosarcoma, but it is not associated with the development of Ewing's sarcoma.

III. GENETICS

The Ewing's sarcoma family of tumors is characterized by a consistent chromosomal translocation fusing the

TABLE I
Comparison of Clinical Features of Ewing's Sarcoma and Osteosarcoma

	Ewing's sarcoma	Osteosarcoma
Peak incidence	Peak incidence in second decade Rare after age 30	Peak incidence in second decade Occurs in adults, particularly in Paget's
Racial predilection	Uncommon in blacks and Chinese	None
Etiologic factors	None	Ionizing radiation
Genetics	A consistent chromosomal translocation is observed	Frequent genetic abnormalities at p53 and retinoblastoma gene loci
Pathology	Small round blue cell tumor	Spindle cell sarcoma with osteoid
Skeletal location	Diaphyses	Metaphyses
Common sites of metastases	Lungs, bone, bone marrow	Lungs, bone
Treatment modalities	Surgery, radiation, chemotherapy	Surgery, chemotherapy

EWS gene on chromosome 22 to a member of the ETS family of transcription factors. In 95% of cases the translocation is t(11;22)(q24;q12) fusing EWS to the FLI1 transcription factor. Much experimental evidence suggests that the aberrant protein produced by this fusion initiates tumorigenesis and is responsible for much of the biological behavior. As Ewing's sarcoma progresses, a number of secondary genetic alterations can be acquired, including mutation of the p53 tumor suppressor gene and INK4A deletion, as well as other cytogenetic abnormalities. Although the basis for its development is unclear, chromosomal translocation appears to be central to the pathogenesis of Ewing's sarcoma. A similar observation has been made in many soft tissue sarcomas, including synovial sarcoma, alveolar rhabdomyosarcoma, and desmoplastic small round cell tumors, among others.

Osteosarcoma, like many other tumors, has no characteristic chromosomal translocation. The consistent cytogenetic abnormalities associated with osteosarcoma are alterations in chromosomal regions, which contain tumor suppressor genes involved in cell cycle control, namely the retinoblastoma and p53 genes. Clinical observations and experimental data suggest that alterations in these two genes are central to the pathogenesis of osteosarcoma. The incidence of osteosarcoma is dramatically increased among survivors of retinoblastoma. In the hereditary

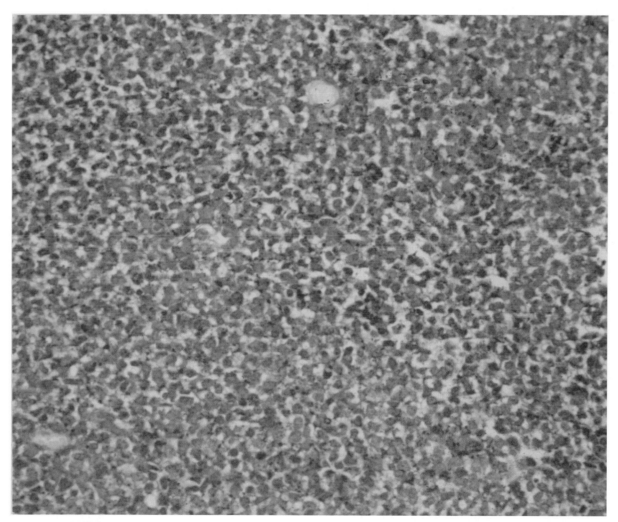

FIGURE 1 Typical histologic appearance of Ewing's sarcoma. The tumor is composed of small round blue cells.

form of this disorder, germline mutations of the retinoblastoma gene are common. Germline mutations in the p53 gene can lead to a high risk of developing malignancies, including osteosarcoma, which has been described as the Li–Fraumeni syndrome. Approximately 3% of patients with osteosarcoma have germline mutations in p53. The p53 and retinoblastoma genes are altered in the majority of osteosarcoma tumor samples. In the majority of tumor samples with intact retinoblastoma and p53 genes, alterations in other genes involved in the same pathways can be found (i.e., MDM2 amplification, cyclin dependent kinase-4 amplification, INK4A deletion). The p53 gene product has a role in the response to DNA damage and the retinoblastoma gene product regulates cell cycle progression, both functions being critical for tumor growth. Numerous other oncogenes are found to be altered in osteosarcoma tumor cells (i.e., fos, HER2/neu, myc, met). Although it is clear alterations in tumor suppressor genes and oncogenes are necessary to produce OS tumors, it is not clear in the majority of patients which of these events occurs first and why or how it occurs.

IV. PATHOLOGY

Ewing's sarcoma appears under light microscopy to be composed of undifferentiated small round blue cells (Fig. 1). The cells have hyperchromatic nuclei and scanty cytoplasm with high mitotic rates and areas of necrosis are common. A distinction of this entity from other small round blue cell tumors, such as lymphoma, rhabdomyosarcoma, neuroblastoma, and other tumor types, is made most commonly through immunohistochemistry. Evidence of the cell surface protein p30/32 mic2 (also referred to as HBA71, 12E7, and O13) is the primary marker used to identify this tumor. Demonstration of the characteristic molecular translocation (described previously) in the tumor tissue through cytogenetics or molecular biology techniques is increasingly relied upon to support the diagnosis. Primitive neuroectodermal tumor is distinguished from Ewing's sarcoma by the presence of neural markers such as S-100 and neuron-specific enolase. Because these two clinical entities are biologically similar, possessing the same characteristic chromosomal translocation, and are treated in almost all studies in an identical manner, the value of distinguishing these two entities is unclear.

Osteosarcoma is diagnosed based on histopathologic criteria, with the radiologic appearance being confirmatory. The pathognomonic feature is the presence of tumor osteoid in association with pleomorphic malignant spindle cells (Fig. 2). When diagnosed in children and adolescents, osteosarcoma is typically high grade, but in adults, low-grade lesions occur frequently as well. Several histologic variants of OS have been described, including osteoblastic, chondroblastic, and telangiectatic. All histologic variants are treated in a similar manner based on grade with similar outcomes. Mixtures of histologic variants within a single tumor are frequently described.

V. CLINICAL PRESENTATION AND DIAGNOSTIC EVALUATION

The most common clinical presentation of Ewing's sarcoma and osteosarcoma is pain frequently associated with a mass. The pain is often attributed to trauma or vigorous physical exercise, both of which are common in the patient population at risk. Trauma is not believed to be involved in the pathogenesis of either tumor. Systemic symptoms can occur, but rarely in patients with localized disease. Symptoms are usually present for several months before the diagnosis is made. The most common nonneoplastic diagnosis that can result in these presenting features is osteomyelitis.

Ewing's sarcoma and osteosarcoma can occur in any bone of the body. Ewing's sarcoma tends to occur more centrally than osteosarcoma, with approximately 40% occurring in the pelvic girdle. Roughly half of all osteosarcomas arise around the knee with an additional 25% occurring in the proximal humerus. Ewing's sarcoma traditionally arises in the diaphyseal regions of the bone, whereas osteosarcoma arises in the metaphyses. On plain radiographs, Ewing's sarcoma typically appears as a poorly marginated, permeative, lytic, or sclerotic lesion with soft tissue extension. Periosteal new bone formation is characteristically referred to as an "onion skin" appearance (Fig. 3). Os-

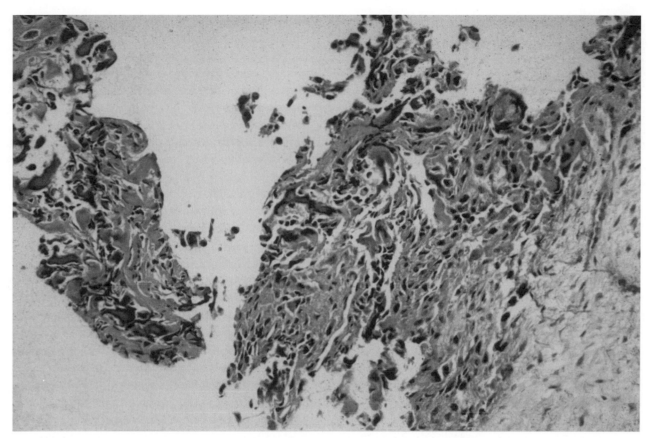

FIGURE 2 Typical histologic appearance of osteosarcoma. The tumor is composed of spindle cells, which are producing osteoid.

teosarcoma can present as a lytic or blastic lesion or as a mixture of these processes, resulting in the classic "sunburst" appearance. Periosteal elevation with soft tissue extension can result in a "Codman's triangle" (Fig. 4). Although suggestive, the diagnosis can never be made from images alone. It is mandatory to obtain a biopsy for pathological confirmation of the diagnosis. The biopsy must be carried out by a physician who is sensitive to the issues of subsequent surgery. A poorly placed or performed biopsy can foreclose important therapeutic options for the orthopedic oncologist at the time of definitive surgical resection. The extent of the tumor in both bone and soft tissue is best appreciated with cross-sectional imaging techniques, such as computed tomography or magnetic resonance imaging. These studies are therefore an essential portion of the initial diagnostic evaluation.

The natural history of these primary tumors is

metastasis very early in their evolution. Approximately 15–40% of patients with Ewing's sarcoma and 10–20% of patients with osteosarcoma present with overt metastases at diagnosis. Virtually all patients with apparently localized disease have subclinical, microscopic metastasis as evidenced by the fact that only 10% of patients treated with surgery alone remain free of disease. The most frequent site for metastatic presentation of both these diseases is the lung. Computerized tomography of the lung is more sensitive than plain films of the chest to detect metastasis and is therefore an essential part of the diagnostic evaluation. Both Ewing's sarcoma and osteosarcoma can present with metastases to other bones, necessitating radionuclide bone scans as part of the diagnostic evaluation (Fig. 5). Lesions in osteosarcoma can occur in close proximity to the primary lesion (i.e., skip metastases) or can be at a distant site. Bone metastases are far less common than the lung.

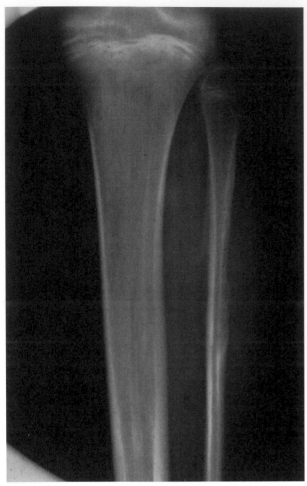

FIGURE 3 Typical radiographic appearance of Ewing's sarcoma involving the fibula. Periosteal elevation leads to an "onion skin" appearance.

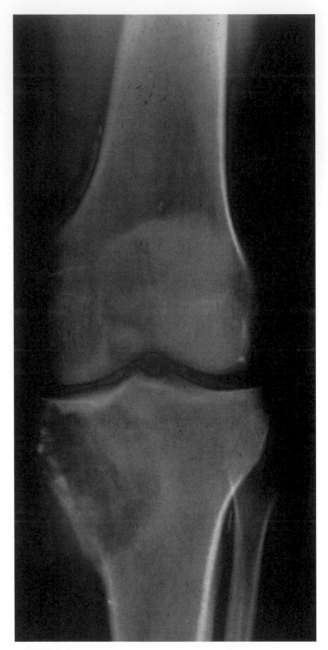

FIGURE 4 Typical radiographic appearance of osteosarcoma involving the proximal tibia. Osteoblastic and osteolytic regions are apparent.

A site of metastases relatively unique to Ewing's sarcoma is the bone marrow, which necessitates multiple site bone marrow aspirates as part of the diagnostic evaluation for this disease. Ewing's sarcoma can involve the central nervous system at diagnosis, particularly the spine and paraspinal region. Osteosarcoma only spreads to the central nervous system when it is widely metastatic. Other imaging modalities that have been utilized in these diseases to evaluate the extent of disease or predict response to therapy include gallium scans for Ewing's sarcoma and thallium scans for osteosarcoma, but these are still investigational.

In addition to defining the extent of disease, the initial evaluation needs to assess the patient's suitability for treatment. It is essential to obtain baseline studies prior to the initiation of chemotherapy so that toxicities can be monitored and appropriate changes in treatment can be made, if necessary. All patients need a baseline evaluation of renal function (usually with a creatinine clearance determination), cardiac function (usually with an echocardiogram or a ra-

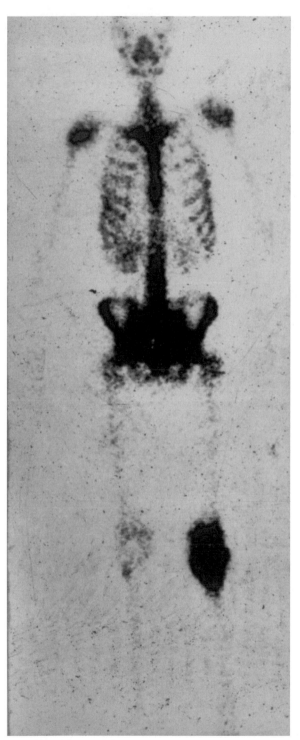

FIGURE 5 Typical appearance of a radionuclide bone scan in a patient with osteosarcoma. The site of the primary tumor, the left proximal tibia, demonstrates intense activity.

dionuclide scan), and an audiogram. Several of the common chemotherapeutic agents can cause permanent sterility in males. All men past the age of puberty should be offered the opportunity to carry out sperm banking. Female infertility is less common, but does occur. Present techniques to preserve female fertility are investigational. As these techniques become routine, they should be offered to female patients as well.

VI. TREATMENT

A. Local Control

The successful treatment of Ewing's sarcoma and osteosarcoma requires local control and systemic chemotherapy. Despite the effectiveness of chemotherapy against microscopic metastatic disease, chemotherapy cannot control clinically detectable disease. Local therapy directed at bulky tumor is required for the primary site as well as sites of metastases. In Ewing's sarcoma, options for local control include radiation therapy and surgery. Which modality is utilized depends on a number of factors, including resectability of the tumor, likely functional consequences of surgery, concern over late affects, and treating physician preferences. To obtain local control, some tumors are treated with both radiation and surgery. In these cases, radiation therapy can be administered as an external beam pre- or postoperatively, intraoperatively, or as radioactive implants. Osteosarcoma is considered resistant to radiation therapy, and the only effective tool for local control is surgery. Historically, this surgery was amputation of the affected extremity, but at present the majority of patients undergo a limb salvage procedure. The limb salvage procedure involves a wide excision of the entire affected region with replacement of the resected area by an autologous graft, allograft, or endoprosthesis. A wide range of surgical techniques and options for the preservation of limbs and limb function are currently available. For the successful treatment of osteosarcoma, all sites of radiographically visible metastatic disease need to be resected as well, including pulmonary metastases. This is usually accomplished through bilateral-staged thoracotomies.

B. Systemic Chemotherapy

The importance of systemic chemotherapy in the treatment of Ewing's sarcoma and osteosarcoma is evidenced by the fact that the tumor will recur in approximately 90% of patients if treated by surgery alone, whereas the majority will remain disease free with the addition of systemic chemotherapy. In osteosarcoma, the Multi-Institution Osteosarcoma Study, reported by Link and others, demonstrated the unequivocal value of adjuvant chemotherapy in the treatment of this disease. Patients who did not receive chemotherapy had a probability of disease-free survival of 11% as compared to 66% for patients who received chemotherapy.

A variety of combination chemotherapy regimens have been used to treat Ewing's sarcoma and osteosarcoma. Ewing's sarcoma is responsive to many individual chemotherapeutic agents. As a single agent in conventional phase II trials, the following drugs showed objective response rates of at least 20%: cyclophosphamide, doxorubicin, ifosfamide, vincristine, etoposide, and melphalan. Table II summarizes some of the combination chemotherapy protocols reported for Ewing's sarcoma. As compared to Ewing's sarcoma, osteosarcoma is responsive to much fewer chemotherapeutic agents. In conventional phase II trials, only doxorubicin, cisplatin, ifosfamide, and high dose methotrexate have demonstrated objective response rates greater than 20%. Table III summarizes some of the combination chemotherapy protocols reported for osteosarcoma. Studies attempting to improve outcomes have focused on intensification of therapy. For patients with Ewing's sarcoma, this has involved the use of high-dose chemotherapy with autologous bone marrow rescue. This approach remains experimental.

C. Induction Chemotherapy

A treatment approach initially pioneered by Rosen and others that has become the standard of care for osteosarcoma and is becoming more frequent in the treatment of Ewing's sarcoma is the use of induction chemotherapy (also referred to as neoadjuvant or preoperative chemotherapy). Induction chemotherapy provides several theoretical and real advantages. By giving chemotherapy prior to the definitive surgical procedure, surgical outcomes are potentially improved and microscopic metastatic disease is treated more rapidly. At the time of definitive surgery, the amount of necrosis (Huvos grade) in the resected tumor is a strong predictor of subsequent patient outcome. In patients with Ewing's sarcoma, the degree of necrosis in the primary tumor following induction chemotherapy also correlates with subsequent event-free survival.

VII. PROGNOSIS

The prognosis for patients with Ewing's sarcoma and osteosarcoma treated with appropriate surgery and systemic chemotherapy depends on several factors, the most important of which is the presence or absence of overt metastatic disease. Reported single institutional studies currently describe a disease-free survival of 50–70% at 3 years for patients who present with localized Ewing's sarcoma. In patients who pre-

TABLE II
Selected Protocols in the Literature for the Treatment of Ewing's Sarcoma

Protocol	Chemotherapy agents utilized[a]
Children's Cancer Study Group—7942	CTX, DOX, VCR, IFOS, ETOP vs more intensive dosing
Memorial Sloan-Kettering Cancer Center—P6	CTX, DOX, VCR, IFOS, ETOP
Intergroup Ewing's Sarcoma Study—1	VCR, CTX, actinomycin D ± DOX ± RT
Instituto Ortopedico Rizzoli	VCR, DOX, CTX
St. Jude Children's Cancer Research Hospital	VCR, DOX, CTX

[a]CTX, cyclophosphamide; DOX, doxorubicin; VCR, vincristine; IFOS, ifosfamide; ETOP, etoposide; RT, radiation therapy.

TABLE III
Selected Protocols in the Literature for the Treatment of Osteosarcoma

Protocol	Chemotherapy agents utilized[a]
Children's Cancer Study Group—7921	HD-MTX, cisplatin, DOX ± ifosfamide ± MTP-PE
Memorial Sloan-Kettering Cancer Center—T10	HD-MTX, VCR, DOX, BCD ± cisplatin
Multi-Institution Osteosarcoma Study	HD-MTX, DOX, BCD, cisplatin vs no chemotherapy
St. Jude Children's Cancer Research Hospital—OSTEO77	HD-MTX, DOX, CTX

[a]HD-MTX, high-dose methotrexate; DOX, doxorubicin; MTP-PE, muramyl tripeptide phosphatidyl-ethanolamine; VCR, vincristine; BCD, bleomycin, cyclophosphamide, actinomycin D; CTX, cyclophosphamide.

sent with metastatic disease, disease-free survival is less than 30% at 3 years, with patients with metastases limited to the lung doing better than patients with metastatic disease in other sites. Reported single institutional studies describe an event-free survival of 60–80% for patients with localized osteosarcoma. Disease-free survival for patients presenting with overt metastatic disease is less than 20%, with patients with single, unilateral pulmonary nodules faring better than those with more extensive metastatic disease.

Other features that have been reported to be prognostically significant in Ewing's sarcoma and osteosarcoma are the site of the primary lesion and tumor size. Tumors that are axial (osteosarcoma) or are more proximal (Ewing's sarcoma) have an inferior prognosis. Tumors that are larger either measured directly on radiographic images (Ewing's sarcoma) or through biochemical measures, such as serum lactate dehydrogenase (Ewing's sarcoma and osteosarcoma) or alkaline phosphatase (osteosarcoma), are associated with an inferior prognosis. In Ewing's sarcoma the specific location of the characteristic chromosomal translocation may be a prognostic factor. In osteosarcoma, no molecular marker with reliable prognostic value has been identified.

In recent years a number of new treatment approaches and agents have been identified. These include approaches such as immunizing patients with peptides produced by the unique chromosomal translocation in Ewing's sarcoma or the use of a biological agent, muramyl tripeptide phosphatidyl ethanolamine, to stimulate macrophages to destroy minimal residual disease in osteosarcoma. These approaches and agents remain investigational, but it is hoped that they will ultimately improve the prognosis of patients inflicted with these diseases.

See Also the Following Articles

EWING'S SARCOMA (EWING'S FAMILY TUMORS) • RHABDOMYOSARCOMA, EARLY ONSET • SARCOMAS OF SOFT TISSUE

Bibliography

Granowetter, L. (1996). Ewing's sarcoma and extracranial primitive neuroectodermal tumors. *Curr. Opin. Oncol.* **8,** 305–310.
Himelstein, B. P. (1998). Osteosarcoma and other bone cancers. *Curr. Opin. Oncol.* **10,** 326–333.
Link, M. P., and Eilber, F. (1988). Osteosarcoma. In "Principles and Practice of Pediatric Oncology" (P. A. Pizzo and D. G. Pollack, eds.), pp. 659–688, Lippincott, Philadelphia.
Link, M. P., Goorin, A. M., Miser, A.W., et al. (1986). The effect of adjuvant chemotherapy on relapse-free survival in patients with osteosarcoma of the extremity. *N. Engl. J. Med.* **314,** 1600–1606.
Malawer, M. M., Link, M.P., and Donaldson, S. S. (1997). Sarcomas of bone. In "Cancer; Principles and Practice of Oncology" (V. T. Devita, S. Hellman, and S. A. Rosenberg, eds.), 5th Ed., pp. 1789–1852, Lippincott-Ravens, Philadelphia.
Meyers, P. A., and Gorlick, R. (1997). Osteosarcoma. *Ped. Clin. North Am.* **44,** 973–990.
Miser, J. S., Triche, T. J., Pritchard, D. J., et al. (1988). Ewing's sarcoma and the nonrhabdomyosarcoma soft tissue sarcomas of childhood. In "Principles and Practice of Pediatric Oncology" (P. A. Pizzo and D. G. Pollack, eds.), pp. 659–688. Lippincott, Philadelphia.
Rosen, G., Marcove, R. C., Caparros, B., et al. (1979). Primary osteogenic sarcoma: The rationale for preoperative chemotherapy and delayed surgery. *Cancer* **43,** 2163–2177.
Yaw, K. M. (1999). Pediatric bone tumors. *Semin. Surg. Oncol.* **16,** 173–183.

Brachytherapy

Harry Quon
Louis B. Harrison
Beth Israel Medical Center and
St. Luke's–Roosevelt Hospital Center

GLOSSARY

activity The number of disintegrations per second a given radioactive source emits over its lifetime.

afterloading The subsequent placement of radioactive sources into a hollow applicator device mimicking the desired position of the radioactive sources. This may be performed manually or remotely by computer control.

dosimetry The topographic distribution of the dose of radiation that is affected by various physical factors, including the activity of the radioactive source.

fractionation The intentional delivery of a planned total dose of radiation over several treatments. The dose per fraction and the interval between each fraction are often parameters of study. Typically, for external beam radiotherapy, once-daily fractions delivering the same dose per day are given. Fractionation is typically used for HDR brachytherapy as a strategy to reduce the risk of late complications.

isodose Regions receiving the same dose of radiation. This is often represented by a line connecting points of equal dose and normalized or expressed as a proportion of the isodose line receiving the prescribed dose of radiation.

The term "brachytherapy" is derived from the Greek word *brachio*, meaning short, and refers to treatment with a radioisotope at a "short distance." The radioactive sources may be sealed or unsealed with the former typically sealed within a metal capsule and inserted into or placed adjacent to a tumor. This article highlights the relative advantages and disadvantages of sealed source brachytherapy and the current indications as applied to various site-based malignancies. Technical aspects of brachytherapy are beyond the scope of this article.

I. PRINCIPLES OF BRACHYTHERAPY

The management of cancer is founded on the underlying principle of achieving an optimal therapeutic ratio due to the recognition that both the probabilities of tumor control and normal tissue complications are a function of treatment dose. Brachytherapy is unique for its ability to influence the therapeutic ratio by way of both physical and biological effects on the probabilities of tumor control and normal tissue complications.

A. Advantages of Brachytherapy

The advantages of brachytherapy implants are summarized in Table I. With a brachytherapy implant, the dose delivered to the surrounding tissues attenuates by the inverse square of the distance, considerably reducing the dose to the surrounding normal tissues. The conformal radiation permits the reirradiation of previously irradiated tissues, as complications are influenced not only by the total dose of radiation received, but by the volume of normal tissue irradiated. As such, high doses may be delivered with acceptable complication rates.

With the physical placement of an implant within the tumor substance, the likelihood of a geographic miss due to patient or organ movement is reduced. Interstitial placement of an implant places the inherent dose inhomogeneities, particularly the relative higher dose regions, within the central relatively hypoxic regions of the tumor. This may be beneficial in overcoming this aspect of radioresistance. As these regions of higher dose inhomogeneity may be manipulated, selected regions within the tumor may receive dose-escalated radiotherapy.

When the implant is loaded with continuous low-dose rate (LDR) radiation, the overall treatment time is reduced, yielding several advantages from both a patient and an economic perspective. Loading a temporary implant with fractionated high-dose rate (HDR) radiation has been the subject of much study due to reduced radiation precaution requirements; hence, the ability to deliver outpatient therapy. HDR implants are remotely afterloaded by computer control, permitting differential stepping source dwell positions and dwell times, resulting in conformal irradiation and the ability to manipulate dose inhomogeneities.

Several radiobiologic advantages unique to continuously irradiating implants may be anticipated. The reduction in the overall treatment time may contribute to reducing the risk of tumor clonogen repopulation. Implants placed at the time of surgical resection may be promptly loaded in the postoperative period, potentially minimizing the risk of tumor repopulation and the adverse effects of hypoxia within the surgical tumor bed. Continuous LDR radiation also allows for the redistribution of tumor cells such that those cells in the less radiosensitive S phase tend to accumulate in the more radiosensitive M phase of the cell cycle. The influence of hypoxia on radioresistance is minimized by LDR irradiation. Finally, the low-dose rate maximally exploits the differential DNA repair capacity that exists between many tumor clonogens and surrounding normal tissues. This is enhanced by a further reduction in the effective dose rate de-

---

TABLE I
Advantages and Disadvantages of Brachytherapy Implants

Advantages	Disadvantages
Rapid dose attenuation sparing surrounding normal tissues and precise conformal irradiation	Radiation exposure hazards, particularly for continuous low-dose rate implants
Regions of high-dose inhomogeneities are placed within the central relatively hypoxic regions of the tumor	Continuous low-dose rate irradiation requires compliant patients with radiation precautions
Overall treatment time may be reduced	High-dose rate implants may increase the risk of late normal tissue complications
May be placed at the time of surgery, allowing for accurate tumor volume and high-risk regions to be delineated. Permits prompt initiation of irradiation	Potential for geographic miss from suboptimal placement of the implant or the adverse effects of organ swelling and movement
Continuous low-dose rate irradiation may radiosensitize tumors through redistribution and reoxygenation mechanisms and minimizes the risk of late normal tissue complications	Invasive procedure with inherent complications

livered to normal tissues due to the inverse square law of dose attenuation.

B. Disadvantages of Brachytherapy

The disadvantages of brachytherapy implants are summarized in Table I. The principle disadvantage, particularly with continuous LDR implants, is the hazard of radiation exposure. This is a particular issue to health care providers and to patients of childbearing age. Appropriate radioisotope selection, meticulous attention to radiation precautions, and remote afterloading technologies have helped reduce this hazard.

For continuous LDR radiation, the need for inpatient therapy, compliance to radiation precautions, and the need for a well-motivated patient able to assist in self-care, particularly in the postoperative setting, are significant barriers with this modality. This has given impetus to the study of outpatient HDR temporary implants for several tumor sites. Concerns remain with regard to the potential for an increased risk of radiation-induced late toxicities with HDR radiation schedules. This modality remains the subject of clinical investigations to define the optimal HDR-fractionated radiotherapy schedule.

The precise delivery of radiation inherent to brachytherapy implants necessitates meticulous and accurate delineation of the tumor volume and hence is subject to the risk of a geographic miss. The application of brachytherapy implants is also subject to the requisite skill and experience of the radiation oncologist. As an invasive procedure, implants are also subject to inherent complications, such as bleeding and infections.

C. Types of Implants

Brachytherapy implants may be categorized by the method in which the implant is inserted, the technique by which the radioisotope is loaded into the implant, and by the duration and dose rate of the irradiation. This is summarized in Table II.

The tumor site and the adequacy of the implant encompassing the tumor volume often dictate the technique selected. Several body orifices, such as the vagina and uterine cavity, lend themselves to intracavitary techniques whereby the sources are placed directly against the cavity surface or, more commonly, afterloaded into hollow applicator systems placed adjacent to the cavity surface. This technique is advantageous when only the cavity surface is involved with cancer due to the rapid dose attenuation. The prescription of dose at a defined depth from the surface may permit larger depths to be treated but is limited by the consequential higher dose to the cavity surface. A similar technique involves the body surface placement of either radioisotopes or an applicator system. Alternatively, the interstitial placement of radioisotopes or plastic catheters for afterloading may be used for larger or more complex volumes or ones inaccessible to intracavitary techniques.

Permanent implants, emitting radiation over the lifetime of its radioactivity, use sources that provide LDR irradiation. This technique may be subject to the permanent consequences of suboptimal placement or the potential adverse dosimetric effects of organ swelling. In this regard, temporary implants are often used with an afterloading applicator system mimicking the desired position of the radioactive sources. This permits optimization of the implant to adequately cover the tumor volume dosimetrically and a more deliberate and accurate placement of the implant without radiation exposure concerns during the placement of a permanent implant. For continuous LDR implants, plastic catheters are commonly used, permitting the afterloading of radioactive seeds embedded at defined positions along a nylon strand

TABLE II
Types of Brachytherapy Implants

Technique	Dose rate	Duration	Loading	Emission type
Intracavitary	Low	Permanent	Manual "hot"	γ
Interstitial	Medium	Temporary	Manual afterloading	β
Surface mold	High		Remote afterloading	Neutron

that may be customized with differential seed activities and seed positions to accomplish this goal. The nylon strand may also be differentially left within the implant to achieve further conformal irradiation of the tumor. For fractionated HDR implants, plastic catheters facilitate remote computer-guided afterloading of a high activity source fixed at the end of a cable wire that moves along the length of the catheter lumen occupying differential positions for differential periods of time.

The radiation dose rate has been categorized as low [0.4–2 Gray per hour (Gy/h)], intermediate, or high (>12 Gy/h). LDR irradiation is commonly given continuously but may be temporary or permanent in duration. HDR irradiation may be given as a single treatment, often for rapid palliative tumor responses, but is often fractionated to reduce the risk of late toxicities. Pulse dose rate (PDR) radiation refers to the use of remote computer-guided afterloading with a medium dose rate source, of about 3 Gy/h, delivering radiation typically every hour for a period of 10–30 min over several days. This has been studied as a technique to exploit the reduced radiation exposure of remote afterloading and the LDR biologic advantages that may be mimicked by this schedule.

II. CLINICAL APPLICATIONS AND INDICATIONS OF BRACHYTHERAPY

The majority of the scientific literature reporting on the role of brachytherapy for various tumor sites is limited by institutional observational studies with many being retrospective in nature. In part, this is the result of the requisite skill and experience limiting the generalized application of brachytherapy and the inherent limitations of more rigorous study designs with skilled interventions. Despite this, studies providing clear delineation of the patient selection criteria employed, consistency in independently reported series, and large patient cohorts with mature follow-up provide confidence in defining specific indications for brachytherapy.

A. Brain Malignancies

For adult brain malignancies, brachytherapy has been extensively studied in the treatment of glioblastoma multiforme (GBM). Several large prospective series have demonstrated an improved median survival and 2-year survival rates compared to historical controls when selected patients were treated with gross total resection, conventional external beam radiotherapy (EBRT) (typically to 60 Gy), and a temporary LDR interstitial iodine-125 implant (50–55 Gy). Selection criteria for these studies included patients with a Karnofsky performance score of at least 70 and a unifocal well-defined supratentorial tumor measuring less than 5 cm involving only one hemisphere. These studies were confounded by the observation that 46–67% of implanted patients required reoperation, with these patients demonstrating improved survival to those not undergoing reoperation. Two randomized trials of temporary interstitial implants in malignant gliomas using similar selection criteria have since been reported with conflicting results. The Brain Tumor Cooperative Group has reported in abstract form only the results of a study of EBRT (60.2 Gy) with carmustine chemotherapy randomizing more than 250 patients (87% with GBM) to an LDR iodine-125 implant (50 Gy). The median survival favored the implanted group (16 months vs 13 months, $p=0.05$). A second study of 140 patients randomized to EBRT (50 Gy) with or without a temporary iodine-125 implant (60 Gy) demonstrated no difference in the median survival observed (13 months). A randomized trial from U.C.S.F. of 112 similarly selected patients with GBM demonstrated a survival advantage for patients receiving hyperthermia before and after a brachytherapy boost to patients receiving a brachytherapy boost alone after conventional postoperative EBRT and hydroxyurea sensitization. Hence, an established indication for brachytherapy implants remains to be defined and may still have a role in dose escalation for larger lesions not amenable to a radiosurgery boost.

Interstitial implants have also been studied for recurrent GBMs previously irradiated, as a boost for malignant astrocytomas, as definitive therapy in the management of low-grade astrocytomas, and in the management of brain metastases. Brachytherapy for these indications remains a subject of study again, especially for lesions too large for radiosurgery.

B. Head and Neck Malignancies

Brachytherapy has a significant role in the management of head and neck squamous cell carcinomas

(HNSCC). This is due to the importance of locoregional control, the desire to minimize treatment-related functional deficits, and the risk of second malignancies in this site.

1. Nasopharynx

The primary indication for a brachytherapy implant is in the management of recurrent disease where several institutional series have reported sustained local control rates of 20–60% with the variability due to the extent of initial disease presentation and at recurrence and the dose of reirradiation. The greatest experience has been with LDR implants. In selected series treating only disease confined to the nasopharynx mucosa amenable to either an intracavitary or an interstitial implant, sustained local control rates of 50–60% may be realized. However, these series have also demonstrated a significant risk of developing late radiation-related complications, including soft tissue and bone necrosis, trismus, fistula formation, and neurologic complications, such as radiation myelitis and temporal lobe necrosis. In a study of over 600 patients reirradiated, the selection of small EBRT fraction size and the use of a brachytherapy implant were associated with a reduced risk of late complications. Hence, a brachytherapy implant is an integral part in treating early disease recurrences either alone or in combination with EBRT to provide a sufficient dose, of at least 60 Gy, while minimizing the risk of late complications.

A limited number of studies have reported on the role of an implant in patients with persistent disease following standard therapy. These studies have suggested that further irradiation in early stage disease, amenable to intracavitary and interstitial techniques (see Fig. 1), results in comparable local control rates as achieved in patients demonstrating a prompt complete response. Hence, dose escalation may be adequate in compensating for tumors demonstrating a low radioresponsiveness. The optimal dose schedule remains to be determined with both 60 Gy LDR and 22.5–25 Gy HDR schedules reported. A confounding factor in these reports is the timing of the diagnosis of persistent disease, as diagnosis early on following EBRT may select for more favorable but slow to regress lesions. Late toxicities do not appear to be increased. In light of the poorer local control rates and survival rates in patients managed for local recurrences, a brachytherapy implant should be considered in the management of patients demonstrating persistent disease.

Several investigators have also examined the value of dose escalation with adjuvant brachytherapy in unselected patients as part of the initial management. Again, implants were limited to T1 and T2 lesions amenable to mainly intracavitary techniques with HDR schedules. Notwithstanding the inherent limitations of retrospective comparative studies, consistent observations of an improvement in local control and survival with a modest increased risk of chronic mucosal complications have been noted. At present, the clinical benefits of an implant may be modest and limited to patients with node negative early stage lesions. Its utility in patients treated with concurrent chemoradiotherapy for advanced lesions is likely to be limited, as a preliminary study of a radiosurgery boost has been demonstrated to be safe, effective, and able to encompass larger tumor volumes.

2. Tonsil and Soft Palate

Several institutions have reported their experience employing a brachytherapy implant to these sites typically as a boost (20–30 Gy) following EBRT (45–50 Gy) due to the risk of lymph node metastases. The predominant experience has been with temporary interstitial LDR implants using iridium-192. In general, when combined with EBRT, local control rates of 85% or greater may be expected for T1 and T2 lesions and 65–70% for T3 lesions. Protracted overall treatment time beyond 7 weeks and a time interval between EBRT and the brachytherapy implant of greater than 20 days may adversely affect treatment outcomes possibly due to the risk of tumor repopulation. Mild to moderate self-healing soft tissue complications are the most common side effects and may be seen in 10–20% of patients with the risk of serious soft tissue complications and the risk of osteoradionecrosis rare in experienced hands. An LDR iridium-192 implant has also been demonstrated to be effective in providing salvage local therapy for selected small recurrences or second primary HNSCC occurring within previously irradiated tissue. Local control rates between 65 and 80% may be expected but do not appear to impact on survival due to competing comorbidities and the risk of further aerodigestive tract malignancies.

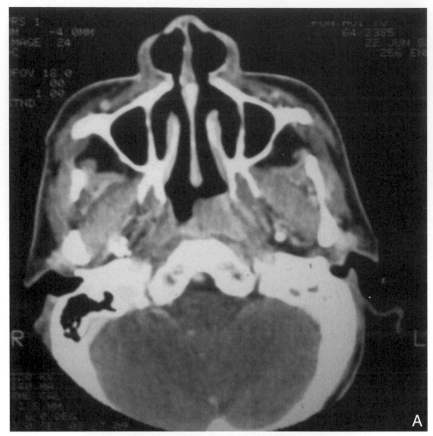

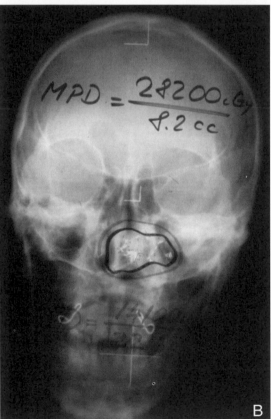

FIGURE 1 Interstitial permanent low-dose rate brachytherapy implant for early stage disease in the left nasopharynx that was amenable to a volume seed implant (A). Plain radiograph demonstrating the seed positions with superimposed isodoses (B).

3. Base of Tongue

The vast majority of patients with base of tongue (BOT) squamous cell carcinomas (SCC) present with advanced disease due to the insidious natural history and rich surrounding lymphatics. Surgical resection unfortunately is associated with significant functional deficits in this site. Several independent investigators have consistently demonstrated that a brachytherapy implant boost (20–30 Gy) following EBRT (45–55 Gy) is associated with effective local control rates with no significant functional deficits as demonstrated in several quality of life domains. The greatest experience has been with temporary interstitial LDR iridium-192 implants. Mature local control rates of 85% or greater may be expected for T1 and T2 lesions and 80–85% with T3 lesions. A retrospective comparative study reported comparable local control rates between EBRT and an implant and surgery followed by postoperative EBRT. In contrast, local control rates with conventional fractionated EBRT alone were noted to be inferior. Hence, compelling data exist to use interstitial implants in the management of BOT HNSCC where effective organ-preserving therapy is

required. Complication rates appear to be acceptable with the use of a looping technique (see Fig. 2).

4. Oral Tongue

Several treatment options exist for oral tongue (OT) SCC and appear to offer comparable rates of local control. Hence, the toxicity and functional impairments often guide treatment selection. In this regard, brachytherapy has been used alone or in combination with EBRT demonstrating local control efficacy with a 10–20% risk of mild–moderate self-limiting soft tissue ulceration and a low risk of mandibular osteoradionecrosis in experienced hands. Custom lead-embedded mandibular prostheses are recommended to reduce the risk of bone complications. This modality also permits the preservation of oral tongue function and a shorter treatment time. The largest experience of over 600 patients from the Curie Institute reported local control rates of 86, 80, and 68% for T1, T2, and T3 lesions, respectively. Early T1 and T2 lesions were treated with temporary interstitial LDR iridium-192 implants alone delivering 70 Gy in 6–9 days. Larger T2 and T3 lesions were treated with

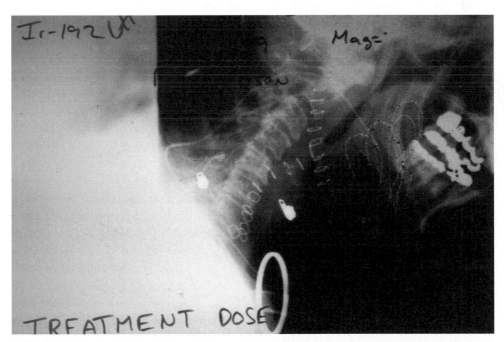

FIGURE 2 Interstitial temporary low-dose rate brachytherapy implant for a base of tongue squamous cell carcinoma. Afterloading catheters are placed percutaneously through a submandibular approach looping over the base of tongue. Dummy ribbons demonstrating the seed positions that may be loaded with radioactive seeds have been placed within the catheters.

EBRT (50–55 Gy) followed by an implant (20–30 Gy). Other investigators have demonstrated similar results. A time interval between EBRT and the implant of greater than 20 days may adversely impact on local control rates. The optimal HDR schedule for treatment alone in early stage OT carcinomas has been the subject of several studies. A small randomized trial has demonstrated comparable local control rates for an HDR schedule of 60 Gy in 10 fractions over 6 days to an LDR implant of 70 Gy over 4–9 days.

A small subset of patients with a close or positive surgical excision margin and no indication for neck irradiation have been treated with a brachytherapy implant alone (iridium-192 LDR to 60 Gy) by several investigators. This obviates the risk of EBRT-related xerostomia. Mature local control rates of 85–90% have been observed.

5. Floor of Mouth

Similar to oral tongue carcinomas, several treatment options exist for floor of mouth (FOM) carcinomas, although surgical resection is often preferred due to minimal functional deficits and high rates of local control achieved. Brachytherapy implants may have a role in the management of FOM but must be judiciously applied due to the proximity of the mandible increasing the risk of osteoradionecrosis complications. Several institutions have demonstrated that an iridium-192 implant alone (60–70 Gy) may yield local control rates of over 90, 70–75, and 50–55% for T1, T2, and T3 lesions, respectively. A small retrospective trial has demonstrated comparable local control rates in early stage lesions with either an HDR or an LDR implant. Iridium-192 implants (60 Gy) have also been demonstrated to offer excellent mature local control rates of 85–90% in lesions with close or positive margins following surgical excision.

6. Lip

Cancer of the lip is the most common malignancy of the oral cavity. Several treatment options exist including surgery, EBRT, and a brachytherapy implant. As with OT lesions, an implant affords minimal functional and cosmetic disabilities, especially for lesions near the commissure with the advantage of a shorter overall treatment time. Several large series, including

one treating over 700 patients, confirm comparable high rates of local control as expected with surgical resection. The vast majority of the reported series have used temporary LDR iridium-192 or iodine-125 implants delivering a typical dose of 60 Gy over 6 days for T1 and T2 lesions with local control rates in excess of 90 and 85%, respectively. A brachytherapy implant boost (20–30 Gy) may be integrated with the management of the neck for selected more advanced T2 and T3 lesions with an expected control rate of approximately 75%. Customized lead-embedded dental prostheses are recommended, especially for large implants lying in close proximity to bony structures.

7. Recurrent HNSCC

The optimal management for recurrent nonnasopharyngeal HNSCC remains to be defined and is complicated by the heterogeneity of patients studied. However, brachytherapy can play an important role, particularly in the setting of tumors occurring within a previously irradiated volume of tissue, including recurrent and second primary HNSCC.

Surgery is offered for resectable lesions in the absence of unacceptable functional and cosmetic sequelae. In this setting, there is often a need for the management of microscopic residual disease with radiotherapy. A planned introduction of nonirradiated tissue flaps and coordination of the implant placement and of the wound reconstruction may reduce the risk of increased late radiotherapy complications. Despite this, complication rates of 30–50% have been reported, which is tempered by local control rates of 44–80%, suggesting a limited therapeutic ratio. Hence, appropriate selection is particularly important for this indication.

Several institutional series have also demonstrated that an implant alone may be effective in providing local control rates of 60% or greater for selected secondary HNSCC with control rates differing by tumor site and lesion size. Small lesions (<3 cm) occurring in the tonsil appear to be well controlled with an implant. The greatest experience has been with temporary interstitial LDR iridium-192 implants delivering 60 Gy. For recurrent HNSCC, an implant alone can be expected to yield local control rates of 20–45% consistent with the treatment of more radioresistant clonogens. Serious complications are significant and may include soft tissue ulceration, bone necrosis, and fistula formation, which may occur in 20–50% of patients treated.

8. Eye

Functional and cosmetic organ preservation considerations are important goals in the management of ocular and orbital malignancies. The use of brachytherapy implants is well suited to this anatomic site due to the close proximity of normal structures and the need to provide precise irradiation. Several large institutional series confirm an established role for plaque surface brachytherapy for several isotopes, including iodine-125, cobalt-60, ruthenium-106, and, most recently, palladium-103 in the management of choroidal malignant melanoma. The greatest clinical experience has been with temporary LDR iodine-125 plaque therapy delivering an apical dose of 75–80 Gy to lesions less than 10 mm in thickness and less than 15 mm in diameter in an eye with potential salvageable vision. Local control rates of 63–80% and 10-year survival rates of 60–65% comparable with those achieved with enucleation have been reported. Vision is well preserved in over 85% of patients achieving local control. Toxicities may include retinitis, optic neuropathy, and cataracts. The need for prospective evaluation has prompted the ongoing National Eye Institute-sponsored Collaborative Ocular Melanoma Study (COMS), a large multi-institutional trial randomizing patients between radiation therapy and enucleation with survival as the major end point. For unilateral medium-sized tumors (height >2.5 mm and ≤10 mm, base diameter ≤ 16 mm), the radiation is with iodine-125 plaque brachytherapy (apical dose 80–120 Gy). Results of these studies remain pending.

C. Skin Malignancies

Treatment options for nonmelanoma skin malignancies may include surgery or radiation therapy with the greatest experience with EBRT. However, in selected situations the use of either a surface mold implant or an interstitial implant may be advantageous, particularly in sharply curving tumor sites where the dosimetry of EBRT techniques may be suboptimal. Various techniques have been described. The greatest experi- ence has been with temporary LDR implants (60 Gy) using interstitial techniques. Excellent and comparable results to those with EBRT or surgery may be achieved. HDR fractionation schedules using surface molds with customized shielding have also been studied. Various schedules have been recommended, although schedules analogous to those with EBRT have often been employed.

D. Breast Malignancies

Standard local therapy may include mastectomy or lumpectomy followed by whole breast EBRT. Traditionally, breast implants have been used selectively to boost deeply located tumor beds, especially in large breasts and in the treatment of gross residual disease. Several institutions have studied the role of breast brachytherapy as the sole form of adjuvant radiotherapy based on the observation that the vast majority of breast recurrences occur within the proximity of the tumor bed. This has been motivated by the ability to promptly initiate and to reduce the overall treatment time, which may be advantageous when a need exists to integrate it with systemic therapy. To date, results from several institutional pilot trials are promising with the longest follow-up based on temporary interstitial volume LDR iridium-192 implants (45–50 Gy). One institutional pilot study has reported no local relapses following a median follow-up of 47 months. Early experiences with temporary interstitial HDR iridium-192 implants have also been reported. Although promising, these results remain preliminary and await longer follow-up. Remote relapses from the tumor bed remain a major concern with this therapeutic strategy; hence these trials reflect a select patient population with lobular carcinomas and lesions with features consistent with multicentric disease excluded from study. A multi-institutional cooperative study has recently closed accrual assessing the reproducibility and efficacy of this treatment strategy. Breast brachytherapy has also been used as part of a multimodality approach for BCT in locally advanced breast cancers and as potential breast-conserving therapy for recurrent lesions in a prior irradiated breast. These indications remain to be established with further study and follow-up.

E. Lung Malignancies

The majority of patients with nonsmall cell lung cancer (NSCLC) require locoregional symptom palliation in the setting of limited pulmonary reserves warranting careful consideration of the dose and volume of lung irradiated. In this regard, temporary LDR or HDR intraluminal brachytherapy (ILBT) has an established role in the management of NSCLC. In general, LDR-ILBT (30–60 Gy in one to two sessions) institutional series have reported effective palliation for various symptoms with rates comparable to HDR-ILRT. HDR-ILBT has been more commonly applied (Fig. 3). As monotherapy, several large patient series have reported palliation of hemoptysis in 55–85%, cough in 60–95%, and dyspnea in 60–85% of patients treated with significant patient, treatment, and end point definition heterogeneity complicating the interpretation of these series. Symptom palliation appears to be durable in the majority of patients responding. The optimal fractionation schedule and prescription point re-

main to be determined with both multiple and single fraction schedules studied. When compared to EBRT in a randomized setting, HDR-ILRT (intraluminal radiotherapy) is comparable regarding symptom palliation but appears to be inferior regarding the durability of palliation, especially for good performance patients. The improved durability likely reflects the ability of EBRT to address the extraluminal bulk of disease, resulting in a modest improvement in survival. For patients with a limited prognosis, a single fraction of 10 Gy has been demonstrated to be effective. Higher single doses (≥15 Gy), particularly when prior laser intervention was used, are associated with higher risks of massive hemoptysis. Significant toxicities of HDR-ILBT may include radiation bronchitis, stenosis, and massive hemoptysis in 5–10% of cases.

Experience with EBRT and HDR-ILBT exists as a planned intervention. A trial randomized 98 untreated patients between EBRT and EBRT with HDR-ILRT demonstrating a trend toward improved local

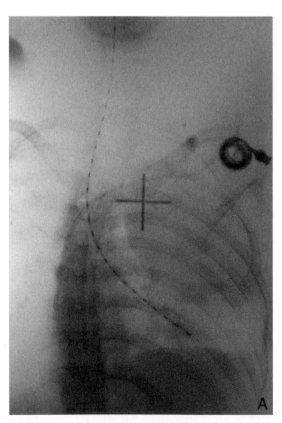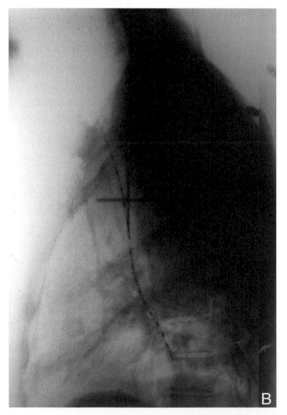

FIGURE 3 Orthogonal plain radiographs demonstrating a temporary high-dose rate intraluminal brachytherapy implant of the left main stem bronchus. A dummy ribbon demonstrates the seed positions that may be occupied by the radioactive source. Courtesy of Juliana Pisch, M.D.

control in the later arm with no improvement in survival. Subgroup analysis suggested significant local control and survival improvement for squamous cell carcinomas. A second similar randomized trial did report that the addition of ILRT improved the durability of dyspnea palliation for obstructing tumors lying in the main bronchus. Institutional series demonstrate palliation of hemoptysis in >85%, cough 50–85%, and dyspnea 50–100% of patients treated. Massive fatal hemoptysis appears in 15–20% of cases and does not appear to be increased with ILRT where the fraction size does not exceed 10 Gy. In general, HDR-ILRT for recurrent previously irradiated lesions appears to have comparable rates of palliation. However, fatal hemoptysis may be as high as 30–50%. Tumor progression, particularly when located in proximity to the pulmonary artery, may also contribute to higher rates of fatal hemoptysis. In part, this may be due to selection of patients with more biologically aggressive disease who fail EBRT. Hence, caution is recommended when large single fractions are used for this indication.

Combined EBRT and LDR-ILRT or HDR-ILRT alone has been reported in several small series as definitive treatment for radiographically occult endobronchial carcinomas. Careful attention to tumor volume definition and dosimetry is recommended. Promising local control and survival rates have been reported. Various intraoperative radiotherapy techniques employing either permanent or temporary LDR implants have been reported to supplement the local control rates in the setting of gross or microscopic residual disease. Further study is awaited to support this indication for an implant.

F. Gastrointestinal Malignancies

1. Esophagus

Locally persistent or recurrent disease remains a significant clinical problem in the management of esophageal carcinoma. For previously untreated patients, HDR-ILRT has commonly been studied in the definitive setting to provide dose escalation. Several retrospective series and a prospective randomized trial have demonstrated that the addition of an intracavitary HDR or LDR-ILRT boost (10 Gy / 2 fractions / over 2 weeks) compared to an EBRT boost (10 Gy / 5 fractions / over 1 week) improves local control and dysphagia. In the subgroup with tumors 5 cm or less, 5-year cause-specific survival was 64% vs 31.5% ($p=0.025$) in favor of ILRT. The role of an ILRT boost for lesions treated with concurrent chemoradiotherapy remains to be defined, as a cooperative study demonstrated a high rate of fistulas, life-threatening toxicity, and treatment-related deaths.

For palliation, the American Brachytherapy Society consensus guideline recommends EBRT (30 Gy) followed by either an HDR-ILRT (10–14 Gy in 1–2 f) or an LDR-ILRT (25–40 Gy at 0.4–1 Gy/h) boost for patients with an expected life expectancy of 3–6 months. For patients with an expected life expectancy of less than 3 months, an ILRT implant is recommended. Palliation of dysphagia may be seen in 60–100% of patients treated with toxicity limited to esophagitis, ulcerations, strictures, and a low risk of fistulae.

2. Extrahepatic Bile Duct Malignancies

Surgical resection is the primary treatment modality for cancers of the extrahepatic biliary tree. Unresectable disease or residual gross or microscopic disease is a common problem with the ability to irradiate cancers in this region limited by surrounding normal tissues. Hence, an extensive body of literature exists examining the role of both LDR- and HDR-ILRT in the management of extrahepatic bile duct carcinomas. Unfortunately, the majority of the patient series are limited by small patient numbers and heterogeneous groups of patients studied. Hence, outcome improvements may be significantly influenced by selection bias. In the postoperative setting following complete gross resection, the addition of EBRT (45–50 Gy) and LDR-ILRT (15–25 Gy at 1 cm) or HDR-ILRT (20 Gy in 4 f at 1 cm) may offer survival improvements. In the setting of unresectable or gross residual disease, the use of EBRT and ILRT appears to improve the patency of biliary drainage and may offer improvements in survival compared to EBRT alone. Complications may include transient cholangitis, fatal sepsis, perihepatic abscesses, and gastrointestinal tract injury. Hence, ILRT must be cautiously applied. A cooperative randomized trial to evaluate the role of EBRT and ILRT has been proposed.

3. Rectum and Anal Canal

A limited number of institutions have reported on the role of transperineal template-guided interstitial temporary LDR iridium-192 implants (15–20 Gy) in combination with pelvic EBRT for rectal adenocarcinomas. Small patient numbers, heterogeneous selection criterias including a mixture of patients with anal canal carcinomas, and the potential for significant complications limit any definitive conclusions regarding the generalizability of this technique. Typically, selected patients refusing a colostomy due to the location or the extent of the tumor have been treated with local control rates of 70–85% reported.

Various brachytherapy techniques have been reported in the treatment of recurrent rectal cancers often failing previous surgery and pelvic radiotherapy. These include transperineal and open-surgical techniques with permanent and temporary implants. Permanent implants for small volumes of gross residual disease may afford local control benefits with minimal toxicities. Intraluminal temporary HDR implants may offer effective palliation.

More recently, intraoperative HDR radiotherapy (HDR-IORT) has been applied with flexible surface HAM applicators following surgical resection for recurrent previously irradiated lesions (see Fig. 4). The applicator is able to conform to the sloping surfaces of most tumor beds in the pelvis typically delivering a dose of 12–15 Gy. This technique has also been studied in combination with preoperative EBRT and chemotherapy for unresectable lesions. To date, early results demonstrate promising local control and disease-free survival rates with the results largely influenced by the ability to completely resect the lesion. It remains to be demonstrated to what extent the selection of favorable tumor biology contributes to the results reported. Peripheral neuropathy appears to be the major toxicity.

For anal canal carcinomas, a temporary interstitial LDR iridium-192 implant boost (typically 20–30 Gy) in combination with EBRT and chemotherapy has been reported by several institutions. These series suggest that for a mixture of tumor stages, local control rates of 75% or greater may be achieved with the risk of severe soft tissue necrosis less than 10%.

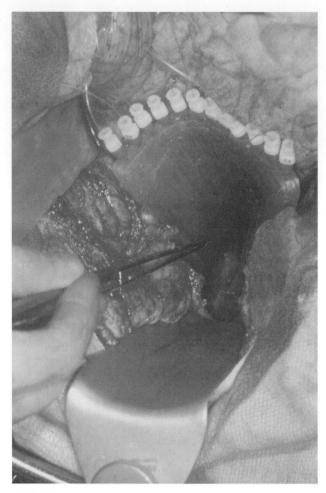

FIGURE 4 An intraoperative temporary high-dose rate surface brachytherapy implant using the flexible HAM applicator. This applicator maintains a uniform intercatheter distance and a distance between the surface and the plane of the catheters. The HAM applicator has been placed in the presacral space to permit reirradiation following resection for a recurrent rectal adenocarcinoma.

G. Genitourinary Malignancies

1. Prostate

Several therapeutic options exist for organ-confined prostate adenocarcinoma, including radiation therapy. Radiation therapy strategies include EBRT alone, permanent interstitial iodine-125 or palladium-103 seed implants alone, or combination EBRT and seed implants. Most recently, experience with temporary interstitial HDR iridium-192 implants in combination with EBRT as a boost have been reported. For each of these options, the addition of androgen ablation has also been studied. No randomized data exist to compare each of these strategies; hence, patient selection criteria are important in assessing the relative efficacy of each treatment option. The definition of risk groups for extracapsular extension (ECE) by PSA, Gleason score, and clinical T stage is well accepted and has provided a basis for relative comparisons of treatment strategies. The recent interest in prostate brachytherapy results from technological innovations and the recognition of improved treatment outcome with radiotherapy dose escalation that is limited by

adjacent critical structures such as the rectum and urethra.

Currently, permanent radioactive seed implants are performed with a transperineal approach under transrectal ultrasound guidance producing axial prostate images (see Fig. 5). These images are referenced to a rigid transperineal template that is used to guide the relative positions of needles used to facilitate the radioactive seed placement. Various techniques have been reported. Institutional experience provides the principal evidence to support therapeutic efficacy, although follow-up with implants is shorter than the

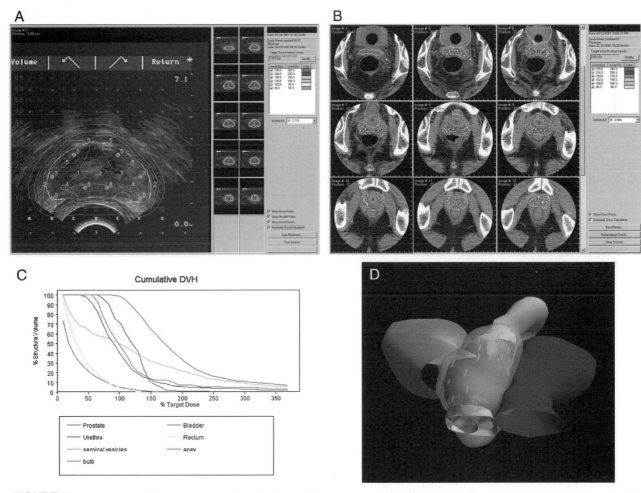

FIGURE 5 Permanent low-dose rate interstitial seed implant of the prostate. (A) Axial ultrasound-derived prostate images used to plan the implant with the superimposed anticipated isodoses covering the prostate. (B) Dosimetry achieved following the implant using CT images of the prostate. (C) The dose–volume histogram for each identified structure, including the prostate. Ninety-nine percent of the prostate volume received 100% of the prescribed dose. (D) A three-dimensional reconstruction of the prostate and surrounding rectum, bladder, seminal vesicles, implanted seeds, and the 100% isodose covering the prostate. Courtesy of Daniel Shasha, M.D.

experiences with EBRT. In general, seed implants in lesions with a low risk of ECE have demonstrated 5-year biochemical control between 85–95%. One study of over 100 patients has reported a 10-year biochemical control rate of 70%. The recommended doses for monotherapy are 145 Gy for iodine-125 and 115–120 Gy for palladium-103.

Implants for intermediate-risk and high-risk groups of patients suggest short-term control rates (4–5 years) of 45–80 and 30–60%, respectively. In the short-term, PSA control appears more likely in patients receiving an implant in combination with androgen ablation than an implant alone. Similarly, treatment with combination EBRT (40–50 Gy) and an implant (125I: 100–110 Gy, 103Pd: 80–90 Gy) for these risk groups is associated with biochemical control rates of 65–75% at 10 years. With the addition of androgen ablation, a 5-year freedom from biochemical failure of 77% has been reported. With seed implants, symptoms include prostatitis and urethritis occurring in approximately 80% of patients with the severity peaking several months after the implant and potentially persisting for 12–24 months. Urinary retention may occur typically in less than 10% of patients treated. Long-term complications may include urinary incontinence, impotency, and radiation proctitis.

Prostate boost radiotherapy with a temporary HDR implant has been studied in several institutions and has been advocated on the basis of dosimetric optimization within the prostate and surrounding normal tissues. In general, various techniques have been described with preliminary results showing promising rates of biochemical control with various fractionation schedules studied to date. Acute and late toxicity has been low with potency preserved in the majority. This promising technique remains the subject of further study to define the optimal technique and fractionation schedule.

2. Bladder

Both permanent seed implants and temporary interstitial LDR implants have been studied in the management of bladder carcinoma. The temporary afterloading iridium-192 implant (30–40 Gy) has been used in selected patients for bladder preservation therapy often in combination with EBRT (30–40 Gy) following a partial cystectomy. Selected lesions have included solitary T1, T2, and T3 tumors <4–5 cm involving a nonfixed portion of the bladder with no evidence of nodal metastases often following a lymph node dissection. Local control rates have ranged from 65 to 85% with low rates of acute and late organ complications based on institutional experiences. The main advantages lie in accurate target delineation, which is an issue in EBRT organ-preserving strategies, providing local dose escalation. In contrast, it is an invasive procedure that is less appealing in a disease where distant metastases remain a therapeutic challenge.

3. Penis

Penis squamous cell carcinoma is a rare cancer. Surgery is an established treatment option for local disease. However, functional organ preservation is often a desired treatment goal. Several institutional series, including one with over 200 patients, have provided consistent evidence demonstrating that local temporary surface mold or interstitial iridium-192 implants (50–60 Gy) are able to achieve local functional organ preservation in 70–85% of selected early stage cases. These have included noninfiltrating or infiltrating tumors of less than 4 cm diameter with minor or no invasion of the corpora cavernosa. Lesions larger than 4 cm or those deeply infiltrating the corpora cavernosa are associated with increased rates of local relapse with limited functional preservation such that surgery has been recommended.

H. Gynecological Malignancies

1. Uterus

Brachytherapy has been extensively studied in the management of endometrial carcinoma. Currently, the major indication includes the use of temporary LDR intracavitary cesium-137 implants or HDR intracavitary iridium-192 implants for adjuvant therapy in pathologic stage I intermediate- and high-risk uterine carcinomas delivering a high dose to the underlying vaginal cuff mucosal lymphatics often with or without pelvic EBRT. Risk selection factors may include depth of myometrial invasion, histologic grade, surgical margin status, and lymph node metastases. Several institutional practices have provided guidance with regard to dose schedules. For LDR intracavitary implants alone (60–70 Gy) or with EBRT (10–20 Gy), paired colpostats are used to deliver the dose to the mucosal surface. For HDR intracavitary implants with a vaginal cylinder or with paired colpostats, various fractionation schedules prescribed at the vaginal surface or typically at a depth of 0.5 cm for implant treatment alone and in combination with EBRT have been reported. To date, high local control rates (>90%) and low complication rates have been observed with adjuvant HDR implants. Late complications have included vaginal stenosis, cystitis, and proctitis. Clinical FIGO stage II lesions with cervical stromal invasion may be treated with preoperative radiation with either an LDR or HDR implant in combination with pelvic EBRT.

Medically inoperable or unresectable advanced endometrial carcinoma may be treated with radiation therapy. Often, the comorbidities that make these patients medically inoperable may also increase the risk of complications arising from prolonged immobilization associated with LDR implants. Hence, institutional preferences have been with HDR intracavitary implants with or without EBRT. Various techniques have been described to accurately delineate and to provide adequate dosimetric coverage of the uterus with intracavitary techniques. Commonly, tandem variations are used in combination with paired colpostats. As the dose delivered is by necessity higher to treat gross disease, accurate and verified displacement of adjacent normal structures, including the bladder and rectum, is critical.

2. Cervix

Brachytherapy has an established role in the management of both early stage and advanced stage cervix carcinomas. The greatest clinical experience has been with LDR temporary intracavitary cesium-137 implants with both manual and remote afterloading techniques reported. Several technical considerations of the implant, the integration with EBRT, and the overall treatment time have been shown to influence local control rates and survival. Early stage lesions, carcinoma in situ, and FIGO IA and IB1 are adequately managed with radiation alone, although many other treatment options exist with comparable results. Where the risk of occult metastases to draining lymph nodes is low, a temporary LDR intracavitary cesium-137 implant alone may be used. For more advanced lesions, a cesium-137 implant boost has been demonstrated to significantly increase local control rates and survival. A dose of 80–85 Gy prescribed to point A and a dose of 85–90 Gy have been recommended for early and advanced lesions, respectively. Similarly, doses to the pelvic sidewall of 50–55 and 55–65 Gy are recommended restricting the dose to the bladder and rectum to 80 and 75 Gy, respectively. Where the tumor geometry does not lend itself to an intracavitary implant, a temporary interstitial implant often with transperineal is indicated with local control rates appearing to improve compared to the use of inadequate intracavitary implants. Reported late complication rates of 15–20% necessitate careful planning.

Several randomized trials and retrospective comparative analyses have suggested that temporary intracavitary HDR implants with iridium-192 may yield at least equivalent efficacy and toxicity results to LDR cesium implants. Complication rates are affected by high dose per fraction. The optimal fractionation schedule remains to be defined, although several institutional experiences and the American Brachytherapy Society Consensus report exist to guide the use of HDR brachytherapy implants.

3. Vagina

Intracavitary and interstitial brachytherapy implants have important roles in the management of vaginal carcinomas permitting local control and functional organ preservation. Several large retrospective institutional series show consistent results demonstrating that a temporary LDR intracavitary cesium-137 or interstitial (80 Gy) iridium-192 implant is sufficient for stage I lesions (<0.5 cm thick). Typically, a transperineal template technique is used for interstitial implants. An LDR intracavitary implant (60 Gy) may also successfully treat in situ disease. Local control rates in excess of 85–90% may be achieved. For high-risk stage I lesions and more advanced stages, EBRT (45–50 Gy) to the pelvis with an interstitial LDR iridium-192 boost (25–30 Gy), for a mimimum dose of 75 Gy, provides better control and survival than either modalities alone. Higher doses appear to be required for more advanced stage II and III lesions.

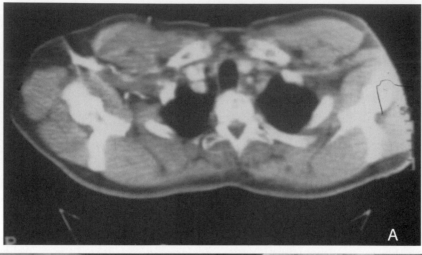

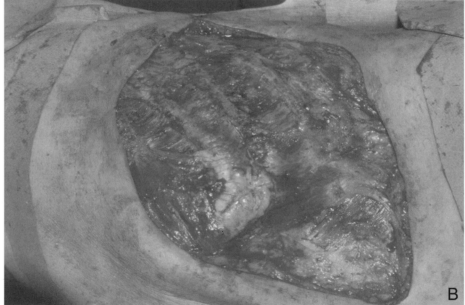

FIGURE 6 An intraoperative temporary high-dose rate surface brachytherapy implant with the HAM applicator for a chest wall sarcoma. The sarcoma is located on the right posterior chest wall (A). The tumor was resected (B) with the HAM applicator applied to facilitate treatment of a complex curved surface (C). As the treatment is delivered intraoperatively, the underlying lung was deflated under controlled conditions during the delivery of the radiation to further minimize any irradiation of the underlying lung.

Pelvic control rates of 55–65 and 25–30% may be expected for stage II–III and stage IV, respectively. As with cervix carcinomas, protracted overall treatment times appear to adversely influence pelvic control rates, mandating close integration. Complications, seen in 15–20% of cases, may include fistula formation, mucosal necrosis, and vaginal stenosis. Experience with temporary HDR implants remains prelimi-

nary and requires further follow-up to define its efficacy and toxicity profile.

4. Urethra

Female urethral carcinoma is rare, with treatment options including surgery and radiation therapy. Institutional experiences support a role for brachytherapy in providing local control with organ preservation when

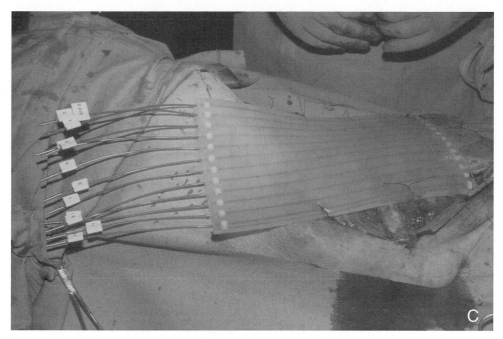

FIGURE 6 *(Continued)*

used alone or in combination with EBRT for advanced lesions. Early T1 distal lesions of the urethra have been treated with temporary LDR interstitial iridium-192 implants (60 Gy). For larger lesions and for more proximal lesions where the risk of inguinal lymph node metastases is increased, EBRT (45–50 Gy) may be given in combination with a temporary LDR iridium-192 implant (30–40 Gy). Local control rates for all lesions considered have ranged from 65 to 85%. Complications may occur in up to 40–50% of patients, reflecting the high mucosal dose, and may include urethral stenosis, necrosis, fistula formation, cystitis, and incontinence.

I. Pediatric Malignancies

External beam radiotherapy is often indicated in the management of various pediatric malignancies. However, late sequelae, including growth abnormalities, organ dysfunction, and the risk of secondary malignancies, are related to the volume of normal tissues exposed to irradiation. Hence, brachytherapy implants have been studied in various tumor sites to characterize the associated efficacy and risk of late sequelae.

Clinical experience has contributed to established indications for brachytherapy implants in the management of retinoblastomas and craniopharyngiomas. Promising results have been reported for selected cases of soft tissue sarcomas, rhabdomyosarcomas, Ewing's sarcoma, and various central nervous system malignancies. The predominant experience has been with temporary LDR implants. The needs for sedation, immobilization, and radiation exposure hazards are major limitations with this technique. Hence, interests have focused on PDR, HDR, and IORT techniques with encouraging results. These require further prospective evaluation to establish their indications in the management of pediatric malignancies.

J. Sarcoma

1. Extremity Sarcoma

The standard therapy for extremity sarcomas has evolved to wide local excision and the application of risk-appropriate adjuvant radiotherapy, with both EBRT and brachytherapy implants demonstrated to be successful. The results of a mature randomized trial comparing no adjuvant therapy and temporary planar interstitial LDR iridium-192 brachytherapy implants (45–50 Gy over 4–5 days) have demonstrated improved rates of local control with the efficacy largely restricted to high-grade lesions (66% vs 89%). Low-grade lesions are more appropriately treated with adjuvant EBRT, possibly due to the slow rate of cellular proliferation limiting the efficacy of an implant during its treatment duration. Deferring the loading of the implant for at least 5 days in the postoperative period permitting sufficient fibrogenesis will significantly reduce wound complications. The efficacy of brachytherapy implants has challenged the EBRT paradigm of generous normal tissue margins around the surgical bed requiring irradiation. The coordination of an implant at the time of surgical resection (see Fig. 5) permits accurate delineation of close or potentially positive resection margins, which has been suggested to further benefit with the use of an implant as a boost (15–20 Gy) compared to adjuvant treatment with EBRT alone for high-grade lesions. The restricted volume of normal tissues that are irradiated is particularly beneficial for extremity sarcomas in ensuring functional status and in the pediatric population. This therapeutic approach has also been reported by several investigators for recurrent extremity sarcomas in areas of prior EBRT permitting a 52–68% local control rate and a 12–15% rate of wound complications severe enough to require surgery. The use of HDR and IORT brachytherapy implants (see Fig. 6) has been limited to date and remains an area of active investigation.

III. CONCLUSIONS

Brachytherapy has an established role in the management of cancer for many different tumor sites in the definitive and salvage treatment scenarios. When appropriately applied for specific indications, it may provide a significant improvement in the therapeutic ratio as a result of both physical and biologic manipulations of the probability of tumor control and the risk of late normal tissue complications, increasing the likelihood of functional organ preservation.

See Also the Following Articles

BRAIN AND CENTRAL NERVOUS SYSTEM CANCERS • DOSIMETRY AND TREATMENT PLANNING FOR THREE-DIMENSIONAL RADIATION THERAPY • HEAD AND NECK CANCER • LATE EFFECTS OF RADIATION THERAPY • LUNG, LARYNX, ORAL CAVITY, AND PHARYNX • PROTON BEAM RADIATION THERAPY • RADIOBIOLOGY, PRINCIPLES OF

Bibliography

Alektiar, K. M., Velasco, J., Zelefsky, M. J., Woodruff, J. M., Lewis, J. J., and Brennan, M. F. (2000). Adjuvant radiotherapy for margin-positive high-grade soft tissue sarcoma of the extremity. Int. J. Radiat. Oncol. Biol. Phys. 48(4), 1051–1058.

Alektiar, K. M., Zelefsky, M. J., Paty, P. B., et al. (2000). High-dose-rate intraoperative brachytherapy for recurrent colorectal cancer. Int. J. Radiat. Oncol. Biol. Phys. 48(1), 219–226.

Gaspar, L. E., Winter, K., Kocha, W. I., Coia, L. R., Herskovic, A., and Graham, M. (2000). A phase I/II study of external beam radiation, brachytherapy, and concurrent chemotherapy for patients with localized carcinoma of the esophagus (Radiation Therapy Oncology Group Study 9207): Final report. Cancer 88(5), 988–995.

Gaspar, L. E., Nag, S., Herskovic, A., Mantravadi, R., and Speiser, B. (1997). American Brachytherapy Society (ABS) consensus guidelines for brachytherapy of esophageal cancer: Clinical Research Committee, American Brachytherapy Society, Philadelphia, PA. Int. J. Radiat. Oncol. Biol. Phys. 38(1), 127–132.

Gerbaulet, A., Panis, X., Flamant, F., and Chassagne, D. (1985). Iridium afterloading curietherapy in the treatment of pediatric malignancies: The Institut Gustave Roussy experience. Cancer 56(6), 1274–1279.

Gollins, S. W., Ryder, W. D., Burt, P. A., Barber, P. V., and Stout, R. (1996). Massive haemoptysis death and other morbidity associated with high dose rate intraluminal radiotherapy for carcinoma of the bronchus. Radiother. Oncol. 39(2), 105–116.

Harrison, L. B., Franzese, F., Gaynor, J. J., and Brennan, M. F. (1993). Long-term results of a prospective randomized trial of adjuvant brachytherapy in the management of completely resected soft tissue sarcomas of the extremity and superficial trunk. Int. J. Radiat. Oncol. Biol. Phys. 27(2), 259–265.

Harrison, L. B., and Janjan, N. (1995). Brachytherapy in sarcomas. Hematol. Oncol. Clin. North Am. 9(4), 747–763.

Harrison, L. B., Lee, H. J., Pfister, D. G., et al. (1998). Long term results of primary radiotherapy with/without neck dissection for squamous cell cancer of the base of tongue. Head Neck 20(8), 668–673.

Harrison, L. B., Minsky, B. D., Enker, W. E., et al. (1998). High dose rate intraoperative radiation therapy (HDR-IORT) as part of the management strategy for locally advanced primary and recurrent rectal cancer. *Int. J. Radiat. Oncol. Biol. Phys.* **42**(2), 325–330.

Huber, R. M., Fischer, R., Hautmann, H., Pollinger, B., Haussinger, K., and Wendt, T. (1997). Does additional brachytherapy improve the effect of external irradiation? A prospective, randomized study in central lung tumors. *Int. J. Radiat. Oncol. Biol. Phys.* **38**(3), 533–540.

Inoue, T., Teshima, T., Murayama, S., Shimizutani, K., Fuchihata, H., and Furukawa, S. (1996). Phase III trial of high and low dose rate interstitial radiotherapy for early oral tongue cancer. *Int. J. Radiat. Oncol. Biol. Phys.* **36**(5), 1201–1204.

Inoue, T., Yamazaki, H., Koizumi, M., *et al.* (1998). High dose rate versus low dose rate interstitial radiotherapy for carcinoma of the floor of mouth. *Int. J. Radiat. Oncol. Biol. Phys.* **41**(1), 53–58.

Lanciano, R. (2000). Optimizing radiation parameters for cervical cancer. *Semin Radiat Oncol.* **10**(1), 36–43.

Langendijk, H., de Jong, J., Tjwa, M., *et al.* (2001). External irradiation versus external irradiation plus endobronchial brachytherapy in inoperable non-small cell lung cancer: A prospective randomized study. *Radiother. Oncol.* **58**(3), 257–268.

Langendijk, J. A., Tjwa, M. K., de Jong, J. M., ten Velde, G. P., and Wouters, E. F. (1998). Massive haemoptysis after radiotherapy in inoperable non-small cell lung carcinoma: Is endobronchial brachytherapy really a risk factor? *Radiother. Oncol.* **49**(2), 175–183.

Laperriere, N. J., Leung, P. M., McKenzie, S., *et al.* (1998). Randomized study of brachytherapy in the initial management of patients with malignant astrocytoma. *Int. J. Radiat. Oncol. Biol. Phys.* **41**(5), 1005–1011.

Lapeyre, M., Hoffstetter, S., Peiffert, D., *et al.* (2000). Postoperative brachytherapy alone for T1-2 N0 squamous cell carcinomas of the oral tongue and floor of mouth with close or positive margins. *Int. J. Radiat. Oncol. Biol. Phys.* **48**(1), 37–42.

Lee, A. W., Law, S. C., Foo, W., *et al.* (1993). Retrospective analysis of patients with nasopharyngeal carcinoma treated during 1976–1985: Survival after local recurrence. *Int. J. Radiat. Oncol. Biol. Phys.* **26**(5), 773–782.

Nag, S. (1997). "Principles and Practice of Brachytherapy." Futura, Armonk, NY.

Nag, S., Erickson, B., Thomadsen, B., Orton, C., Demanes, J. D., and Petereit, D. (2000). The American Brachytherapy Society recommendations for high-dose-rate brachytherapy for carcinoma of the cervix. *Int. J. Radiat. Oncol. Biol. Phys.* **48**(1), 201–211.

Pierquin B., and Marinello, G. (1997). "A Practical Manual of Brachytherapy." Medical Physics, Madison, WI.

Selker, R. G., Shapiro, W. R., and Green, S. (1995). A randomized trial of interstitial radiotherapy (IRT) boost for the treatment of newly diagnosed malignant glioma (glioblastoma multiforme, anaplastic astrocytoma, anaplastic oligodendroglioma, malignant mixed glioma): BTCG study 87-01. *In* "Congress of Neurological Surgeons 45th Annual Meeting Program, pp. 94–95. [Abstract].

Sneed, P. K., Stauffer, P. R., McDermott, M. W., *et al.* (1998). Survival benefit of hyperthermia in a prospective randomized trial of brachytherapy boost +/− hyperthermia for glioblastoma multiforme. *Int. J. Radiat. Oncol. Biol. Phys.* **40**(2), 287–295.

Stout, R., Barber, P., Burt, P., *et al.* (2000). Clinical and quality of life outcomes in the first United Kingdom randomized trial of endobronchial brachytherapy (intraluminal radiotherapy) vs. external beam radiotherapy in the palliative treatment of inoperable non-small cell lung cancer. *Radiother. Oncol.* **56**(3), 323–327.

Stock, R. G., and Stone, N. N. (1999). Permanent radioactive seed implanatation in the treatment of prostate cancer. *Hematol. Oncol. Clin. North Am.* **13**(3), 489–501.

Vicini, F., Kini, V. R., Chen, P., *et al.* (1999). Irradiation of the tumor bed alone after lumpectomy in selected patients with early-stage breast cancer treated with breast conserving therapy. *J. Surg. Oncol.* **70**(1), 33–40.

Brain and Central Nervous System Cancer

Melissa Bondy
Randa El-Zein
M.D. Anderson Cancer Center, Houston, Texas

Margaret Wrensch
University of California, San Francisco

GLOSSARY

brain tumors Brain tumors are tumors that grow in the brain and can be either benign or malignant. A benign brain tumor consists of benign (harmless) cells and has distinct boundaries, but may occur in a vital area of the brain and be malignant. A malignant brain tumor is life-threatening, has uncontrolled growth, and poor prognosis.

cancer family syndrome (Li–Fraumeni syndrome) A syndrome first described by Li and Fraumeni in 1969 showing a familial association of breast cancer, sarcoma, leukemia, and brain tumors. It has been shown that this association is vertically transmitted in a dominantly inherited pattern. Germline *p53* mutations have also been identified with this syndrome.

glioma The general term for a tumor that arises from the supportive tissue of the brain (glial cells). Approximately 90% of brain tumors are gliomas. Examples of these include astrocytoma, oligodendroglioma, and glioblastoma multiforme.

hereditary syndrome An inherited condition (or new mutation) that predisposes an individual to developing a brain tumor. Some of these syndromes include neurofibromatosis, tuberous sclerosis, and Turcot's syndrome.

mutagen sensitivity A measure of interindividual differences in DNA repair activity, measured by the rate at which chromatid breaks are repaired. Mutagen sensitivity is associated with an increased risk for cancer and may reflect the presence of an altered DNA repair pathway.

B rain cancer accounts for approximately 9% of all cancers and 90% of these are gliomas. The incidence of brain cancer has been rising, and much of this rise could be a result of more accurate and comprehensive diagnoses rather than changing or more extensive exposures. Although the etiology of brain tumors is unclear, environmental exposures, family history, and genetic susceptibility are possible explanations for this disease. This article reviews and discusses each of these.

I. INTRODUCTION

Environmental concerns, media, and questionable research methodologies complicate progress toward understanding the etiology of brain cancer and obscure the truism that, at the molecular level, all cancer is genetic. We here first emphasize and discuss the achievement of consensus that the etiology of tumors requires random, inherited, or induced initiation in genes. We review putative risk studies, which point to a need for genetic epidemiology, with sensitive statistical methods as the best hope for an explanation of brain cancer etiology.

Brain cancer, accounting for approximately 1.4% of all cancers and 2.3% of cancer deaths, is never truly benign, as slight impairments of brain or central nervous system (CNS) function, from cancer or its treatment, may have dramatic consequence. The incidence of brain cancer has been rising, and much of this rise could be a result of more accurate and comprehensive diagnoses rather than changing or more extensive exposures. Accurate and complete reporting and the construction of relevant databases required in epidemiology develop only slowly, as can be seen in the limited coverage or catchment area of the best U.S. collections of cancer cases. National monitoring of brain cancer is lacking, as are even universally agreed upon classifications of types and grades of invasiveness of brain tumors. Primary brain tumors are currently classified in a manner that reflects their histological appearance and location. The common typology includes the following.

Gliomas arise from the glial tissues, accounting for 40% of CNS neoplasms and is a general category that includes astrocytomas, oligodendrogliomas, and ependymomas. According to the World Health Organization (WHO), there are four major grades of as-

trocytoma so denoted by their cellular star-like appearance and the most invasive of the tumors in children and adults.

Astrocytomas are subdivided into grade I or pilocytic astrocytomas and are the most frequent brain tumors in children. These tumors rarely undergo neoplastic transformation. Grade II or low-grade astrocytomas account for 25% of all gliomas and are infiltrative in nature. Grade III or anaplastic malignant astrocytomas are highly malignant gliomas and have an increased tendency to progress to glioblastoma. Grade IV or glioblastoma multiforme is a highly malignant brain tumor and typically affects adults. This type of glioma has poor prognosis, largely because the tumor rapidly spreads to other regions of the brain.

Oligodendrogliomas account for less than 10% of intracranial tumors. Oligodendrogliomas take their name and arise from the oligodendrocytes in the brain. Oligodendrogliomas are less aggressive than astrocytomas but are invasive and can traverse the cerebral spinal fluid (CSF). The ability of oligodendrogliomas to metastasize complicates their surgical removal, but because they are limited to the brain and CSF, some patients have a better prognosis and longer survival.

Ependymomas are tumors arising from cells lining the brain ventricles or ependymal cells. Their growth may block the flow of CSF, causing notable swelling of the ventricle or hydrocephalus. Although ependymomas may move along the CSF, they characteristically do not infiltrate normal brain tissue and are sometimes amenable to surgical treatment, especially surgery of the spinal cord.

Meningiomas arise from the sheaths surrounding the brain. The growth of meningiomas and the pressure they produce lead to the symptoms of brain tumors. Meningiomas are quite common, accounting for about 50% of primary central nervous system tumors. Because meningiomas are usually near the surface of the brain, they are often operable and are usually benign.

Medulloblastomas include primitive neuroectodermal tumors that arise in the cerebellum. Medulloblastomas replicate quickly but can be treated with radiation because of their site specificity and early age of onset. They occur most commonly in children and frequently spread throughout the CSF.

Ganglioglioma are tumors containing both neurons and glial cells. They have a high rate of cure by surgery alone or surgery combined with radiation therapy.

Schwannomas (neurilemomas) arise from Schwann cells, which surround cranial and other nerves. Schwannomas are usually benign tumors and often form near the cerebellum and in the cranial nerves responsible for hearing and balance.

Chordomas are spinal tumors that preferentially arise at the extremities of the spinal column and usually do not invade brain tissues and other organs. They are amenable to treatment but stubbornly recur over a span of 10–20 years.

Geneticists, molecular biologists, and epidemiologists are seeking methods for identifying and characterizing brain cancer genes for a clearer understanding of cancer etiology and to develop prevention strategies. Of special interest in carcinogenesis are *protooncogenes*, initiating carcinogenesis by activating cell division, and *suppressor genes*, inhibiting tumors. Epigenetic processes may also inhibit or stimulate tumor growth. Equally essential information under scrutiny is the mechanism of gene–environment interaction. Guiding characterization and gene–environment investigations are studies of known heritable syndromes associated with CNS tumors. These studies also indicate the potential of further collection and use of genetic data.

II. CONGENITAL CONDITIONS

Original studies of CNS tumor-associated syndromes, as well as hereditary conditions associated with CNS tumors, parallel in method and implication the studies of other congenital anomalies. These, and follow-ups, associate congenital medulloblastoma with gastrointestinal and genitourinary system anomalies, congenital ependymoma with multisystem anomalies, astrocytoma with arteriovenous malformation of the overlying meninges, and glioblastoma multiforme with adjacent arteriovenous angiomatous malformation and pulmonary arteriovenous fistula. CNS tumors commonly arise in individuals with Down's syndrome, a disorder involving trisomy 21, and gliomatous tumors with syringomyelia, a disorder possibly of genetic origin. Mental retardation may also be associated with familial brain cancer, as children with astrocytomas had a mentally retarded sibling three times more frequently than controls ($p = 0.04$), whereas mentally retarded sibs, nieces, and nephews occurred in families of adult males 4.8 times more often than in families of controls.

Many reports note cooccurrence of CNS tumors and hereditary syndromes. They are described briefly here.

Tuberous sclerosis, or Bourneville's disease, is an autosomal dominantly inherited progressive disorder occurring in 1 per 10,000–150,000 persons. It is characterized by hamartomas and hamartias of the skin, CNS, and kidneys and results in sebaceous adenomas of the skin, muscle and retinal tumors, epileptic seizures, mental retardation, and nodes or tubers of abnormal glial fibers and ganglion cells in the brain. Its association with CNS tumors is anecdotal, although one hospital study reported seven CNS tumors in 48 cases (15%) of tuberous sclerosis, whereas another found 22 cases of subependymal giant cell astrocytoma in 345 patients (6.4%) with tuberous sclerosis. Astrocytoma, ependymoma, and glioblastoma multiforme have been associated with tuberous sclerosis in up to 5% of cases. Contradictory studies, some reporting linkage to the long arm of chromosome 9q32-34 and others linkage to loci on 11q, indicate that tuberous sclerosis may be genetically heterogeneous.

Neurofibromatosis (NF-1), or von Recklinghausen's disease, occurring in 1 of 3000 live births and showing an autosomal-dominant pattern of heredity, is regarded as among the most common single gene disorders. Paternal origin of the mutation was found in one study in 12 of 14 families, but single gene etiology has yet to be firmly established, as the spontaneous mutation rate of large populations has been put at 50%. NF-1 characteristics are cutaneous pigmentation (cafe-au-lait spots) and multiple neurofibromas involving the skin and possibly deeper peripheral nerves and neural roots. NF-1 patients (94%) present with Lisch nodules or pigmented iris hamartomas and commonly experience optic nerve gliomas, astrocytomas, ependymomas, acoustic neuromas, neurilemmomas, meningiomas, and neurofibromas. Of NF-1 patients, 4–45% experience brain tumors.

Neurofibromatosis type 2, or bilateral acoustic

neurofibromatosis, occurs with one-tenth the frequency of NF-1. NF-2 presents the clinical characteristics of multiple tumors, usually schwannomas of the cranial and spinal nerve roots. Multiple ependymomas, meningiomas developing from arachnoidal cells in the cranial cavity and spinal canal, and spinal cord or brain stem astrocytic gliomas occur in individuals with NF-2. These are often low-grade malignancy but with devastating neurological effects. NF-2 is caused by a deletion in the long arm chromosome 22 associated with meningiomas, gliomas, and spinal neurofibromas.

Nevoid basal cell carcinoma syndrome, or Gorlin syndrome, an autosomal-dominant disorder, presents with multiple basal cell carcinomas having arisen early in life and jaw cysts, characteristic facies, skeletal anomalies, intracranial calcifications of the falx, and ovarian fibromas. The syndrome, but not its rate of co-incidence, was associated with medulloblastoma. Loss of heterozygosity at the chromosomal location examined, particularly in hereditary tumors, implies that the gene, normally functioning as a tumor suppressor, is homozygously inactivated. Bare and colleagues found loss of heterozygosity on chromosome 1q22.

Turcot's syndrome, Gardner's syndrome, and familial polyposis, characterized by adenomatous polyps, have been associated with medulloblastoma and glioblastoma. Because of their marked similarity, some authorities consider Turcot's syndrome, Gardner's syndrome, and classical adenomatous polyposis variations of a single genetic defect. Investigators associate chromosome 5q with these three syndromes.

Sturge–Weber disease is an inherited neurocutaneous syndrome characterized by facial and leptomeningeal angiomas and, frequently, facial and optical port wine lesions. Computer-assisted tomography and magnetic resonance imaging of Sturge–Weber cases show cerebral lobar atrophy, brain calcification, choroid plexus enlargement, and venous abnormalities.

Von Hippel–Lindau disease, a rare autosomal-dominant multisystem disorder, involves cerebellar hemangioblastoma of the CNS and visceral organs, retinal angiomatosis, pancreatic cysts, and benign and malignant renal lesions. Several studies link von Hippel–Lindau disease to the short arm of chromosome 3 (3p13-14.3 and 3p25-26). These findings strongly suggest that a tumor suppressor gene is in-

volved in the disease, and discovery of the gene(s) should enable a reliable diagnostic test to screen family members.

III. FAMILIAL ASSOCIATIONS OF BRAIN TUMORS

In addition to the association of hereditary syndromes with CNS tumors, investigation of brain cancer etiology focuses on families of CNS tumor patients aggregating CNS and other cancers. Tumors of patients and their relatives in these "cancer families" are histologically and biologically similar, and well documented, although the precise relationship between genetics and CNS neoplasms remains unknown. Methodologic constraints unfortunately limit the authority of many of these studies, also obscured by the confounding factor of common familial exposure to environmental agents potentially contributing to neoplasia induction, but they consistently report the presence of similar brain or other tumors in siblings and the cancer family syndrome. With regard to etiology, two possible explanations of family occurrence emerge: a genetic factor may in itself cause family clustering of CNS tumors or a hereditary vulnerability to exposures may produce the clusters.

A. CNS Tumors among Twins

A problem in the area of family studies is the lack of, or yet undiscovered finding of, concordance of CNS tumors in twins. Incidence studies of concordance of twins with CNS tumors in twins have not shown that twins' tumors are histologically identical. In a review of childhood cancer deaths in 145,708 twins and singletons born between 1940 and 1964, Norris and Jackson found 54 instances of solid tumors, 21 were brain tumors. Neither Harvald and Hauge nor Miller found evidence of concordance of CNS neoplasms in twins. To our knowledge, no recent reports discuss the etiologic significance of lack of concordance of CNS tumors in twins.

B. CNS Tumors among Siblings

Surveys of childhood cancer registries reveal a high frequency of siblings concordant for brain tumors, siblings with childhood brain tumors and leukemia, and siblings with brain tumors and other childhood cancers. Miller's national survey of children's death certificates from 1960 to 1967 found a significant excess of brain and bone cancers and leukemia among patients' siblings. The lack of adequate numbers in some early surveys was overcome by Farwell and Flannery using the Connecticut Tumor Registry to compare cancer incidence in parents, siblings, and children of 643 patients with CNS tumors in childhood. They used controls selected from Connecticut birth certificate files matched to cases by sex, age, and birth place and found no case-control cancer risk differential but a significantly higher risk of brain cancer in case siblings. Similarly, Draper and colleagues used the Marie Curie/Oxford Survey of Childhood Cancers in England, Scotland, and Wales to review more than 20,000 cases of malignant neoplasms. They found 11 sib pairs with brain tumors and 21 sib pairs with dissimilar cancers. They, as the other sibling researchers, concluded that sibs of patients are at increased risk and, further, susceptibility to cancer might be genetic.

C. CNS Tumors and Cancer Family Syndrome

Going beyond twin and sibling studies, family studies derived pedigrees of brain and other tumors consistent with a dominantly inherited disorder. In 1988, Li and co-workers described this cancer family syndrome in 24 kindred that had both childhood and adult onset cancers of diverse sites. Fourteen (9%) of the 151 cancers that occurred before age 45 were brain tumors. The Li–Fraumeni cancer syndrome has since been linked to a p53 mutation on chromosome 17p in some families.

Additional evidence for a family syndrome comes from many epidemiologic comparisons of family medical histories of brain tumor cases to those of controls. These report a relative risk of 1 to 1.8 for any cancer in families of brain tumor cases and relative risks of brain tumors in these families of 1 to 9. Two case-control studies further suggest that risks for other types of cancer may be elevated in family members of brain cancer patients; one found elevated risk of leukemia and liver cancers, and another identified elevated breast and respiratory tract cancer in families. Relatives of children with brain tumors are reported at increased risk for colon cancer, whereas families with colon polyposis of the colon experience elevated frequencies of gliomas. Also of interest are reports of familial clustering of brain tumors with Hodgkin's disease.

IV. GENETIC SUSCEPTIBILITY

A. Metabolic Susceptibility

A refinement of heritability investigations is those into genetic susceptibility, which are genetic alterations that influence oxidative metabolism, carcinogen detoxification, and DNA stability and repair. Genetic technology has described the role of genetic polymorphisms (altered forms of genes established in populations) in modulating susceptibility to carcinogenic exposures. Such a role has been explored in some detail for tobacco-related neoplasms but much less so for other neoplasms, including gliomas. Epidemiology is making widespread use of this technology to examine potentially relevant polymorphisms, including genes involved in carcinogen detoxification, oxidative metabolism, and DNA repair. Earlier studies of a role of genetic susceptibility in the development of brain tumors found variants of cytochrome P450 2D6 (CYP2D6) and glutathione transferase (GSTT1) significantly associated with an increased risk and a significant threefold increased risk for oligodendroglioma associated with the GSTT1 null genotype. The latter study did not find an association between adult onset glioma with either the GSTT1 null genotype or homozygosity for the CYP2D6 variant poor metabolizer genotype. However, when they stratified data by histologic subtype, there was a significant threefold increased risk for oligodendroglioma associated with the GSTT1 null genotype. Negative findings can be fruitful, too, as with Trizna and colleagues, considering the insignificant association of the null genotypes of glutathione transferase μ, GSTT1, and CYP1A1 and the risk of adult gliomas. The observed pattern of N-acetyltransferase acetylation status proved intriguing, where rapid acetylation produced nearly a twofold increased risk and the intermediate acetylation produced a 30% increased risk. It is unlikely that any single polymorphism will be sufficiently predictive of brain tumor risk. Therefore, a panel of relevant markers integrated with epidemiologic data should be assessed in a large number of study participants to clarify the role of genetic polymorphisms and brain tumor risk.

A more precise estimation of the impact of shared genes, environment, or gene–environment interaction on familial aggregation awaits segregation analysis in population-based studies to test hypotheses of the genetic basis of the aggregation. The sole segregation analysis study of childhood brain tumors rejected the hypothesis that chance explains case families' cancer patterns; a multifactorial model best explained the data.

B. Mutagen Sensitivity

Cytogenetic assays of peripheral blood lymphocytes have been extensively used to determine response to genotoxic agents. The basis for these cytogenetic assays is that genetic damage reflects critical events in carcinogenesis in the affected tissue. To test this hypothesis, Hsu and colleagues developed a mutagen sensitivity assay in which the frequency of *in vitro* bleomycin-induced breaks in short-term lymphocyte cultures is used to measure genetic susceptibility. This assay was modified using γ radiation to induce chromosome breaks because radiation is a risk factor for brain tumors and can produce double-stranded DNA breaks and mutations. γ radiation-induced mutagen sensitivity is one of the few significant independent risk factors for brain tumors. DNA repair capability and predisposition to cancer are hallmarks of rare chromosome instability syndromes and are related to differences in radiosensitivity. An *in vitro* study showed that individuals vary in lymphocyte radiosensitivity, which correlates with DNA repair capacity. Therefore, it is biologically plausible that an increased sensitivity to γ radiation results in an increased risk of developing brain tumors because of individuals' inability to repair radiation damage. However, this finding needs to be tested in a larger study to determine the roles of mutagen sensitivity and radiation exposure in the risk of developing gliomas. The mutagen sensitivity assay has been shown to be an independent risk factor for other cancers, including head and neck and lung, suggesting that the phenotype is constitutional. The breaks are not affected by smoking status or dietary factors (micronutrients).

C. Chromosome Instability

A number of chromosomal loci have been reported to play a role in brain tumorigenesis because of the numerous gains and losses in those loci. For example, Bigner and co-workers reported gain of chromosome 7 and loss of chromosome 10 in malignant gliomas and structural abnormalities involving chromosomes 1, 6p, 9p, and 19q; Bello and colleagues reported involvement of chromosome 1 in oligodendrogliomas and meningiomas; and Magnani and colleagues demonstrated involvement of chromosomes 1, 7, 10, and 19 in anaplastic gliomas and glioblastomas. Loss of heterozygosity for loci on chromosome 17p and 11p15 has also been reported. There are little data on chromosomal alterations in the peripheral blood lymphocytes of brain tumor patients. Information on such changes might shed light on premalignant changes that lead to tumor development. We have investigated whether glioma patients have increased chromosomal instability that could account for their increased susceptibility to cancer. Using fluorescent *in situ* hybridization methods, background instability in these patients was measured at hyperbreakable regions in the genome. Reports indicate that the human heterochromatin regions are frequently involved in stable chromosome rearrangements. Smith and Grosovsky (1993) and Grosovsky and co-workers reported that breakage affecting the centromeric and pericentromeric heterochromatin regions of human chromosomes can lead to mutations and chromosomal rearrangements and increase genomic instability.

Our study demonstrated that individuals with a significantly higher level of background chromosomal instability have a 15-fold increased risk of development of gliomas. A significantly higher level of hyperdiploidy was also detected. Chromosome instability leading to aneuploidy has been observed in many cancer types. Although previous studies have demonstrated the presence of chromosomal instability in brain tumor tissues, our study was the first study to investigate the role of background chromosomal instability in the peripheral blood lymphocytes of patients with gliomas. This suggests that accumulated chromosomal damage in peripheral blood lymphocytes may be an important biomarker for identifying individuals at risk of developing gliomas.

V. ETIOLOGY AND RISK FACTORS

A. Ionizing Radiation

Research consensus holds that therapeutic, not diagnostic, ionizing radiation is a strong risk factor for intracranial tumors. Even relatively low doses (averaging 1.5 Gy) for ringworm of the scalp (tinea capitis) have been associated with relative risks of 18, 10, and 3 for nerve sheath tumors, meningiomas, and gliomas, respectively. Other studies report a prevalence of prior therapeutic radiation among (17%) patients with glioblastoma or glioma and increased risk of brain tumors in children after radiation for acute lymphoblastic leukemia. Shorter term, diagnostic radiation apparently plays no role; three case-control studies of exposure to dental X rays reported relative risks of 0.4, 1.2, and 3.0 for gliomas. For meningioma, three of four studies reported risks higher than 2, but because the results all issue from one site, they invite authentication from other geographic areas.

Risk due to prenatal or occupational radiation exposure remains unknown, as studies of *in utero* exposure to atomic bomb or occupational radiation have found standard brain tumor incidence or results that are confounded or contradictory. Small-scale prenatal exposure studies are statistically insignificant, and the slightly elevated risk associated with a comparatively uncommon radiation exposure would not explain most childhood brain tumors. The study finding a small but statistically significant elevated risk of 1.2 for brain tumors in nuclear facility employees and nuclear materials production workers allows for the possibility of confounding or effect modification by chemical exposures. A study reporting increased mortality from brain tumors among airline pilots, possibly implicating exposure to cosmic radiation at high altitudes, is contradicted by another study reporting standard morbidity rates in pilots.

B. Electromagnetic Fields

Despite largely negative findings, the debate on the impact of electromagnetic fields on brain cancer continues, prolonged by methodological difficulties with some studies and popular media warnings about consumer products inviting personal exposures. In 1979, Wertheimer and Leeper described an apparent increased risk of brain tumors and leukemia in Denver children living near high-current versus low-current wiring. Their report set off widespread public and scientific interest in the potential health effects of electromagnetic fields and electronic devices, but positive findings came into question after contrary outcomes and reviews of sample sizes and method.

Among the studies reducing suspicion about electricity was a meta-analysis showing an insignificant increased childhood brain tumor risk for residents in homes coded for high current. In a meta-analysis of 29 studies of adult brain tumors in relation to occupational exposures to electric and magnetic fields, apparently adding to the weight of evidence against electricity, Kheifets and colleagues reported a significant (10 to 20%) increased risk for brain cancer among electrical workers, but could not show a consistent dose–response relationship or different outcomes for electrical workers at different exposure levels. Nor could risk be shown in large population or epidemiologic studies of the relation of brain tumor to EMF. In a San Francisco study, 492 adults with glioma and 463 controls were equally likely to have lived in homes with high wire codes during the 7 years before diagnosis. Spot measurements in the homes also showed that cases and controls experienced the same level of electromagnetic fields at home.

EMF investigation continues in the quest of reliable risk determination, but exposure research reveals inconsistencies. Electromagnetic field measurement in the home is inexact because of varying wire codes and the spot measurement snapshots usually taken for studies and, as well, the neglect of long-term exposure measurement or factoring in additional potential exposures from internal wiring, appliances, and gadgets. Temporal, intensity, and external influences may overshadow domestic exposures. The complexity required by further investigation is suggested by a Swedish study reporting increased risks of adult leukemia and central nervous system tumors after both residential and occupational exposure but not after either separately. The study used detailed EMF information preserved over decades from Swedish power suppliers recording levels of exposure. Such information is unavailable in the United States, but, again, the study lacked specificity about the exact daily experience of its subjects. The difficulties of quantification in EMF research pale compared to the main problem in this field of investigation: electromagnetic fields are incapable of inducing mutations that in turn might promote tumorigenesis. The EMF studies, as well as several occupational or environmental reports and many cluster reports, lack the criteria for causal relationships proposed by Bradford Hill, among which are specificity, consistency, and plausibility

C. Diet

Studies of the susceptibility of primates and other mammals to chemically induced brain tumors have prompted extensive study of diet and brain tumors. Experimental animal studies find N-nitroso compounds are clearly neurocarcinogens; other investigations describe mechanisms involving DNA damage through which N-nitroso compounds might cause brain tumors. These compounds can initiate neurocarcinogenesis through both prenatal and postnatal exposure, although in animals, more tumors result from fetal than postnatal exposures. The lag reported between exposure and tumor formation opens the possibility of the implication of early exposure in adult tumors. However, the ubiquity of N-nitroso compounds complicates human dietary studies, nonetheless eagerly pursued, especially into the salutary effects of vitamins. N-nitroso compounds arise in the digestive system in a promoting enzymatic milieu when common amino compounds from fish, other foods, or drugs contact a nitrosating agent, such as nitrites in cured meats. Some vegetables also contain nitrates convertible to nitrites but, as well, contain vitamins that block the formation of N-nitroso compounds. Despite great effort, human diet studies have achieved no consensus and provide only limited support for their motivating hypothesis, that dietary N-nitroso compounds heighten the risk of both childhood and adult brain tumors. However, some studies find that brain tumor cases or their mothers consumed more nitrosamines than controls, whereas others note lower tumor rates after a comparatively elevated consumption of fruits and vegetables or vitamins that might block nitrosation or harmful effects of nitrosamines.

Ambiguities are evident. For example, a case control study by Lee and co-workers found that adults with glioma were more likely than controls to consume diets high in cured foods or nitrites and low in vitamin C, but the effect only achieved statistical significance in men. The finding is compatible with the hypothesis that N-nitroso compounds play a role in human neurooncogenesis, but the observed patterns also support the hypothesis of oxidative burden and antioxidant protection.

Also, despite much searching, particularly in connection with pediatric brain tumors, neither alcohol nor tobacco has been clearly implicated in brain tumors. Their demonstrable impacts, especially fetal, require concern. Beer and malt liquors alone among alcoholic beverages are suspect due to the oxidation of malt, a nitrosamine derivative. Despite its other dangers and the polycyclic aromatic hydrocarbons and nitroso compounds in its smoke, tobacco has not been established as a causative agent in primary brain tumors, although two studies claim increased glioma risk lies in unfiltered cigarettes. The risk for secondhand smoke seems more clearly established; reports support an elevated risk of near 1.5, roughly equal to the elevated risks in passive smokers for adult lung cancer or cardiovascular disease. Most frequently associated with maternal smoking or passive smoke exposure are childhood brain tumors and leukemia–lymphoma, with risks going up to two or more in selected studies. Paternal as well as maternal smoking produces risk, suggest some. Even in the absence of definitive findings in human studies, the demonstrations of fetal genotoxicity from metabolites of tobacco smoke, and the demonstrable presence of adducts, should lead to strong recommendations for mothers to reduce fetal and infant exposure to tobacco smoke.

D. Industry and Occupation

Attempts to link specific chemicals to human brain tumors in specific work groups, hampered by small numbers and the difficulties of segregating one of the many agents in the workplace, as well as inherent problems in retrospective studies, have proven inconclusive. Findings from animal experiments may be inapplicable or irreproducible in humans. Chemical implantation shown to provoke tumors in animals differs from inhalation or dermal exposures in occupational settings. Nor are factors clearly altering animal susceptibility such as strain, gestational age, and fetal versus adult status useful for occupational studies. Follow-up studies of occupationally induced brain cancer usually consist of too few affected subjects to establish or pinpoint causal chemicals, physical agents, work processes, or interactions.

Thus, suspect chemicals and occupations listed in 1986 by Thomas and Waxweiler, despite many more recent studies, retain their ambiguous status, although among them are agents with undoubted animal neurocarcinogenicity, such as organic solvents, lubricating oils, acrylonitrile, formaldehyde, polycyclic aromatic hydrocarbons, phenols, and phenolic compounds. Cancer clusters, forming no risk pattern, have been found in chemical, automotive, and textile industries. Possibly the strongest case can be made against vinyl chloride, lethal in rats, and in 9 of 11 studies of human workers associated with as much as a twofold increased relative risk of dying of brain tumors.

Animal studies usually involve implantation of a single chemical rather than skin or lung exposures to many substances at the same time that workers experience. Thus, because of the problem, no definitive link has been established between brain tumors and even strongly suspected carcinogens. For example, organochlorides, alkyl ureas, and copper sulfates compounds that induce cancer in laboratory animals only randomly produce risk in agricultural workers. Study design faults and small numbers plague the occupational studies, so far unable to agree on risks involved in manufacturing pesticides or fertilizers, but reporting in four of five studies of pesticide applicators a nearly threefold risk elevation.

Because they involve the production of many suspect carcinogens, synthetic rubber production and processing have received careful scrutiny by investigators who generally found a median increase in brain tumors of as much as 90%. The by-products of synthetic rubber processing, such as coal tars, carbon tetrachloride, N-nitroso compounds, and carbon disulfide, might appear to account for this increased risk of brain tumors. However, several studies showed no increased risk or a decreased risk of brain tumors in this industry, and studies have usually failed to show a link with a single chemical.

With formaldehyde, another long-suspected compound, the numbers are greater but conclusions are similarly elusive. Formaldehyde, to which nearly two million U.S. workers are exposed, causes cancer in laboratory animals. However, Blair and co-workers, in evaluation of 30 epidemiological studies of segments of this large group, concluded that the risk was 50% elevated for those exposed in professional roles such as embalmers, pathologists, and anatomists but not for industrial workers with formaldehyde exposure. Blair and colleagues therefore rejected a causal role for formaldehyde in human brain tumorigenesis, a finding with impact in the workplace. Other unknown cofactors may obscure the true risk in industrially exposed workers and create a skewed estimate of risk in occupational groups.

E. Viruses

Certain viruses, like the suspect chemicals, have been found to induce brain tumors in animal studies. As in chemical studies, small numbers and negative findings hinder epidemiological evaluation. Repeatedly, calls have been made for aggressive studies addressing the role of viruses (and other infectious agents) in causing human brain tumors. Unfortunately, very few epidemiological studies have addressed the virus–tumor relationship, probably because of the difficulties in designing meaningful studies. Viruses and infectious agents could be an explanation for a proportion of brain tumors, and therefore intriguing as virology advances.

Contamination by the simian virus of the widely distributed Salk vaccine for polio offered the numbers from which to derive significant statistics, as 92 million United States residents received it. However, as with other risk exposure studies, investigations of SV40 were flawed, often anecdotal, based on questionable recall, or amenable to confounding factors. They offered hints, clues, or perhaps merely coincidences. Generally no association between virus and cancer could be established, although it may not be ruled out because the level of contamination varied among lots and manufacturers and was not taken into account in the United States and in Germany. Association was found small to none in a variety of studies, including a cohort study of the risk of ependymoma, osteosarcoma, and mesothelioma and a rare case-control study in England. Maternal contaminated vaccination risks for childhood cancer and brain cancer in particular are from sketchy and possibly confounded reports.

Viral disease investigations for protective or heightened risk effects are similarly contradictory. After reports that mothers of children with medulloblastoma were exposed in pregnancy to chicken pox, a herpes virus, Wrensch and colleagues found that mothers of glioma cases had lower rates than controls of chicken pox or shingles. This observation was supported by serologic evidence that cases were less likely than controls to have antibody to varicella zoster virus, the agent for chicken pox and shingles. There is some plausibility that viruses and infectious agents could be an explanation for a proportion of brain tumors, and therefore intriguing as they are still in their earliest stages.

The JC virus has come under scrutiny because it is excreted in the urine of immunosuppressed, immunodeficient, and pregnant women and was found associated with medulloblastoma in children and other tumors. However, the JC virus exists in cancer-free subjects and its connection, if any, to tumorigenesis is only a surmise.

F. Drugs and Medications

Preliminary studies have generally reported an insignificant association between tumors and medications, including pain, headache, sleep, fertility drugs, oral contraceptives, tranquilizers, antihistamines, and diuretics. Ryan and colleagues found that diuretics have a nonsignificant protective association against meningioma, which is opposite for adult glioma. They also found little association between antihistamine use and adult glioma, but a 60% increased relative risk for meningioma. Prenatal exposure to diuretics was half as common among children with brain tumors than among controls in two studies, but twice as common in one study. Prenatal exposure to barbiturates has not been consistently or convincingly linked to childhood brain tumors. As nonsteroidal antiinflammatory drugs may be protective against certain cancers, the role of these drugs in brain tumors should be investigated.

G. Cellular Telephones

The use of cellular telephones has grown remarkably over the last decade, and it is estimated that more than 500 million individuals worldwide use handheld cellular devices. The telephones contain a small transmitter that emits radio frequency radiation next to the head, and there has been great public concern that individuals exposed to radiation emitted from wireless communication technologies might have an increased risk of developing tumors of the brain and nervous system. To date, six papers have been published, none of the studies support the hypothesis of an association between use of these telephones and tumors of the brain or other cancers.

Rothman and colleagues reviewed mortality among more than 250,000 customers of a large cellular phone operator in the United States and did not find an increased risk after a follow-up of only 1 year. The numbers of brain cancers ($n = 6$) and of leukemias ($n = 15$) were small, and there were no statistically significant associations with number of minutes of phone use per day or years of phone ownership. The second study, a case-control study from Sweden by Hardell, reported a statistically nonsignificant increased risk for brain tumors on the side of the head on which cellular telephones were used. However, the risk for brain tumors overall was not increased, and there were methodologic concerns related to the ascertainment of cases. The fourth report was a case-control study from five academic institutions in the United States with 469 patients with primary brain cancer and 422 matched controls between 18 and 80 years of age. They found no association with brain cancer by duration of use ($p = 0.54$). In some cases, cerebral tumors occurred more frequently on the same side of the head where cellular telephones had been used (26 vs 15 cases; $p = 0.06$), but in cases with temporal lobe cancer, a greater proportion of tumors occurred in the contralateral than ipsilateral side (9 vs 5 cases; $p = 0.33$). The fifth study was also a hospital-based case-control conducted by investigators at the National Cancer Institute. They included 782 patients and 799 controls. The relative risks associated with cellular phone use for more than 100 h was 0.9 for gliomas [95% confidence interval (CI) = 0.5–1.6] and 0.7 for meningioma (95% CI = 0.3–1.7); 1.4 for acoustic neuroma (95% CI = 0.6–3.0). They found no evidence that the risks were higher among persons who used cellular phones for more than 5 years, nor did they observe more tumors on the side of the head the phone was typically used.

The sixth study was a retrospective cohort study of cancer incidence conducted in Denmark using subscriber lists from the two Danish operating companies. They identified 420,095 cellular telephone users during the period from 1982 through 1995 and linked the list with the Danish Cancer Registry. They observed 3391 cancers overall and expected 3825 cases (SIR = 0.89; 95% CI = 0.86 to 0.92); the risk cancers of the brain or nervous system were also lower than expected (SIR = 0.95; 95% CI = 0.81–1.12).

In addition, a large occupational cohort mortality study among 195,775 employees of Motorola, a manufacturer of wireless communication products, did not support an association between occupational radio frequency exposure and brain cancers or lymphoma/leukemia.

To date, the studies all seem to support the hypothesis that there is no association between use of these telephones and tumors of the brain or other cancers.

VI. CONCLUSIONS

The most generally accepted model, and productive of the most fruitful research, of carcinogenesis holds that cancers develop through the accumulation of genetic alterations allowing the cells to escape regulatory mechanisms and/or destruction by the immune system. Some inherited alterations in crucial cell cycle control genes, such as p53, as well as chemical, physical, and biologic agents that damage DNA, are therefore considered candidate carcinogens. Although rapid advances in molecular biology, genetics, and virology promise to help elucidate the molecular causes of brain tumors, continued epidemiologic work will be necessary to clarify the relative roles of different mechanisms in the full scope of human brain tumors. Genetic and familial factors implicated in brain tumors have been the subject of many studies.

In summary, the etiology of brain tumors remains largely unknown. We now know that primary brain tumors have many causes. Because not one cause thus far identified accounts for a very large proportion of cases, many possibilities remain that will enable us to discover important risk factors. Moreover, in the continuing search for explanations for this devastating disease, new concepts about neurooncogenesis might emerge, making the study of brain tumor epidemiology particularly exciting. The family studies conducted thus far suggest some role for inherited susceptibility to CNS tumors. Until the gene or genes for brain tumors are identified, genetic counseling in families at high risk of brain tumors is not possible. However, individuals with specific hereditary syndromes that predispose to brain tumors can be told their genetic risks.

Acknowledgments

This work was supported in part by Grants RO1-CA52689 and PO1-CA55261A from the National Cancer Institute.

See Also the Following Articles

Brain Cancer and Magnetic Resonance Spectroscopy • Li–Fraumeni Syndrome

Bibliography

Berleur, M. P., and Cordier, S. (1995). The role of chemical, physical, or viral exposures and health factors in neurocarcinogenesis: Implications for epidemiologic studies of brain tumors. *Cancer Causes Control* **6**, 240–256.

Blatt, J., Jaffee, R., Deutsch, M., *et al.* (1986). Neurofibromatosis and childhood tumors. *Cancer* **57**, 1225.

Bondy, M. L., Lustbader, E. D., Buffler, P. A., *et al.* (1991). Genetic epidemiology of childhood brain tumors. *Genet. Epidemiol.* **8**, 253.

Bondy, M., Wiencke, J., Wrensch, M., *et al.* (1994). Genetics of primary brain tumors: A review. *J. Neuro-Oncol.* **18**, 69–81.

Choi, N. W., Schuman, L. M., and Gullen, W. H. (1970). Epidemiology of primary central nervous system neoplasms. II. Case-control study. *Am. J. Epidemiol.* **91**, 467.

Draper, G. J., Heaf, M. M., and Kinnier Wilson, L. M. (1977). Occurrence of childhood cancers among sibs and estimation of familial risks. *J. Med. Genet.* **14**, 81.

Grosovsky, A. J., Parks, K. K., Giver, C. R., and Nelson, S. L. (1996). Clonal analysis of delayed karyotypic abnormalities and gene mutations in radiation-induced genetic instability. *Mol. Cell. Biol.* **16**, 6242–6262.

Kleihues P, Cavenee W. K. (eds.) (1997). Tumors of the central nervous system: pathology and genetics. International Agency for Research on Cancer, Lyon, France.

Kuijten, R. R., Bunin, G. R., Nass, C. C., et al. (1990). Gestational and familial risk factors for childhood astrocytoma: Results of a case-control study. Cancer Res. 50, 2608.

Li, F. P., and Fraumeni, J. F., Jr. (1975). Soft tissue, breast cancer and other neoplasms. Ann. Int. Med. 83, 833.

Lynch, H. T., Guirgis, H. A., Lynch, P. M., et al. (1977). Familial cancer syndromes: A survey. Cancer 39, 1867.

Magnani, C., Pastore, G., Luzzatto, L., Carli, M., Lubrano, P., and Terracini, B. (1989) Risk factors for soft tissue sarcomas in childhood cancer: A case-control study. Tumori 75, 396–400.

Muscat, J. E., Malkin, M. G., et al. (2000). Handheld cellular telephone use and risk of brain cancer. JAMA 284, 3001–3007.

Preston-Martin, S., and Mack, W. J. (1996). Neoplasms of the nervous system. In "Cancer Epidemiology and Prevention" (D. Schottenfeld and J. F. Fraumeni, eds.), 2nd Ed., pp. 1231–1281. Oxford Univ. Press, New York.

Rothman, K. J., Loughlin, J. E., Funch, D. P., and Dreyer, N. A. (1996). Overall mortality of cellular telephone customers. Epidemiology 7, 303–305.

Ryan, P., Lee, M. W., North, J. B., et al. (1992). Risk factors for tumors of the brain and meninges: Results from the adelaide adult brain tumor study. Int. J. Cancer 51, 20–27.

Schwarz, B., and Schmeiser-Rieder, A. (1996). Epidemiology of health problems caused by passive smoking. Wien. Klin. Wochenschr. 108, 565–569.

Seizinger, B. R., Rouleau, G. A., Ozeluis, L. J., et al. (1987). Genetic linkage of von Reckinghausen neurofibromatosis to the nerve growth factor receptor gene. Cell 49, 589.

Weinberg, R. A. (1991). Oncogenes, tumor suppressor genes, and cell transformation: Trying to put it all together. In "Origins of Human Cancer" (J. Brugge, T. Curran, E. Harlow, et al., eds.), Cold Spring Harbor Laboratory Press, Cold Spring Harbor, NY.

Wrensch, M., Bondy, M. L., Wiencke, J., et al. (1993). Environmental risk factors for primary malignant brain tumors: A review. J. Neurooncol. 17, 47–64.

Brain Cancer and Magnetic Resonance Spectroscopy

Jeffry R. Alger

Ahmanson-Lovelace Brain Mapping Center,
University of California, Los Angeles

GLOSSARY

N-acetylaspartate MRS signal A prominent MRS signal produced by the neuronal component of brain tissue.

choline MRS signal A prominent MRS signal produced by neoplastic tissue in the brain that has been attributed to altered phospholipid and membrane metabolism.

localized MRS A method wherein a specific tissue volume is anatomically defined from a previously acquired reference image, and the MRS signals are obtained from this tissue volume.

magnetic resonance spectroscopic imaging A method wherein a tissue volume is defined and the topographic variation of the MRS signals generated by this volume is imaged.

magnetic resonance spectroscopy A technique wherein magnetic fields and radio technologies are used to detect electronic signals produced by atomic nuclei that are naturally present within living tissues.

Brain cancer has been studied with magnetic resonance spectroscopy (MRS) since the early 1990s. This research is now leading to the regular use of MRS for the routine clinical evaluation of brain cancer patients. This article summarizes the present state of knowledge related to MRS and brain cancer and illustrates likely future areas of development and application.

I. MAGNETIC RESONANCE SPECTROSCOPY (MRS) FUNDAMENTALS IN RELATION TO BRAIN CANCER

A. Background Physics

Nuclear magnetic resonance (NMR) spectroscopy involves the interaction between atomic nuclei and magnetic fields. Individual atomic nuclei within molecules can produce unique NMR signal frequencies and unique NMR signal-splitting patterns that are characteristic of the electronic orbital structure surrounding the atomic nuclei. In this manner, NMR spectrum features can be identified with reference to the molecular framework of which the nuclei are a part. NMR spectroscopy provides a readily detected and unique signature of individual molecular structures that has been used extensively in chemical and biochemical studies. This signature is obtained nondestructively using radio wave technology when the sample is placed in a strong and spatially homogeneous static magnetic field. The nondestructive nature of the NMR signal detection, together with the ability of radio waves to penetrate deep within the living body, in principle, permits one to detect the presence of specific molecular signatures in living tissue using NMR spectroscopy. In the 1980s many of the practical impediments associated with realizing this expectation were overcome. This was, in part, due to the contemporaneous development of magnetic resonance imaging (MRI), an ingenious methodology by which the NMR spectrum of tissue water is used to create images depicting the internal structure of the human body at millimeter resolution. By analogy with MRI, NMR spectroscopy, when applied to a living organism for the purpose of detecting particular molecules from within tissue, became known as MRS for magnetic resonance spectroscopy.

B. Physical Limitations

The ability to detect MRS signals from molecules within tumors and cancer cells nondestructively *in situ* would seem to open the door to exceedingly intricate studies of the biochemistry and metabolism of these entities. Unfortunately, three key physical limitations inherent to MRS limit this realization to a very great extent.

The first limitation is that MRS signals generated by molecules having molecular weights greater than a few thousand daltons tend to produce signals that decay appreciably faster than can be detected using currently available instrumentation. This effectively means that macromolecules and supermolecular aggregates, such as proteins, nucleic acid polymers,

and membranes, fail to produce a readily detectable MRS signal. Typically, only small molecules, some of which are involved in intermediary metabolism, are detected in MRS. Accordingly MRS is often said to detect "tissue metabolites" or, specifically in the case of brain cancer, "tumor metabolites." From this comes the generalization that MRS measures metabolism. In this light, MRS is frequently discussed in association with nuclear imaging procedures, such as fluorodeoxyglucose positron emission tomography (FDG-PET), which are designed to measure metabolic rates through the use of radioactively labeled tracer molecules. Radiotracer imaging technologies and MRS do not sense metabolism in precisely the same manner. MRS detects the presence of certain metabolite signals that are inherently present in the tumor tissue. With appropriate calibration, these measures can be used to obtain the tissue concentration of certain specific tumor metabolites. However, radiotracer imaging techniques measure the steady-state rate of a metabolic pathway. In typically complex pathways, metabolite concentrations and metabolite fluxes are not always related in simple ways and, therefore, nuclear medicine imaging and MRS offer distinct and complementary views of tumor metabolism.

The second limitation of MRS relates to the inherently low sensitivity of the NMR signal detection process, which, in essence, is a consequence of the inherent innocuity of NMR. The MRS sensitivity limitation has two important ramifications. First, only a few of the most heavily concentrated tumor metabolites are easily detected with MRS. Second, appreciable tissue volumes must be sampled to attain sufficient sensitivity to detect even the most heavily concentrated metabolites. For human brain cancer the minimal volume that can be evaluated with MRS has been about 0.2 cm^3. The majority of studies evaluate larger volumes. The norm is 1–8 cm^3. In the MRS evaluation of cancers, it is important to consider that tumors usually display a substantial degree of microscopic disorganization. Edema and necrosis are often present and the cells are not as closely packed, as is the case for normal organized brain tissue. This disorganized cellular ultrastructure further limits the sensitivity with which intracellular tumor metabolites can be detected because there tend to be fewer cells per unit volume in comparison to normal tissue.

The third limitation relates to the strict requirement for a spatially homogeneous magnetic field having a strength of approximately 1.5 Tesla (30,000 times the earth's magnetic field) or greater. In order to detect an MRS metabolite signal, it is necessary that the applied magnetic field intensity vary by less than approximately 100 parts per billion over the intended sampling volume. Brain and tumor anatomy can distort the shape and intensity of the applied magnetic field beyond this extent, introducing problems with the detection of MRS signals from certain brain regions, such as the anterior brain stem or the inferiomedial aspects of the frontal lobes. Tumors also sometimes produce microhemorrhages that contain hemoglobin-derived magnetic iron particles and these may also distort the magnetic field homogeneity to an appreciable extent. Patients who have previously undergone neurosurgical procedures also tend to have a significant amount of magnetic particles near the surgical site, and MRS is sometimes unable to detect the metabolite signal in the vicinity of the magnetic field distortions produced by these particles.

C. Signal Localization

MRS studies of brain cancer have employed two complementary methodologies for attaining volume localization of the MRS signal. In localized single volume MRS, a conventional MR image is used to identify a location of interest, which is typically defined as a rectilinear "voxel," and the MRS signal is acquired from only this location. If it is desired to obtain MRS from other locations, the process is repeated. In magnetic resonance spectroscopic imaging (MRSI), MRS signals are acquired from a large number of rectilinear voxels simultaneously. Each localization methodology has drawbacks and attributes. Localized single volume MRS offers a high degree of spectroscopic specificity. Often, more metabolite signals can be detected when localized MRS is used compared to MRSI. However, MRSI provides a broad view of the entire neoplastic lesion and the surrounding brain with significantly greater time efficiency than is possible with localized single volume MRS.

II. THE MRS APPEARANCE OF BRAIN TUMORS

A. MRS Sensitive Nuclei

MRS signals can be obtained from many naturally occurring nuclear isotopes having biological significance. These include ^{1}H, ^{2}H, ^{3}H, ^{19}F, ^{13}C, ^{31}P, and ^{23}Na. Early MRS studies of brain cancer used ^{31}P MRS because this could detect key metabolites of the energy-transducing pathways (e.g., adenosine triphosphate and inorganic phosphate) and components of the phospholipid metabolism pathways. ^{31}P MRS studies of intracranial cancers have become less frequent during recent years because there are relatively few commercially available human-sized MRI scanners that have the technical capability for ^{31}P signal detection and because the volume resolution in ^{31}P studies is rarely less than 20 cm^3. The majority of the subsequent research studies and the resultant everyday clinical use have been mostly based on ^{1}H (proton) MRS because it offers significantly better volume resolution compared to ^{31}P and can be performed with the majority of standard clinical MRI scanners. For this reason, the remainder of this article focuses on the use of ^{1}H-MRS in relation to brain cancer.

B. Typical 1H-MRS Patterns: Primary Brain Tumor

Figure 1 provides an example of typical MRS findings obtained from a frequently encountered variety of primary brain tumor. Data were obtained from a patient who was suffering from glioblastoma multiforme. They were taken a few days before the patient underwent surgical resection of the tumor. During the operation, biopsies were taken and these were examined microscopically to obtain the diagnosis. The tumor location in the patient's left (displayed on the viewer's right) frontoparietal area is displayed as high signal on the postcontrast T1-weighted MRI and as high signal on the T2-weighted MRI (Fig. 1a). Figures 1b–1d illustrate voxel spectra sampled from an ^{1}H-MRSI study. Here white squares that represent the voxel location are drawn on the MRI. Corresponding spectra are plotted to the right. The voxel spectrum obtained from normal-appearing tissue (Fig. 1d) at

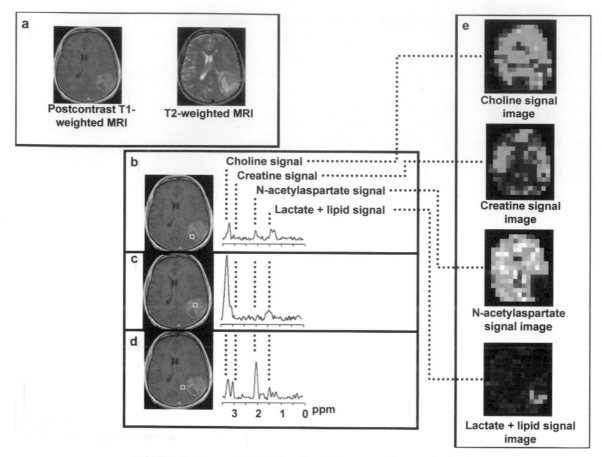

FIGURE 1　A typical 1H-MRSI study of a brain tumor. See text for details.

the tumor periphery shows the typical signal patterns of choline signal, creatine signal, and *N*-acetylaspartate (NAA) signal. The voxel spectrum obtained from a contrast-enhancing portion of the tumor mass (Fig. 1c) shows an intensely elevated choline signal and no apparent NAA signal. The creatine signal may be identified as a shoulder on the right side of the elevated choline signal in this spectrum. The voxel spectrum obtained from the nonenhancing fluid-filled cystic cavity (Fig. 1b) displays a lactate signal, although this overlaps with, and often cannot be distinguished from, signals generated by relatively small lipid molecules. These spectroscopic features can also be appreciated in the color spectroscopic images (Fig. 1e), which convey the relative strengths of the various signals using a color scale in which the red represents high signal and dark blue represents low signal. It is important to emphasize that these images illustrate only general features. Several studies have emphasized that there can be a substantial degree of variability in the MRS patterns expressed by two individual tumors, even when the two tumors have similar histopathological features. The general rules of thumb are as follows. Choline signal elevation generally coincides with the tumor mass except in regions that have become necrotic. The creatine signal tends to be evenly distributed in the tumor, but is not as substantially elevated as the choline signal is, although its level tends to show some degree of variability. The NAA signal is generally reduced throughout the lesion. The lactate signal is elevated to some extent in neoplastic tissues. However, this elevation tends to be variable and is often seen to coincide with the necrotic–cystic components.

C. Metabolic and Physiological Interpretations of MRS Features

A complete and systematic understanding of the metabolic and physiological underpinnings of the MRS signal alterations seen to coincide with intracranial neoplasia has yet to be completely attained. Alterations seen in the tumor signals from choline, creatine, NAA, and lactate are often "explained" within the context of our limited knowledge of the neoplastic metabolism that involves these compounds or biological tissue properties. Neoplastic choline signal elevation has been attributed to metabolic alterations that accompany active cell proliferation. Free choline and phosphorylcholine contribute to the choline signal seen in the MRS spectrum. These molecules are metabolic precursors of the phospholipids that are used for membrane construction. It is thought that their levels are high in tumors because biosynthetic pathways related to membrane synthesis are activated in proliferating cells and because neoplastic choline signal increases are often attributed to enhanced membrane turnover. However, it must also be remembered that these signal-generating molecules are found within the tumor cells and, therefore, one must consider that the presence of a substantial necrotic component may attenuate the choline signal elevation. The NAA molecule is found only within neurons, including the axonal components of white matter. The neoplastic NAA signal reduction is therefore attributed to the neuronal death or functional impairment as the neurons become engulfed by neoplastic tissue. The creatine signal includes contributions from both phosphocreatine and creatine and one cannot discern the relative contributions of these two contributors from the measure of the total signal provided by ^{1}H-MRS. The relative consistency in the level of creatine signal seen in tumor compared to normal tissues is thought to reflect that all cells maintain a relatively fixed total creatine level. Because of this, some investigators have argued that the creatine signal intensity may be used as an internal standard and, therefore, one frequently sees the levels of the NAA signal, the choline signal, or the lactate signal expressed as a ratio to the level of the creatine signal. Lactate signal elevation is generally attributed to the tendency of neoplastic tissue to consume glucose using only the anaerobic metabolic pathways.

III. CLINICAL USES OF MRS FOR BRAIN TUMOR MANAGEMENT

The majority of MRS studies of brain tumors have emphasized the possible clinical applications. Several of these have been moderately large studies or multicenter efforts. As a result of this background research, MRS is now being used in many of the more advanced medical centers throughout the world for the routine evaluation of brain tumor cases.

A. Diagnosis

Tumor histopathological classification and tumor grade have important implications for clinical management. Survival probability and course of therapy are usually defined to a substantial extent by these parameters. Making the histopathological diagnosis requires biopsy during an open or stereotactic neurosurgical procedure. Considerable effort has been expended toward applying noninvasive MRS technology for obtaining the needed information without biopsy. The very first MRS study of cerebral neoplasia by Bruhn and colleagues in 1989 suggested that the MRS signal patterns served to identify tumor type and grade. Subsequent studies have generally supported this concept. Hence, strong evidence suggests that MRS can provide a clinically important preoperative diagnosis. However, this result has yet to see widespread practical application. This is undoubtedly related to the fact that patients receive other benefits (e.g., cytoreduction, genetic tumor profiling) from neurosurgical procedures, and for these reasons, clinicians rarely proceed to conventional therapies without a surgical resection or biopsy.

B. Neurosurgical Planning

Depending on their location, brain tumors can cause sensory, motor, or speech functional impairment or can produce neuropsychiatric symptoms. A tumor in the dominant (usually the left) hemisphere at the temporofrontal junction can have a significantly different clinical manifestation compared to an otherwise identical lesion at the same location in the nondominant (usually the right) hemisphere. The latter lesion can be resected more effectively, whereas the former cannot be resected without risk of speech loss. MRS is sometimes looked to as a means for identifying the extent of tumoral infiltration in order to provide the patient with a more optimal and safe resection. Here the significance is that the contrast used in conventional MRI is inadequate to delineate the extent of tumoral infiltration in many cases. For instance, many intracranial tumors or portions thereof fail to enhance with the contrast agents that are commonly employed in conventional MRI or computed tomography examinations. While MRS has not been proven to have sufficient contrast to unequivocally delineate tumor from normal brain, the significant MRS pattern differences between normal and neoplastic tissue indicate that MRS will at least augment conventional MRI in the delineation of lesion extent. The principal criticism of MRS in this regard has been its limited spatial resolution.

C. Longitudinal Evaluation of Brain Tumor with MRS

There have been exploratory studies in a number of additional clinically significant areas. For instance, studies have demonstrated that progressive or recurrent glioma manifests itself through a pronounced change in choline signal elevation. Accordingly, many clinicians hope to use MRS as a means of distinguishing recurrent or progressing glioma from radiation necrosis. Others have shown in preliminary work that effective treatment reverses the abnormal MRS patterns to some extent. In this context, it is hoped that MRS can play a larger role in defining whether chemotherapies are being effective on a case-by-case basis.

IV. SUMMARY

The body of existing knowledge related to the MRS characteristics of brain tumors supports the following potential clinical uses of MRS within the context of neuro-oncological management. (1) MRS shows promise of providing accurate diagnosis without surgical tissue sampling. (2) MRS can conceivably be used as a adjunct to conventional neuroimaging for the planning of neurosurgical procedures to enhance the probability of representative biopsy sampling or of maximizing cytoreduction while maintaining safety. (3) MRS can be used to longitudinally follow patients who are being treated to evaluate whether treatment is having an effect. (5) MRS can be used for detecting recurrent or progressing disease and for differentiating this from radiation necrosis. These potential areas of clinical utility have not been fully substantiated. MRS capability is now becoming available in a large number of centers because virtually any conventional MRI scanner that operates at a field strength of greater than 1 Tesla has the needed technical capability. Accordingly, MRS is being used to an ever greater extent for evaluating individual brain tumor cases. As this development occurs, we will gain more experience regarding the extent to which MRS will have everyday applicability for neuro-oncologic management.

See Also the Following Articles

BRAIN AND CENTRAL NERVOUS SYSTEM TUMORS • MAGNETIC RESONANCE SPECTROSCOPY AND MAGNETIC RESONANCE IMAGING, INTRODUCTION • MAGNETIC RESONANCE SPECTROSCOPY OF CANCER: CLINICAL OVERVIEW • MAGNETIC RESONANCE STUDIES OF TUMORS: EXPERIMENTAL MODELS • METABOLIC DIAGNOSIS OF PROSTATE CANCER BY MAGNETIC RESONANCE SPECTROSCOPY • PET IMAGING AND CANCER

Bibliography

Alger, J. R., and Cloughesy, T. F. (2000). Structural and functional imaging of cerebral neoplasia, *In* "Brain Mapping: The Disorders" (A. Toga and J. C. Mazziotta, eds.). Academic Press, San Diego.

Bruhn, H., Frahm, J., Gyngell, M. L., Merboldt, K. D., Hanicke, W., Sauter, R., and Hamburger, C. (1989). Noninvasive differentiation of tumors with use of localized H-1 MR spectroscopy in vivo: Initial experience in patients with cerebral tumors. *Radiology* **172,** 541–548.

Leeds, N. E., and Jackson, E. F. (1994). Current imaging techniques for the evaluation of brain neoplasms. *Curr. Opin. Oncol.* **6,** 254–261.

Negendank, W. G., Sauter, R., Brown, T. R., Evelhoch, J. L., Falini, A., Gotsis, E. D., Heerschap, A., Kamada, K., Lee, B. C., Mengeot, M. M., Moser, E., Padavic-Shaller, K. A., Sanders, J. A., Spraggins, T. A., Stillman, A. E., Terwey, B.,

Vogl, T. J., Wicklow, K., and Zimmerman, R. A. (1996). Proton magnetic resonance spectroscopy in patients with glial tumors: A multicenter study. *J. Neurosurg.* **84,** 449–458.

Preul, M. C., Caramanos, Z., Collins, D. L., Villemure, J. G., Leblanc, R., Olivier, A., Pokrupa, R., and Arnold, D. L. (1996). Accurate, noninvasive diagnosis of human brain tumors by using proton magnetic resonance spectroscopy. *Nature Med.* **2,** 323–325.

Sijens, P. E., Knopp, M. V., Brunetti, A., Wicklow, K., Alfano, B., Bachert, P., Sanders, J. A., Stillman, A. E., Kett, H., and Sauter, R. (1995). 1H MR spectroscopy in patients with metastatic brain tumors: a multicenter study. *Magn. Reson. Med.* **33,** 818–826.

Brain Tumors: Epidemiology and Molecular and Cellular Abnormalities

Shoichiro Ohta
Mark A. Israel
University of California, San Francisco

Fred G. Barker II
Massachusetts General Hospital, Boston

GLOSSARY

anaplastic astrocytoma A tumor thought to be derived from astrocytic glial cell precursors, which is characterized by an intermediate degree of histologic and clinical malignancy.

astrocytoma A tumor thought to be derived from astrocytic glial cell precursors, which is characterized by a low degree of histologic and clinical malignancy.

ependymoma A tumor thought to be derived from ependymal glial cell precursors.

glioblastoma multiforme A tumor thought to be derived from astrocytic glial cell precursors, which is characterized by a high degree of histologic and clinical malignancy.

medulloblastoma A primitive neuroectodermal tumor that is located in the posterior fossa of children.

meningioma A predominantly benign tumor that arises from the cerebral meninges.

oligodendroglioma A tumor thought to be derived from oligodendrocytic glial cell precursors.

primitive neuroectodermal tumor A tumor composed of small cells with scanty cytoplasm that arises most frequently in the cerebellum of children (see medulloblastoma).

Brain tumors are a diverse group of neoplasms. Brain tumors that arise as primary tumors of central nervous system (CNS) tissues or metastatic foci of tumors from other locations are difficult to treat and remain a particularly problematic management challenge. Approximately 35,000 new primary brain tumors are diagnosed each year corresponding to an incidence of just under 13 brain tumor patients per 100,000 people in the United States. Metastatic spread of tumors arising in areas of the body other than the brain is much more common and is estimated to occur in up to 15% of all patients with cancer. This would correspond to over 150,000 cases per year. Brain tumors are the most common solid tumor occurring in children, and second only in frequency to leukemia and lymphoma. Approximately 2500 new brain tumors are diagnosed in children each year. While a possible increase in the incidence of both pediatric and adult brain tumors has been a topic of considerable interest in the recent past, it is currently thought that in both age groups improvements in diagnosis made possible through better imaging modalities is the most likely explanation for this apparent change.

pearance. The most recent World Health Organization (WHO) classification schema retains this strategy (Table I), but incorporates a characterization of the genetic and cell biological features of different tumors in their description. This will be helpful in the future if the genetic alterations that occur in different tumors can be recognized as being responsible for specific pathologic features of tumor growth and pathology.

Today it is recognized that classification of brain tumors by histologic criteria can allow successful prognostication and can guide treatment. Presumably this results from shared molecular mechanisms of oncogenesis between histologically similar tumors. The different tumors that arise in the brain occur with varying frequency in patients of different ages and sex and have characteristic clinical behaviors. Over 90% of all primary brain tumors arise in glia or the meninges, and not in the neuronal elements of the CNS. This article describes these tumors and primitive neuroectodermal tumors that typically occur in children.

I. INTRODUCTION

Primary tumors of the brain were initially classified by surgeons and pathologists on the basis of histologic ap-

II. GLIOMA

Glioma, the most common primary brain tumor of both children and adults, arises in glial cells of the

---

TABLE I

Pathological Classification of Central Nervous System Tumors According to the World Health Organization

Tumors of neuroepithelial tissue	Lymphomas and hemopoietic neoplasm
Astrocytic tumors	Malignant lymphoma
Oligodendroglial tumors	Plasmacytoma
Ependymal tumors	Granulocytic sarcoma
Mixed glioma	Germ cell tumors
Choroid plexus tumors	Germinoma
Glial tumors of uncertain origin	Embryonal carcinoma
Neuronal and mixed neuronal–glial tumors	Yolk sac tumor
Neuroblastic tumors	Choriocarcinoma
Pineal parenchymal tumors	Teratoma
Embryonal tumors	Mixed germ cell tumors
Tumors of peripheral nerves	Tumors of the sellar region
Schwannoma	Craniopharyngioma
Neurofibroma	Granular cell tumor
Malignant peripheral nerve sheath tumor	Metastatic tumors
Tumors of the meninges	
Tumors of meningothelial cells	
Mesenchymal, nonmeningothelial tumors	
Primary melanocytic lesions	
Tumors of uncertain histogenesis	

brain. Glial cells (astrocytes, oligodendrocytes, and other less well-defined glia) occur throughout the brain, and tumor behavior has not been recognized to vary significantly in different parts of the brain. Glial tumors are usually malignant in that they are invasive, grow relatively rapidly, and are life-threatening if not treated. These account for about 60% of primary brain tumors in adults. Astrocytic tumors occurring in adults are graded by histologic appearance (see later). In order of increasing malignancy, astrocytic tumors are graded as pilocystic astrocytoma, astrocytoma (WHO grade I), diffuse astrocytoma (WHO grade II), anaplastic astrocytoma (WHO grade III), or glioblastoma multiforme (GM) (WHO grade IV). Low-grade astrocytoma, especially the special variant of astrocytic tumor known as pilocystic astrocytoma, which arises most commonly in the cerebellum or optic nerves and has a characteristically benign behavior, can often be cured by complete surgical excision. Astrocytic tumors in adults are virtually always malignant tumors and are rarely cured after surgical excision, radiotherapy, and chemotherapy. Other less commonly encountered glioma include oligodendroglioma and ependymoma (see later).

A. Astrocytic Tumors of Adulthood: Astrocytoma, Anaplastic Astrocytoma, and Glioblastoma Multiforme

1. Epidemiology

Glial tumors that arise in adults are most commonly astrocytoma, AA, and GM, in order of increasing malignancy. Within this spectrum, the more malignant tumors are more common in older patients. The median age of patients with astrocytoma, AA, and GM is approximately 35, 45, and 55 years, respectively. Although some higher grade tumors arise from known preexisting lower grade tumors that recur after treatment, other high-grade tumors appear to arise *de novo*, especially in older patients. At all ages there is a slight tendency for men to be more commonly affected. Although familial inheritance of astrocytic tumors has been described, nearly all cases appear to be sporadic, and environmental exposures predisposing to glioma development have not been identified.

Some complex inherited syndromes carry a risk of glioma development, although brain tumors occur rather infrequently in such patients. The Li–Fraumeni syndrome can result from inheritance of a mutated copy of the *P53* tumor suppressor gene. Affected individuals have a high risk of breast cancer, soft tissue sarcoma, and glioma. Patients with Turcot syndrome, which is characterized by multiple colorectal adenoma and a brain tumor, carry a germline mutation of the *APC* gene or a mutation in one of the DNA mismatch-repair genes, *hMLH1* or *hPMS2*. Glioblastoma is the most common brain tumor in patients who have mutations in genes important for DNA repair. In patients with neurofibromatosis type 1, a defective copy of the *NF1* tumor suppressor gene causes the development of multiple peripheral nerve tumors, as well as an increased risk of malignant glioma. Patients with tuberous sclerosis develop a rare type of glioma known as subependymal giant cell astrocytoma: two genetic loci for this disease have been mapped, and candidate genes for these loci (*TSC1* and *TSC2*) have been isolated.

2. Cytogenetic Abnormalities

Extensive chromosomal abnormalities are unusual in low-grade glioma but occur with increasing frequency in glioma of higher grades. Low-grade glioma most often have a normal karyotype or simple gain or loss of single chromosomes. Gain of chromosome 7 or loss of chromosomes 10, 19, or 22 has been noted most frequently. In high-grade glioma near-trisomy or near-tetraploidy chromosomal patterns are sometimes observed. Characteristic patterns of loss of chromosomal material in multiple examples of a particular tumor type are often hypothesized to indicate the location of tumor suppressor loci within the chromosomal region that is preferentially lost. Loss of chromosomal material may be detected by techniques that can detect the loss of large chromosomal regions, such as karyotyping and comparative genomic hybridization (CGH), or may be detectable only by methods that detect the loss of smaller chromosomal regions, such as fluorescence *in situ* hybridization (FISH) or microsatellite analysis.

In addition to the gain or loss of entire chromosomes, there are other forms of genetic instability leading to the increased gene copy numbers that occur in primary brain tumors. Double minute chromosomes are observed in some glioblastoma. These represent amplification of portions of chromosomes containing one or more genes that have been selected for during tumor growth, presumably because the proteins they encode provide a growth advantage. The gene most commonly amplified in glial tumors is *EGFR*, which encodes the epidermal growth factor receptor. When *EGFR* is amplified in glial tumors, it frequently is mutated in a manner that renders it constitutively active. Some glioblastoma contain an amplicon that encompasses several genes from the 12q13-14 regions, including the *GLI* oncogene, the *CDK4* cyclin-dependent kinase gene, and other genes of potential importance for oncogenesis. Which of these genes is important in the pathogenesis of glial tumors is not known.

3. Genetic Abnormalities

Tumor suppressor genes encode proteins that regulate or suppress cell growth or promote cell death. Both copies of a tumor suppressor gene must be inactivated for its phenotype to become manifest. The *INK4A/ARF* locus encodes two separate proteins through differential splicing of alternative first exons. Use of exon 1α produces p16-INK4a, and use of exon 1β leads to the expression of p14-ARF. The p16-INK4a protein inhibits cyclin-dependent kinases that control phosphorylation of the retinoblastoma protein (pRb), and p14-ARF complexes with MDM2 protein within the nucleus, leading to activation of the p53 protein. The *INK4A/ARF* gene was initially isolated based on its ability to bind a cyclin-dependent kinase, and some patients from kindreds with familial melanoma carry a defective copy of the *INK4A/ARF*.

Although point mutations in the region of *INK4A/ARF* encoding p16-INK4a are uncommon in astrocytic neoplasms, deletion of both copies of *INK4A/ARF* has been reported to occur in approximately 25–50% of AA and 40–70% of GM. Loss of p16-INK4 is an uncommon event in low-grade astrocytoma. Loss of p14-ARF has also been found to occur in high-grade astrocytoma, and interestingly, p14-ARF deletions and p53 mutations appear mutually exclusive, providing strong evidence for their presumed functionally redundant roles in glioma tumor development. *INK4A/ARF* is located on chromosome 9p, and its loss may account for the frequently described observation of 9p deletions in high-grade astrocytoma.

The *RB1* tumor suppressor gene is located on chromosome 13q. Patients who inherit a defective copy of the *RB1* gene have a strong predisposition to develop retinoblastoma, a malignant tumor of the retina. Loss of *RB1* function resulting from homozygous deletion or mutation has been reported in about 30% of high-grade glioma, but appears to be rare in low-grade astrocytoma. When the *RB1* gene protein product (Rb) is unphosphorylated, it suppresses cell growth. Phosphorylation of Rb, which is dependent on the activity of a complex of CDK4 and cyclin D, results in loss of this growth suppression. Because p16-INK4 is an inhibitor of CDK4, it is possible that defects in both p16-INK4 and Rb convey no additional growth advantage to a cell in comparison to a defect in either p16-INK4 or Rb alone. It has been reported that most GM have a defect in either p16-INK4 or Rb, but that both genes together are only rarely inactivated in these tumors. Interestingly, some of the rare GM that do not have inactivation of either p16-INK4 or Rb have been found to have amplification of CDK4, presumably a third way in which GM cells lose the function of this evidently critical pathway for cell growth regulation.

Another tumor suppressor gene frequently implicated in glial oncogenesis is the *P53* gene, located on chromosome 17p. The p53 protein has been found to influence multiple cellular functions, including progression through the cell cycle, DNA repair after radiation damage, genomic stability, and the tendency for a cell with genomic damage from radiation or chemotherapeutic agents to undergo apoptosis, programmed cell death. p53 acts as a transcription factor, which induces or represses the transcription of multiple genes through sequence-specific interaction with DNA. There are five regions of the protein that have been highly conserved throughout evolution. Inactivating mutations of *P53* that occur in human cancers appear to be clustered in these conserved domains, which are known to be required for the binding of p53 to DNA.

P53 mutations have been found in many types of human cancers, including malignant astrocytoma. *P53* mutations have been reported in astrocytic tumors of all grades, occurring in approximately 40% of astrocytoma, in 32% of AA, and in 27% of GM. This may indicate that *P53* mutations are associated principally with the change from normal tissue to low-grade neoplasia rather than with the progression from low-grade to high-grade tumors. However, some groups have reported the development of a *P53* mutation as a low-grade glial tumor progressed to a higher degree of malignancy. There is no sex predilection for *P53* mutations in human astrocytic tumors, but interestingly, the age of a patient with astrocytoma may correlate with the frequency of *P53* mutation: patients aged 18 to 39 years have a significantly higher rate of *P53* mutation than those aged 40 years or greater. Children are an exception. *P53* mutations have not been observed in hemispheric astrocytic tumors arising in patients aged 1 to 18 years. The prognostic implication of a *P53* mutation in astrocytic tumors with respect to resistance to radiation and chemotherapy, as measured by the time to tumor recurrence after treatment, is not yet clearly defined.

Patients with the Li–Fraumeni syndrome, caused by an inherited, constitutional *P53* mutation, have a predisposition for the development of brain tumors. Astrocytic tumors are the most frequent histologic type noted in these kindreds: tumors tend to begin as low-grade astrocytoma and frequently present in younger patients (before age 50). In addition to members of Li–Fraumeni kindreds, other classes of patients with glial tumors may be more likely to carry a constitutional *P53* mutation. These include younger patients, those with multifocal gliomas, or patients with second neoplasms in addition to their glioma.

Patients with neurofibromatosis type 1, which is caused by a germline mutation in the *NF1* tumor suppressor gene, are predisposed to the development of glial neoplasms. However, the majority of patients with this syndrome do not develop malignant glioma, and studies to date have found mutations or deletions of *NF1* to be rare in sporadic malignant glioma.

Protooncogenes are normal cellular genes whose protein product functions normally to promote cell growth. Protooncogenes can be "activated" in many ways, including overexpression or mutation, to form oncogenes. The protein product of an oncogene promotes unregulated cell growth. Many oncogenes have been implicated in the complex process of glial oncogenesis. Some protooncogenes function normally as

growth factors or growth factor receptors. The epidermal growth receptor gene (*EGFR*) is the gene most frequently found to be amplified in malignant astrocytoma. The protein product of *EGFR* is a receptor that contains an extracellular domain that binds epidermal growth factor, a transmembrane domain, and an intracellular domain with tyrosine kinase activity. *EGFR* amplification is reported in about 3% of astrocytoma, 7% of AA, and 36% of GM, indicating that this molecular change is principally associated with the progression from low- or intermediate-grade neoplasia to high-grade astrocytic neoplasia. *EGFR* genes amplified in GMs are frequently mutated, encoding a shortened protein product. The portion of the gene deleted appears to be nonrandom because several tumors examined contained very similar deletions in the extracellular portion of the EGFR molecule. These mutated receptors typically lack EGF-binding ability and have constitutive tyrosine kinase activity. A common form of deletion in this molecule leads to a novel extracellular peptide sequence that is shared by about 10–15% of GMs. Other growth factor receptor molecules have been reported to be overexpressed or amplified in some glioma. One such growth factor/receptor pair is platelet-derived growth factor subunits (PDGF) and their receptor (PDGFR). Many GM express platelet-derived growth factor, and the simultaneous expression of PDGF and PDGFR by a tumor can form an autocrine loop that enhances tumor growth.

It is clear that not all astrocytic tumors have acquired the same molecular alterations in the same order. For example, many GM display loss of chromosome 10, but have no evidence of *P53* inactivation. These GM are sometimes assumed to have followed a different "pathway" to malignancy than those known to have arisen from low-grade astrocytoma. It is not yet clear whether the molecular alterations frequently observed in high-grade astrocytic tumors require any earlier, still uncharacterized mutations for their transforming action to be manifested.

4. Pathology

All glioma are characterized by proliferation, and typically the amount of detectable apoptosis in these tumors is very low. Higher grade tumors are characterized by the presence of nuclear atypia, mitoses, necrosis, and endothelial proliferation within the tumor. Important angiogenic factors secreted by malignant astrocytoma include vascular endothelial growth factor (VEGF), transforming growth factor α, PDGF-A, PDGF-B, and HGF/SF. Highly malignant astrocytoma secrete large amounts of VEGF, up to 50-fold higher levels than low-grade tumors or normal brain. In addition, endothelial cells from vessels within high-grade astrocytoma express both of the two known high-affinity VEGF receptors, FLT1 and FLK1. These are not expressed by endothelial cells in normal brain.

Another characteristic aspect of glioma growth is the migration of tumor cells through adjacent normal brain. Some migratory glioma cells retain the ability to divide and may elude local treatments such as surgery or focused radiotherapy. Even though normal brain tissue lacks the organized extracellular matrix characteristic of other tissues, migration of tumor cells through the brain is associated with the secretion of proteolytic enzymes. Cells from high-grade glioma secrete several metalloproteinases, such as gelatinase A and B, type IV collagenase, and matrilysin. Secretion of these enzymes by glioma cells presumably facilitates their passage through the brain. Malignant glioma almost never metastasize outside the brain, but the reason for this is unclear.

5. Clinical Features and Treatment

Brain tumors typically are recognized as the result of patients developing symptoms of either a focal neurologic disorder or generalized symptoms such as headache, dementia, or personality change. Metastatic tumors are more commonly associated with systemic symptoms such as malaise and weight loss. Focal neurologic deficits typically are progressive. Because these result from the compression of neurons, they can sometimes help identify the location of the tumor, although imaging technologies now make possible easy identification of the precise location of most brain tumors on a routine basis. Focal symptoms can include hearing problems or hearing loss, altered vision, difficulty with speech, decreased lack of muscle coordination, and weakness or paralysis. Seizures may result from stimulation of excitatory circuits or interference with inhibitory mechanisms.

Generalized neurologic dysfunction usually reflects increased intracranial pressure, hydrocephalus, or diffuse tumor spread. Headache may result from focal irritation or displacement of pain-sensitive structures. Headaches arising from increased intracranial pressure are frequently characterized as involving the entire head and occurring most frequently upon becoming upright in the morning. They may be precipitated by coughing, sneezing, or straining. These headaches are typically intense but last only a short time, 20 to 40 min, and subside quickly. Frontal lobe tumors may present with personality change, dementia, or depression. The Karnofsky performance scale is useful in assessing and following brain tumor patients. A score of 70 or greater indicates that the patient is ambulatory and independent in self-care activities.

Treatment for primary brain tumors, especially malignant astrocytic tumors, is typically multimodality. Virtually all tumors are initially evaluated by surgical biopsy and, when possible, the widest possible resection of the primary tumor is attempted. There is an established role for irradiation in the treatment of malignant astrocytic tumors, and some studies have shown that nitrosourea-based chemotherapeutic regimens have antitumor activity.

B. Oligodendroglioma

Oligodendroglioma are uncommon glioma (3–5% of all intracranial tumors) that appear to arise from oligodendrocytes. They occur most frequently in the white matter of the adult cerebrum, with a peak incidence of age at diagnosis between 26 and 46 years. Oligodendroglial tumors frequently contain a malignant astrocytic component, in which case the tumor is called a mixed oligoastrocytoma. Cytogenetic studies of oligodendroglioma occasionally show loss of chromosomes 9p and 22 or a gain of chromosome 7, but the most characteristic cytogenetic findings in oligodendroglioma are loss of chromosomes 1p and 19q. These cytogenetic changes are of particular importance in that patients whose tumors have these changes are more responsive to chemotherapy combinations that include nitrosoureas. Other molecular genetic events common in astrocytic tumors seem to be rare in oligodendroglioma: P53 mutations and EGFR amplification are infrequently present. LOH for chromosome 9p loci, observed in some oligodendroglioma, suggests the possible loss of the INK4A/ARF in some oligodendroglial tumors, and other data suggest that loss of *INK4A/ARF* is associated with a poorer outcome for patients with oligodendroglioma. Patients with oligodendroglioma frequently present for care following many years of minor nervous system complaints. Treatment typically includes surgery, radiation therapy, and chemotherapy.

C. Ependymoma

Ependymoma are uncommon tumors (1.9–7.8% of intracranial neoplasms) that usually affect young children. Ependymoma are thought to arise in ependymal cells, the cells that line the cerebral ventricles and the central canal of the spinal cord. Patients with neurofibromatosis type 2 are predisposed to develop ependymoma, among other tumors, including vestibular schwannoma and meningioma (see later). The gene defective in this syndrome, *NF2*, has been mapped to chromosome 22q. Chromosome 22q losses have been reported in 30% of sporadic ependymoma, and *NF2* mutations in association with the loss of the nonmutated *NF2* allele have been reported in a small minority of sporadic ependymoma. However, the majority of these tumors do not have detectable *NF2* mutations. *P53* inactivation is very uncommon in ependymoma, although *P53* mutations have been observed in a few anaplastic ependymoma. Amplification of *EGFR* or other oncogenes has not been found in the small number of ependymoma screened to date. Chromosomal abnormalities reported in small subsets of ependymoma include loss of chromosomes 10, 17p, 6q, 9p, 13q, and 19q.

III. MENINGIOMA AND VESTIBULAR SCHWANNOMA

We have grouped meningioma and vestibular schwannoma together because they affect similar patient populations and seem to share some mechanisms of oncogenesis. Meningioma are tumors that arise in the dura, the membrane that encloses the brain, and vestibular schwannoma arise in the vestibular nerve at the base of the brain. Both are benign tumors that affect women more frequently than men. Elderly patients are most frequently affected. A small percentage of

meningioma appear histologically to be malignant: these tumors are more aggressive in their local growth pattern and may metastasize. Malignant transformation of vestibular schwannoma is very rare.

Patients with neurofibromatosis type 2 may be affected by multiple meningiomas and bilateral vestibular schwannoma, as well as by spinal schwannoma and ependymoma. Because deletion of loci on chromosome 22q is a frequent event in both vestibular schwannoma and meningioma, the *NF2* gene (located at chromosome 22q12) may be important in the pathogenesis of both of these tumors. The protein product of the *NF2* gene, known as merlin, is a member of the protein 4.1 family of cytoskeletal proteins. This protein participates in linking the cytoskeleton to the cell membrane. Both loss of heterozygosity (LOH) for loci near *NF2* and mutations in the *NF2* gene have been reported in sporadic meningioma and vestibular schwannoma. The majority of reported *NF2* mutations predict a truncated protein product due to frame-shift mutations, creation of a new stop codon, or mutations affecting normal RNA splicing. In addition, there is evidence for a second tumor suppressor locus on chromosome 22q that is relevant to meningioma formation.

Amplification or high-level expression of oncogenes and deletion or mutation of *P53* appear to be infrequent events in the development of meningioma and schwannoma. One exception may be expression of the *ROS1* receptor tyrosine kinase oncogene, which has been reported in as many as 55% of meningioma. Malignant meningioma may be associated with deletion of loci on chromosomes 1p, 6p, 9q, 10q, 14q, and 17p, and *P53* mutations have also been reported in malignant meningioma. Patients with the Gorlin syndrome, mapped to *PTCH* on chromosome 9q, are very susceptible to radiation-induced meningioma, suggesting that the 9q losses observed in malignant meningioma may have the Gorlin locus as their target.

Some patients have multiple meningioma at separate locations on the dura, and commonly such patients have a recognizable genetic predisposition. These tumors are almost invariably benign. Less than 1% of meningiomas are frankly malignant, and therefore surgery is a key therapeutic modality typically able to cure the tumors without further therapy.

IV. PRIMITIVE NEUROECTODERMAL TUMORS OF THE CENTRAL NERVOUS SYSTEM

Primitive neuroectodermal tumors (PNET) consist of small round malignant cells with scant cytoplasm. They arise most frequently in the cerebellum of children, where they are referred to as medulloblastoma and account for approximately 20% of all childhood brain tumors. They can also occur in the cerebellum of adults or in the cerebrum at any age. It has not yet been possible to discern with any confidence significant genetic, biological, or therapeutic differences among tumors of similar histology occurring in these disparate locations.

Medulloblastoma occurs in two inherited cancer syndromes: Turcot syndrome and Gorlin syndrome. In Turcot syndrome, familial adenomatosis of the colon is combined with CNS tumors. Medulloblastoma is probably the most frequent CNS tumor in this syndrome, although astrocytic tumors occur in some kindreds. Germline mutations in the APC gene, which is mutated in patients with adenomatous polyposis coli, have been reported in Turcot syndrome patients who develop medulloblastoma. In the Gorlin syndrome, multiple basal cell carcinoma are associated with jaw cysts and other less frequent tumors, including medulloblastoma. The gene for this syndrome, PTCH, has been mapped to chromosome 9q22.3-9q31. Although LOH for these loci is infrequent in sporadic medulloblastoma, it has been reported to be associated with a specific histologic subclass of medulloblastoma, the desmoplastic medulloblastoma. A second gene, PTCH2, similar in structure to PTCH, has also been found to be altered in medulloblastoma.

Cytogenetic studies of medulloblastoma have identified chromosome 17p as a frequent site of deletions. The P53 locus, located on 17p, has been examined in sporadic medulloblastoma by several groups: mutations at this locus are uncommon, despite the occasional occurrence of medulloblastoma in Li–Fraumeni families. A second locus on 17p13, telomeric to P53, is suspected to harbor a tumor suppressor gene, which is deleted in medulloblastoma. Deletions at this locus have been associated with an aggressive clinical course. Other molecular genetic changes sometimes found in medulloblastoma are deletions of chromosomes 2p, 6q, 8p, 10q, 11p, 11q, and 16q and rare amplification of CMYC and NMYC. Expression of high levels of the TRKC neurotrophin receptor mRNA in medulloblastoma has been reported to be associated with a favorable outcome in a small series of patients. The PAX5 gene, a member of the PAX family of homeobox genes, has been reported to be expressed in proliferating portions of medulloblastoma, but not in normal cerebellar tissue, suggesting a possible role for this gene in the growth regulation of these tumors.

Medulloblastoma typically appears as densely packed sheets of small, round, undifferentiated cells. Occasionally, tumors show regions of desmoplasia and apparent nodularity. Medulloblastoma can be easily confused with another embryonal tumor of the CNS, the atypical teratoid/rhabdoid tumor. This tumor has been recognized to develop in association with inactivation of INI1, a gene on chromosome 22. Patients typically present with nonspecific, nonlocalizing symptoms resulting from increased intracranial pressure. Of all tumors arising in the CNS, medulloblastoma has the greatest propensity to spread throughout the neuroaxis, and patients are routinely staged at the time of presentation. Current therapy is similar for patients of all stages and includes surgery and chemotherapy. Radiation therapy is also widely used, although in younger children, efforts to delay and minimize the amount of radiation are a constant focus of research in efforts to limit exposure of the developing nervous system.

See Also the Following Articles

Bibliography

Berger, M. S., and Wilson, C. B. (eds). (1996). "Textbook of Gliomas." Saunders, Philadelphia.

Greenlee, R., Murray, T., Bolden, S., and Wingo, P. (2000). "Cancer Statistics, 2000," Vol. 50, No. 1, pp. 12, 13, and 23. American Cancer Society, CA.

Kleihues, P., and Cavenee, W. K. (eds.) (2000). "Pathology and Genetics of Tumors of the Nervous System." IARC Press, Lyon.

Breast Cancer

Catherine Van Poznak
Andrew D. Seidman
Memorial Sloan-Kettering Cancer Center

GLOSSARY

adjuvant therapy Treatment after primary therapy to increase the chances of cure. Adjuvant therapy may include chemotherapy, radiotherapy, and/or hormonal therapy.

biomarkers Substances sometimes found in an increased amount in the blood, other body fluids, or tissues and that may suggest the presence of some types of cancer. Also called tumor markers.

biopsy The removal of cells or tissues for examination under a microscope. When only a sample of tissue is removed, the procedure is called an incisional biopsy or core biopsy. When an entire tumor or lesion is removed, the procedure is called an excisional biopsy. When a sample of tissue or fluid is removed with a needle, the procedure is called a needle biopsy or fine-needle aspiration.

BRCA1 A gene located on chromosome 17 that normally helps suppress cell growth. Inheriting an altered version of BRCA1 predisposes an individual to breast, ovarian, or prostate cancer.

BRCA2 A gene on chromosome 13 that normally helps suppress cell growth. A person who inherits an altered version of the BRCA2 gene has a higher risk of getting breast, ovarian, or prostate cancer.

breast-conserving surgery An operation to remove the breast cancer but not the breast itself. Types of breast-conserving surgery include lumpectomy (removal of the lump), quadrantectomy (removal of one quarter of the breast), and segmental mastectomy (removal of the cancer as well as some of the breast tissue around the tumor and the lining over the chest muscles below the tumor).

metastasis The spread of cancer from one part of the body to another. Tumors formed from cells that have spread are called "secondary tumors" and contain cells that are like those in the original (primary) tumor. The plural is metastases.

monoclonal antibodies Laboratory-engineered molecules that can locate and bind to cancer cells. Many monoclonal antibodies are used in cancer detection or therapy; each one recognizes a different protein on certain cancer cells. Monoclonal antibodies can be used alone or can be used to deliver drugs, toxins, or radioactive material directly to a tumor.

Breast cancer is the most common cancer diagnosis in American women and has an incidence of more than 180,000 invasive cases and 25,000 noninvasive cases per year. Over the past several decades, there has been a steady increase in the incidence. Fortunately, the death rates between the years 1992 and 1996 have shown a decrease, although approximately 42,000 American woman die annually from this disease. Breast cancer is one of the tumors for which there is conclusive evidence that screening can substantially decrease mortality. Patients with breast cancer now have more treatment options and a better chance of long-term survival than ever before. In addition, hormonal and surgical interventions are able to prevent some breast cancer within high-risk populations. This article provides an overview of breast cancer, with discussion of epidemiology and risk factors, screening, diagnosis, pathology and prognostic and predictive factors, treatment modalities, and guidelines for the follow-up of patients.

I. PATHOLOGY

Nearly all breast cancers arise from the glandular tissue (adenocarcinoma). Most invasive breast cancers (>80%) are of the ductal type; infiltrating lobular carcinomas constitute approximately 10%. Medullary, mucinous, or tubular histologies occur less often and carry a better prognosis. Other breast cancers, such as cystosarcoma phylloides, sarcomas, squamous cell carcinomas, and carcinosarcomas, are rare. Ductal carcinoma *in situ* (DCIS) is characterized by malignant epithelial cells within the mammary ductal system without evidence of invasion and is considered an early stage carcinoma. DCIS is generally treated by either mastectomy or breast-conserving therapy followed by adjuvant tamoxifen. Lobular carcinoma *in situ* typically lacks both clinical and mammographic signs; it is often present as an incidental finding on breast biopsy performed for another reason. Currently, lobular carcinoma *in situ* (LCIS) is considered a marker for increased breast cancer risk and the lesion itself is not treated as a cancer. The subsequent risk of breast cancer is equal for both the biopsied breast that demonstrated LCIS and the contralateral side.

II. EPIDEMIOLOGY AND RISK FACTORS

Epidemiologic studies indicate that the incidence of breast cancer is influenced by familial, endocrine, and environmental factors; other significant risk factors include a personal history of either breast cancer or benign proliferative breast disease. However, despite the recognition of these risk factors, the majority of patients developing breast cancer have no identifiable risk factor beyond being female and aging. Breast cancer affects patients in a female-to-male ratio of approximately 100:1. Table I illustrates the Surveillance, Epidemiology, and End Result Program (SEER) lifetime risk assessment of breast cancer by age of diagnosis for women. Mathematical models of risk assessment have been created; the most commonly used is the Gail model, which is available through links from the National Cancer Institute at http://www.cancer.gov.

A. Genetic

An important risk factor for developing breast cancer is a family history of the disease. It appears that there

TABLE I
SEER Lifetime Risk Breast Cancer
Diagnosed by Age

By age	Risk of breast cancer
30	1 out of 2212
40	1 out of 235
50	1 out of 54
60	1 out of 23
70	1 out of 14
80	1 out of 10
Ever	1 out of 8

are two categories of breast cancer risk associated with a family history of breast cancer: those with a specific germline mutation derived from either maternal or paternal relatives and those without a link to a germline mutation. It is estimated that 5–10% of all women with breast cancer may carry mutations in one of two such genes: BRCA1 and BRCA2. These mutations are associated with a risk of developing breast cancer ranging between 40 and 85%, are most often found within the Ashkenazi Jewish population, affect both sexes, and may be associated with cancers other than breast. Patients with mutations in the p53 tumor suppressor gene and familial syndromes (i.e., Li–Fraumeni) may also have an increased risk of breast cancer. Patients whose personal history and or family history suggest a genetic mutation may be referred to genetic counseling and, if appropriate, genetic testing. Potential medical, psychological, and socioeconomic risks need to be addressed before testing. The optimal methods of screening and treating patients with known genetic mutations are an area of intense investigation.

B. Endocrine

The risk of breast cancer is increased in women who have had long periods of uninterrupted estrogen exposure by early menarche (before age 12), late menopause (after age 55), nulliparity, or age of first-term pregnancy after age 30. In addition, hormonal exposure from hormonal replacement therapy for long duration, high-dose estrogen oral contraceptives in women who carry BRCA1 or BRCA2 mutations, or exposure to diethylstilbestrol may place a woman at an increased risk for breast cancer. In women with a personal history of breast cancer, the use of hormonal replacement therapy is controversial and the risks and benefits of this intervention need to be weighed on an individual basis. Although experimental data suggest that estrogens have a role in the development of breast cancer, the mechanism has not been completely elucidated.

C. Environmental

It has been suggested that a lower incidence of breast cancer in certain countries is related to dietary influences, particularly dietary fat consumption. To explore this, a randomized trial of low-fat intervention among breast cancer patients is ongoing. Dietary intake of phytoestrogens, as found in soy products, may act like selective estrogen receptor modulators (SERMs) by competing with the action of endogenous estrogen, although they do so with less avidity than estradiol. However, there is the possibility that phytoestrogens may increase overall estrogenic (i.e., potentially carcinogenic) activity in postmenopausal women, and further formal investigation of phytoestrogens should take place prior to recommending use of this as a dietary supplement. Ionizing radiation, as seen in young women who received mantle radiation for Hodgkin's disease and those who survived the atomic bomb blasts of World War II and the Chernobyl nuclear accident, creates an increased risk of breast cancer.

Over 50 epidemiologic studies have investigated the effect of alcohol on the risk of breast cancer without definitive results. Pooled analysis from 6 cohort studies demonstrated that women who drank 30–60 or more grams of alcohol a day had a 40% increased risk of breast cancer regardless of the alcohol source. Epidemiologic studies relating physical activity to the risk of breast cancer show inconsistent results. One study demonstrated that women whose lifetime average of 3.8 h or more of physical activity per week had a relative risk of 0.42 (95% CI 0.27 to 0.64). Environmental factors that may have an association with breast cancer support the recommendations that patients follow a "heart healthy" diet, limit alcohol consumption, and regularly exercise as a means of reducing the risk of breast cancer.

III. PREVENTION

Tamoxifen is a SERM that has been used for over 20 years in the treatment of breast cancer and is the first drug shown to reduce the incidence of breast cancer in healthy women. The Breast Cancer Prevention Trial (NSABP P-1) demonstrated the value of tamoxifen as a chemoprevention. In this prospective clinical trial, patients were randomized to tamoxifen versus placebo for 5 years. The tamoxifen group demonstrated an approximate reduction of 50% for both invasive estrogen/progesterone receptor-positive invasive breast cancer and noninvasive breast cancer, although no difference in overall survival has yet been observed. Two European randomized controlled trials of tamoxifen did not show a similar benefit. However, the European trials differed from the NSABP P-1 trial in that they were statistically underpowered, had high rates of noncompliance, and included women who were currently using hormonal replacement therapy. Another SERM, raloxifene, which is currently FDA approved for the treatment of osteoporosis, is undergoing study as a breast cancer prevention agent in the Study of Tamoxifen and Raloxifene (STAR) clinical trial (NSABP P-2).

Prophylactic mastectomy reduces the risk of breast cancer by approximately 90% in women with a family history of breast cancer. When prophylactic mastectomy is undertaken, the procedure should be similar to a therapeutic mastectomy. This prophylactic procedure should be discussed with patients at very high risk for breast cancer; however, patient satisfaction is noted only when the patients themselves have suggested prophylactic mastectomy as the treatment of choice.

IV. EVALUATION

A. Asymptomatic (Screening)

Screening offers the opportunity for early detection of cancer and thereby reduces the morbidity and mortal-ity associated with advanced disease. The main methods for early detection of breast cancer are clinical breast examination (CBE) by a trained health professional and mammography. Self-breast examination (SBE) has not yet been demonstrated to affect mortality, although approximately 50% of breast cancer patients report having found the breast mass themselves, and women who perform SBE are more likely to have smaller tumors and less likely to have axillary lymph node metastases than those who did not (Table II).

Screening mammography is performed on asymptomatic patients to detect occult breast cancer, whereas the diagnostic mammogram is performed in patients who have a breast abnormality. Mammography has a sensitivity of 85–90%, therefore missing 10–15% of breast cancers. This fact confirms the need to fully evaluate all palpable lesions for diagnosis, whether by additional imaging study or by obtaining tissue (see Section V). The risk of false-positive screening breast exam and/or false-positive screening mammogram was evaluated in a retrospective study where approximately one-third of women screened over a 10-year period required an addition evaluation, although no breast cancer was present.

The screening mammogram is universally recommended for women over the age of 50, and most cancer associations recommend screening to begin at age 40. Although controversial in both younger women and women over 75 years old, the screening mammography in women ages 50–75 has been shown to significantly decrease the death rate from breast can-

TABLE II
American Cancer Society's Screening Guidelines[a]

Age in years	Recommendations[b]	Benefit
20–39	SBE every month CBE every 3 years High-risk patients: consider additional screening	No data
40–49	SBE every month CBE every year Mammogram every year	Reduce risk of dying from breast cancer by 18%
>50	SBE every month CBE every year Mammogram every 1 year	Reduce risk of dying from breast cancer ~30%

[a]From Leitch *et al.* (1997) and Tabar *et al.* (1995).
[b]SBE, self-breast examination; CBE, clinical breast examination.

cer. Young women with a strong risk of familial breast cancer may begin screening at 5–10 years prior to the youngest age that a first-degree relative was diagnosed with breast cancer. The optimal method of screening patients with genetic mutations is not yet known, and mammography in younger women may be difficult to interpret due to the density of the breast tissue.

Digital mammography is a computerized technique that displays an infinite scale of gray tones allowing for an enhanced quality of imaging as well as magnifying the view of specific areas of the breast. This technique is undergoing clinical investigation, as is computer-assisted diagnosis (CAD). Ultrasound is commonly used to define cystic breast structures or guide biopsies and it is also being explored in clinical trials as a screening technique. Magnetic resonance imaging (MRI) is a highly sensitive imaging modality undergoing investigation as a screening technique for high-risk women. Unfortunately, neither ultrasound nor MRI is as consistent as mammography at detecting microcalcifications. Techniques of obtaining breast tissue for screening purposes are under investigation; these include nipple aspiration, ductal lavage, and fiber-optic ductoscopy. These minimally invasive techniques obtain cells for cytologic examination from breast ducts for histologic assessment.

B. Presenting Symptoms and Signs

Once a patient has developed a breast symptom or sign, the workup that ensues is not one of screening, but one of diagnosing the complaint or finding. Breast signs and symptoms may include a mass, breast pain, skin changes, nipple discharge, and change in the breast size or nipple. Any suspicious lesion warrants an investigation.

When a dominant breast mass is noted and the history and physical are consistent with the lesion representing a cyst (changes with menstrual cycle and a well-demarcated, mobile, firm lesion on examination of a premenopausal women), then aspiration of the lesion is an appropriate evaluation, either with or without ultrasound evaluation and guidance. If nonbloody fluid is obtained and the lesion disappears completely, then the patient requires no further immediate evaluation, although follow-up is required to confirm that the lesion has remained completely re-solved. Cytologic assessment of nonbloody fluid from a cyst that resolves is not recommended. Should the cyst recur after repeated aspiration or should aspiration demonstrate bloody fluid or incomplete resolution of the mass, then surgical biopsy is recommended. Failure to aspirate the cyst suggests a solid mass.

Evaluation of a solid mass may be performed with mammography, fine needle aspiration (FNA), or biopsy. The decision to observe a breast mass that appears to be benign should only be made after careful clinical, radiologic, and cytologic/pathologic examination, as the false-negative rates of the individual modalities are high. Fibroadenomas comprise approximately 50% of breast biopsies. On physical examination, fibroadenomas are rubbery, round, or lobulated masses that are nontender and mobile. Sonographic criteria to diagnose a fibroadenoma include shape, contour, echo texture, echogenicity, sound transmission, and surrounding tissue. Fibroadenomas themselves are benign but carry with them a small increased risk (1.2–3.0 relative risk) for the development of breast cancer. Treatment of a fibroadenoma includes either excision of the lesion (gold standard for diagnosis) or clinical close follow-up with recording of the lesion size over time.

A solid breast mass that is not consistent with a fibroadenoma warrants a tissue diagnosis. Tissue may be obtained by FNA, core needle biopsy, incisional biopsy, or excisional biopsy; however, FNA for cytology should only be relied upon if an experienced cytologist is available and if all suspicious or negative lesions have a definitive biopsy procedure. Nonpalpable lesions may require needle localization or biopsy under stereotactic guidance. Radiographic assessment of the nonpalpable lesion after biopsy is required to confirm that the abnormality has been removed. Prior to definitive surgery, the entire breast in question, as well as the contralateral breast, should have undergone a thorough assessment for additional foci of breast cancer.

V. DIAGNOSIS

The majority of breast biopsies do not yield cancer. Approximately 30% of biopsies demonstrate no disease, 40% fibrocystic changes, 7% fibroadenoma, and

13% contain miscellaneous benign breast lesions. Benign proliferative lesions, particularly if atypia is present, confer an increased risk of breast cancer. Only 10% of breast biopsies contain carcinoma. After a patient is diagnosed with cancer, the next step is the clinical staging of the cancer followed by definitive therapy, if possible. Of note is a recent study that demonstrated that hospitals treating >25 breast cancer cases annually have better survival rates than those treating fewer cases across all strata of treatment conditions.

A. Staging

Prior to definitive surgery, the breast cancer patient should undergo clinical staging with a thorough history and physical examination to identify any contraindications to breast-conserving therapy (BCT) or immediate breast reconstruction, as well as to identify any metastases. Barring any element of history or finding on physical examination that dictates further investigation, the extent of disease evaluation for a primary, operable breast cancer includes complete blood count, liver function testing, chest X-ray, and bilat-

TABLE III
TNM Staging System for Breast Cancer

Primary tumor (T)

Tx	Primary tumor cannot be assessed
T0	No evidence of primary tumor
Tis	Carcinoma *in situ*: intraductal, LCIS, or Paget's disease of the nipple with no tumor
T1	Tumor ≤2 cm
Tmic	Microinvasion of ≤0.1 cm in greatest dimension
T1a	Tumor >0.1 but ≤0.5 cm in greatest dimension
T1b	Tumor >0.5 but ≤1 cm in greatest dimension
T1c	Tumor >1 but ≤2 cm in greatest dimension
T2	Tumor >2 but ≤5 cm in greatest dimension
T3	Tumor >5 cm in greatest dimension
T4	Tumor of any size, with direct extension to (a) chest wall (b) skin only, as below
T4a	Extension to chest wall
T4b	Edema (including peau d'orange) or ulceration of the skin or satellite skin nodules confined to the same breast
T4c	Both T4a and T4b
T4d	Inflammatory carcinoma

Regional lymph nodes (N)

NX	Regional lymph nodes cannot be assessed (e.g., previously removed)
N1	No regional lymph nodes metastases
N2	Metastasis to ipsilateral axillary lymph node(s) fixed to one another or other structures
N3	Metastasis to ipsilateral internal mammary lymph node(s)

Distant metastases

MX	Distant metastases cannot be assessed
M0	No distant metastases
M1	Distant metastases, including metastasis to ipsilateral supraclavicular lymph node(s)

Staging grouping

Stage 0	Tis	N0	M0
Stage I	T1	N0	M0
Stage IIA	T0	N1	M0
	T1	N1	M0
	T2	N0	M0
Stage IIB	T2	N1	M0
	T3	N0	M0
Stage IIIA	T0	N2	M0
	T1	N2	M0
	T2	N2	M0
	T3	N1–2	M0
Stage IIIB	T4	Any N	M0
	Any T	N3	M0
Stage IV	Any T	Any N	M1

eral mammogram. Additional testing may be indicated by an individual patient's symptoms and the results of the extent of disease evaluation, i.e., an elevated alkaline phosphatase or bone pain, which may warrant a bone scan to rule out osseous metastases. Also, for patients found to be at high risk of metastasis after definitive surgery, e.g., due to extensive axillary lymph node involvement, other imaging studies, such as nuclear bone scintography and computerized tomography or ultrasound of the liver, should be considered to rule out occult metastatic disease. The most widely used system to stage breast cancer is the American Joint Committee on Cancer (AJCC) classification, which is based on tumor size (T), the status of regional lymph nodes (N), and the presence of distant metastases (M). Table III demonstrates the TNM staging of breast cancer.

B. Pathology: Prognostic and Predictive Factors

A prognostic factor is one that influences the outcome independently of treatment and a predictive factor is one with a relationship to the response to a particular therapy. The most important prognostic factors include axillary lymph node status, tumor size, estrogen and progesterone receptor status, and HER2/neu protein overexpression or gene amplification. Other factors that have been used to predict outcome include, but are not limited to, histologic grade, mitotic index, lymphovascular invasion, S-phase fraction, ploidy, the tumor suppressor gene p53, p27, cathepsin D, and microvessel density.

VI. TREATMENT

A. Early Stage Disease

Treatment planning involves selecting the optimal sequence of procedures and interventions to maximize the patients' outcome and minimize toxicity. Classically, treatment for invasive carcinoma is initiated with surgery, followed by adjuvant chemotherapy, radiotherapy, and hormonal therapy as indicated. Situations exist where a patient may not be a candidate for immediate surgery, such as cases of inflammatory carcinoma or those patients who desire neo-

adjuvant chemotherapy either to improve the opportunity for breast-conserving therapy or as part of a clinical trial. Treatment planning requires the integration of many factors, including the patient's general health and attitude toward treatment. For patients not receiving preoperative systemic therapy, after completing surgery, the estimated risk of recurrence can be calculated. Then an estimate of the anticipated absolute risk reduction in recurrence and survival for the patient's and the tumor's characteristics can be calculated for discussion of the risks and benefits of the adjuvant therapy.

B. Surgery

1. Primary Treatment

The extent of surgery performed depends on multiple factors, including histology (invasive versus *in situ* disease or a favorable histology), status of the margins, the patient's comorbid conditions and ability to tolerate surgery and adjuvant treatment, and patient preference for breast-conserving therapy versus modified radical mastectomy (with or without reconstruction). Age alone is not prima facie a factor on which to make treatment decisions, but individual patient characteristics are crucial to the planning of surgery. Consideration should be given to neoadjuvant therapy and local control of disease should be optimized by the least invasive means. The sentinel lymph node dissection technique, when performed by an experience surgeon, should be strongly considered. This procedure is still undergoing clinical trials for assessment against the standard full axillary lymph node dissection.

Patients with operable breast cancer receive local therapy with complete removal of tumor. Most patients will receive either a modified radical mastectomy or breast-conserving therapy with some form of lymph node sampling (sentinel or complete axillary dissection). Absolute contraindications to breast-conserving therapy include first or second trimester of pregnancy, multifocal disease with involvement of separate quadrants of the breast, diffuse microcalcifications, and prior breast irradiation. Relative contraindications include a large tumor-to-breast ratio, tumor location beneath the nipple, a history of collagen vascular disease, and large breast size, which can be a relative contraindication due to technical limitations of obtaining adequate radiation dose homogeneity. Ductal carcinoma *in situ* without evidence of microinvasion does not warrant exploration of a clinically negative axilla, and certain patients with small *in situ* carcinoma may be appropriate candidates for treatment with breast-conserving therapy with wide margin resection alone.

2. Reconstruction

Reconstructive surgery, either immediate or delayed, should be offered to all patients undergoing modified radical mastectomy. A variety of reconstructive options exist, and selection of the procedure is based on the patient's habitus as well as preference. Options include placement of an implant or transposition of muscle, blood supply, and soft tissue from either the latissimus dorsi or the rectus abdominus muscle. In addition, patients may opt for contralateral breast surgery to obtain symmetry. Patients who undergo breast-conserving therapy may also desire breast revision for an improved sense of body integrity.

C. Adjuvant Therapy for Early Stage Breast Cancer

Both local and distant control of disease must be addressed to minimize the risk of recurrence. The current prevailing biologic concept is that occult systemic micrometastases may be present at the time of diagnosis. Systemic adjuvant therapy is therefore administered to eradicate occult micrometastatic disease. Adjuvant systemic therapy for operable breast cancer includes chemotherapy, hormonal therapy, or both. This usually begins 4–8 weeks after definitive surgery, allowing the patient sufficient time for wound healing. Numerous individual randomized clinical trials as meta-analyzed by the Early Breast Cancer Trialists' Collaborative Group (EBCTCG) have demonstrated that chemotherapy and hormonal therapy add to local treatment to favorably alter the natural history of breast cancer. The magnitude of this benefit varies with both patient and tumor-specific characteristics.

1. Adjuvant Chemotherapy

Chemotherapy has been shown to substantially improve the long-term, relapse free, and overall survival in both premenopausal and postmenopausal women with node-positive and node-negative disease. The November 2000 Consensus Development Conference Statement indicates that accepted practice is to offer chemotherapy to most women with lymph node metastases or with a primary tumor greater than 1 cm in diameter, noting that the consideration of adjuvant chemotherapy should be further individualized. The use of polychemotherapy regimens has been shown to be superior to single-agent regimens for adjuvant chemotherapy. The optimal regimen, with selection of drugs, doses, schedule, and duration of treatment, is still a matter of clinical investigation, and a variety of chemotherapeutic regimens have been proven effective. The contribution of each drug versus the contribution of duration of therapy is still being explored. Presently, adjuvant chemotherapy is administered over 3 to 6 months; the EBCTCG meta-analysis suggests no additional benefit for prolonged (e.g., 1 year) polychemotherapy regimens. In addition, anthracycline-containing regiments have demonstrated an incremental advantage over nonanthracycline-containing regimens. Current clinical trials are investigating the emerging role of the taxanes in the adjuvant setting and the role of trastuzumab (monoclonal antibody targeting the HER2/neu receptor). The roles of dose density and dose intensity are also being explored. To date, there is no convincing evidence that dose-intensive treatment regimens requiring stem cell support result in improved survival when compared to standard doses of polychemotherapy, although improved disease-free survival has been observed in some studies.

2. Adjuvant Hormonal Therapy

The decision to recommend adjuvant hormonal therapy is based on the presence of hormone receptors assessed during review of the tumor's pathology. Patients with estrogen- and progesterone-receptor positive tumors may obtain benefit from adjuvant hormonal manipulation regardless of age, menopausal status, involvement of axillary lymph nodes, or tumor size. There is no evidence that patients with hormone receptor-negative tumors receive any benefit from adjuvant hormonal therapy. The goal of hormonal therapy is to prevent occult breast cancer cells from receiving stimulation from estrogen, a known growth factor for tumors that express either of the hormonal receptors. Estrogen deprivation may be achieved by use of pharmaceutical agents, and in premenopausal women, consideration may be given to chemical or surgical ovarian ablation.

Tamoxifen is the most commonly used form of hormonal therapy in the adjuvant setting, and newer antiestrogens and aromatase inhibitors are being evaluated in clinical trials. Randomized trials have demonstrated that 5 years of tamoxifen use is superior to 1–2 years; however, whether 5 years is the optimal duration is still unknown and is the subject of clinical investigation. Presently the recommended duration of adjuvant tamoxifen use is 5 years. The EBCTCG meta-analysis has shown that the 10-year proportional reductions in recurrence and mortality associated with 5 years of tamoxifen use were 47 and 26%, respectively. An additional benefit was the approximately 50% decrease in the incidence of contralateral breast cancer noted in women receiving tamoxifen, regardless of hormonal receptor status of the primary tumor. Adjuvant hormonal therapy may be the most active component of the adjuvant treatments in some patient subsets. Tamoxifen is generally not administered simultaneously with chemotherapy as there is an additive risk of thromboembolic events and no clear therapeutic benefit. Therefore, if chemotherapy is given, it should be completed prior to initiating tamoxifen.

3. Adjuvant Radiation Therapy

Adjuvant radiotherapy is administered to those patients who have undergone breast-conserving therapy and postmastectomy patients with primary tumors greater than 5 cm or more than four positive lymph nodes. Postmastectomy patients with less advanced disease may also be candidates for adjuvant radiotherapy, as two clinical trials have demonstrated a survival advantage for postmastectomy radiotherapy, although confirmatory trials are awaited. Radiotherapy significantly adds to local control in these circumstances and its role in other settings, such as routine use postmastectomy; its use in small ductal carcinoma *in situ* lesions with wide surgical margins is controversial. Adjuvant chemotherapy is administered prior to radiotherapy to address the potential systemic element of the disease. These two treatment modalities are generally not used concurrently due to the potential for increased locoregional toxicities.

VII. TREATMENT OF RECURRENT AND METASTATIC DISEASE

A. Locoregional Relapse

Patients who experience a locoregional relapse should be considered for treatment modalities that could render them without evidence of disease. Unfortunately, ipsilateral breast tumor recurrence is associated with an approximate 20–50% chance of systemic disease. Those recurrences that did not occur within the residual breast tissue, but rather as local skin, chest wall involvement, or distant lesions, represent blood or lymphatic-borne metastases.

B. Metastatic Disease

Patients may initially present with metastatic disease or they may relapse after primary therapy. Once metastases have developed, breast cancer is rarely, if ever, a "curable" condition, although metastatic breast cancer frequently is responsive to a variety of hormonal and chemotherapeutic manipulations. When managing metastatic disease, the treatment objectives are to optimize treatment response, improve survival, and balance these goals with maintaining quality of life. Assessing prognosis and devising treatment options require knowledge of the patient's pathologic predictive factors and extent of metastases. Evaluation of the extent of disease includes physical examination, complete blood count, comprehensive biochemical profile with liver function tests and alkaline phosphatase, tumor markers (typically CEA and CA15.3 or CA27.29), and imaging studies with computerized tomography of the chest, abdomen, and pelvis, as well as a bone scan. Additional imaging with magnetic resonance (MR), ultrasound (US), positron emission tomography (PET), and plain radiographs are obtained as clinically indicated.

1. Hormonal Therapy for Metastatic Disease

Patients whose tumors express the estrogen and/or the progesterone receptor should be considered for hormonal manipulation of their metastatic breast cancer. Hormonal therapy is less toxic than most chemotherapies and therefore is typically employed first. Response to hormonal therapy may be slow (up to 12 weeks) and patients may experience a "flare" with the initiation of hormonal therapy, where there may be a brief period of increased bone pain, elevation of tumor markers, or increased uptake of the bone lesions seen on bone scan.

The choice of hormonal therapy depends on a patient's menopausal status as well as the prior exposure to hormonal manipulation. For the postmenopausal woman, treatment options include antiestrogen therapy (tamoxifen, toremifene), aromatase inhibitors (anastrozole, letrozole), aromatase inactivators (exemestane), progestins (megestrol acetate, medroxyprogesterone acetate), or androgen (fluoxymesterone) therapy. Premenopausal women may be made menopausal by luteinizing hormone releasing hormone (LHRH) analog, oophorectomy, or radioablation of the ovaries; once castrate, then all treatment options available to postmenopausal women should be considered. Klijn and colleagues performed a meta-analysis of four randomized trials and demonstrated that combined estrogen blockage with both LHRH analog and tamoxifen was superior to LHRH analog alone in premenopausal women. The meta-analysis resulted in both a clinically relevant and a statistically significant reduction in the risk of dying or progression of disease/death. Hormonal therapies are used sequentially, with a trial of one drug in each class, until there is progression of disease, drug-related toxicity, or indication to initiate chemotherapy. Hormonal therapies are generally well tolerated, and side effects vary with the agent selected; in general, this treatment modality is associated with hot flashes, mild nausea, and thrombophlebitis. Tamoxifen is associated with an increased risk of uterine cancer in women over age 50 (1 in 500) whether used for metastatic disease, adjuvant therapy, or chemoprevention. Patients on tamoxifen need to be followed for evidence of dysfunctional uterine bleeding; a proven role for sonographic screening for endometrial cancer has not been demonstrated.

2. Chemotherapy for Metastatic Disease

Patients with metastatic disease are considered candidates for chemotherapy if they are symptomatic (secondary to visceral involvement), have rapidly progressing or bulky disease, or are inappropriate candidates for hormonal therapy either because of negative hormonal receptor status or progression of disease on hormonal therapies. The selection of chemotherapy must take into consideration the patients' prior exposure to chemotherapy in the adjuvant setting and time from adjuvant therapy. Chemotherapy agents that are very active in breast cancer include anthracyclines (doxorubicin and epirubicin) and taxanes (docetaxel and paclitaxel). Other active agents include cyclophosphamide, capecitabine, fluorouracil, gemcitabine, methotrexate, and vinorelbine. Cisplatin and carboplatin have significant activity in chemotherapy-naive and minimally treated patients; these agents are presently being revisited, in part due to the potential for clinical synergism with trastuzumab in HER2-overexpressing metastatic breast cancer. As a generality, combination chemotherapies may offer a faster and increased response rate; however, this may be associated with increased toxicities in a patient population that is being treated for palliation. To date, there is no evidence that high-dose chemotherapy with stem cell rescue improves outcome over standard therapy. Like hormonal therapy, patients are often treated with a chemotherapy regimen until progression of disease, or prohibitive toxicity, at which time the therapy is changed to a second or a third line therapy.

3. Monoclonal Antibody Therapy

The HER2/neu gene product is a transmembrane tyrosine kinase receptor belonging to a family of epidermal growth factor receptors structurally related to the human epidermal growth factor receptor. HER2/neu is overexpressed or amplified in approximately 30% of human breast cancers and is a poor prognostic feature. However, it predicts for a positive response to a monoclonal antibody, trastuzumab, targeted against the HER2/neu receptor. Trastuzumab has activity as a single agent and has been shown to improve response rate and overall survival when used in combination chemotherapy regimens. Trastuzumab demonstrated a significantly increased incidence of symptomatic cardiac toxicity when used simultaneously with anthracycline-based chemotherapy and therefore this combination is contraindicated outside of a clinical trial until further safety data are available.

4. Supportive Therapies

Patients with metastatic disease may become symptomatic from either the disease itself or from the toxicities of therapy. Supportive measures are used as indicated. These measures include radiation therapy to control localized sites of relapse, supplemental oxygen for decreased pulmonary function, bisphosphonate therapy in patients with osteolytic metastases to decrease bone pain, fracture or hypercalcemia, and analgesics such as COX2 inhibitors or narcotics prescribed for pain control. Other supportive measures include antiemetics for nausea related to either therapy or disease; antidepressants for mood disturbance or control of hot flashes; and hematopoietic growth factor support with either GCSF or erythropoietin as required to support myelo- and erythropoiesis, as needed. In addition, psychological and social services for both the patient and that of the caregivers are important elements of supportive therapy. Many patients and physician researchers are interested in complimentary medicine as an adjunct to the therapies presently considered the standard of care. In a study by Burstein and co-workers, the use of alternative medicines in patients with early stage breast cancer was associated with increased stress levels and a decrease in the quality of life. Further study is necessary to scientifically define the risks and benefits with each alternative intervention.

IX. FOLLOW-UP OF BREAST CANCER PATIENTS

Patients with a history of early stage breast cancer continue with regular follow-up with specific attention to the potential for recurrence and treatment-related complications. Most recurrences present within the first 5 years; however, it is not uncommon for breast cancer to recur long after this time. Women with a history of breast cancer have an approximate 0.5–1% per year risk of developing a second primary breast cancer, although the risk is higher in certain subsets. Patients with a history of breast cancer have several unique health issues that may have developed from breast cancer therapy, such as postmastectomy or reconstruction pain, lymphedema, cellulitis in the ipsilateral arm, cardiac dysfunction, pulmonary fibrosis, premature menopause, cognitive dysfunction, arthropathy, osteoporosis, and treatment-related secondary malignancies.

Recommended follow-up care of early stage breast cancer includes a physician visit with history and physical examination every 3–6 months for the first 3 years, every 6–12 months for the next 2 years, and then annually for life. The patient should perform a self-breast examination monthly, as well as undergo an annual clinical breast examination and mammography in addition to age-appropriate cancer screening. The use of routine laboratory testing or radiographic studies is not recommended unless directed by symptoms or physical examination. Age-appropriate screening for other cancers is recommended as directed for the general population. It is unknown whether patients who are at very high risk for breast cancer due to family history and genetic predisposition require more intensive follow-up and these patients may be referred to a high-risk clinic. Follow-up of patients with metastatic disease is dictated by the patients' needs and therapy.

IX. SPECIAL PROBLEMS

A. Emergencies

Patients with breast cancer are at increased risk for a wide range of emergencies that may be secondary to either the cancer or its therapy. Table IV illustrates some of these potential emergencies.

B. Paget's Disease

Paget's disease of the breast is characterized by red, scaling patches over the areola, nipple, or accessory breast tissue. Paget's disease is associated with breast cancer. The diagnosis of Paget's disease is made by pathologic assessment of biopsy or nipple scrape cytology. Physical examination and mammography are performed to identify multicentric disease or coexistent invasive breast cancer; preoperative breast MRI may be useful. Treatment is primarily with surgery, either mastectomy (commonly) or breast conservation with consideration to radiotherapy; additional adjuvant therapy may be considered.

TABLE IV
Emergencies Relating to Either Breast Cancer or Its Therapy

Cardiovascular: Tamponade (effusion, extrinsic compression) restrictive pericarditis, congestive heart failure (cardiotoxic agents)

GI: Obstruction, perforation, liver failure

GU: Hemorrhage, obstruction

Hematologic: Bleeding, thrombosis

Infection: Neutropenic fevers, central nervous system infections

Metabolic: Hypercalcemia, hyponatremia, lactic acidosis (liver disease/dysfunction), acute tumor lysis syndrome (rare)

Neurologic: Epidural or spinal cord compromise, raised intracranial pressure, and intracerebral hemorrhage, seizure; cranial nerve palsy/paralysis, phrenic nerve/recurrent laryngeal nerve paralysis

Orthopedic: Fracture, spinal cord compression

Respiratory: Superior vena cava syndrome, pulmonary embolism, lymphangitic disease, large pleural effusion(s)

C. Breast Cancer During Pregnancy

Breast cancer diagnosed during pregnancy occurs in 1:3,000 to 1:10,000 pregnancies. Overall, pregnancy-associated breast cancer is associated with a worse prognosis as the patient usually presents with more advanced disease. Management of breast cancer during pregnancy involves the patient, the unborn fetus, the family of the patient, the obstetrician, the neonatologist, and the oncology team of radiologists, surgeons, radiotherapists, and medical oncologists.

X. AREAS OF ACTIVE RESEARCH

Investigation is ongoing in every aspect of breast cancer. Prevention and early detection remain the ultimate goal. Biomarkers with increased prognostic and predictive value are being sought, and the new technology of gene arrays may aid in identifying such markers. Novel therapies with hormones, chemotherapies, cell cycle regulators, biologic agents, and vaccines are being studied. Underserved populations of minority status and the growing elderly populations warrant additional investigation. Additionally, methods to minimize the complications of therapy are being explored. Increased patient education and patient advocacy have positively created improved dynamics among patient, physician, and researcher.

See Also the Following Articles

ESTROGENS AND ANTIESTROGENS • HEREDITARY RISK OF BREAST CANCER AND OVARIAN CANCER

Bibliography

Burstein, H. J., Gelber, S., Guadagnoli, E., and Weeks, J. C. (1999). Use of alternative medicine by women with early-stage breast cancer. N. Engl. J. Med. **340,** 1733–1739.

Burstein, H. J., and Winer, E. P. (2000). Primary care for survivors of breast cancer. N. Engl. J. Med. **343,** 1086–1094.

Clemons, M., and Goss, P. (2001). Estrogen and the risk of breast cancer. N. Engl. J. Med. **344**(4), 276–285.

Cotran, R. S., Kumar, V., and Robbins, S. L. (eds.) (1989). "Robbins Pathologic Basis of Disease," 4th Ed. Saunders, Philadelphia.

Early Breast Cancer Trialists' Collaborative Group (1998). Polychemotherapy for early breast cancer: An overview of the randomised trials. Lancet **352,** 930.

Early Breast Cancer Trialists' Collaborative Group (1998). Tamoxifen for early breast cancer: An overview of the randomised trials. Lancet **351,** 1451.

Elmore, J. G., Barton, M. B., Moceri, V. M., Polk, S., Arena, P. J., and Fletcher, S. W. (1998). Ten-year risk of false positive screening mammograms and clinical breast examinations. N. Engl. J. Med. **338,** 1089–1096.

Fisher, B., Costantino, J. P., Wickerham, D. L., Redmond, C. K., Kavanah, M., Cronin, W. M., Vogel, V., Robidoux, A., Dimitrov, N., Atkins, J., Daly, M., Wieand, S., Tan-Chiu, E., Ford, L., and Wolmark, N. (1998). Tamoxifen for prevention of breast cancer: Report of the National Surgical Adjuvant Breast and Bowel Project P-1 Study. J. Natl. Cancer Inst. **90,** 1371–1388.

Fossati, R., Confalonieri, C., Torri, V., Ghislandi, E., Penna, A., Pistotti, V., Tinazzi, A., and Liberati, A. (1998). J. Clin. Oncol. **16,** 3439–3460.

Gapstur, S. M., Morrow, M., and Sellers, T. A. (1999). Hormone replacement therapy and risk of breast cancer with a favorable histology: Results of the Iowa Women's Health Study. JAMA **281,** 2091–2097.

Grabrick, D. M., Hartmann, L. C., Cerhan, J. R., Vierkant, R. A., Therneau, T. M., Vachon, C. M., Olson, J. E., Couch, F. J., Anderson, K. E., Pankratz, V. S., and Sellers, T. A. (2000). Risk of breast cancer with oral contraceptive use in women with a family history of breast cancer. JAMA **284,** 1791–1798.

Hartmann, L. C., Schaid, D. J., Woods, J. E., Crotty, T. P., Myers, J. L., Arnold, P. G., Petty, P. M., Sellers, T. A., Johnson, J. L., McDonnell, S. K., Frost, M. H., Jenkins, R. B., Grant, C. S., and Michels, V. V. (1999). Efficacy of bilateral prophylactic mastectomy in women with a family history of breast cancer. N. Engl. J. Med. **340,** 77–84.

Klijn, J. G. M., Blamey, R. W., Boccardo, F., Tominaga, T., Duchateau, L., Sylvester, R., for the Combined Hormone

Agents Trialists' Group and the European Organization for Research and Treatment of Cancer (2001). Combined Tamoxifen and luteinizing hormone-releasing hormone (LHRH) agonist versus LHRH agonist alone in premenopausal advanced breast cancer: A meta-analysis of four randomized trials. *J. Clin. Oncol.* **19**(2), 343–353.

Leitch, A. M., Dodd, G. D., Costanza, M., Linver, M., Pressman, P., McGinnis, L., and Smith, R. A. (1997). American Cancer Society guidelines for the early detection of breast cancer: Update 1997. *CA Cancer J. Clin.* **47**, 150–153.

Morrow, M., Stewart, A., Sylvester, J., and Bland, K. (2000). Hospital volume predicts outcomes in breast cancer: A National Cancer Data Base (NCDB) Study. *Proc. Am. Clin. Oncol.* **19**. [Abstract 309.]

Overgaard, M., Jensen, M. B., Overgaard, J., Hansen, P. S., Andersson, M., Kamby, C., Kjaer, M., Gadeberg, C. C., Rasmussen, B. B., Blichert-Toft, M., and Mouridsen, H. T. (1999). Randomized controlled trial evaluation postoperative readiotherapy in high-risk post-menopausal breast cancer patients given tamoxifen: Report from the Danish Breast Cancer Cooperative Group DBCG 82c Trial. *Lancet* **353**, 1641–1648.

Powles, T., Eeles, R., Ashley, S., Easton, D., Chang, J., Dowsett, M., Tidy, A., Viggers, J., and Davey, J. (1998). Interim analysis of the incidence of breast cancer in the Royal Marsden Hospital tamoxifen randomised chemoprevention trial. *Lancet* **352**(9122), 98–101.

Ragaz, J., Jackson, S. M., Le, N., Plenderleith, I. H., Spinelli, J. J., Basco, V. E., Wilson, K. S., Knowling, M. A., Coppin, C. M. L., Paradis, M., Coldman, A. J., and Olivotto, I. A. (1997). Adjuvant radiotherapy and chemotherapy in node-positive premenopausal women with breast cancer. *N. Engl. J. Med.* **337**, 956–962.

Schairer, C., Lubin, J., Troisi, R., Sturgeon, S., Brinton, L., and Hoover, R. (2000). Menopausal estrogen and estrogen-progestin replacement therapy and breast cancer risk. *JAMA* **283**(4), 485–491.

Silverstein, M., Lagios, M. D., Groshen, S., Waisman, J. R., Lewinsky, B. S., Gamagami, M. S., and Colburn, W. J. (1999). The influence of margin width on local control of ductal carcinoma in situ of the breast. *N. Engl. J. Med.* **340**(19), 1455–1461.

Slamon, D. J., Leyland-Jones, B., Shak, S., Fuchs, H., Paton, V., Bajamonde, A., Fleming, T., Eiermann, W., Wolter, J., Pegram, M., Baselga, J., and Norton, L. (2001). Use of chemotherapy plus a monoclonal antibody against HER2 for metastatic breast cancer that overexpresses HER2. *N. Engl. J. Med.* **344**, 783–792.

Smith-Warner, S. A., Spiegelman, D., Yaun, S. S., van den Brandt, P. A., Folsom, A. R., Goldbohm, R. A., Graham, S., Holmberg, L., Howe, G. R., Marshall, J. R., Miller, A. B., Potter, J. D., Speizer, F. E., Willett, W. C., Wolk, A., and Hunter, D. J. (1998). Alcohol and breast cancer in women: A pooled analysis of cohort studies. *JAMA* **279**(7), 535–540.

Stadtmauer, E. A., O'Neil, A., Goldstein, L. J., Grilley, P. A., Mangan, K. F., Ingle, J. N., Brodsky, I., Martino, S., Lazarus, H. M., Erban, J. K., Sickles, C., and Glick, J. H. (2000). Conventional-dose chemotherapy compared with high-dose chemotherapy plus autologous hematopoietic stem-cell transplantation for metastatic breast cancer. Philadelphia Bone Marrow Transplant Group. *N. Engl. J. Med.* **342**(15), 1069–1076.

Tabar, L., Fagerberg, G., Chen, H.-H., Phil, C. M., Duffy, S. W., Smart, C. R., Gad, A., and Smith, R. A. (1995). Efficacy of breast cancer screening by age. New results from the Swedish Two-County Trial. *Cancer* **75**, 2507–2517.

Thune, I., Brenn, T., Lund, E., and Gaard, M. (1997). Physical activity and the risk of breast cancer. *N. Engl. J. Med.* **336**(18), 1269–1275.

Veronesi, U., Maisonneuve, P., Costa, A., Sacchini, V., Maltoni, C., Robertson, C., Rotmensz, N., and Boyle, P. (1998). Prevention of breast cancer with tamoxifen: Preliminary findings from the Italian randomised trial among hysterectomised women. *Lancet* **352**, 93–97.

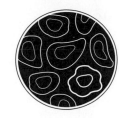

Camptothecins

Chris H. Takimoto

University of Texas Health Science Center at San Antonio

I. Historical Background
II. Mechanism of Action
III. Mechanisms of Resistance
IV. Specific Camptothecin Analogs
V. Conclusions

GLOSSARY

camptothecins A class of antitumor agents derived from the parent compound, camptothecin, a natural product found in the Chinese tree *Camptotheca acuminata*.

DNA–topoisomerase I cleavable complex Normally transient intermediate in the reaction catalyzed by topoisomerase I in which the protein is covalently bound to the DNA at the site of a single-stranded DNA break. Cleavable complexes are stabilized in the presence of camptothecin derivatives.

fork collision model Proposed mechanism by which camptothecins produce cell lethality. Drug-stabilized cleavable complexes interact with active DNA replication forks to generate cytotoxic DNA damage.

irinotecan A camptothecin derivative approved for the treatment of colorectal cancer.

irinotecan carboxylesterase-converting enzyme Carboxylesterase enzyme responsible for converting the prodrug irinotecan to the active agent, SN-38.

topoisomerase I Unique molecular target of camptothecin derivatives. An essential enzyme in mammalian cells that can relax supercoiled double-stranded DNA.

topotecan A water-soluble camptothecin derivative approved for the treatment of ovarian and small-cell lung cancer.

UGT1A1 Uridine diphosphate glucuronosyl transferase isoform responsible for glucuronidating the active metabolite of irinotecan, SN-38. Proposed as the rate-limiting step in the elimination of this metabolite.

Camptothecin derivatives are a novel group of antitumor agents with clinical utility in the treatment of human malignancies, including colorectal, lung, and ovarian tumors. Camptothecins uniquely target topoisomerase I, an enzyme that catalyzes the relaxation of torsionally strained double-stranded DNA. Camptothecins stabilize the binding of topoisomerase I to DNA and, in the presence of ongoing DNA synthesis, can generate potentially lethal DNA damage. Two camptothecin derivatives, topotecan and irinotecan, are commercially available for the treatment of human solid tumors in the United States. Several other camptothecins, including 9-aminocamptothecin, 9-nitrocamptothecin, GI47211, DX-8951f, homocamptothecin, and karenitecin, have been tested in clinical trials. Research on characterizing new agents that target topoisomerase I is an active area of anticancer drug development.

I. HISTORICAL BACKGROUND

In the 1950s, National Cancer Institute-sponsored screening studies found that extracts of the wood of the Chinese tree *Camptotheca acuminata* inhibited the growth of tumor cells (Table I). However, not until 1968 did Drs. Wani and Wall isolate and identify the active agent in these extracts as camptothecin (Fig. 1). In preclinical testing, camptothecin was active against a wide variety of tumors; however, its poor aqueous solubility required its formulation as the less active sodium salt for initial clinical testing. In early clinical trials in the 1970s, unpredictable and severe gastrointestinal toxicities and hemorrhage cystitis halted the further clinical development of camptothecin.

In the 1980s, a resurgence of interest in this class of agents was fueled by the discovery that camptothecins had a unique molecular target, the enzyme topoisomerase I. This key enzyme relaxed torsionally strained supercoiled DNA and it was postulated to be important for allowing normal DNA processes such as

transcription and replication to proceed. Even today, camptothecins remain the best-characterized inhibitors of this enzyme. At this same time, the new water-soluble camptothecin analogs, topotecan and irinotecan, were synthesized and formulated for intravenous use (Fig. 1). When early clinical trials of these agents in the late 1980s showed predictable dose-related toxicities and impressive antitumor activity, research on this novel class of drugs intensified.

In 1996, the U.S. Food and Drug Administration approved two camptothecin compounds for clinical use. Topotecan (Hycamtin) was approved for use as second-line therapy for advanced ovarian cancer, and irinotecan (Camptosar) was approved for use as second-line therapy for advanced colorectal cancer. Thus, in a single year, an entirely new class of drugs became available to the oncologist for the treatment of human solid tumors, thereby establishing topoisomerase I as an important target for cancer chemotherapy. Today, the use of camptothecin derivatives is increasing as their clinical activity is recognized in the treatment of a growing number of different human neoplasms.

II. MECHANISM OF ACTION

Human DNA topoisomerase I is a 100-kDa protein composed of 765 amino acids encoded for by a gene located on human chromosome 20. Expression of topoisomerase I is essential for all mammalian cells; however, yeast mutants completely lacking topoisomerase I have been identified. Interestingly, topoisom-

---

TABLE I
Camptothecin Developmental Time Line

1958	Extracts of the wood of the Asian tree *Camptotheca acuminata* are found to have antitumor activity in NCI screening studies
1966	Camptothecin identified by Drs. Wani and Wall
1971	Camptothecin induces reversible single-strand DNA breaks and inhibits DNA and RNA synthesis by unknown mechanisms
1970–1972	Phase I trials of the water-soluble camptothecin sodium salt demonstrate antitumor activity and unpredictable gastrointestinal and bladder toxicity, especially hemorrhagic cystitis
1985	Identification of topoisomerase I as the cellular target for camptothecin
1989	Synthesis of water-soluble camptothecin derivatives, such as CPT-11 (irinotecan) and topotecan, with promising preclinical activity in nude mouse/human tumor xenograft studies
1991	Phase I clinical trials of CPT-11 and topotecan demonstrate antitumor activity and mild toxicity
1993	Initiation of phase I clinical trials of 9-aminocamptothecin
1996	Topotecan and irinotecan approved by U.S. Food and Drug Administration

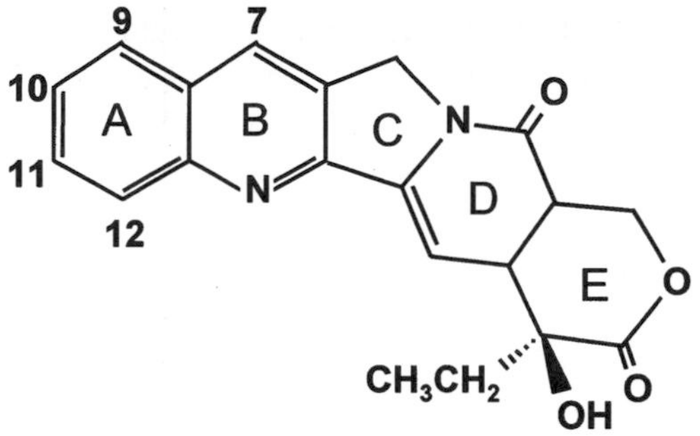

	C-11	C-10	C-9	C-7
Camptothecin	H	H	H	H
Topotecan	H	OH	$(CH_3)_2NCH_2$	H
9-AC	H	H	NH_2	H
9-NC	H	H	NO_2	H
SN-38	H	OH	H	CH_3CH_2
Irinotecan	H	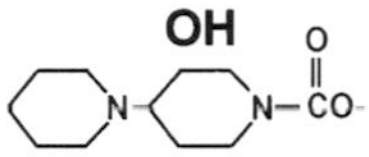 (piperidine-N—N-CO-O)	H	CH_3CH_2

FIGURE 1 Camptothecin chemical structures.

erase I has been recognized as the major antigenic epitope responsible for the autoimmune disease scleroderma.

Human topoisomerase I catalyzes the relaxation of both positively and negatively supercoiled double-stranded DNA. Unwinding of the double helix during DNA replication or RNA transcription generates torsional strain above and below the region of strand separation. Topoisomerase I can relax this localized super coiling, thereby allowing these important DNA functions to proceed in an orderly fashion. Topoisomerase I may be particularly important in facilitating RNA transcription. Supporting evidence comes from immunohistochemical studies demonstrating high levels of topoisomerase I in the nucleolus, which is actively involved in RNA synthesis. Furthermore, topoisomerase I associates intracellularly with RNA polymerase II and with other transcriptionally active proteins. Treatment of cell with camptothecin interferes with these processes and causes topoisomerase I to redistribute to nonnucleolar regions of the nucleus.

Human DNA topoisomerase I preferentially binds to torsionally strained supercoiled double-stranded DNA, resulting in cleavage of one of the phosphodiester backbones, causing a single-stranded nick in the DNA (Fig. 2). During this process, a transient intermediate, called the cleavable complex, is formed in which the topoisomerase I enzyme is temporarily bound at a tyrosine residue at position 723 to the 3′ end of the single-stranded break in the DNA. The structure of the cleavable complex allows for relaxation of the strain in the supercoiled DNA, either by passage of the intact single strand through the gap in the nicked DNA or by free rotation of the DNA about the noncleaved strand. Finally, religation and dissociation restore the integrity of the now relaxed DNA helix. Unlike type II topoisomerases, no energy-dependent cofactors are required for this reaction. Topoisomerase I cleavage sites do not occur randomly throughout the genome; instead, weak consensus DNA sequences exist.

Camptothecins noncovalently interact with DNA-bound topoisomerase I and inhibit the religation step, resulting in a drug-induced stabilization of the cleavable complex. However, the accumulation of stabilized cleavable complexes and the resulting persistence of single-stranded breaks in the DNA are not inherently toxic to the cell because these lesions are highly reversible and can disappear rapidly on drug removal. However, if DNA synthesis is ongoing, the interaction of a DNA replication fork with a stabilized cleavable complex can potentially generate lethal cytotoxic double-stranded breaks in the DNA. According to this "fork collision model," first proposed by Liu and colleagues, cleavable complex formation is necessary but not sufficient for

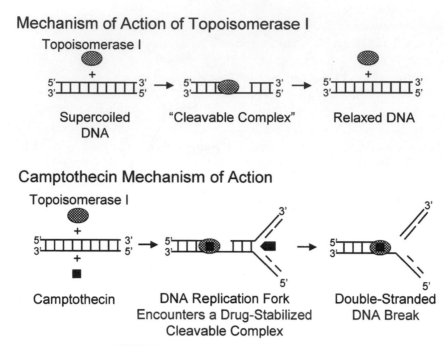

FIGURE 2 Camptothecin mechanism of action.

camptothecin-induced cytotoxicity. Inhibition of DNA synthesis by agents such as aphidicolin or hydroxyurea, can protect cells from camptothecin-induced cell death. The unique mechanism of action of camptothecins has important clinical consequences. First, because of the need for ongoing DNA synthesis, camptothecins are, by definition, predominantly S-phase cell cycle-specific agents, which has been confirmed in most experimental studies. Cell cycle-specific agents generally require more prolonged cell exposures times to drug concentrations above a minimum threshold in order to maximize the fractional cell kill. Thus, one would predict a priori that camptothecins should be relatively schedule-dependent agents. Furthermore, the presence of topoisomerase I protein is an absolute requirement for the generation of drug-induced cytotoxicity. Mutant yeast cells lacking functional DNA topoisomerase I are completely resistant to camptothecins. However, transfection of topoisomerase I into these mutant cells can restore drug sensitivity.

Thus, camptothecins are distinct from classic antimetabolite enzyme inhibitors that strive to eliminate the function of key essential enzymes, such as methotrexate inhibition of dihydrofolate reductase or fluoropyrimidine metabolites that inhibit thymidylate synthase. Instead, camptothecins are biologically active because they convert a normal endogenous cellular protein, topoisomerase I, into a potent molecular poison. Consequently, some investigators have suggested that the term topoisomerase I poisons be used for this class of drugs instead of topoisomerase I inhibitors.

III. MECHANISMS OF RESISTANCE

Little is known about the mechanisms of camptothecin resistance in clinical tumors; however, in laboratory cell lines, several different mechanisms of drug resistance have been characterized. Numerous point mutations in topoisomerase I have been identified that confer a relative resistance to camptothecins without abolishing its enzymatic catalytic activity. These single amino acid substitutions can span a large portion of the protein. However, no topoisomerase I mutations have been identified in drug-resistant tumors obtained from patients. Insensitivity to camptothecins can also result from decreased topoisomerase I activity resulting from decreased enzyme expression, although the regulatory mechanisms responsible for altering the topoisomerase I content of cells have not been clearly identified.

Drug efflux out of the cell may be important for camptothecin sensitivity. The P-glycoprotein-associated multidrug resistance (MDR) phenotype may play a partial role in the resistance to some camptothecins analogs, such as topotecan, which are modestly active substrates for this drug efflux pump. Other camptothecins, such as the active metabolite of irinotecan (SN-38), appear to be relatively poor substrates for P-glycoprotein or other well-characterized drug efflux systems. Interestingly, a recently discovered new membrane drug transporter was identified in mitoxantrone-resistant tumors cells that conferred cross-resistance to numerous camptothecin analogs. Further studies of the clinical relevance of this drug transporter are in progress.

IV. SPECIFIC CAMPTOTHECINS ANALOGS

A. Topotecan (Hycamtin)

Topotecan [(S)-10-[(dimethylamino)methyl]-4-ethyl-4,9-dihydroxy-1H-pyrano[3',4':6,7] indolizino [1,2- b] quinoline-3,14-(4H,12H)-dione monohydrochloride] is a water-soluble camptothecin derivative containing a basic side chain at position C-9 on the A ring of 10-hydroxycamptothecin (Fig. 1). Phase I trials of topotecan were initiated in 1989 by SmithKline Beecham in collaboration with the National Cancer Institute, and in 1996 it was approved for use in the United States as second-line chemotherapy in patients with advanced ovarian cancer. In 1998, it was also approved for the treatment of recurrent small cell lung cancer.

In preclinical studies, topotecan showed a broad range of activity in human tumor xenografts, including activity in colon, ovarian, central nervous system tumors, rhabdomyosarcoma, osteosarcoma, and medulloblastoma tumors. Its excellent water solubility allowed it to be easily administered intravenously. Like most camptothecins, topotecan contains a terminal α-hydroxy lactone ring that is unstable in aqueous solutions and can undergo a rapid, nonenzymatic

hydrolysis to form the less active, open-ring hydroxy carboxylic acid. Following intravenous administration, the majority of the circulating drug is in the carboxylate form and it is not highly protein bound. In animal studies, penetration into the cerebrospinal fluid (CSF) resulted in CSF concentrations of topotecan that were about 32% of the simultaneously generated plasma concentrations. Thus, topotecan penetration into the CNS is relatively higher than most other camptothecins. Hepatic metabolism is thought to be responsible for the formation of an N-desmethyl plasma metabolite, but the clinical relevance of this is not clear because the major route of drug excretion appears to be via the kidneys. Most of the clinical experience with topotecan has been as an intravenous administration, although oral preparations have been tested clinically. Because of its predominant renal clearance, dose adjustments are warranted for patients with decreased glomerular filtration rates. In contrast, dose adjustments in hepatic dysfunction are less important and not routinely recommended.

The major dose-limiting toxicity of topotecan is noncumulative, reversible neutropenia. The greatest clinical experience has been administering topotecan intravenously on a daily times five schedule, and the median time to blood count nadir is about 9 days after the initiation of therapy. Most patients can be treated every 3 weeks. Thrombocytopenia and anemia occur less frequently, and most other toxicities are generally mild and well tolerated, consisting of nausea, vomiting, mild diarrhea, fatigue, alopecia, occasional skin rash, and elevated liver function tests. In leukemia patients treated at very high doses, mucositis and diarrhea were dose limiting. Interestingly, topotecan does not appear to cause the hemorrhagic cystitis that was observed in the early clinical trials of the parent compound, camptothecin. In addition, severe and profound diarrhea, such as that seen with irinotecan, is also uncommon.

Randomized phase III trials have demonstrated the utility of topotecan single-agent therapy in patients with advanced ovarian cancer who progress following treatment with prior platinum-based chemotherapy. Overall, antitumor efficacy activity was not significantly different than single-agent paclitaxel therapy for these patients. In lung cancer, topotecan has proven activity in recurrent small cell lung cancer with equivalent efficacy compared to the three-drug combination regimen of cyclophosphamide, doxorubicin, and vincristine in patients previously treated with etoposide and cisplatin. Lesser degrees of activity have been reported in nonsmall cell lung cancer patients. Topotecan also has promising activity in hematologic malignancies, including the difficult to treat myelodysplastic syndromes, and research on its activity in pediatric malignancies is ongoing. In contrast to irinotecan, topotecan has not demonstrated meaningful clinical activity in gastrointestinal tumors.

Combination chemotherapy regimens with topotecan have been performed with a wide variety of agents. These include two drug combinations with drugs such as cisplatin, paclitaxel, doxorubicin, etoposide, cyclophosphamide, and cytarabine. None of these topotecan combinations are firmly established as standard regimens for the treatment of any specific cancers to date. Nonetheless, there is great optimism that the use of these topotecan combinations up front as first-line therapy for diseases such as ovarian or small cell lung cancer may ultimately improve clinical outcomes.

B. Irinotecan

Irinotecan [(S)-4,11-diethyl-3,4,12,14-tetrahydro-4-hydroxy-3,14-dioxo-1H-pyrano13',4':6,7]-indolizino[1,2-b]quinolin-9-yl-[1,4'-bipiperidine]-1'-carboxylate, monohydrochloride, or CPT-11] was originally developed in Asia by the Yakult Honsha and Daiichi pharmaceutical companies. Irinotecan is unique among the camptothecin derivatives in that it is a prodrug that must first be converted by a carboxylesterase-converting enzyme to the active metabolite, SN-38 (Fig. 3). It was first approved in Japan for the treatment of nonsmall cell lung cancer and later for the treatment of small cell lung, cervical, gastric, and ovarian cancers. In Europe and North America, irinotecan was predominantly developed for the treatment of gastrointestinal malignancies, and in 1996 it was approved in the United States for use in patients with advanced colorectal cancer following 5-fluorouracil (5-FU) chemotherapy. This was the first new anticancer agent to become available for the treatment of this disease in the United States in over 35 years. In 2000, it was approved for use in newly diagnosed patients with metastatic colorectal cancer when combined with 5-FU and calcium leucovorin.

In preclinical studies, irinotecan was active in human tumor xenografts, including colon, mammary, gastric, and lung cancers. The most common route of administration is as a short intravenous infusion either weekly for 4 out of 6 weeks or every 3 weeks. Because it is a prodrug, relatively short infusions of irinotecan can generate plasma concentrations of SN-38 that persist over a longer period of time than most other camptothecins. However, the efficiency of enzymatic conversion of irinotecan to SN-38 is low, with the to-

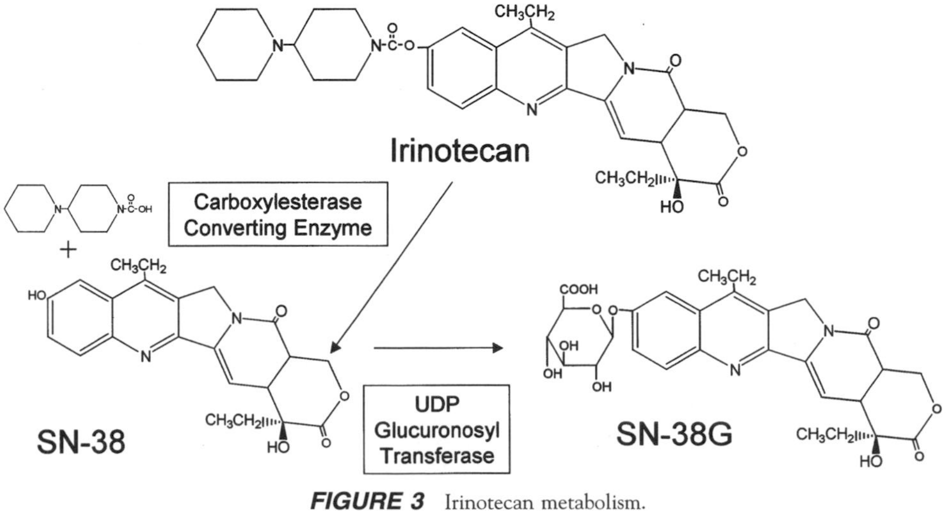

FIGURE 3 Irinotecan metabolism.

tal systemic exposure to the metabolite comprising only about 3–4% of the corresponding parental drug on the typical weekly or every 3-week schedule. Marked variation in the plasma concentrations of the active metabolite is thought to result from enzymatic variations in both the metabolic activation of irinotecan and the hepatic glucuronidation and biliary excretion clearance pathways. Interestingly, the active lactone species of SN-38 is more stable than most other camptothecin lactone derivatives, suggesting that a relatively larger portion of the circulating drug in plasma is biologically active. SN-38 is relatively highly protein bound, and its predominant mechanism of clearance is via the liver. In exact contrast to topotecan, irinotecan dose modification appears to be very important for patients with impaired liver function, especially those with hyperbilirubinemia. Unfortunately, formal guidelines for the treatment of patients with hepatic function impairment with irinotecan have not yet been developed.

The predominant site of drug activation is not known, but it is thought to be in the liver and the gastrointestinal tract, which are relatively rich in carboxylesterase activity. Irinotecan is also catabolized by the hepatic cytochrome P450 system to form several mostly inactive metabolites. Pharmacogenetic variation may be an important predictor of clinical drug toxicity. For example, the uridine diphosphate glucuronosyl transferase enzyme, isoform UGT1A1, is known to be the rate-limiting step in converting SN-38 to the glucuronide, SN-38G. Patients with Gilbert's syndrome are genetically deficient in this enzyme, and preliminary evidence suggests that they may be at risk for severe toxicity following standard doses of irinotecan chemotherapy. Research into the value of pharmacogenetic screening for this condition is ongoing. Thus, the overall pharmacology of irinotecan is quite complex (Fig. 3) due to its enzymatic activation and clearance and due to the number of different metabolites generated.

The major clinical dose-limiting toxicity of irinotecan is severe delayed diarrhea. This side effect can be ameliorated somewhat by the use of an intensive oral loperamide antidiarrheal regimen that is now a standard supportive therapy for irinotecan chemotherapy. Irinotecan can also induce an acute onset cholinergic syndrome associated with acute secretory diarrhea, flushing, nausea, and possible hypertension. This symptom complex is thought to be related to the anticholinesterase activity of the parent compound; however, it is usually easily treated with atropine. Myelosuppression, especially neutropenia, is also frequently observed with irinotecan, with thrombocytopenia and anemia being less common. Other toxicities include mild-to-moderate nausea and vomiting, mucositis, elevated liver function tests, fatigue, and mild-to-moderate alopecia. Rare pulmonary interstitial infiltrates have also been observed.

In 1996, the demonstration that second-line therapy with irinotecan could improve survival in patients with advanced colorectal cancer after treatment with 5-fluorouracil and leucovorin led to the initial approval of this agent in the United States. More recently, a randomized study comparing the combination of irinotecan and 5-FU plus leucovorin to either agent alone was conducted in untreated patients with advanced colorectal cancer. An overall modest survival advantage was seen in the combination arm, leading to the adoption of this regimen as standard treatment for newly diagnosed patients with colorectal cancer in 2000. In small cell lung cancer, preliminary reports suggest that a small survival advantage exists for newly diagnosed patients treated with irinotecan and cisplatin compared to standard therapy with etoposide and cisplatin. Thus, it is highly likely that the use of irinotecan will further expand to other tumors besides colorectal cancer in the near future. Combination trials of irinotecan and agents such as gemcitabine, carboplatin, paclitaxel, oxaliplatin, and etoposide have all been performed. Irinotecan is probably the most clinically useful camptothecin analogue that has been developed to date.

C. 9-Aminocamptothecin

9-Aminocamptothecin (9-AC) is a water-insoluble camptothecin derivative (Fig. 1) with impressive preclinical activity in human xenograft models of malignant melanoma, prostate, breast, ovarian, bladder, and especially colon cancer. In three human colon cancer xenografts, 9-AC was highly active with minimal systemic toxicity and produced the best antitumor response compared to a panel of nine anticancer agents, including 5-fluorouracil, doxorubicin, melphalan, methotrexate, vincristine, vinblastine, and several nitrosourea compounds.

In pharmacokinetic studies, the amount of 9-AC present in plasma relative to total drug (lactone + carboxylate) levels is quite low, with most reported being values below 10%. This observation is consistent with earlier studies demonstrating greater instability of 9-AC lactone in human plasma compared with other camptothecin derivatives, such as topotecan or irinotecan. Urinary clearance accounted for about one-third of the administered drug, and no metabolites of 9-AC have been identified.

Clinical testing of 9-AC began in 1993 with initial phase I trials using a 72-h infusion every 2 or 3 weeks. Later trials examined various different schedules, including prolonged 120-h infusions weekly for 3 and 4 weeks. On all schedules, the major dose-limiting toxicities were neutropenia and, to a lesser extent, thrombocytopenia. Other common toxicities included anemia, fatigue, nausea and vomiting, diarrhea, alopecia, and mucositis. 9-AC is not associated with pulmonary toxicity or hemorrhagic cystitis, and the diarrhea it produces is much less severe than that seen with irinotecan.

In phase II studies of 72-h infusions of 9-AC, no meaningful activity was seen in colorectal or non-small cell lung cancer and only modest responses were seen in ovarian, small cell lung, and malignant lymphoma. Thus, despite its impressive preclinical activity in human colon cancer xenografts models, 9-AC has not shown effective antitumor activity in the clinical studies completed to date. One potential explanation for this discrepancy may be the inability to achieve the necessary plasma drug concentrations needed for antitumor efficacy. Because of the greater sensitivity of human bone marrow stem cells to 9-AC compared with murine bone marrow, dose-limiting myelosuppression made it impossible to achieve the same plasma drug concentrations in humans that were associated with optimal antitumor efficacy in the preclinical animal models. At present, the development of 9-AC has largely been halted.

D. 9-Nitrocamptothecin

9-Nitrocamptothecin (9-NC) is an inherently active camptothecin analog (Fig. 1) that is also converted

in vivo into the active metabolite, 9-AC. In preclinical studies, it has excellent activity in nude mice bearing human tumor xenografts, including melanoma, breast, and ovarian cancers. 9-NC is predominantly being developed as an oral agent, and its principal toxicities are myelosuppression, alopecia, and hemorrhagic cystitis. Interestingly, after oral dosing of 9-NC, plasma concentrations of 9-AC above 200 nM were achieved and sustained for several hours, suggesting a promising pharmacokinetic profile. Phase III trials in advanced pancreatic cancer are ongoing.

E. GI47211

GI47211 [7-(methylpiperazinomethylene)-10,11-ethylene-dioxy-20(S)] camptothecin dihydrochloride is a water-soluble synthetic analog of camptothecin that has also undergone clinical testing. The principal dose-limiting toxicities of GI47211 were neutropenia and thrombocytopenia, with most other toxicities, such as nausea and vomiting, headaches, alopecia, and fatigue, being mild in severity. Although some antitumor activity has been observed, the free drug is not currently in large-scale clinical development. Phase I testing of a liposomal formulation of this agent is in progress and may improve the therapeutic index.

F. Newer Agents

Several newer camptothecin derivatives are currently in clinical testing. These include DX-8951f (Exotecan), homocamptothecin, and kareniticin. DX8951f is highly potent and has promising activity in pancreatic cancer and other tumors. Homocamptothecin is a novel camptothecin with a modified terminal lactone ring with increased chemical stability. Kareniticin is a lipophilic silicon-containing camptothecin derivative that also is very stable in aqueous solutions.

V. CONCLUSIONS

Camptothecin topoisomerase I-targeting agents now have an established role in the treatment of human tumors, and their use is growing in the treatment of an increasing number of different types of malignancies. Major areas of ongoing clinical research include testing these agents as front-line treatments for newly diagnosed cancers and developing new clinically useful camptothecin-containing combination chemotherapy regimens. In addition, many new and promising camptothecin derivatives are also in clinical development. Thus, although substantial advances have been achieved since the first camptothecin derivatives became available in 1996, we are still quite far from reaching the full potential of this important class of antitumor agents.

See Also the Following Articles

Colorectal Cancer • Lung Cancer • Ovarian Cancer • Resistance to Topoisomerase-Targeting Agents

Bibliography

Bjornsti, M. A., Benedetti, P., Viglianti, G. A., and Wang, J. C. (1989). Expression of human DNA topoisomerase I in yeast cells lacking yeast DNA topoisomerase I: Restoration of sensitivity of the cells to the antitumor drug camptothecin. *Cancer Res.* **49**(22), 6318–6323.

Doyle, L. A., Yang, W., Abruzzo, L. V., Krogmann, T., Gao, Y., Rishi, A. K., and Ross, D. D. (1998). A multidrug resistance transporter from human MCF-7 breast cancer cells. *Proc. Natl. Acad. Sci. USA* **95**(26), 15665–15670.

Giovanella, B. C., Stehlin, J. S., Wall, M. E., Wani, M. C., Nicholas, A. W., Liu, L. F., Silber, R., and Potmesil, M. (1989). DNA topoisomerase I: Targeted chemotherapy of human colon cancer in xenografts. *Science* **246**(4933), 1046–1048.

Hsiang, Y. H., and Liu, L. F. (1988). Identification of mammalian DNA topoisomerase I as an intracellular target of the anticancer drug camptothecin. *Cancer Res.* **48**(7), 1722–1726.

Iyer, L., Hall, D., Das, S., Mortell, M. A., Ramirez, J., Kim, S., Di Rienzo, A., and Ratain, M. J. (1999). Phenotype-genotype correlation of in vitro SN-38 (active metabolite of irinotecan) and bilirubin glucuronidation in human liver tissue with UGT1A1 promoter polymorphism. *Clin. Pharmacol. Ther.* **65**(5), 576–582.

Juan, C. C., Hwang, J. L., Liu, A. A., Whang-Peng, J., Knutsen, T., Huebner, K., Cruce, C. M., Zhang, H., Wang, J. C., and Liu, L. F. (1988). Human DNA topoisomerase I is encoded by a single-copy gene that maps to chromosome region 20q12-13.2. *Proc. Natl. Acad. Sci. USA* **85**(23), 8910–8913.

Nitiss, J. L., and Wang, J. C. (1996). Mechanisms of cell killing by drugs that trap covalent complexes between DNA topoisomerases and DNA. *Mol. Pharmacol.* **50**(5), 1095–1102.

Saltz, L. B., Cox, J. V., Blanke, C., Rosen, L. S., Fehrenbacher, L., Moore, M. J., Maroun, J. A., Ackland, S. P., Locker, P. K., Pirotta, N., Elfring, G. L., and Miller, L. L. (2000). Irinotecan plus fluorouracil and leucovorin for metastatic colorectal cancer: Irinotecan Study Group. *N. Engl. J. Med.* **343**(13), 905–914.

ten Bokkel Huinink, W., Gore, M., Carmichael, J., Gordon, A., Malfetano, J., Hudson, I., Broom, C., Scarabelli, C., Davidson, N., Spanczynski, M., Bolis, G., Malmstrom, H., Coleman, R., Fields, S. C., and Heron, J. F. (1997). Topotecan versus paclitaxel for the treatment of recurrent epithelial ovarian cancer. *J. Clin. Oncol.* **15**(6), 2183–2193.

von Pawel, J., Schiller, J. H., Shepherd, F. A., Fields, S. Z., Kleisbauer, J. P., Chrysson, N. G., Stewart, D. J., Clark, P. I., Palmer, M. C., Depierre, A., Carmichael, J., Krebs, J. B., Ross, G., Lane, S. R., and Gralla, R. (1999). Topotecan versus cyclophosphamide, doxorubicin, and vincristine for the treatment of recurrent small-cell lung cancer. *J. Clin. Oncol.* **17**(2), 658–667.

Wall, M. E., Wani, M. C., Cook, C. E., Palmer, K. H., McPhail, H. T., and Sim, G. A. (1966). Plant antitumor agents. I. The isolation and structure of camptothecin, a novel alkaloidal leukemia and tumor inhibitor from *Camptotheca acuminata*. *J. Am. Chem. Soc.* **88**, 3888–3890.

Wasserman, E., Myara, A., Lokiec, F., Goldwasser, F., Trivin, F., Mahjoubi, M., Misset, J. L., and Cvitkovic, E. (1997). Severe CPT-11 toxicity in patients with Gilbert's syndrome: Two case reports. *Ann. Oncol.* **8**(10), 1049–1051.

Cancer Risk Reduction (Diet/Smoking Cessation/ Lifestyle Changes)

Peter Greenwald
National Cancer Institute, National Institutes of Health, Bethesda, Maryland

Darrell E. Anderson
Sharon S. McDonald
Scientific Consulting Group, Inc., Gaithersburg, Maryland

GLOSSARY

enzyme A protein molecule produced by living organisms that catalyzes chemical reactions of other substances without itself being destroyed or altered upon completion of the reactions.

epidemiology The science concerned with the study of factors determining and influencing the frequency and distribution of disease and other health-related events and their causes in a defined human population.

gene–nutrient interaction The influence exerted by genes and nutrients on each other. The action may be unilateral or reciprocal and usually involves the alteration of metabolic pathways or products.

micronutrient A vitamin or mineral that the body must obtain from outside sources. Micronutrients are essential to the body in small amounts because they are either components of enzymes (the minerals) or act as coenzymes in managing chemical reactions.

oncogene Mutated and/or overexpressed version of a normal gene that in a dominant fashion can release the cell from normal restraints on growth and thus, alone or in concert with other changes, convert a cell into a tumor cell.

pharmacotherapy The treatment of diseases or conditions by medicines.

polymorphism The occurrence of different forms (alleles) of a gene (typically greater than 1%) in individual organisms or in organisms of the same species, independent of sexual variations.

primary prevention The identification, control, and avoidance of environmental factors related to cancer development.

randomized, controlled trials A clinical trial that uses a control group of people given an inactive substance (placebo) and an intervention group given the substance or action under study.

sunscreen A substance applied to the skin to protect it from the effects of the sun's rays; sunscreens act by either absorbing ultraviolet (UV) radiation or reflecting incident light. Their effectiveness is rated by their sun protection factor (SPF); e.g., a sunscreen with an SPF of 15 allows only 1/15 of the incident UV radiation or light to reach the skin.

$\mathbf{M}$any cases of cancer can be prevented. Generally, people can reduce their risks for developing cancer by making wise lifestyle choices such as eating low-fat, high-fiber diets that include a variety of vegetables and fruits, avoiding tobacco use, being physically active, and minimizing sun exposure. Specific genetic susceptibilities, however, can influence cancer risk associated with certain lifestyle factors, and variation in risk exists among individuals. Guidelines for implementing lifestyle choices to reduce cancer risk have been formulated to help people adopt cancer-protective behaviors.

I. INTRODUCTION

The risk of developing cancer, a disease that affects many millions of people worldwide, can be reduced markedly by approaches that encourage primary prevention. A landmark report by Doll and Peto in 1981 summarized the evidence relating lifestyle choices, including diet, tobacco use, and sun exposure, as well as other environmental factors (e.g., occupation, ionizing radiation), to cancer risk. The report suggested that 75–80% of cancer cases were potentially avoidable and that dietary factors, tobacco use, and sun exposure were associated with approximately 35, 30, and 1–2%, respectively, of all cancers. Scientists now recognize that the effects of environmental factors, including lifestyle choices, on cancer risk can be influenced by a person's genetic susceptibility.

II. DIET

A. The Diet–Cancer Relationship

A considerable body of evidence—experimental, epidemiologic, and clinical—indicates that dietary factors, both individual food constituents and dietary patterns, play a major role in determining cancer risk. Generally, the evidence supports inverse associations between cancer risk and intakes of vegetables, fruits, whole grains, dietary fiber, certain micronutrients, and certain types of fat (e.g., n-3 fatty acids, particularly n-3/n-6 fatty acid ratios), as well as direct associations between cancer risk and intakes of excessive calories, alcohol, total fat, and certain types of fat (e.g., saturated fat). To illustrate, epidemiologic studies have provided consistent and convincing evidence for increased cancer risk when migrants from countries with a low-fat, high-fiber diet adopt the high-fat, low-fiber diet characteristic of Western countries. The Western countries also have higher rates of obesity. Of interest is the possible cancer-protective Mediterranean diet, which emphasizes a high intake of vegetables, fruits, whole grains, fish (high in n-3 fatty acids), and olive oil (high in monosaturated fatty acids). Interactions likely occur among many dietary constituents. However, neither these interactions nor their influence on cancer risk is well understood. Thus, at present it is difficult to tease out the specific effects of individual dietary components from diet and cancer research data.

Randomized, controlled trials (RCTs) offer one of the best means for testing diet and cancer hypotheses developed from the insights provided by epidemiologic and experimental studies. Among specific dietary constituents investigated in RCTs, vitamins A, C, and E, folic acid, calcium, and selenium have shown promise in reducing cancer risk at certain sites (e.g., vitamin E and selenium for prostate cancer). Some diet and cancer trials include efforts to modify certain lifestyle choices other than diet, such as smoking and level of physical activity, that also could influence cancer risk and thus influence study results.

B. Gene–Nutrient Interactions

Cancer risk reduction by dietary modification likely will depend, in part, on increased understanding of both gene–nutrient interactions and the role of genetic differences (polymorphisms) among individuals. Genes involved in carcinogenesis influence metabolic activation/detoxification, DNA repair, chromosome stability, activity of oncogenes or tumor suppressors, cell cycle control, signal transduction, hormonal pathways, vitamin metabolism pathways, immune function, and receptor or neurotransmitter action. Exposure to the same quantitative level of dietary factor(s) or dietary carcinogens can increase cancer risk in one individual but not in another, depending on specific susceptibilities to gene–nutrient interactions. For example, an intake of heterocyclic amines (HAs), produced by grilling of meat, increases the risk of colorectal cancer. However, people with polymorphic forms of the enzymes N-acetyltransferase type 2 (NAT2) and cytochrome P4501A2 (CYP1A2), which cause rapid activation of HAs, have a greater risk of colorectal cancer than people with polymorphic forms that cause a slow activation of HAs. Folate, found in green, leafy vegetables, is also associated with polymorphisms and cancer risk. A specific polymorphism in the gene that codes for methylenetetrahydrofolate reductase—an enzyme critical to DNA methylation and synthesis—can reduce colorectal cancer risk by altering cellular responses to dietary folate and methionine.

Understanding gene–nutrient interactions and individual differences in genetic susceptibilities may lead to future dietary intervention strategies to reduce cancer risk. Focusing on polymorphisms in intervention studies allows investigators to develop study designs, stratify participants, and analyze results based on genetic differences within the study population. For example, polymorphisms in genes affecting the use of vitamin D confer different levels of risk for prostate cancer—a fourfold increase in risk among individuals with one polymorphism and a 60% reduction in risk among individuals with another. This kind of information is important for researchers designing trials to investigate the role of vitamin D, or its analogs, in prostate cancer risk. As more knowledge is gained about how genetic polymorphisms influence cancer risk through specific dietary constituents or patterns, researchers can refine recommendations for healthful eating regimens to reduce cancer risk.

TABLE I
National Cancer Institute Dietary Guidelines

Reduce fat intake to 30% or less of calories

Increase fiber intake to 20 to 30 g daily, with an upper limit of 35 g

Include a variety of vegetables and fruits in the daily diet

Avoid obesity

Consume alcoholic beverages in moderation, if at all

Minimize consumption of salt-cured, salt-pickled, and smoked foods

C. Dietary Guidelines

As research continues into the role of specific dietary constituents in cancer risk, it is important that clinicians and the public be advised about the importance of modifying diets to reduce cancer risk. Since the mid-1970s, various scientific organizations around the world, including the World Cancer Research Fund (WCRF) in association with the American Institute for Cancer Research (AICR), the American Cancer Society (ACS), and the U.S. National Cancer Institute (NCI), have developed dietary guidelines to promote cancer risk reduction as a population strategy. The guidelines of the NCI, outlined in Table I, are in agreement with dietary guidelines developed by other organizations. The average American, according to the latest national health assessment, consumes too much fat (too much saturated fat, too little monosaturated fat), too little fiber, and too few vegetables, fruits, and whole grains. This pattern is seen in many developed countries worldwide. People should be encouraged to adhere to dietary guidelines that promote good health. It is incumbent that physicians, nutritionists, and registered dietitians play a key role in advocating healthful diets that have the potential to reduce cancer risk and are beneficial overall.

III. SMOKING CESSATION

A. Smoking and Cancer Risk

Lung cancer is the most common cancer in the world, accounting for almost 13% of all cancers (18% for men, 7% for women). Smoking is the single most important lifestyle factor contributing to lung cancer incidence worldwide. In fact, at least 20 carcinogens that are components of tobacco smoke cause lung tumors in either animals or humans. In addition to lung cancer, smoking substantially increases the risk for cancers of the larynx, oral cavity, and esophagus and contributes to risk for cancers of the pancreas, uterine cervix, kidney, and bladder. People may have different susceptibilities to developing smoking-related cancers because of genetic variations in their metabolism of tobacco smoke carcinogens. Furthermore, the adverse effects of smoking on cancer risk can be enhanced by alcohol consumption and by the presence of other environmental carcinogens, particularly radon and asbestos.

In many areas of the world, particularly in third-world countries, tobacco use is rising. Although it is estimated that as many as 30% of cancers in developed counties are tobacco related, tobacco use in these countries remains high. In the United States, about one-fourth of adults currently smoke, and tobacco use among high school students has increased steadily since the early 1990s. Results of a national 1999 survey show that almost 35% of high school students smoke.

Nonsmokers exposed to environmental tobacco smoke (ETS), as a result of either household or occupational exposure, inhale and metabolize components of the smoke and thus also may be at increased risk for lung cancer. An analysis of 37 case-control and cohort studies indicated that, for men and women combined, the risk of lung cancer increased by 23% for a nonsmoker who lived with a smoker; also, risk appeared to be directly related to the number of cigarettes smoked by the spouse and the duration of exposure.

Educational strategies to prevent the start of smoking by adolescents and smoking cessation approaches to stop tobacco use by smokers permanently are among the most effective ways to reduce cancer risk. Although 70% of smokers claim to be interested in quitting smoking, most of them have no immediate plans to quit. When smokers try to quit on their own, relapse in the majority occurs within days, and only about 7% achieve long-term success. However, long-term success rates can be increased to 15–30% if interventions such as pharmacotherapies and intensive counseling are used. A combination of pharmacotherapy and counseling should be used for adult smokers trying to quit, except for light smokers (< 10 cigarettes/day), women who are either pregnant or breastfeeding, or when pharmacotherapy is medically contraindicated.

B. Pharmacotherapies for Smoking Cessation

Nicotine, present in all tobacco products, is an addictive substance. For most users, tobacco use results in true drug dependence. Not all smokers, however, have the same level of nicotine dependence; a high number of cigarettes smoked each day, frequent smoking in the morning, and smoking while ill indicate a high dependence level. Evidence demonstrating that pharmacotherapies can help people addicted to nicotine quit smoking is strong and consistent, and several pharmacotherapies—primarily nicotine replacement therapies (NRTs)—have been approved for smoking cessation by the U.S. Food and Drug Administration (Table II). All currently approved pharmacotherapies approximately double the chances that an attempt to quit smoking will be successful. Abundant evidence confirms that both nicotine gum and nicotine patches are safe and effective aids to smoking cessation. Nicotine nasal spray, which delivers larger doses of nicotine more rapidly than nicotine gum and patches, is also an effective smoking cessation aid. The nicotine inhaler, a plastic rod containing a plug impregnated with nicotine, is designed to combine pharmacologic and behavioral substitution

TABLE II
Pharmacotherapies for Smoking Cessation

Pharmacotherapy	Availability	Side effects
Nicotine gum	Over-the-counter only	Mouth soreness Indigestion
Nicotine patch	Over-the-counter and prescription	Skin reaction at patch site Insomnia
Nicotine nasal spray	Prescription only	Nasal/throat irritation Sneezing, coughing
Nicotine inhaler	Prescription only	Mouth/throat irritation Coughing
Bupropion	Prescription only	Dry mouth Insomnia

strategies; it results in blood levels of nicotine similar to those from use of nicotine gum. Bupropion, an antidepressant and the only approved nonnicotine pharmacotherapy, appears to be an effective aid to smoking cessation and is safe even when used jointly with NRT. Although bupropion likely does not influence smoking cessation via its antidepressant effect, its mechanism of action is unclear.

C. Behavioral Interventions

Behavioral interventions can range from minimal intervention, such as a 3-min intervention during a routine visit to a physician, to intensive group or one-on-one counseling using multiple sessions. In the United States, more than 70% of smokers visit a healthcare setting every year, providing an excellent opportunity for brief advice and counseling. In fact, patients who smoke expect their physician to inquire into their smoking habits and advise them regarding cessation techniques. Studies show that brief physician advice to quit smoking can produce cessation rates of 5–10% each year. Simple intervention strategies that can be used by physicians to help their patients stop smoking are outlined in Table III. Effective counseling is essential to help a smoker who is willing to quit achieve long-term success in smoking cessation. Practical counseling that provides coping strategies and basic information about smoking/quitting, social support offered as part of treatment, and social support arranged outside of treatment (e.g., community resources) all are important components of effective counseling.

IV. LIFESTYLE CHANGES

A. Physical Activity

Regular physical activity is associated with reduced all-cancer mortality through various mechanisms, including altering hormone levels and increasing immune system activity, energy expenditure, and antioxidant activity. Of particular interest is the role of

---

TABLE III

Synopsis for Physicians: How to Help Your Patients Stop Smoking[a]

Ask about smoking at every opportunity
  a. "Do you smoke?" If so, "How much?"
  b. "How soon after waking do you have your first cigarette?"
  c. "Are you interested in stopping smoking?"
  d. "Have you ever tried to stop before?" If so, "What happened?"

Advise all smokers to stop
  a. State advice clearly, e.g., "As your physician, I must advise you to stop smoking now."
  b. Personalize the message to quit. Refer to the patient's clinical condition, smoking history, family history, personal interests, or social roles.

Assist the patient in stopping
  a. Set a quit date. Help the patient pick a date within the next 4 weeks.
  b. Provide self-help materials. Review the materials with the patient, if desired.
  c. Consider prescribing nicotine replacement therapy, especially for highly addicted patients (smoke one pack or more a day or smoke within 30 min of waking).
  d. Consider signing a stop-smoking contract with the patient.
  e. If the patient is not willing to quit now, provide motivating literature and ask again at the next visit.

Arrange follow-up visits
  a. Set a followup visit within 1 to 2 weeks after the quit date.
  b. Contact the patient within 7 days after the initial visit; reinforce the decision to stop and remind the patient of the quit date and the follow-up visit.
  c. At the first follow-up visit, discuss the patient's smoking status to provide support and help prevent relapse. Relapse is common; if it happens, encourage the patient to try again immediately.
  d. Set a second follow-up visit in 1 to 2 months. For patients who have relapsed, discuss the circumstances of the relapse and other special concerns.

---

[a]Adapted from Glynn, T., and Manley, M. (1993). "How to Help Your Patients Stop Smoking: A National Cancer Institute Manual for Physicians." NIH Publication No. 93-3064. Public Health Service.

physical activity in reducing weight and body fat and the possible subsequent effect on cancer risk reduction. For example, being overweight or obese is associated with an increased risk of hormone-related cancers. Losing weight and body fat reduces circulating levels of estrogen and progesterone, hormones related to breast and colorectal cancer. Studies suggest that moderate physical activity can reduce breast cancer risk in both premenopausal and postmenopausal women. For colorectal cancer, leanness and regular physical activity have been consistently associated with reduced risk in both men and women. Numerous studies have reported that when caloric intake exceeds energy output, there is an increased risk of cancer of the colon, rectum, prostate, endometrium, breast, and kidney.

The amount of physical activity needed to maintain a healthy weight, lose weight, and promote good health, including reducing cancer risk, is recommended by various organizations in the United States, including the NCI and ACS, to be 30 min of moderate physical activity on most days of the week. This level of activity might include walking briskly (3–4 miles per hour) for about 2 miles, gardening and yard work, jogging, or swimming. The activity does not need to be continuous; the key is to exercise on a regular basis.

B. Sun Exposure

Exposure to sunlight, the main source of ultraviolet (UV) radiation, is implicated as a causative factor in the development of skin cancer—the most common form of cancer, with about 1.3 million new cases each year in the United States. People with red or blond hair and fair skin that freckles or burns easily are at especially high risk for skin cancer. Basal cell and squamous cell carcinomas, both highly curable, account for the majority of skin cancers. However, the incidence of malignant melanoma, the most dangerous form of skin cancer, is increasing. Total worldwide incidence increased about 15% between 1985 and 1990 estimates. In the United States, the lifetime risk of developing melanoma was 1 in 1500 in the 1930s. Now, the risk is 1 in 74, and there will be an estimated 47,700 new cases in the year 2000.

Abundant evidence has established that skin cancer risk can be reduced by limiting exposure to sun-

light and, thus, to UV radiation. Generally, effective protective behaviors include avoiding the sun during midday (especially between 10 AM and 2 PM), wearing protective clothing and broad-brimmed hats, wearing sunglasses, avoiding tanning beds and sun lamps (these are also sources of UV radiation), and using sunscreen that has a sun protection factor (SPF) of 15 or higher, even on hazy or cloudy days.

The relationship between sunscreen use and melanoma risk is somewhat controversial. Many epidemiologic studies investigating the association between melanoma risk and sunscreen use have found either reduced risk or no clear association. However, findings in others have suggested that sunscreen use is associated with an increased risk for melanoma, leading some to question the advisability of widespread recommendations for its use. It has been hypothesized that people who use sunscreen primarily to avoid sunburn during intentional sun exposure, such as sunbathing, might increase their sun exposure time when using sunscreen, thus increasing their exposure to UV radiation and risk for melanoma. At present, accumulated evidence on sun exposure and skin cancer still warrants using sunscreen as part of an overall sun protection strategy, during both intentional and unintentional exposures (e.g., in gardening or hiking).

See Also the Following Articles

Chemoprevention, Principles of • Chemoprevention Trials • Nutritional Supplements and Diet as Chemopreventive Agents • Tobacco Carcinogenesis

Bibliography

Doll, R., and Peto, R. (1981). The causes of cancer: Quantitative estimates of avoidable risks of cancer in the United States today. *J. Natl. Cancer Inst.* **66,** 1191.

Fiore, M. C. (2000). A clinical practice guideline for treating tobacco use and dependence: A U.S. Public Health Service report. *J. Am. Med. Assoc.* **283,** 3244.

Hackshaw, A. K., Law, M. R., and Wald, N. J. (1997). The accumulated evidence on lung cancer and environmental tobacco smoke. *Br. Med. J.* **315,** 980.

Heber, D., Blackburn, G. L., and Go, V. L. W. (eds.) (1999). "Nutritional Oncology." Academic Press, New York.

Hein, D. W., Doll, M. A., Fretland, A. J., Leff, M. A., Webb, S. J., Xiao, G. H., Devanaboyina, U. S., Nangju, N. A., and

Feng, Y. (2000). Molecular genetics and epidemiology of the NAT1 and NAT2 acetylation polymorphisms. *Cancer Epidemiol. Biomark. Prev.* **9,** 29.

Pandey, M., Mathew, A., and Nair, M. K. (1999). Global perspective of tobacco habits and lung cancer: A lesson for third world countries. *Eur. J. Cancer Prev.* **8,** 271.

Perera, F. P. (1996) Molecular epidemiology: Insights into cancer susceptibility, risk assessment, and prevention. *J. Natl. Cancer Inst.* **88,** 496.

Reif, A. E., and Heeren, T. (1999). Consensus on synergism between cigarette smoke and other environmental carcinogens in the causation of lung cancer. *Adv. Cancer Res.* **76,** 161.

Rigel, D. S., and Carucci, J. A. (2000). Malignant melanoma: Prevention, early detection, and treatment in the 21st century. *CA Cancer J. Clin.* **50,** 215.

Sinha, R., and Caporaso, N. (1999) Diet, genetic susceptibility and human cancer etiology. *J. Nutr.* **129,** 556S.

U.S. Department of Health and Human Services (1996). "Physical Activity and Health: A Report of the Surgeon General." U.S. Department of Health and Human Services, Centers for Disease Control and Prevention, National Centers for Chronic Disease Prevention and Health Promotion, Atlanta, GA.

U.S. Department of Health and Human Services (2000). "Reducing Tobacco Use: A Report of the Surgeon General." U.S. Department of Health and Human Services, Centers for Disease Control and Prevention, National Center for Chronic Disease Prevention and Health Promotion, Office on Smoking and Health, Atlanta, GA.

Weinstock, M. A. (1999). Do sunscreens increase or decrease melanoma risk: An epidemiologic evaluation. *J. Invest. Dermatol. Symp. Proc.* **4,** 97.

World Cancer Research Fund (1997). "Food, Nutrition and the Prevention of Cancer: A Global Perspective." American Institute for Cancer Research, Washington, DC.

Cancer Vaccines: Gene Therapy and Dendritic Cell-Based Vaccines

James W. Young
Jean-Baptiste Latouche
Michel Sadelain
Memorial Sloan-Kettering Cancer Center

GLOSSARY

antigen presentation The display of peptide fragments bound to MHC molecules on a cell surface in a manner required by T lymphocytes for recognition and response.

chemokine Small cytokine that influences migration and activation of cells, especially phagocytes and lymphocytes, but also dendritic cells.

cytokine Protein made by one cell that affects the development or function of another cell by interacting with a specific cell surface signaling receptor.

major histocompatibility complex A highly polymorphic gene cluster on human chromosome 6 (mouse chromosome 17) composed of codominant alleles that encode specialized membrane proteins for binding and presenting peptide antigens to $CD8^+$ (class I MHC) and $CD4^+$ (class II MHC) T lymphocytes.

transduction Gene transfer in mammalian cells mediated either by nonviral vectors or by viral vectors. Vector entry is an infectious process in the latter case, albeit not followed by viral replication when using a replication–defective viral vector.

transfection In mammalian cells, refers to gene transfer mediated by physical or chemical means, e.g., electroporation, calcium-phosphate precipitation, and lipofection.

viral vector (adenoviral, retroviral, etc.) Usually, replication–defective viral vectors are minimal recombinant viral genomes that retain *cis*-acting sequences required for permitting efficient transduction.

I. INTRODUCTION

Immunologists have long tried to exploit the immune system to control human disease, in many cases with great success. The prevention of viral diseases by immunizations that stimulate durable antibody responses is a cardinal example. Cancer and certain other infections have proven more elusive, however. Among the myriad reasons for this are that most tumor antigens (Ags) are self or differentiation Ags to which the immune system is not responsive, the tumor microenvironment itself may be inhibitory, and tumor cells lack the other surface molecules required for immunogenicity.

The stimulation of an immune response also requires more than just tumor Ags and lymphocytes. T lymphocytes in particular will only respond to Ag bound to special cell surface molecules that comprise the major histocompatibility complex (MHC) and are abundantly expressed by specialized Ag-presenting cells (APCs). Moreover, the sensitization of resting or naïve T cells to Ag requires multiple additional costimulatory and adhesive ligands expressed on the APC surface together with the Ag and MHC. The dendritic cell (DC) is a specialized type of leukocyte, rare in the steady state, which provides a means of orchestrating all of these various requirements for initiating cellular immunity.

Tumors express antigens, and DCs possess everything else needed to stimulate T cell immunity. The challenge now is how best to combine the two, given that investigators can now generate sufficient numbers and purity of DCs for large-scale experimental and clinical applications. Various methods for loading tumor Ag(s) onto DCs are under evaluation, especially those that ensure durable expression and stimulation of T cells, which in turn target tumors expressing the same Ags. This article discusses the various genetic approaches used to transfer Ag into highly immunostimulatory DCs.

II. THE DENDRITIC CELL SYSTEM

A. DCs *in Vivo*

Dendritic cells are widely distributed throughout the body, notably at peripheral sites of Ag exposure. The physiologic process of antigen capture, followed by maturation and migration to secondary lymphoid organs where DCs select and stimulate Ag-specific, resting T cells, parallels an inducible increase in accessory molecule expression and stimulatory function. This segregates antigen uptake from antigen presentation, both physically and functionally, which are the two components of the afferent or sensitization arm of the immune response. T cells activated in secondary lymphoid organs then exit into the periphery to perform the effector functions of the efferent arm of the immune response.

DCs reside in epidermal and mucosal surfaces as Langerhans cells (LCs) and in the dermis and interstitia as dermal or interstitial DCs (DDC-IDCs). DCs at various degrees of maturation are also found migrating in afferent lymph and in draining secondary lymphoid organs, but DCs are never found in efferent lymph. DCs are not identifiable in fresh blood, e.g., in peripheral blood smears, without immunocytochemical detection of surface markers, which in the aggregate distinguish DCs from other leukocytes. Freshly isolated DCs do not exhibit their unique, stellate, veiled cytoplasmic extensions unless first activated in some way. Nonlymphoid, mononuclear leukocytes, or monocytes are now recognized as precursors of at least one type of DC; these are readily found in peripheral blood.

B. Generation of DCs *ex Vivo*

Prior methods for isolating these specialized APCs from circulating blood were laborious, lengthy, technically demanding, and of low yield. Methods for the generation of DCs *ex vivo* using defined precursors and cytokine conditions have fostered a much greater understanding of the heterogeneity of DCs. The complexity of the DC system is proving useful, given the resultant variety of important T-cell responses that can be stimulated.

Like all leukocytes, all DCs develop initially from $CD34^+$ as well as more primitive hematopoietic progenitor cells (HPCs). Hematopoiesis is inherently a stochastic process, but cytokines can skew this process, especially *in vitro*. With increasing differentiation down a particular pathway, there is decreasing opportunity for differentiation into alternative progeny.

While it is now recognized that myeloid (or nonlymphoid) DCs, as well as so-called lymphoid or plasmacytoid DCs, constitute the two broad types of DCs, this article focuses on myeloid DCs because their immunogenic capacities are better established (Fig. 1).

1. Monocyte-Derived DCs

CD14$^+$ peripheral blood monocytes are the most accessible precursors for generating DCs. These precursors are postmitogenic and capable only of further differentiation, which bears directly on the type of gene transfer that can target these cells. Despite their more restricted differentiation potential, blood monocytes yield more highly purified populations of DCs with fewer enrichment steps than needed for generating DCs from multipotent CD34$^+$ HPCs.

The granulocyte–macrophage colony-stimulating factor (GM-CSF) has consistently been the critical cytokine for supporting DC growth, differentiation, and survival from all precursors, including blood monocytes. Interleukin (IL)-4 has also proven essential for suppression of the alternative monocyte differentiation pathway into macrophages. By themselves, GM-CSF and IL-4 will only generate immature monocyte-derived DCs (moDCs). Upon removal of cytokines, these may revert to a precursor form or even differentiate into macrophages. Immature moDCs can also have the effect of stimulating a regulatory or suppressor type of T-cell response rather than a preferred immunogenic response. Exposure of immature DCs to a mixture of inflammatory cytokines and/or CD40 ligand ensures that these DCs achieve irreversible maturation and/or activation before exposure to T cells.

2. CD34$^+$ HPC-Derived DCs

CD34$^+$ HPCs can give rise to two types of myeloid, or nonlymphoid, DCs. Langerhans cells (LCs) develop in the presence of GM-CSF and transforming growth factor (TGF)-β. In the absence of TGF-β, dermal-interstitial DCs (DDC-IDCs) develop. Investigators now avoid fetal calf serum (FCS) supplementation of culture media, even for preclinical work in the laboratory, but especially for cultures generating progeny for administration to humans. The absence of FCS compromises the total expansion and yield, but this is

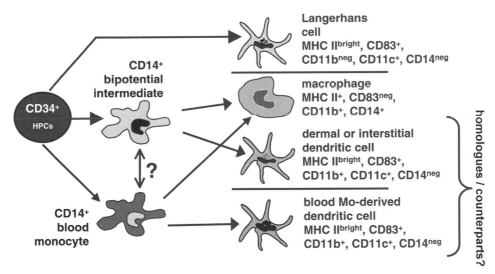

FIGURE 1 Hematopoietic development of human myeloid dendritic cells. Human DCs are all originally derived from CD34$^+$ hematopoietic progenitor cells (HPCs), but follow alternative differentiation pathways depending on cytokine exposure. GM-CSF is the pivotal cytokine for all DC growth and differentiation. IL-4 is useful for the suppression of macrophage differentiation. TGF-β supports the differentiation of Langerhans cells. Stem cell factor (c-*kit*-ligand) and FLT-3L are useful for progenitor expansion but do not affect differentiation. Inflammatory cytokines (e.g., TNF-α, IL-1, IL-6, PGE-2, and type I IFNs) and/or CD40L has proven useful for terminal maturation or activation. All terminally matured DCs are MHC bright, CD14 negative, and CD83$^+$. Myeloid DCs are always CD11c$^+$. Langerhans cells are CD11b negative, whereas the other myeloid DCs are CD11b$^+$.

an acceptable concession for avoiding the introduction of xenogeneic antigens into a highly immunogenic system.

Cytokines like FLT-3L and/or stem cell factor (c-kit-ligand) are useful for recruiting progenitors into the cell cycle and for expanding these clonogenic progenitors. These precursor populations then remain sensitive to the differentiating effects of cytokines like GM-CSF, tumor necrosis factor (TNF)-α, and IL-4 in the case of DDC-IDCs or to GM-CSF, TNF-α, and TGF-β in the case of LCs. Several lines of evidence support differentiation of DDC-IDCs, but not LCs, through a CD14$^+$ intermediate. DDC-IDCs and moDCs are very similar, but simultaneous evaluations have not established whether these DCs are exactly homologous, albeit derived from different starting populations.

3. Phenotypic and Functional Characterization of DCs

There are consistent and reliable characteristics that distinguish DCs from other leukocytes, and specifically from other APCs. Most of these features are useful both in situ and in vitro, and they characterize all the different DC types.

The unique, circumferential, cytoplasmic, dendritic extensions, which are eponymous for DCs, are readily identified in situ, in epidermal sheets for example. These morphologic characteristics develop in vitro as well, becoming most pronounced with maturation and activation.

Mature myeloid DCs lack significant phenotypic expression of any epitopes specific to lymphocytes or macrophages, e.g., CD3, CD14, CD16, CD19, and CD20. Mature DCs increase expression of MHC, especially class II, and CD83. CD83 is unique to DCs among myeloid cells, can be detected intracellularly before terminal maturation and surface expression, and indicates commitment to the DC differentiation pathway. Its surface expression is the best available marker of maturation, and its function is under study. DC maturation also increases the expression of all costimulatory and adhesive molecules (e.g., CD40, CD50, CD54, CD58, CD80, and CD86, among others) for interacting with and stimulating T cells. These epitopes are not restricted to DCs, however, so they cannot be used alone for DC identification. Differential expression of chemokines and chemokine receptors are being increasingly recognized as important components of the migratory and maturational stages of DCs.

The most straightforward and reliable assay of DC function in vitro, compared with that of other candidate APCs, is the allogeneic mixed leukocyte reaction (alloMLR). Terminally matured DCs are consistently the most potent stimulators of allogeneic T cells, including naïve or resting populations, by one to two logs compared with any other candidate, physiologic APCs like B lymphocytes or macrophages. Dose–response titrations of DCs versus other APCs are especially revealing on this point. More sensitive assays (e.g., ELISpot, tetramer staining) in vitro are now available for monitoring responses stimulated in vivo by the clinical administration of DCs. Careful dose titrations still support the superior potency of DCs as stimulators of cellular immunity.

III. GENE TRANSFER IN DENDRITIC CELLS AND THEIR PRECURSORS

A. Rationale for a Genetic Approach to Express Antigens in DCs

The origin of DCs and their requirements for differentiation and activation are critical determinants of their biological activity and hence their therapeutic efficacy. Another essential consideration is how and when to provide relevant antigens to DCs or their precursors. Gene transfer in DCs provides a means of enhancing presentation and immunogenicity of tumor antigens, as well as optimizing DC maturation and function.

Following generation ex vivo, DCs can be activated and loaded with antigen in a controlled manner. This is essential to assessing the function of well-defined cellular reagents and establishing proof of principle of their therapeutic efficacy. Loading DCs with antigen is classically performed using protein extracts, purified or recombinant proteins, or synthetic peptides. Pulsing DCs with necrotic or apoptotic cells, or peptides bound to chaperones like heat shock proteins, are alternative ways of providing tumor antigens. Genetic approaches to antigen loading are based on the transduction of DCs or their precursors with cDNA or mRNA encoding the antigen.

In principle, gene transfer may offer several advantages over pulsing with peptide or cellular extracts.

a. A set of selected, pure (recombinant) proteins can be expressed, either alone or in defined combinations.
b. The level of antigen expression can be controlled at the transcriptional level.
c. Antigens can be processed into HLA-restricted peptides, irrespective of the HLA type of each individual, allowing an individual's own cells to process those peptides best suited for presentation on its own MHC molecules.
d. Antigen presentation may be more sustained if the antigen is expressed endogenously rather than pulsed onto the cell surface.
e. Genetic alterations (point mutations, gene fusions) can be easily introduced in the cDNA encoding the antigen in order to augment antigenicity or facilitate processing.
f. The generation of DCs from their genetically modified precursors could greatly facilitate the production of effective DCs ex vivo or, perhaps, in vivo.
g. Genetic approaches offer attractive means to codeliver antigens and signals designed to enhance immune stimulation, e.g., CD40 ligand, cytokines, or chemokines.

B. Vectors Used for DC Transduction

Various strategies to generate and transduce DCs, using an expanding repertoire of available vector systems, are currently under investigation. Most use viral vectors (see Table I). Nonviral methods using RNA or DNA transfection are also actively investigated.

1. Stable Transduction Systems

Strategies for modifying HPCs genetically require stable gene delivery systems. Stable gene transfer can be achieved with viral vectors that integrate into host cell chromosomes. Oncoretroviral vectors stably transduce $CD34^+$ HPCs from bone marrow, cord blood, and cytokine-elicited peripheral blood. As oncoretroviral vectors require division of the infected cell to integrate (Table I), their efficacy is restricted to progenitor cells that proliferate before differentiation into DCs. This approach is thus not applicable to moDCs.

Lentiviruses, however, are able to integrate stably into certain nondividing cells. Wild-type human immunodeficiency virus-1 (HIV-1) in particular is capable of infecting moDCs in the absence of cell proliferation. Recombinant vectors derived from HIV-1 have been used successfully for transduction in vivo or in vitro of terminally differentiated cells like neurons, hepatocytes, retinocytes, and macrophages. To improve the safety of lentiviral-mediated gene transfer, one or more of the four accessory genes vpr, vpu, vif, and nef, which contribute to viral pathogenicity, have been removed in the second generation of lentiviral vectors. Such multiply attenuated vector systems efficiently transduce moDCs.

2. Transient Expression Systems

Because DCs can prime T cells in a few hours (or days), transgene integration is not necessary to obtain an immune response. Other gene transfer approaches are then possible using nonintegrating viral vectors, plasmid DNA, or mRNA.

TABLE I
Viral Vectors Used to Transduce DCs or Their Precursors

Vector type	Prototypic virus	Packaging size	Vector immunogenicity	Required target cell division	Lytic activity	Example
Replication defective (RD) adenovirus	Human adenovirus	8 kb[a]	+++[a]	No	No	Dietz (1999)
RD lentivirus	Human immunodeficiency virus-1	8–9 kb	+	No	No	Dyall (2001)
RD oncoretrovirus	Murine leukemia virus	8 kb	+	Yes	No	Szabolcs (1997)
Vaccinia	Vaccinia (poxvirus)	>30 kb	+++	No	Yes	Chaux (1999)

[a]Second generation.

a. Nonviral Approaches Plasmid DNA and mRNA transfection can be performed in DCs by electroporation, lipofection, or passive pulsing. On the one hand, transfection with plasmid DNA, especially in nondividing cells, has proven extremely difficult and is further complicated by the high immunogenicity of plasmid backbones. On the other hand, mRNA can be easily transfected and has been shown to be very efficient at priming T cells.

A principal advantage of using mRNA is that the antigen does not need to be known. T cells can then be primed against several tumor antigens at the same time, avoiding the risk of escape that could occur with the use of a single protein or peptide. mRNA is also relatively easy to obtain, even from a very limited number of tumor cells. A promoter can be added to the primers used to generate tumor-derived libraries without recombinant DNA intermediates. Finally, the half-life of the mRNA is a few hours, and no insertional mutagenesis can occur, rendering the procedure very safe.

Nevertheless, the main concern is that the use of total mRNA obtained from tumor cells could elicit a deleterious autoimmune response. mRNA could, in principle, be selected by substraction techniques to avoid such a problem, but the logistics would be complicated. Two other relative disadvantages of this approach are that access to tumor tissue is required for every patient and it may not be possible to immunize against antigens encoded by rare mRNA molecules.

b. Viral Vectors Several viral vector systems have been used to transduce moDCs, including those based on adenovirus and poxvirus (Table I). Expression from these vectors is relatively short-lived, ranging from a few days in rapidly dividing cell populations to several weeks in nonreplicating cells. This is not an obstacle to expressing antigens in DCs that have a limited lifespan, however. Of greater concern is the expression of viral proteins encoded by these vectors, which may perturb DC differentiation and activation or alter the immunogenicity of the transduced DCs. Expression of viral antigens may sometimes prove to be beneficial, e.g., by providing helper epitopes, or detrimental, e.g., by providing dominant epitopes that blunt the response to tumor antigens. The presence of highly immunogenic viral antigens may also prove to be problematic upon repeated administration of transduced DCs.

IV. CONCLUSION

DCs are currently viewed as ideal adjuvants for immunizing against tumor antigens. Advances in the definition of DC subtypes and their requirements for activation hold the promise of generating effective DCs for clinical investigation. There are nonetheless a number of remaining questions about how best to use DCs for cancer immunotherapy.

In principle, genetic strategies offer a number of advantages in terms of introducing known or unknown antigens into DCs. Tumor-derived or genetically engineered recombinant antigens can be expressed using a range of technologies based on electroporation, chemical transfection, or viral vector-mediated transduction. A number of vector systems appear promising in terms of transduction efficiency in either moDCs or their hematopoietic progenitors.

Viral vectors differ in terms of their molecular requirements for successful transduction, duration of antigen expression, inherent immunogenicity, and safety. The availability of multiple vector systems for transducing moDCs and CD34[+] HPC-derived DCs will allow for systematic investigation of the biological activity and therapeutic efficacy of different DC subsets. Comparisons between different antigen combinations and vector types will most certainly yield valuable information on the induction of potent immune responses against tumor antigens.

See Also the Following Articles

Adeno-Associated Virus • Anti-Idiotypic Antibody Vaccines • Cancer Vaccines: Peptide- and Protein-Based Vaccines • Carbohydrate-Based Vaccines • Cytokines • DNA-Based Cancer Vaccines • Retroviral Vectors • Targeted Toxins • Tumor Antigens

Bibliography

Banchereau, J., Schuler-Thurner, B., Palucka, A. K., and Schuler, G. (2001). Dendritic cells as vectors for therapy. *Cell* **106,** 271–274.

Banchereau, J., and Steinman, R. M. (1998). Dendritic cells and the control of immunity. *Nature* **392,** 245–252.

Bell, D., Young, J. W., and Banchereau, J. (1999). Dendritic cells. *Adv. Immunol.* **72,** 255–322.

Gilboa, E., Nair, S. K., and Lyerly, H. K. (1998). Immunotherapy of cancer with dendritic cell-based vaccines. *Cancer Immunol. Immunother.* **46,** 82–87.

Hart, D. N. J. (1997). Dendritic cells: Unique leukocyte populations which control the primary immune response. *Blood* **90,** 3245–3287.

Kay, M. A., Glorioso, J. C., and Naldini, L. (2001). Viral vectors for gene therapy: The art of turning infectious agents into vehicles of therapeutics. *Nature Med.* **7,** 33–40.

Young, J. W. (1999). Dendritic cells: Expansion and differentiation with hematopoietic growth factors. *Curr. Opin. Hematol.* **6,** 135–144.

Cancer Vaccines: Peptide- and Protein-Based Vaccines

Paul F. Robbins

National Institutes of Health, Bethesda, Maryland

I. Major Histocompatibility Complex Class I- and Class II-Restricted T-Cell Recognition
II. Identification of Antigens Recognized by Class I-Restricted, Tumor-Reactive T Cells
III. Identification of Antigens Recognized by Tumor-Reactive, Class II-Restricted T Cells
IV. Identification of Shared Epithelial Tumor Antigens
V. Clinical Vaccine Trials
VI. Future Directions

GLOSSARY

adjuvant Material used to enhance the immunogenicity of a protein or peptide.

cytokines Secreted proteins involved in the activation and proliferation of immune cells.

cytotoxic T lymphocytes Immune cells capable of lysing targets expressing the appropriate antigen.

epitope Short peptide sequence bound to MHC gene product that serves as the target recognized by the antigen-specific T-cell receptor.

immunogenicity Ability of a particular molecule to elicit a specific immune response.

major histocompatibility complex (MHC) Locus encoding polymorphic genes utilized by the immune systems for antigen presentation and for self/nonself recognition.

melanocyte Skin cell responsible for the production of the pigment melanin.

transfection Introduction of DNA into a cell using physical manipulation.

Methods developed over the last several years have allowed tumor antigens that are recognized by MHC class I- and class II-restricted T cells to be readily identified. The screening of patient sera against tumor cell cDNA expression libraries has also resulted in the identification of a large number of antigens, some of which were also found to be recognized by tumor-reactive T cells. These antigens, as well as proteins that appear to be overexpressed in tumors, represent targets that can potentially be used for the development of cancer vaccines.

The availability of a wide variety of targets has led to a number of clinical vaccine trials. Melanoma patients have been immunized with peptides that appear to represent dominant T cell epitopes from a number of melanoma antigens, including MAGE-3, MART-1, and gp100. Additional targets now being evaluated in clinical trials include peptides derived from proteins that are overexpressed in particular tumors, such as HER-2/neu, as well as peptides from oncogenes such as ras that are frequently mutated in a variety of tumor types. The human papilloma virus (HPV) is associated with the development of cervical carcinoma, and peptide epitopes identified from viral proteins represent additional targets for vaccine therapies. A variety of methods have been used for peptide delivery; peptides have been administered in soluble form, emulsified in adjuvants, and pulsed on antigen-presenting cells (APC) such as dendritic cells (DC). A variety of cytokines, including interleukin (IL)-2, granulocyte/monocyte colony-stimulating factor (GM-CSF), and IL-12, have also been administered in attempts to enhance immune responses to peptide immunization.

In these primarily phase I trials, while the lack of toxicity of these treatments has been demonstrated, substantial tumor regressions have only been observed in a limited number of patients. Nevertheless, a critical feature of these trials, as well as future clinical trials, is the development of effective strategies for monitoring immune responses in vaccinated patients, which include *in vivo* as well as *in vitro* assays. It is hoped that the careful evaluation of immune responses to vaccination, in conjunction with animal model studies, will result in the development of effective vaccines for the treatment of cancer patients.

I. MAJOR HISTOCOMPATIBILITY COMPLEX CLASS I- AND CLASS II-RESTRICTED T-CELL RECOGNITION

Cytotoxic T lymphocytes (CTL) recognize short peptides in association with class I MHC molecules. Peptide titration studies, as well as studies carried out with peptides of varying lengths, have demonstrated that the optimal peptides generally have ranged between 8 and 10 amino acids. Studies carried out in the early 1990s by Rammensee and others demon-

strated that peptides eluted from class I MHC molecules, in addition to ranging between 8 and 10 amino acids in length, contained characteristic amino acids at particular positions in the sequence. For example, peptides that bound to the human HLA-A2 class I gene product generally possessed an aliphatic residue such as L or M at position 2 (P2) and a V or L residue at the carboxy terminus of the peptide (P9 or P10) (Table I). The amino acids at these positions, which have been termed primary anchor residues, appear to be critical residues for binding to class I MHC molecules, and the solution of the crystal structure of MHC class I gene products containing bound peptides has confirmed these findings. As a result of these studies, binding motifs have now been defined for multiple HLA class I alleles.

Extensive studies have also been carried out to define the nature of CD4[+] helper T-cell epitopes, which are recognized in association with MHC class II molecules. The length of MHC class II-binding peptides varies more than class I-binding peptides, and it has been more difficult to establish binding motifs for class II alleles. Nevertheless, minimal epitopes of 9 or 10 amino acids have been identified for a number of MHC class II antigens. Compilations of these sequences have also resulted in the identification of two or three primary anchor residue positions that appear to be involved in binding to particular HLA alleles, and determination of the crystal structure of class II MHC molecules bound to peptides has confirmed these results.

II. IDENTIFICATION OF ANTIGENS RECOGNIZED BY CLASS I-RESTRICTED, TUMOR-REACTIVE T CELLS

In the early 1990s, efficient methods were developed for the isolation of genes that encode antigens recognized by tumor reactive T cells. Tumor-specific T-cell lines and clones were initially identified from tumor-infiltrating lymphocytes (TIL), as well as peripheral blood mononuclear cells (PBMC) that had been stimulated *in vitro* sensitization with tumor cells. The genes that encode tumor antigens were primarily

TABLE I

Melanoma Antigen T-Cell Epitopes: Comparison with the HLA-A2-Binding Motif

	Position									
	1	2	3	4	5	6	7	8	9	
Anchors or auxiliary anchors[a]		L				V			V	
	M							L		
Preferred residues				E				K		
				K						
Other residues	I	A	G	I	I	A	E			
	L	Y	P	K	L	Y	S			
	F	F	D	Y	T	H				
	K	P	T	N						
	M	M		G						
	Y	S		F						
	V	R		V						
				H						
HLA-A2-restricted melanoma antigen epitopes										
MART-1 27–35	A	A	G	I	G	I	L	T	V	
gp100 154–162	K	T	W	G	Q	Y	W	Q	V	
gp100 209–217	I	T	D	Q	V	P	F	S	V	
gp100 280–288	Y	L	E	P	G	P	V	T	A	
gp100 619–627	R	L	M	K	Q	D	F	S	V	
gp100 639–647	R	L	P	R	I	F	C	S	C	
gp100 457–466	L	L	D	G	T	A	T	L	R	L
gp100 476–485	V	L	Y	R	Y	G	S	F	S	V
Tyrosinase 1–9	M	L	L	A	V	L	Y	C	L	
Tyrosinase 369–377	Y	M	D	G	T	M	S	Q	V	
TRP-2180-188	S	V	Y	D	F	F	V	W	L	

[a]Data indicating primary and secondary anchor residues and residues and preferred residues, as well as other residues commonly observed in HLA-A2-binding peptides, were obtained from the internet site www.uni-tuebingen.de/uni/kxi/database.html.

identified through the screening of cDNA libraries generated from tumor cell mRNA. This was carried out by transfecting DNA that was isolated from pools of cDNA clones into antigen-negative target cells that expressed the appropriate MHC restriction element. The transfected target cells were then assayed for their ability to stimulate the release of cytokines such as interferon-γ (IFN-γ), tumor necrosis factor α (TNF-α), or GM-CSF from tumor-specific T cells. Positive pools were then subdivided and screened using an iterative process until an individual positive cDNA clone encoding the tumor antigen was identified. The majority of antigens identified were isolated following screening with melanoma reactive T cells; however, T cells isolated from other tumor types, such as renal and squamous carcinomas, have also been utilized to identify antigens expressed in these tumors.

These antigens have been sorted into several general categories on the basis of their expression patterns. Melanocyte differentiation antigens represent a family of proteins that are limited in their expression to normal melanocytes and melanomas. T cells have been shown to recognize nonmutated epitopes derived from several members of this family, including MART-1, gp100, TRP-1, TRP-2, and tyrosinase. One epitope appears to predominate in the HLA-A2-restricted T-cell response to MART-1, but for certain gene products, such as gp100, several epitopes have been identified. Based on the frequency of responsiveness of HLA-A2-restricted TIL, as well as sensitized PBMC, three peptides appear to predominate in the response to this antigen: gp100:209-217 (ITDQVPFSY), gp100:280-288 (YLEPGPVTA), and gp100:154-162 (KTWGQYWQV).

Members of a second family of antigens, the

cancer-testis antigens, are limited in their expression in normal tissues to the testis. These include members of the MAGE, BAGE, GAGE, and NY-ESO-1 protein families. These gene products, in contrast to melanocyte differentiation antigens, are expressed in a variety of tumor types, including breast, lung, bladder, and prostate cancers. The NY-ESO-1 gene product was initially identified by screening the reactivity of patient sera against a λ phage cDNA expression library. The NY-ESO-1 product is expressed in about 30% of patients with these cancers, and subsequent studies have shown that the majority of these patients possess antibody directed against this gene product.

Mutated antigens have been identified in melanoma as well as a number of additional tumor types. Examples of mutated epitopes that are expressed in more than a single tumor have been described; however, only a small minority of all the tumors of a particular type express a particular mutation. These antigens, which represent foreign epitopes, thus may be more immunogenic than normal self-peptides identified from antigens such as MART-1 and gp100; however, only a small percentage of patients can be treated with these vaccines.

Unique mechanisms appear to be involved in maintaining self-tolerance toward certain antigens that are expressed in a variety of normal tissues. A T-cell clone directed against the PRAME melanoma antigen expressed an NK inhibitory receptor that recognized a product of the HLA-C gene products. In addition, evidence shows that professional antigen-presenting cells may fail to efficiently present certain melanoma T-cell epitopes as a result of altered processing.

Additional studies have focused on the identification of analogs of tumor antigen epitopes with enhanced immunogenicity. Results of *in vitro*-binding assays indicate that the immunodominant HLA-A2 MART-1 epitope, as well as a majority of the gp100 epitopes recognized in the context of HLA-A2, possesses a relatively low affinity for this HLA allele. In addition, these peptides contain residues that fail to conform to the binding motif at one of the primary anchor residue positions. As described further later, peptides with enhanced binding to HLA-A2, as well as with enhanced immunogenicity, can be derived by substituting an optimal for a nonoptimal anchor residue.

III. IDENTIFICATION OF ANTIGENS RECOGNIZED BY TUMOR-REACTIVE, CLASS II-RESTRICTED T CELLS

Antigens that are recognized by class II-restricted, tumor reactive T cells have been identified using a number of methods, including the screening of cDNA libraries using techniques similar to those used to identify genes that encode class I-restricted antigens. Class II-restricted, melanoma-reactive T cells have also been examined for their ability to recognize target cells that have been transfected with genes that encode known class I-restricted melanoma antigens. Using this approach, class II-restricted epitopes from tyrosinase, gp100, TRP-1, and TRP-2 have been identified. Multiple HLA class II-restricted T-cell epitopes have also been identified from the MAGE-3 protein by carrying out *in vitro* sensitizations using antigen-presenting cells that had been pulsed with candidate peptides.

Antigens that are recognized in the context of HLA class II alleles can be processed through either an endogenous pathway or an exogenous pathway resulting from endocytosis in antigen-presenting cells such as monocytes, dendritic cells, and B cells. Epitopes from the NY-ESO-1 and MAGE-3 cancer-testis antigens have been identified by stimulating with APC that have been pulsed with purified recombinant proteins, followed by screening either candidate peptides identified using HLA class II-binding motifs or a library of overlapping peptides.

IV. IDENTIFICATION OF SHARED EPITHELIAL TUMOR ANTIGENS

Several attempts have been made to generate T-cell responses against candidate antigens that are expressed in common tumor types, such as breast and ovarian cancer, as many of the antigens recognized by melanoma reactive T cells are limited in their expression to cells of this tissue type. The HER-2/neu oncogene, a member of the epidermal growth factor receptor family, has been shown to be widely overexpressed in breast, colorectal, and ovarian adenocarcinomas, and overexpression appears to be correlated with poor prognosis in patients. The peptide KIFGSLAFL, representing amino acids 369–377 (p369), has been shown by a number of groups to be recognized by HLA-A2-restricted T-cells clones and lines isolated from patients with breast and ovarian cancer; however, additional epitopes have also been identified from this molecule.

Viral antigens, which are expressed in certain tumor types, represent attractive targets for vaccine therapies. The HPV is expressed in over 90% of cervical carcinomas, and the HPV 16 genotype is found in 50% of squamous carcinomas of the cervix. HPV E6 and E7 proteins appear to be involved in tumorigenesis, and selective pressure to maintain expression of these products may prevent the generation of antigen loss variants. Studies carried out in HLA-A2 transgenic mice resulted in the identification of several candidate epitopes from these gene products. The peptide corresponding to amino acids 86–93 of the HPV E7 protein (TLGIVCPI) has been shown to bind with high affinity to HLA-A2, and the stimulation of human lymphocytes with this peptide appears to be capable of raising tumor-reactive CTL.

Antigens that are overexpressed in particular tumor types represent potential targets for the development of anticancer vaccines. The carcinoembryonic antigen (CEA) is a tissue-specific gene product that is expressed in a high percentage of colon tumors as well as breast carcinomas. Although a low level of CEA expression has been observed in normal colon tissue, this gene product appears to be overexpressed in tumor cells, and thus may represent a target for vaccine therapies. Several closely related gene products, which include normal cross-reacting antigen (NCA) and biliary glycoprotein (BGP), are expressed in a variety of normal tissues. Studies described in more detail later have resulted in the identification of an HLA-A2-restricted T-cell epitope that is expressed in the CEA, but not in the NCA or BGP gene products. Differentiation antigens whose expression is restricted to prostate tissue also represent candidate antigens for tumors of this histology. The prostate-specific antigen (PSA), as well as prostate-specific membrane antigen (PSMA), is highly restricted in its expression to normal prostate and appears to be highly expressed by the majority of tumors of this histology. Increased expression of these markers in patient serum

is associated with progressive disease, and clinical trials utilizing peptides derived from these proteins are detailed in the following section.

V. CLINICAL VACCINE TRIALS

A. Melanoma Antigens

Peptide vaccine trials were initially carried out in melanoma patients utilizing epitopes from MAGE-1 and MAGE-3 antigens that are recognized in the context of the HLA-A1 class I allele. Patients that expressed this HLA allele and whose tumors were shown to express MAGE-3 by RT-PCR were immunized with the MAGE-3 peptide EVDPIGHLY in soluble form. In one of the initial clinical trials, 12 melanoma patients were treated with this peptide, which was administered subcutaneously as well as intradermally in saline. This peptide was injected monthly, but 6 of the 12 patients were withdrawn after one or two injections because of the rapid progression of the disease. Partial regressions were reported in 3 of the 6 remaining patients, but cells in the peripheral blood of immunized patients did not show evidence for increased reactivity to the MAGE-3 peptide.

Another melanoma clinical trial has involved intradermal injection of a total of six HLA-A2-restricted peptides, two derived from each of the melanocyte differentiation antigens MART-1, gp100, and tyrosinase. All of the peptides utilized in this trial had previously been shown to be recognized by melanoma-reactive CTL. Six patients with metastatic melanoma were immunized with 100 μg of each of these peptides weekly for 4 weeks, and delayed type hypersensitivity (DTH) responses were assessed by examining skin induration 24–48 h following peptide injection. In five out of the six patients, some evidence for a specific DTH response was seen with one of the tyrosinase peptides, but not with the other peptides. Some evidence was found for increased reactivity against the MART-1 peptides and one of the tyrosinase peptides following vaccination; however, no tumor regression was observed in any of the immunized patients. In an attempt to further boost tumor-specific immune responses, GM-CSF was administered to patients that were vaccinated with five peptides derived from MART-1, tyrosinase, and gp100. Injection of GM-CSF appeared to increase the CTL activity directed against tyrosinase peptides in the three patients that were examined and appeared to enhance reactivity against MART-1 in one out of three patients; however, no significant clinical responses were observed in this trial.

Vaccinations have also been carried out using APC that have been pulsed with peptides identified from tumor antigens. A clinical trial carried out in melanoma patients involved intradermal injections of cultured monocytes that had been pulsed with the MAGE-1 HLA-A1 peptide. The results of patient monitoring, which was carried out by testing skin reactions to intradermal peptide inject, indicated that MAGE-1-specific immune responses were not induced in vaccinated patients. When assays were carried out on T cells that had been expanded *in vitro* using peptide-pulsed target cells, a low level of peptide reactivity, as well as tumor reactivity, appeared to be present in postimmunization, but not preimmunization samples from some patients. No specific therapeutic responses were observed in this trial. In a separate clinical trial, melanoma patients were immunized with APC that had been pulsed with MAGE-1:161-169 and MAGE-3:168-176 HLA-A1-restricted epitopes, along with MART-1:27-35, tyrosinase 1-9, and gp100:154-162 HLA-A2-restricted peptides. The pulsed target cells were injected into an uninvolved inguinal lymph node at weekly intervals, and patients were evaluated for clinical responses as well as DTH responses to the peptides. One complete and one partial response were observed in the six HLA-A2+ patients that were immunized with the HLA-A2 restricted peptides, and one out of the six HLA-A1+ patients that had been immunized with the MAGE peptides demonstrated a partial response. The results of skin testing indicated that the majority of patients had been primed by immunization with the peptide-pulsed dendritic cells.

A recent report has detailed the results of a clinical trial in which melanoma patients received intradermal as well as subcutaneous injections of dendritic cells that had been pulsed with the MAGE-3 HLA-A1-restricted epitope. Vaccination appeared to result in the expansion of MAGE-3 peptide reactive T cells in 8 out of 11 patients, as determined by semiquantitative precursor frequency analysis. Complete regression of individual metastases was observed in 6 out of the 11 patients; however, disease progression was seen in all of the patients.

Studies carried out in the Surgery Branch of the National Cancer Institute focused initially on immunization with the MART-1:27-35 peptide (AAGIGILTV). Immunization of 18 patients with metastatic melanoma with this peptide was carried out subcutaneously in incomplete Freund's adjuvant (IFA) at 3-week intervals. In 15 of the patients, evidence for an increase in the precursor frequency of T cells reactive with the MART-1:27-35 peptide was seen following immunization. No evidence was obtained for a difference in the response of patients to doses that varied from 0.1 to 10 mg per injection. In 1 of the patients that appeared to respond to immunization, a partial response was observed that is ongoing for 4 years, but significant tumor regression was not observed in the other patients. A minimum of three *in vitro* stimulations appeared to be required to elicit significant responses from both immunized and nonimmunized PBMC samples, indicating that the precursor frequency of MART-1-reactive T cells was similar in both nonimmunized and immunized patients.

Peptides from the gp100 antigen have also been tested for their ability to stimulate immune responses in HLA-A2 melanoma patients. Patients were immunized with gp100:209-217 (ITDQVPFSY), gp100:280-288 (YLEPGPVTA), or gp100:154-162 (KTWGQYWQV), and *in vitro* responses to the peptides were analyzed following several *in vitro* stimulations. The patients were immunized subcutaneously with antigen emulsified in IFA at 3-week intervals. One of the patients that received the gp100:209-217 peptide had a complete response that lasted 4 months, but not other significant clinical responses were seen. Evidence for *in vivo* priming was found in patients that had received the gp100:209-217 and 280-288 peptides, but not in patients that had received the gp100:154-162 peptide.

Several studies have focused on the identification of modified T-cell epitopes with enhanced immunogenicity. The immunodominant MART-1 epitope, as well as the three immunodominant HLA-A2-binding epitopes from gp100, does not appear to conform to the optimal HLA-A2-binding motif. Immunization with the modified gp100:209-217(2M) peptide, containing a substitution of an optimal M residue for T at the P2 position, appeared to significantly enhance HLA-A2 binding, as well as the *in vitro* immunogenicity of this peptide. Modification of the gp100:280-288 peptide by the substitution of V, which represent the optimal C-terminal anchor residue, for A at the P9 position similarly enhanced peptide binding to HLA-A2 and *in vitro* immunogenicity.

These results led to clinical trials involving vaccination with modified tumor antigen peptides. In one trial carried out in the Surgery Branch of the National Cancer Institute, melanoma patients were immunized with the modified gp100:209-217(2M) peptide in IFA. The peptide-specific, as well as tumor-specific, responses of PBMC isolated from immunized patients were assessed following a single *in vitro* stimulation with peptide. Specific responses were elicited in 10 out of 11 patients immunized with the gp100:209-217(2M) peptide, but only 2 out of 8 patients immunized with the parental peptide. Results indicate that PBMC obtained before the *in vivo* immunization failed to respond to a single *in vitro* peptide stimulation, in agreement with previous results (Table II). In contrast, PBMC from the majority of

the patients that were obtained following the *in vivo* immunizations demonstrated a vigorous *in vitro* response to peptide-pulsed targets, as well as HLA-A2+ melanoma cells (Table II). Significant clinical responses were not, however, seen in patients that received either the native or the modified gp100 peptide alone in IFA. An additional group of 31 patients were immunized with the modified gp100:209-217 peptide in IFA along with high-dose IL-2, and in this group, 42% demonstrated a partial or complete response. Although the response rate to high-dose IL-2 seen in previous clinical trials was only 17%, a larger randomized trial will be needed to determine the significance of these results.

Curiously, the frequency of T cells reactive with the gp100:209-217 peptide appeared to be lower in patients that received injections of the modified peptide plus IL-2 than in patients that received injections of the peptide alone. This may have resulted from the redistribution of specific T cells from the blood to the site of tumor, as well as from apoptosis of the injected T cells resulting from stimulation by tumor cells. As discussed earlier, the majority of the clinical responses were actually observed in patients that received injections of peptide plus IL-2. Additional studies are needed to help resolve this issue.

TABLE II
Reactivity of PBMC from Patients Immunized with the 209-2M Peptide

Patient	No. of immunizations	T2 —	T2 (280)	T2 (209)	Stimulator[a] 501 mel (A2+) (pg/ml IFN-γ)	SK23 mel (A2+)	888 mel (A2−)	624.28 mel (A2−)
7	0	169	175	220	28	72	84	51
	2	209	243	2,445	1,211	2,037	98	60
8	0	528	691	729	70	640	933	806
	2	202	284	13,600	11,580	14,720	408	489
9	0	13	13	10	ND[b]	ND	ND	ND
	2	229	590	3,987	67	889	291	235
10	0	117	147	150	19	90	39	42
	2	15	18	24,040	23,860	21,580	2	4
11	0	46	50	47	11	39	14	17
	2	29	30	106	5	43	4	10

[a]PBMC were incubated with 1 μM gp100:2092M peptide for 13 days and tested for their response to T2 cells that were pulsed with the native gp100:209 peptide, the irrelevant gp100:280 peptide, and melanoma cell lines that either did or did not express HLA-A2. Data taken from Rosenberg *et al.* (1999). *J. Immunol.* **163,** 1690.
[b]Not done.

Peptide variants of the MART-1 epitope with enhanced immunogenicity than the native peptide have also been described. Modified peptides containing a substitution of leucine or methionine for the alanine residue at the P2 anchor residue position in the MART-1 10-mer EAAGIGILTV, as well as a peptide containing a substitution of methionine for alanine at the P2 position in the MART-1 9-mer AAGIGILTV, possessed a higher HLA-A2 binding affinity than the parental peptides. The results of *in vitro* sensitization studies indicated that the modified MART-1 9-mer and 10-mer peptides could generate tumor-reactive T cells more efficiently than the parental peptides. Clinical trials are now being carried out to evaluate the *in vivo* efficacy of these modifications.

B. Epithelial Tumor Cell Antigens

Previous observations have indicated that stimulation with the HLA-A2-restricted p369 peptide derived from HER/2-neu resulted in the generation of tumor-reactive T cells. In a trial carried out in the Surgery Branch of the National Cancer Institute, four HLA-A2+ patients with metastatic breast, ovarian, or colorectal adenocarcinomas were immunized with the p369 peptide in IFA. Peptide-reactive T cells were generated following a single *in vitro* stimulation of PBMC from three of the four immunized patients, and this response appeared to be dependent on *in vivo* priming. These T cells recognized antigen-negative HLA-A2+ target cells that were pulsed with as little as 1 ng/ml of the specific peptide; however, multiple HLA-A2+ tumor cells that expressed high levels of HER-2/neu were not recognized. In addition, HLA-A2+ target cells that were infected with a vaccinia virus construct encoding HER-2/neu, and which consequently expressed high levels of this gene product, were not recognized by the peptide-reactive T cells. It is possible that T cells with a relatively low affinity for this peptide–MHC complex were generated by *in vivo* immunization and that only low levels of the p369 epitope are naturally processed and presented on the tumor cell surface. The multiple *in vitro* stimulations carried out by previous investigators may have resulted in the stimulation of T cells with a higher affinity than those generated from immunized patients. Further investigation is needed to resolve the discrepancies between these findings, but these results indicate potential difficulties that may be associated with the use of candidate peptides.

A clinical trial carried out in 51 prostate cancer patients involved immunizations with two HLA-A2-binding peptides from PSMA. Immunizations were carried out by an intravenous injection of either the peptides alone or peptide-pulsed autologous dendritic cells. Injections of between 10^6 and 2×10^7 peptide-pulsed autologous dendritic cells were carried out at 6- to 8-week intervals, with patients receiving between four and five cell injections. An increase in the *in vitro* response to PMSA was reported in immunized patients, and the circulating levels of PSA were reported to decrease; however, only limited evidence for objective clinical responses has been presented. Candidate epitopes have also been identified in the PSA antigen. A single 30-mer peptide comprising two HLA-A2-binding peptides, as well as an HLA-A3-binding peptide, all derived from PSA, has been tested *in vitro* as a multivalent vaccine candidate. Following *in vitro* stimulation of PBMC with the 30-mer peptide, CTL were generated that appeared to recognize targets pulsed with each of the individual peptides as well as tumor cells.

In another clinical trial, multiple injections of a recombinant vaccinia virus encoding CEA were administered to colon cancer patients. A peptide from CEA termed CAP-1 (YLSGANLNL), which appeared to possess a relatively high binding affinity for HLA-A2, was then used to stimulate PBMC from HLA-A2+-vaccinated patients. Peptides derived from a similar region of the closely related NCA and BGP proteins, which are expressed in a variety of normal tissues, contained several substitutions from the CAP-1 peptide. Following several rounds of *in vitro* stimulation with the CAP-1 peptide, CTL lines generated from vaccinated patients appeared to recognize peptide-pulsed targets, as well as HLA-A2+, CEA-expressing tumors. Significantly weaker responses were elicited when PBMC obtained prior to vaccination were stimulated with the CAP-1 peptide. Additional studies have indicated that a substitution of D for N at position 6 of this peptide resulted in the generation of a peptide with enhanced *in vitro* immunogenicity, which will be tested in future clinical trials.

C. Mutated Oncogenes and Viral Antigens

Tumors have been shown to express a wide variety of mutated gene products, and although many of these appear to be restricted in their expression to either one or a relatively small number of tumors, a number of common mutations have also been identified. Common point mutations in the ras and p53 oncogenes have been identified in a variety of tumor types, and the identification of mutated T-cell epitopes derived from these gene products could lead to the development of widely applicable vaccines. Codon 12 of the ras oncogene is frequently mutated in epithelial tumors, and over 90% of the mutated ras gene products contain a substitution of alanine, valine, or cysteine for the normal glycine residue at this position. In one study, ras mutations were identified in tumors obtained from patients with pancreatic adenocarcinomas. Synthetic peptides comprising amino acids 5–21 of the mutated ras gene product were used to pulse autologous PBMC, which were then injected intravenously into patients with pancreatic adenocarcinomas on days 14 and 35 and subsequently at an interval of 4 to 6 weeks. In 2 of the 5 patients injected with the mutated ras peptide, transient peptide-specific proliferative responses were observed. Peptide-specific class I as well as class II-restricted T cells appeared to be elicited by *in vitro* stimulation of PBMC obtained from one of the patients vaccinated with the mutated ras peptide. In another study, ras mutations were initially identified in tumors isolated from patients with colon, lung, or pancreatic adenocarcinomas. Patients were immunized with mutated ras peptides whose sequences corresponded to those found in autologous tumor cells. Peptides were administered in Detox, an adjuvant composed of an oil in water emulsion with an added bacterial cell wall and lipid A components. In 3 out of the 8 vaccinated patients, T-cell lines were generated following *in vitro* stimulation of PBMC. These T-cell lines recognized the mutated ras peptide, but failed to respond to the nonmutated peptide. In a second study carried out by the same group, 15 patients were immunized with mutated ras peptides that had been emulsified in Detox adjuvant, and immune responses were evaluated in 10 patients that received a full course of three immunizations. Peptide-specific responses, which consisted of either CD4+ or CD8+ T cells, could be generated by

in vitro stimulation of PBMC obtained from 3 of the 10 immunized patients. Clinical antitumor responses were noted in these trials, which may be a result of the advanced state of disease in these patients.

The association of HPV 16 and 18 with cervical cancer has led to clinical trials involving vaccination with candidate epitopes derived from the viral E6 and E7 sequences. Initial studies suggested that peptide as well as tumor-reactive T cells could be elicited by *in vitro* stimulation of PBMC from HLA-A2 cervical carcinoma patients with a peptide consisting of amino acids 11 to 20 of the HPV16-E7 protein (E711-20:YMLDLQPETT). In another report, an *in vitro* culture of PBMC with DC that had been pulsed with recombinant E7 protein appeared to result in the generation of both class I- and class II-restricted T cells reactive with this antigen. Patients with cervical carcinoma were immunized with two HPV16 CTL epitopes, the E7:11-20 peptide discussed earlier and a second peptide comprising amino acids 86 to 93 of the E7 protein. These peptides were administered in combination with a pan-class II peptide, termed PADRE, that is capable of eliciting T-cell help in patients that express a variety of HLA haplotypes. Strong responses to the PADRE peptide could be generated in 4 out of the 12 immunized patients, indicating that at least some of the patients were immunocompetent. Decreased responses were also observed with PBMC from the majority of the cervical carcinoma patients following *in vitro* challenge with an HLA-A2-restricted influenza peptide, as well as with the other recall antigens. A number of the patients in this study had received prior treatments, such as chemotherapy, which may have had an impact on their response to these antigens.

Evidence for depressed immune responses that are not related to therapy has been obtained in studies of patients with certain cancers, as well as in some mouse model systems. As cited earlier, however, immunization of cancer patients with peptides from the gp100 and HER-2/neu antigens appears to result in the generation of brisk peptide-specific responses. Evaluation of the role of general as well as specific suppression in modulating antitumor responses may lead to the development of strategies that result in enhanced tumor regression.

VI. FUTURE DIRECTIONS

Use of the vaccine strategies described earlier have resulted in clinical responses in only a small minority of the treated patients. These clinical trials are predominantly in phase I testing, however, and the lack of response may have been due to the advanced stage of cancer present in these patients. Future trials directed toward prevention of recurrence in patients with no or minimal disease may demonstrate the efficacy of these approaches. Further evaluation of a variety of additional approaches to tumor vaccine therapy approaches is also needed. Vaccination with multiple class I- and class II-restricted tumor peptides may be more effective than treatment with individual epitopes. In addition, immunization with purified recombinant tumor antigen proteins may elicit cell-mediated as well as humoral responses against multiple epitopes and may be more effective at mediating tumor regression than immunization with peptides from these antigens.

See Also the Following Articles

ANTI-IDIOTYPIC ANTIBODY VACCINES • CANCER VACCINES: GENE THERAPY AND DENDRITIC CELL BASED VACCINES • CARBOHYDRATE-BASED VACCINES • DNA-BASED CANCER VACCINES • TARGETED TOXINS • TUMOR ANTIGENS

Bibliography

Boon, T., and Van den Eynde, B. J. (2000). Shared tumor-specific antigens. *In* "Biologic Therapy of Cancer" (S. A. Rosenberg, ed.), 3rd Ed., p. 493. Lippincott Williams & Wilkins.

Coulie, P. G., Brichard, V., Van Pel, A., Wolfel, T., Schneider, J., Traversari, C., Mattei, S., De Plaen, E., Lurquin, C., Szikora, J. P., Renauld, J.-C., and Boon, T. (1994). A new gene coding for a differentiation antigen recognized by autologous cytolytic T lymphocytes on HLA-A2 melanomas. *J. Exp. Med.* **180,** 35.

Kawakami, Y., Eliyahu, S., Delgado, C. H., Robbins, P. F., Rivoltini, L., Topalian, S. L., Miki, T., and Rosenberg, S. A. (1994). Cloning of the gene coding for a shared human melanoma antigen recognized by autologous T cells infiltrating into tumor. *Proc. Natl. Acad. Sci. USA* **91,** 3515.

Nestle, F. O., Alijagic, S., Gilliet, M., Sun, Y., Grabbe, S., Dummer, R., Burg, G., and Schedendorf, D. (1998). Vaccination of melanoma patients with peptide- or tumor lysate-pulsed dendritic cells. *Nature Med.* **4,** 328.

Robbins, P. F. (2000). Differentiation antigens. *In* "Biologic Therapy of Cancer" (S. A. Rosenberg, ed.), 3rd Ed., p. 504. Lippincott Williams & Wilkins.

Rosenberg, S. A., Yang, J. C., Schwartzentruber, D. J., Hw, P., Marincola, F. M., Topalian, S. L., Restifo, N. P., Dudley, M. E., Schwarz, S. L., Spiess, P. J., Wunderlich, J. R., Parkhurst, M. R., Kawakami, Y., Seipp, C. A., Einhorn, J. H., and White, D. E. (1998). Immunologic and therapeutic evaluation of a synthetic vaccine for the treatment of patients with metastatic melanoma. *Nature Med.* **4,** 321.

van der Bruggen, P., Traversari, C., Chomez, P., Lurquin, C., De Plaen, E., Van den Eynde, B., Knuth, A., and Boon, T. (1991). A gene encoding a tumor antigen recognized by cytolytic T lymphocytes on human melanomas. *Science* **254,** 1643.

van der Bruggen, P., Traversari, C., Chomez, P., Lurquin, C., De Plaen, E., Van den Eynde, B., Knuth, A., and Boon, T. (1996). Generation of cytotoxic T-cell responses with synthetic melanoma-associated peptides in vivo: Implications for tumor vaccines with melanoma-associated antigens *Int. J. Can.* **66,** 162.

Carbohydrate-Based Vaccines

Philip O. Livingston
Govindaswami Ragupathi
Memorial Sloan-Kettering Cancer Center

GLOSSARY

adjuvant Assisting or aiding; after surgical resection of all known disease, a treatment administered to prevent recurrence; any substance mixed with an antigen to increase immunogenicity.

conjugate vaccine A vaccine containing the relevant antigen covalently linked to an immunogenic carrier molecule.

ganglioside A sialic acid containing glycosphingolipid.

keyhole limpet hemocyanin A large highly immunogenic respiratory chromprotein obtained from the blood of the keyhole limpet (a mollusk) and frequently used as a carrier protein.

mucin A glycoprotein that is extensively o-glycosylated.

polyvalent vaccine Vaccines containing multiple antigenic epitopes.

saponin A class of compounds extracted from plants with potent adjuvant activity containing a hydrophilic carbohydrate moiety and a hydrophobic triterpene moiety.

trimer or cluster Three antigenic epitopes (i.e., TF, Tn, or sTn) linked to three threonines with a terminal linker.

Carbohydrate antoantigens have proven to be suitable targets for immune recognition and attack against cancer cells, because of their abundance at the cell surface and their unexpected immunogenicity. Carbohydrates play key roles in intracellular interactions as targets for selectins and adhesins, which may be crucial, not discretionary, to tumor cell survival and the metastatic process. Passively administered and vaccine-induced antibodies in preclinical models are capable of interfering with these processes directly, inducing complement-mediated inflammation and lysis and mediating opsonization, inflammation, and tumor cell death by other Fc-mediated mechanisms. In clinical studies, conjugate vaccines have induced antibodies against a variety of carbohydrate antigens on glycolipids and mucins, and these antibodies are correlated with an improved prognosis. Phase III clinical trials with monovalent and phase II clinical trials with polyvalent carbohydrate antigen vaccines are ongoing.

I. ANTIBODIES CAN ELIMINATE EARLY CANCER SPREAD

The effect of all commonly used vaccines against infectious agents is thought to be primarily a consequence of antibody induction. Antibodies eliminate viral or bacterial infections by preventing their spread through the bloodstream and by eliminating early tissue invasion. Antibodies are also ideally suited for eliminating circulating tumor cells and micrometastasis.

A. Evidence in Experimental Animals

The basis for vaccines that induce only antibodies is well documented in experimental animals. Experiments by Zhang involving the administration of monoclonal antibody (mAb) 3F8 against the ganglioside GD2 have been particularly informative. Administration of 3F8 prior to or up to 4 days after intravenous tumor challenge with EL4 lymphoma (which expresses GD2) results in cure of most mice. Vaccination with GD2–keyhole limpet hemocyanin (KLH) conjugate vaccine achieves the same effect. This timing is comparable to treatment in the adjuvant setting after surgical resection of the primary malignancy or lymph node metastasis, as in both cases the target is circulating tumor cells and micrometastasis. The adjuvant setting in the clinic has been more closely modeled by injecting EL4 cells into the footpad on day 1 and amputating the visible tumor on day 25. Treatment at that point with 3F8 or GD2–KLH once again protects most mice from tumor recurrence, while untreated mice expire with nodal, hepatic, and other systemic metastases.

B. Evidence in Patients

Naturally acquired or passively administered antibodies are also associated with a more favorable prognosis in the clinic.

1. Patients with resected melanoma having natural antibodies against GM2 ganglioside had an 80–90% 5-year survival compared to the expected 40% rate in studies from the John Wayne Cancer Center and Memorial Sloan-Kettering Cancer Center (MSKCC).

2. Patients with small-cell lung cancer (SCLC) and naturally acquired antibodies against SCLC had a prolonged survival compared to antibody-negative patients.

3. Paraneoplastic syndromes in cancer patients have been associated with high titers of natural antibodies against onconeural antigens expressed on neurons and certain malignant cells. The antibodies were apparently induced by tumor growth and have been associated with autoimmune neurologic disorders but also with delayed tumor progression and prolonged survival.

4. Patients with resected Dukes C colon cancer who were treated with mAb 17-1A in the adjuvant setting had a significantly prolonged disease free and overall survival compared to randomized controls. This is the only randomized clinical trial of mAb therapy conducted in an adjuvant setting reported to date.

C. Mechanism of Action

Some antibodies may have direct effects, such as by inhibiting tumor cell attachment or inhibiting growth hormone receptors, but in general the interaction of antibody and antigen is without consequence unless Fc-mediated secondary effector mechanisms are activated. Binding of antibody to antigen results in a functional change in the Fc portion of the antibody and activation of several effector mechanisms. For cancer carbohydrate antigens, IgM bound to antigen is the most active complement activator in the intravascular space, and in humans, IgG1 and IgG3 are the most important complement activators extravascularly. Complement activation mediates inflammatory reactions, opsonization for phagocytosis, clearance of antigen–antibody complexes from the circulation, and membrane attack complex-mediated lysis (CDC). Opsonization for ingestion and destruction by phagocytosis or cytotoxic mechanism can occur through complement activation, but can also occur directly as a consequence of Fc receptors on phagocytic cells [antibody-dependent cell-mediated cytotoxicity (ADCC)].

II. BASIS FOR FOCUSING ON CARBOHYDRATE ANTIGENS AS TARGETS FOR ANTIBODIES

A. Abundant Expression at the Cancer Cell Surface

Cancer cells may occasionally express as many as 10^6 copies of individual protein antigens at the cell surface, as has been described in some cell lines for epidermal growth factor and HER2/neu, but most protein antigens are expressed in far smaller numbers. The number of carbohydrate epitopes expressed at the cell surface, however, is often far greater. Thus the median number of glycolipid molecules, such as gangliosides GM2 and GD2, on melanoma cells is close to 10^7 and for sarcomas and neuroblastomas is over 5×10^7. The median number of GD3 molecules expressed on melanoma and sarcoma cells is also approximately 5×10^7. The number of copies of a given glycoprotein carbohydrate epitope on cancer cells is less well defined. However, each mucin molecule has 30–100 tandem repeats, each of which can express 5–15 carbohydrate epitopes. Because the surface of epithelial cancer cells is covered by a dense glycocalyx of various mucins, most epithelial cancer cells are probably covered by at least 100,000 mucin molecules. Consequently, the number of small carbohydrate epitopes, such as TF, Tn, or sTn, on mucins at or near the cell surface is probably well in excess of 10^7.

B. Effective Targets for Immune Attack

In our series of 110 patients immunized with melanoma cell or melanoma cell lysate vaccines mixed with various adjuvants and in the series of patients immunized with allogeneic melanoma cell vaccines described by Tai, gangliosides GM2 and GD2 were the only antigens recognized by multiple patients. Gangliosides are acidic glycosphingolipids overexpressed at the cell sur-

face of melanomas, sarcomas, and other tumors of neuroectodermal origin. Gangliosides have also been shown to be effective targets for immunotherapy with mAbs with major responses seen in patients after treatment with mAbs against GM2, GD2, and GD3. The experience with mono- or disaccharide epitopes Thomsen–Friedenrich antigen (TF), Tn, and sialyl Tn (sTn), which are expressed on mucins in a great variety of epithelial cancers, has been similar. Fung and Singhal have demonstrated that immunization with TF and sTn protects mice from a subsequent challenge with cancer cells expressing these antigens. Springer and MacLean have increased antibodies against TF and sTn in cancer patients by vaccination. Patients with naturally increased or vaccine-induced antibodies against GM2 and sTn had a more favorable prognosis. Hence, active and passive immunotherapy trials have identified carbohydrate epitopes on glycolipids and glycoproteins as uniquely effective targets for cancer immunotherapy. The simplified chemical structure of these carbohydrate antigens is demonstrated as they appear at the cell surface in Fig. 1.

C. Biological Roles of Cell Surface Carbohydrates

The great majority of the molecules of the mammalian plasma membrane are glycosylated such that glycan structures form a dense forest covering the cell surface. These glycan chains are found on glycolipids and integral membrane glycoproteins, as well as on more specialized glycoproteins, such as mucins and proteoglycans. To some extent, these carbohydrates serve structural, protective, and stabilizing roles, but it is becoming increasingly recognized that they can have information-bearing functions as selectins and adhesins in cell–cell recognition and adhesion as well. Carbohydrate structures on glycoproteins and glycolipids have been implicated in such normal cell functions as proliferation, interaction with endothelial cells, leukocytes, and platelets, embryogenesis, neural cell adhesion, and the biology and metastatic potential of tumor cells. All tumors studied have changes in the expression of carbohydrate structures, which are characteristic of the tissue of origin of the tumor. As a general rule, tumors of neural crest origin (e.g., melanoma, sarcoma and neuroblastoma) exhibit overexpression of gangliosides (sialylated glycolipids),

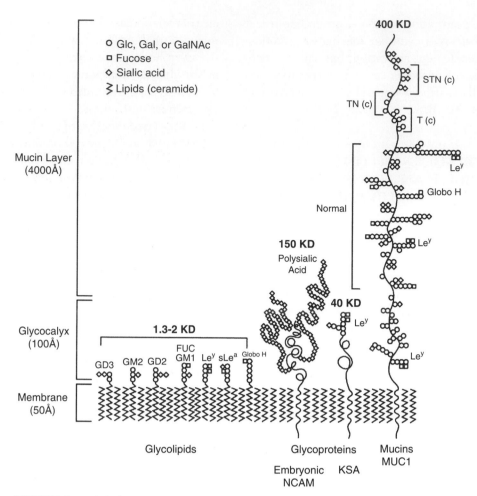

FIGURE 1 Carbohydrate epitopes on cell membrane glycoconjugates. Glc, glucose; Gal, galactose; GalNAc, *N*-acetyl galactosamine; NCAM, neural cell adhesion molecule; KSA, a panepithelial cancer antigen also referred to as 17-1A and GA733.

whereas epithelial cancers (carcinomas) have altered fucosylated structures and mucin core structures (TF, Tn, sTn) as their characteristic antigens. Numerous studies have shown a correlation between high expression of certain carbohydrate specificities (including Le^y, sTn, and Tn blood group antigens) and metastatic potential and decreased patient survival.

III. SELECTION OF CARBOHYDRATE ANTIGENS FOR VACCINE CONSTRUCTION

Using panels of mAb against carbohydrate antigens Zhang screened a variety of malignant and normal tis-

sues by immunohistochemistry. In general, ganglioside antigens have a very different distribution on various malignancies than the other carbohydrate antigens. Melanomas, sarcomas, and neuroblastomas express GM2, GD2, and GD3 but none of the other antigens, whereas epithelial cancers express a broad range of carbohydrate antigens but not GD2 or GD3. Carbohydrate antigens expressed on 50% or more of tumor cells in 60% or more of biopsy specimens of some of the most common types of cancers are listed in Table I.

Each of these antigens is also expressed on some normal tissues. GM2, GD2, and GD3 are all expressed in the brain, especially GD2, which is also expressed on some peripheral nerves and, unexpectedly, a subpopulation of B lymphocytes in the spleen and lymph

TABLE I
Carbohydrate Targets for Vaccine Construction

Tumor	Antigens[a]
Melanoma	GM2, GD2, GD3
Neuroblastoma	GM2, GD2, GD3, polysialic acid
Sarcoma	GM2, GD2, GD3
B-cell lymphoma	GM2, GD2
Small-cell lung cancer	GM2, fucosyl GM1, polysialic acid, globo H, sialyl Le[a]
Breast	GM2, globo H, Le[y], TF
Prostate	GM2, Tn, sTn, TF, Le[y]
Colon	GM2, Tn, sTn, TF, sialyl Le[a], Le[y]
Ovary	GM2, globo H, sTn, TF, Le[y]
Stomach	GM2, Le[y], Le[a], sialyl Le[a]

[a]Present on at least 50% of cancer cells in at least 60% of biopsy specimens.

nodes. Also unexpectedly, GM2, as defined by mAb 696, is expressed at the secretory borders of most epithelial tissues. GD2 and GD3 are also expressed at low levels in connective tissues of multiple organs, and GD3 is known to be expressed on some human T lymphocytes. Fucosyl GM1 is expressed on occasional cells in the islets of Langerhans and in some sensory neurons in the dorsal root ganglia. Polysialic acid is expressed significantly in brain and some bronchial epithelial cells. Globo H, Le[y], TF, Tn, and sTn are expressed at the secretory borders of a variety of epithelial tissues. Le[x] and sialyl Le[x] are expressed at the secretory border of many epithelial tissues and also on polymorphonuclear leukocytes.

The broad expression of most of these carbohydrate antigens on normal tissues raises concern over suitability as targets for immunotherapy. However, there is now sufficient experience from clinical trials with mAbs against GD2, GD3, Le[x], and sTn and with vaccine-induced antibody responses against GM2, GD2, GD3, TF, Tn, sTn, globo H, and Le[y] to draw conclusions about the consequences of antigen distribution on various normal tissues. Expression of gangliosides in the brain and expression of many of these antigens at the secretory borders of epithelial tissues have induced neither immunological tolerance nor autoimmunity once antibodies were present, suggesting that they are sequestered from the immune system. The known expression of Le[x] and sialyl Le[x] on

polymorphonucleocytes, in addition to epithelial surfaces, and the granulocytopenia seen after the treatment of patients with mAb FC-2.15 (later found by to recognize Le[x]) exclude these two carbohydrates as candidates for vaccine construction and so they have been omitted from Table I. The expression of fucosyl GM1 on subpopulations of cells in the islets of Langerhans and the dorsal root ganglia was initially of concern, but no evidence of autoimmunity has been detected in nine patients vaccinated with fucosyl GM1 who produced high titers of IgM and IgG antibodies against fucosyl GM1. Administration of high doses of some, but not other, IgG mAbs against GD2 has been associated with peripheral neuropathy in melanoma patients. High, but not lower, doses of anti-Le[y] mAb BR96 conjugated to doxorubicin have resulted in vomiting, hematemesis, and amylase elevations in some patients, whereas BR55, a second mAb against Le[y] studied by the same investigators, resulted in no such toxicity. With regard to vaccines, trials with vaccines against GD2, fucosyl GM1, and Le[y] have addressed these questions more directly. Moderate to high titers of IgM and IgG antibodies have been induced and have not been associated with any evidence of autoimmunity or other adverse clinical effects. Consequently, Table I, which lists carbohydrate antigens expressed at the cell surface of each of the common solid tumors, has served as a guide as single antigen or polyvalent antigen vaccine trials were planned.

IV. APPROACHES FOR AUGMENTING THE IMMUNOGENICITY OF CARBOHYDRATE ANTIGENS: RESULTS OF PRECLINICAL STUDIES

Vaccination of mice with irradiated melanoma cells selected for GD3 expression plus adjuvants was able to induce low levels of IgM antibodies against GD3, but this could be accomplished more effectively and simply by immunizing with purified GD3 plus immunological adjuvants. While GD3 alone induced no response at all, GD3 adherent to *Salmonella minnesota* mutant R595 or liposomes containing monophosphoryl lipid A (MPL) induced moderate titers of IgM antibodies in most mice. Attempts by Ritter at augmenting the immunogenicity of GD3 by making minor structural modifications to the GD3 so it would be foreign and not recognized as self were unsuccessful.

Based on progress with conjugate vaccines against bacterial polysaccharide antigens, Helling systematically compared the immunogenicity of conjugate vaccines constructed with different carriers and adjuvants using GD3 as antigen. KLH was the best of the six immunogenic carrier molecules tested, the conjugation method was important, and a potent immunological adjuvant was required. GD3 conjugated to KLH by the ceramide double bond and mixed with immunological adjuvant QS-21 (a purified saponin fraction obtained from the bark of the *Quillaja saponaria* Molina tree) was optimal, inducing higher titers of antibody (1/1280) and, for the first time, consistent IgG antibodies (median ~1/160). A simple mixture of GD3 and QS-21 or GD3, KLH, and QS-21 induced no antibodies. These results have been confirmed more recently using a series of other antigens, including the gangliosides GM2 and fucosyl GM1, the neutral glycolipids globo H and Le^Y, and the carbohydrate epitopes expressed on mucins Thompson Freidenreich antigen (TF), Tn, and sialyl Tn (sTn). The KLH conjugate vaccines induced antibodies that reacted with the synthetic antigens and with tumor cells expressing these antigens in all cases except in the case of Tn, TF, and sTn. Trimers of these antigens resulted in a more efficient induction of antibodies reactive with the cancer cell surface.

V. CLINICAL TRIALS WITH CARBOHYDRATE ANTIGEN VACCINES

A. Results of Serological Studies

The availability of reliable serological assays to serve as surrogate markers in clinical trials has greatly speeded progress in developing consistently immunogenic vaccines against carbohydrate antigens. A series of clinical trials with vaccines containing purified carbohydrate antigens has been conducted with TF as target by Springer, with sTn as target by MacLean, and with these and other carbohydrate antigens by Livingston, Helling, Ragupathi, and collaborators at MSKCC. Results demonstrating the progress made in trials at MSKCC are demonstrated in Table II. Trials

TABLE II
Summary of Serological Results in Vaccinated Patients: The MSKCC Experience

| Antigen | Median ELISA | | IgG subclass | Median FACS | | Median IA[b] | Median CDC | % patients positive[a] | References |
	IgM	IgG		IgM	IgG				
GM2	640	320	IgG1 + 3	+++	++	++	++	>90	Livingston *et al.* (1994), Livingston and Ragupathi (1997)
GD3	80	16		+	+	+	+	60	Ragupathi, G. (2000), *Int. J. Can.*
Fucosyl GM1	320	640	IgG1	+++	++		++	>90	Dickler,k M.H. (1999), *Clin Ca. Res.*
Globo H	640	40	IgG1 + 3	++	+	++	+	75	Ragupathi, G. (1999), *Angewardte Chem.* Slovin, S. (1999), *Proc. Natl. Acad. Sci.*
Lewis^Y	80	0		++	+	+	+	50	Sabbatini, P. (2000), *Int. J. Can.*
Tn(c)	1280	1280		++	−	+	−	60	
STn(c)	1280	160	IgG3	+++	−	+	−	>90	
TF(c)	1280	1280		+	−	+	−	50	

[a]Percentage of KLH conjugate plus QS-21-vaccinated patients positive by ELISA and FACS or CDC.
[b]IA, Immune adherence.

with other antigens, including vaccines containing unconjugated ganglioside vaccines, GD3 congeners, and unclustered sTn or TF conjugates, are not shown because the antibodies induced failed to react with antigen-positive tumor cells. The conjugate vaccines shown in Table II are currently able to induce antibodies reactive with purified antigens and tumor cells expressing these antigens in essentially 100% of cases for GM2, fucosylated GM1, and sTn(c) and 50% or more of cases for vaccines containing GD2, GD3, globo H, LeY, Tn(c), and TF(c).

B. Clinical Impact

Vaccine-induced antibody responses against GM2 and sTn have been associated with a more favorable clinical course. A randomized trial with GM2/BCG was conducted in 122 AJCC stage III melanoma patients who were free of disease after resection of metastatic disease in regional lymph nodes. This trial was based on the previous demonstration that immunization with GM2/BCG induced IgM antibodies in 85% of patients and that the production of these antibodies correlated with a more favorable prognosis. Patients were randomized to receive five immunizations over a 6-month period with BCG alone (64 patients) or BCG with GM2 adherent to the BCG surface (58 patients). Fifty-seven patients had GM2 antibody, which was present naturally or vaccine induced, and these patients had a significantly increased disease free ($p = 0.004$) and overall ($p = 0.02$) survival. Comparing the GM2/BCG and BCG groups, exclusion of all patients with preexisting GM2 antibodies (1 in the GM2/BCG group and 5 in the BCG group) resulted in differences of 23% (from 27% of patients remaining disease free to 50%) in disease-free survival and 14% in overall survival at 50 months with a minimal follow-up of 50 months. However, when all patients in the two treatment groups were compared as randomized, these increases were 18 and 11% for disease-free and overall survival in favor of vaccination with GM2/BCG, with neither difference achieving statistical significance. Antibody responses were predominately IgM, of moderate titer, and short lived (returning to baseline within 3 months of the final immunization).

A correlation between vaccine-induced antibody responses and clinical course has also been seen after immunization with sTn-KLH plus Detox. In a series of 113 patients with various types of epithelial cancers treated at the Cross Cancer Institute by MacLean, the 51 patients with high sTn antibody responses after vaccination survived significantly longer than the 62 patients with lower antibody responses. Antibody responses against KLH showed no such correlation. In a separate study, improved survival was also seen in 25 patients with advanced breast cancer who had a high antibody response to the sTn vaccine in combination with intravenous cyclophosphamide compared to 25 patients with a low antibody response and who did not receive the intravenous cyclophosphamide. The median survival increased from 13.3 months in patients with low anti-sTn antibody titers compared to 26.5 months in those with high titers.

VI. PHASE II/III RANDOMIZED TRIALS WITH CARBOHYDRATE VACCINES

Based on the progress described earlier, a series of randomized phase III trials with antibody-inducing single antigen vaccines against GM2 and sTn have been initiated (see Table III). Patient accrual in the stage III NED (no evidence of disease) GM2 trial (850 patients) has been completed. Follow-up data, accumulated at a median period of 16 months, show that the GMK vaccine does not improve relapse-free survival over IFN-α2b. And at this early time point, disease-free and overall survival were significantly lower in the GMK group compared with the interferon group. Further follow-up is needed to show whether the overall survival rates are equivalent. These trials involve (1) GM2 or sTn attached covalently to KLH for optimal induction of T-cell help and enhanced presentation to the immune system; (2) the use of a potent immunological adjuvant to further augment immunogenicity; and (3) immunization in the adjuvant or limited disease setting based on the preclinical and clinical studies described previously.

Although there is every indication that immunization with these single antigen vaccines may prove beneficial when administered in the adjuvant setting, in the long run, polyvalent vaccines offer greater promise. As described earlier, we have now induced

TABLE III
Phase II or Randomized Phase III Trials with Carbohydrate-Based Cancer Vaccines

Vaccine	Patients	Sponsor[a] (clinical centers)	Status	Trial design
Monovalent vaccines				
GM2-KLH+QS-21	Melanoma, stage III NED	PP, BMS ECOG, SWOG, CALGB, NCTP	Completed	Randomized phase III
GM2-KLH+QS-21	Melanoma, stage II NED	PP EORTC	Ongoing	Randomized phase III
sTn-KLH+Detox	Breast cancer, CR or PR to chemotherapy	Biomira Multicenter	Ongoing	Randomized phase III
Polyvalent vaccines (PV[b])				
PV	Ovarian cancer, first remission, NED	MSKCC	Ongoing	Phase I/II
PV-Tn(c)-KLH	Prostate cancer, rising PSA, NED	MSKCC	Ongoing	Phase II
PV	Breast cancer, high-risk stage, NED	MSKCC	Ongoing	Phase I/II

[a]PP, Progenics Pharmaceuticals Inc. (Tarrytown, NY); BMS, Bristol-Myers Squibb Co. (Wallingfold, CT); Biomira, Biomira Inc. (Edmonton, Alberta); MSKCC, Memorial Sloan-Kettering Cancer Center (New York, NY); ECOG, Eastern Cooperative Oncology Group (Boston, MA); SWOG; Southwestern Oncology Group (San Antonio, TX); CALGB, Cancer and Leukemia Group B (Chicago, IL); NCTG, North Central Treatment Group (Rochester, MN); EORTC, European Organization for Research and Treatment of Cancer (Brussels, Belgium).
[b]GM2-KLH, globo H-KLH, Le^Y-KLH, TF(c)-KLH, Tn(c)-KLH, sTn(c)-KLH, MUC1-KLH plus QS-21.

antibodies against GM2, fucosyl GM1, and sTn in close to 100% of patients and against GD3, GD2, Globo H, Le^y, Tn, and TF in 50–80% of patients. In all cases, these antibodies have been demonstrated to react with the cell surface of antigen-positive cancer cells and to activate complement. Consequently, phase I/II or phase II trials with polyvalent vaccines in the adjuvant setting have been initiated at MSKCC in patients with prostate cancer, ovarian cancer, and breast cancer. The antigens included in these vaccines and other aspects of these trials are listed in Table III.

See Also the Following Articles

ANTIBODIES IN THE GENE THERAPY OF CANCER • ANTI-IDIOTYPIC ANTIBODY VACCINES • CANCER VACCINES: GENE THERAPY AND DENDRITIC CELL BASED VACCINES • CANCER VACCINES: PEPTIDE- AND PROTEIN-BASED VACCINES • DNA-BASED CANCER VACCINES • RESISTANCE TO ANTIBODY THERAPY • TUMOR ANTIGENS

Bibliography

Livingston, P. O. (1998). The case for melanoma vaccines that induce antibodies. In "Molecular Diagnosis, Prevention and Treatment of Melanoma" (J. M. Kirkwood, ed.), pp. 139–157. Dekker, New York.

Livingston, P. O., and Ragupathi, G. (1997). Carbohydrate vaccines that induce antibodies against cancer. II. Previous experience and future plans. *Cancer Immunol. Immunother.* **45,** 10–19.

Livingston, P. O., Wong, G. Y. C., Adluri, S., Tao, Y., Padavan, M., Parente, R., Hanlon, C., Helling, F., Ritter, G., Oettgen, H. F., and Old, L. J. (1994). Improved survival in AJCC stage III melanoma patients with GM2 antibodies: A randomized trial of adjuvant vaccination with GM2 ganglioside. *J. Clin. Oncol.* **13,** 1036–1044.

Livingston, P. O., Zhang, S., and Lloyd, K. O. (1997). Carbohydrate vaccines that induce antibodies against cancer. I. Rationale. *Cancer Immunol. Immunother.* **45,** 1–9.

MacLean, G. D., Reddish, M. A., Koganty, R. R., and Longenecker, B. M. (1996). Antibodies against mucin-associated sialyl-Tn epitopes correlate with survival of metastatic adenocarcinoma patients undergoing active specific immunotherapy with synthetic sTn vaccine. *J. Immunol.* **9,** 59–68.

Riethmuller, G., Schneider-Gadicke, E., Schlimok, G., Schmiegel, W., Raab, R., Hoffken, K., Gruber, R., Pichlmaier, H., Hirche, H., Pichlmayr, R., Buggisch, P., Witte, J., and the German Cancer Aid 17-1A Study Group (1994). Randomised trial of monoclonal antibody for adjuvant therapy of resected Dukes' C colorectal carcinoma. *Lancet* **343,** 1177–1183.

Springer, G. F. (1984). T and Tn, general carcinoma autoantigens. *Science* **224,** 1198–1206.

Carcinogen–DNA Adducts

Alan M. Jeffrey
Columbia University, New York, New York

M. I. Straub
Veteran's Administration Medical Center, West Haven, Connecticut

---

I. Introduction
II. Types of Interactions with DNA
III. Detection of DNA Adducts in Biological Systems
IV. Isolation and Structure Determination of DNA Adducts
V. Applications of DNA Adduct Analysis
VI. Summary

GLOSSARY

bay region The bay-like structure formed in some tricyclic and greater polycyclic aromatic hydrocarbons (PAHs) by the nonlinear linkage of the aromatic rings, e.g., the 10–11 positions in benzo[a]pyrene (B[a]P). Many PAHs are metabolically activated to bay region diol epoxides, an example of which is shown for B[a]P.

biochemical monitoring The measurement of biochemical endpoints of exposure, such as DNA or protein adducts, that reflect an individual's difference in response to exposure to the same ambient concentrations.

carcinogen–DNA adduct The addition product between two molecules, in this case a carcinogen and DNA, involving one or more covalent bonds.

cytochrome P450 A member of a superfamily of closely related heme-containing oxygenase that oxidizes a wide variety of substrates.

diol epoxides Metabolites of some PAHs in which a single aromatic ring undergoes an initial epoxidation followed by hydrolysis of the epoxide and a second epoxidation of the remaining isolated double bond of the aromatic ring. These metabolites are often unstable in aqueous solution and hydrolyze to tetraols (see Fig. 1).

environmental monitoring The measurement of chemical in the environment to determine ambient exposure.

immunohistochemistry The use of specific antisera for the visualization of DNA adducts in histological slides.

metabolic activation The metabolism of a compound lacking the ability to react covalently with DNA (or proteins) to a product(s) that does.

pulse field gel electrophoresis A technique used to separate very high molecular weight fragments of DNA that cannot be resolved by conventional electrophoresis.

xenobiotic Describing or relating to a foreign compound.

Carcinogen–DNA adducts result from the covalent interaction of electrophilic chemical carcinogens with nucleophilic sites on DNA. This unifying concept for initiating carcinogens was proposed by Drs. James and Elizabeth Miller. Genotoxic carcinogens may have intrinsic reactivity with DNA or this reactivity may result from metabolic or photochemical activation of otherwise unreactive compounds. The former category most often results from products of the chemical and pharmaceutical industries or pyrolysis where very reactive chemical may be expected to be formed. Metabolic and photochemical activation of both natural and synthetic chemicals can generate reactive species capable of binding covalently to DNA. Additional sources of DNA damage include changes caused by reactive oxygen species and photochemical rearrangements of the bases. More energetic photons, such as X-rays, cause strand breaks in the DNA. All of these types of damage can influence the progress of a cell from its normal state to one which is malignantly transformed. With improved understanding of these processes, it is now recognized that DNA damage is critical at several points along this transformation process. Interactions with nongenotoxic chemicals are critical at other steps. Once a carcinogen–DNA adduct is formed, irrevocable damage does not necessarily follow. Many of these adducts can be successfully removed by one of a variety of pathways involved in DNA repair before replication of the damaged DNA occurs which may result in a mutation and, in that sense, fixation of the lesion. It is an axiom of pharmacology and toxicology that the critical concentration of a drug is that which is present at the receptor. In the case of genotoxic carcinogens that concentration is best represented by the level of DNA adduct formed at target sites in key genes. Despite the recognition that the distribution of DNA adducts on the two strands, or transcribed and untranscribed regions of DNA, may be different and that mutation of only certain genes is critical in carcinogenesis, it is difficult to measure such variations from the level of adducts in bulk DNA with precision in most instances. Adduct measurements in biomonitoring studies, therefore, generally quantitate overall levels of damage in the isolated DNA. The greatest extents of resolution are normally either by immunohistochemical analysis or through fractionation of different cell types before DNA isolation.

I. INTRODUCTION

Over 10 million compounds have been catalogued by the American Chemical Society's Chemical Abstracts. Of these, we are routinely only exposed to less than 1%. Conversely, many potentially carcinogenic plant and microbial metabolites have yet to be identified. Only 44 compounds, including a few inorganic and specific biological agents, have been classified by the fairly rigorous standards of the International Agency for Cancer Research as human carcinogens. In addition, 12 mixtures, such as shale oil, and 13 processes, such as aluminum production, have been added to this category. This number increases significantly if animal carcinogens, or those which have been shown to be mutagenic in one or other of a variety of test systems, are included. Although most compounds have not been investigated, it is probable that only a relative few pose a carcinogenic risk: most either do not react with DNA even after metabolic activation or these reactions are secondary to other toxicities. One of the reasons that it is difficult to be more definitive is the problem of proving a negative. The potency of a carcinogen can vary widely from species to species due to, for example, differences in metabolic capabilities, hormonal status, anatomical differences, or the need for exposure to multiple chemicals, not all of which are genotoxic. Most often chemicals are tested singly due to the obvious explosion of permutations if two or more were to be tested in combination. This approach is clearly imperfect since, for example, when low doses of benzo[a]pyrene (B[a]P), inadequate alone to produce tumors, are given in the presence of other noncarcinogenic polycyclic aromatic hydrocarbons (PAHs), significant yields of tumors result.

II. TYPES OF INTERACTIONS WITH DNA

Two main types of interactions of chemical carcinogens with DNA have been recognized: noncovalent and covalent. The former can have devastating effects on DNA. For example, bleomycin forms a complex with DNA and, together with chelated iron and oxygen, causes base loss. B[a]P, a PAH (Fig. 1), intercalates between the base pairs of DNA but, based on the minimal effects this has on cells without metabolic activation, this does not appear to be critical in the carcinogenicity of this compound. Covalent interactions of carcinogens with DNA may result from the intrinsic reactivity of a particular chemical with DNA. This most often happens with pharmaceuticals, including many of the antineoplastic agents that are designed for this property, or with reactive industrial chemicals. Other compounds, of both natural and synthetic origins, which lack this intrinsic reactivity, need metabolic activation by one or more enzymes to products that do. This led to the classification of carcinogens as either precarcinogens or ultimate carcinogens. A wide variety of enzymes, generally of broad substrate specificity, are involved in these metabolic transformations. They have been divided into two groups. Phase I includes the cytochrome P450 enzymes and epoxide hydrolyases as well as a variety of other oxidative and hydrolytic enzymes. These enzymes produce functional groups on previously generally hydrophobic molecules. These metabolites are then subject to further transforma-

tions by Phase II enzymes which add polar moieties, such as glucuronic or sulfuric acids or glutathione, which assist in excretion. The combined activity of these enzymes helps prevent bioaccumulation in the food chain seen with many heavily halogenated compounds, such as DDT, dioxin, and PCBs, which resist metabolism.

While these enzymes play an essential role in the elimination of hydrophobic components of our diet or contaminants in the water and air to which we are exposed, they sometimes generate highly reactive intermediates which can react with nucleophilic sites in cells, including DNA and proteins. As such, this process of xenobiotic metabolism has been described as a double-edged sword. Examples exist for almost every one of these enzymes in which they are involved in a critical step in the activation of a particular xenobiotic. While historically the cytochrome P450 and epoxide hydrolase enzymes have received the most attention, considerable effort is now being directed toward glutathione (GSH) S-, N-, or O-acetyl, sulfo, and glucuronyl transferases. GSH often provides a nucleophilic site for the inactivation of reactive metabolites but, as with most other pathways,

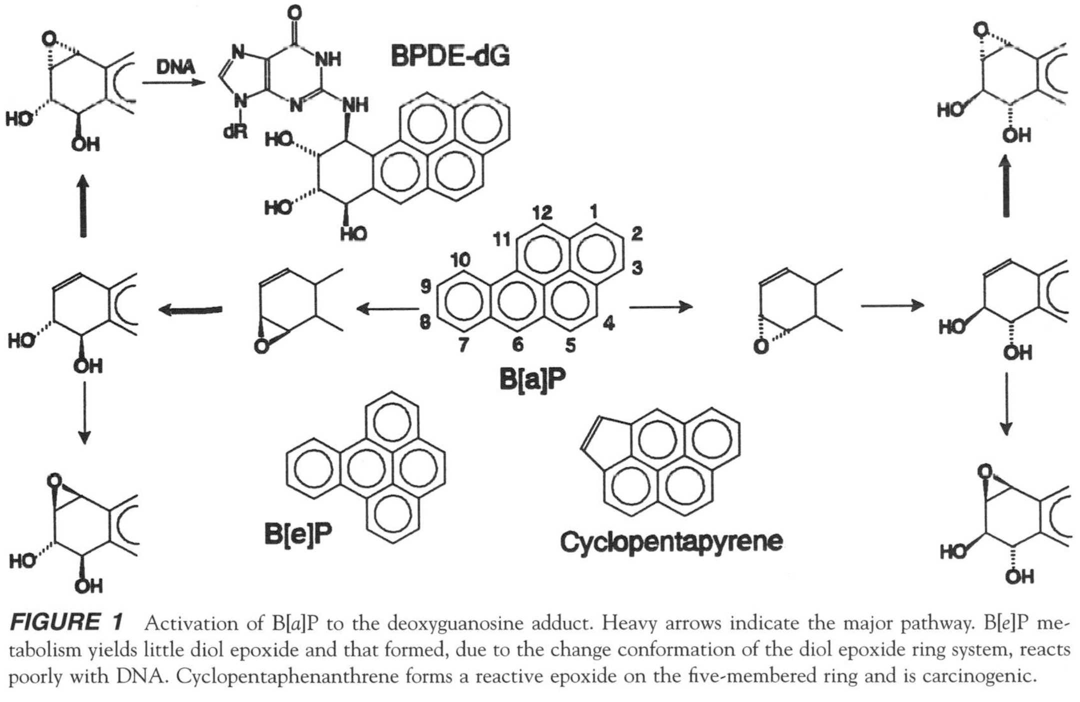

FIGURE 1 Activation of B[a]P to the deoxyguanosine adduct. Heavy arrows indicate the major pathway. B[e]P metabolism yields little diol epoxide and that formed, due to the change conformation of the diol epoxide ring system, reacts poorly with DNA. Cyclopentaphenanthrene forms a reactive epoxide on the five-membered ring and is carcinogenic.

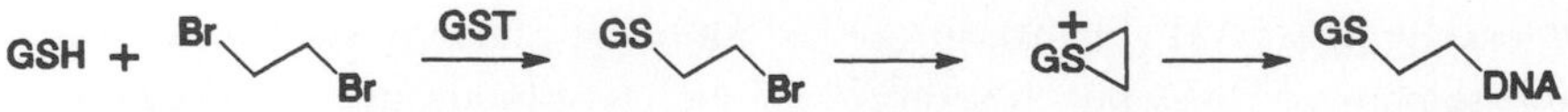

FIGURE 2   Example of activation involving GSH and GSH transferase to DNA formation.

reactions have been seen in which it can play a key role in the activation process and even becomes cross-linked to DNA itself (Fig. 2). NAD(P)H:quinone oxidoreductase has been shown to prevent specifically B[a]P quinone–DNA adduct formation, although the process is likely to be more general. However, such redox cycling can result in oxidative damage to DNA.

A very active area of research is the investigation of polymorphisms in xenobiotic metabolism which help explain interindividual differences in susceptibility to similar exposures to chemical carcinogens. Many of the enzymes involved in xenobiotic metabolism have been, or are being, cloned and probes are being developed to investigate these polymorphisms. This approach of genotyping an individual has advantages over phenotyping since drugs do not have to be administered and coexposure to other compounds, which could influence the phenotype, is not of concern. However, to obtain a comprehensive picture of an individual's ability to metabolize a xenobiotic the regulation of these enzymes also needs characterization.

Besides the metabolic capabilities of the host, the gastrointestinal tract is full of organisms capable of a wide variety of metabolic transformations. It has been long recognized that cycasin, the β-glycoside of methylazoxymethanol (Fig. 3), which occurs in the cycad nut, is only carcinogenic when hydrolyzed to the aglycone by the bacterial gut flora. In contrast, the aglycone is carcinogenic in both conventional and germfree animals by decomposition, through a methyldiazonium ion and loss of nitrogen to form an alkylating carbonium ion. N^7-Methylguanine is the major adduct formed. More recent studies have shown that the bacterial gut flora is involved in the specific activation of several nitroarenes and more generally by causing enterohepatic circulation of conjugates

eliminated in the bile. Interest was raised a few years ago in compounds found in human fecal samples which were highly mutagenic in the Ames bacterial mutagenesis assay. Fecapentaenes were isolated and characterized. It was found that they are an extremely unstable series of compounds, especially in the presence of oxygen. This instability hampered their testing as carcinogens and both positive and negative data have been obtained. Their possible role in the etiology of colon cancer is still unclear. Although reaction products with thiols have been characterized, none with DNA has been identified. However, bacteria of the gut flora clearly play an important role in the overall metabolism of potential carcinogens and efforts, often based on their DNA sequences, are being made to characterize them better.

With the aim of chemoprevention of DNA adduct formation the role of compounds able to modulate the levels of DNA adducts is also being intensely investigated. Some of these compounds, such as indole-3-carbinol (Fig. 4), a constituent of cruciferous vegetables, include a variety of Phase I and II drug-metabolizing enzymes. Because of the complexity of the responses they induce, and therefore the possibility of both beneficial and detrimental consequences depending on the carcinogen to which an individual is exposed, it is unclear how wide an application such compounds could have as specific chemopreventive supplements to our diets. Thus, while specific supplements such as isothiocyanates, organosulfides, polyphenols, and monoterpenes inhibit particular carcinogenesis models in animals, the recent surprise that β-carotene appears to increase the risk associated with cigarette smoking under certain circumstances is a sign that such compounds can act as double-edged swords depending on the specific

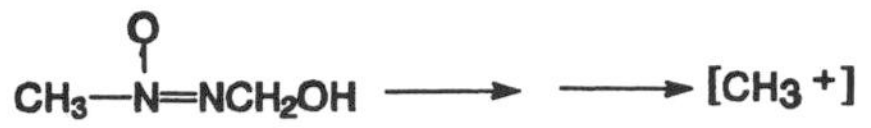

FIGURE 3   Decomposition of cycasin aglycone to a methylcarbonium ion.

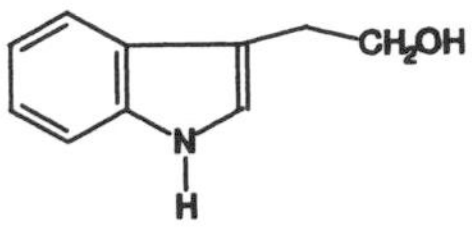

FIGURE 4   Indole-3-carbinol.

chemicals interacting. Diallylsulfide is known, for example, to be a suicide substrate for cytochrome P450 2E1 while 2B1 activity is enhanced by this compound. Thus, it should be possible to design experiments in which it can act as either an inhibitor or a potentiator of carcinogenesis depending on the carcinogen used. Humans, despite significant geographical and cultural differences, are exposed to a wide variety of carcinogens which must eventually be excreted. In general, therefore, slowing the rate of metabolism to avoid peak concentrations in adduct formation may be beneficial by allowing a steady repair of damage.

Once the ultimate carcinogens are formed, numerous factors can influence their reactivity with DNA. These parameters include the reaction mechanism (S_N1 or S_N2), the hardness of the nucleophilic center (oxygen generally being hard and poorly reactive in contrast to nitrogen, which is intermediate, and sulfur, which is soft and reactive), and the presence of adjacent groups which can influence the reactivity of a compound. Most alkylating reagents modify the purine ring nitrogens, especially N^7, and both purine and pyrimidine oxygens. Arylhydroxylamines, formed by the reduction of nitroarenes or oxidation of arylamines, most often react at the C-8 position of purines, possibly by rearrangement of transient N^7 adducts (Fig. 5). PAH diol epoxides react mainly with the exocyclic amino groups. DNA is chiral and therefore any reactive carcinogen containing one or more chiral centers may show preferential isomeric reactivity. The drug-metabolizing enzymes described earlier, while often having broad substrate specificity, can show remarkable specificity in the chirality of products formed, e.g., B[*a*]P metabolites (Fig. 1). No proteins have been described which specifically assist in the binding of the ultimate carcinogens to DNA, although numerous enzyme systems are involved in the repair of such damage. Consequently, shortly after exposure, patterns of DNA adducts formed *in vivo* and *in vitro* are generally similar. Exceptions oc-

cur most often when unusual polymers or solvents are used for the *in vitro* modification.

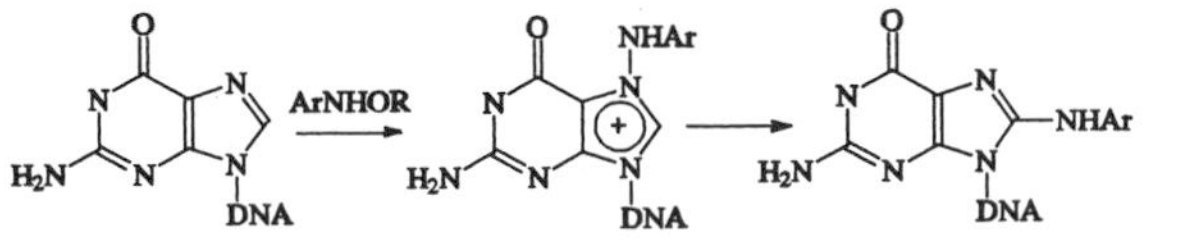

The reactivity of PAH diol epoxides with DNA, compared to hydrolysis to tetraols by water, varies considerably. In a series of the *R,S*-dihydrodiol *S,R*-epoxides, from BPDE to the sterically hindered fjord diol epoxide of benzo[c]phenanthrene, binding ranged from only about 10 to 75% of the diol epoxide added. The increased binding was also reflected in the pattern of adducts changing from only minor quantities of adenine adducts being formed from BPDE to being the major adducts with benzo[c]phenanthrene. Not surprisingly, within a given PAH the various isomeric diolepoxides showed marked differences in their DNA binding and ratios of guanine and adenine adducts.

III. DETECTION OF DNA ADDUCTS IN BIOLOGICAL SYSTEMS

One approach used is to allow biological amplification of the damage. An example of this is the Ames assay which depends on the inability of *Salmonella typhmurium* strains to grow without histidine. DNA damage can result in a back mutation to an organism which regains its ability to grow without histidine. Thus, on a plate containing a lawn of bacteria the few individuals in which such a change has occurred will develop as visible colonies. This test is well suited to the incorporation of enzymes capable of activating premutagens and producing the error-prone repair of adducts. Despite vigorous criticism of this assay regarding its ability to predict the carcinogenicity of a chemical, compounds found positive in this and similar bacterial and mammalian short-term mutagenicity test system are considered more likely to be carcinogenic.

Other indirect methods of detection include measurements of unscheduled DNA synthesis, single or double stand breaks by sedimentation, alkaline elution, or other techniques used to determine the molecular weight of the modified DNA such as pulse field gel electrophoresis or base sequencing methods.

A. Radioactive Labels

In animal and other test systems, most work has used ^{3}H- or ^{14}C-labeled carcinogens, although, for a few

FIGURE 5 Addition of arylamine to the N^7 position of the guanine residue followed by rearrangement to the stable C-8 adduct.

compounds, other potential radioisotopes are available. The advantage of ^{3}H is that it is relatively easily introduced into the carcinogens and can be obtained at higher specific activities than ^{14}C because of the former's shorter half-life. However, it is also very susceptible to loss during metabolism or by exchange reactions. This can result in the formation of tritiated water which in turn may become incorporated into nonexchangeable positions in newly synthesized DNA. Although now at very low specific activity, this tritium can contribute significantly to the overall level of apparent binding. The use of tritium-labeled compounds allow detection down to a level of a few fentomoles or, depending on the amount of DNA that is available, one adduct per 10^9 bases. This is about 200 times more sensitive than can be obtained with ^{14}C analogs, although the latter generally circumvents the exchange problems described earlier. In a few instances where the carcinogen can be degraded to molecules containing a single carbon atom, reincorporation is still possible. Adduct identification is made by chromatographic, normally high-performance liquid chromatography (HPLC), comparison with synthetic standards. Such comparisons should be undertaken carefully by analysis on different columns or with derivatization to ensure chromatographic identity since many adducts are difficult to separate. With the improved resolution of HPLC systems, isotopic separations may become significant, particularly for tritiated compounds. A recent alternative approach to the detection of ^{14}C compounds is by accelerator mass spectrometry. This provides high sensitivity (1 adduct in 10^{12} based), but unfortunately is unlikely to achieve wide spread application since the instrument is currently of warehouse rather than laboratory proportions. It provides no information on the chemistry of the adduct present, only their levels. This approach still requires that radiolabeled carcinogens be used and is limited by the natural background of ^{14}C. The latter can be reduced by growing animals or cells on ancient carbon sources but adds to the cost and complexity of experiments.

^{32}P-postlabeling of DNA (Fig. 6) is particularly suited to the evaluation of complex mixtures or hu-

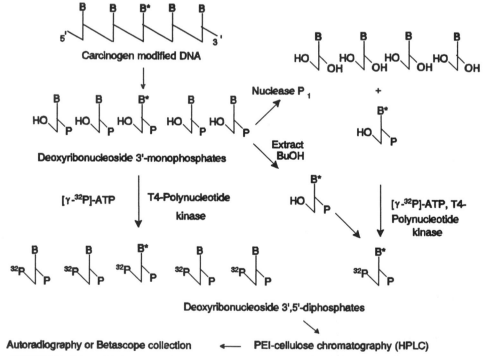

FIGURE 6 ^{32}P-postlabeling DNA (B* indicates the modified base) is digested and phosphorylated by polynucleotide kinase. Two enhancements of the procedure include nuclease P_1 digestion, which hydrolyzes most of the unmodified nucleotides to nucleosides, which are not kinase substrates. Mainly bulky DNA adducts, not linked through the C-8 purine position, are resistant to this enzyme. Butanol extracts mainly hydrophobic adducts.

man exposures where the administration of labeled carcinogen is impossible. DNA, isolated from the source of interest, is digested enzymatically to deoxyribonucleoside 3′-phosphates which are then phosphorylated with $[\gamma\text{-}^{32}P]$-ATP in their 5′ positions. ^{32}P can be obtained at about 300 times higher specific activity than ^{3}H and can be counted with higher efficiency due to the higher energy of the emitted β particle. This allows the method to be intrinsically much more sensitive. However, the major difficulty is the separation of the overwhelming excess of radioactivity associated with residual ATP, inorganic phosphate, the normal nucleotides which also become phosphorylated, and any radiochemical decomposition products that might have been formed. Clearly, depending on the level of modification of the DNA by the carcinogen, which may be the range of one adduct per 10^{6-10} bases, only about that fraction of the disintegrations will be those of interest. This assumes that the kinase will work equally on modified and unmodified 3′-phosphates which appears to be only partially true: in some instances the adduct is preferentially phosphorylated. An elaborate separation technique was therefore developed. The mixture of products was placed in the center of a PEI polyethylimine cellulose thin-layer chromatography (TLC) plate, and the plate was washed first in one direction, cutting away the edge of the plate into which the bulk of the unwanted radioactivity moved. The final two directions of chromatography allow for separation of the carcinogen-modified bases. This approach works quite well providing the carcinogen is hydrophobic, such as the PAHs, but is much less sensitive when simple alkylating agents are investigated. Enhanced sensitivity is achieved by a variety of approaches before the kinase reaction: separation of the unmodified bases by HPLC or immunoaffinity chromatography, if suitable antibodies are available; nuclease P_1 digestion to remove the 3′-phosphate group, which is essential for the kinase reaction, from unmodified nucleotide (best suited for bulky PAH adducts but not simple alkylating agents or C-8 adducts which are often digested); or butanol extraction of hydrophobic adducts using phase transfer reagents. Preseparation of the phosphorylated modified and unmodified bases from the kinase reaction by reverse-phase TLC before final transfer and separation of the adducts by PEI cellulose TLC has also

been used. Appropriate enhancements increase the sensitivity but also increase the effort per assay and can result in a lose of accuracy in quantitation. HPLC has been used, either prior or subsequent to the initial isolation of adduct spots. In the former case, precolumns have been used with flow diverters so that the bulk of the radioactivity does not pass through the analytical column and detectors. Capillary liquid chromatography and capillary zone electrophoresis (CZE) are very promising techniques and ones ideally suited to provide a high resolution of trace quantities and allow interface with mass spectrometers. The difficulty, however, to date with CZE has been the introduction of the sample since the application volumes are normally in the nanoliter range rather than the microliter range in which the postlabeled samples are typically dissolved. Stacking techniques are making progress toward overcoming this limitation. The recent introduction of ^{33}P which, due to its lower energy, can be counted in the presence of ^{32}P allows for the cochromatography of samples and standards when both have been prepared by postlabeling. This has advantages when the ultimate reactive metabolite of a carcinogen has not been made synthetically and so is not readily available for the preparation of adequate quantities of standards for detection by their UV absorption. Generally, for PAH detection, levels of one adduct per 10^{9} can be obtained, although Dr. Randerath and his group, who developed this method, have been able to obtain positive results down to one adduct per 10^{10} bases.

A number of adducts are now being detected at background levels including those from acrolein, crotonaldehyde (Fig. 7), and 4-hydroxynonenal and malondialdehyde, products of lipid oxidation. As animals age, additional spots often appear on the chromatograms. Because they are formed in such small quantities, their chemical identification has been impossible. However, because they add significantly to

R′= OH, R″=H: AC1+2

R′= H, R″=OH: AC3

R′= Me, R″=OH: CA1

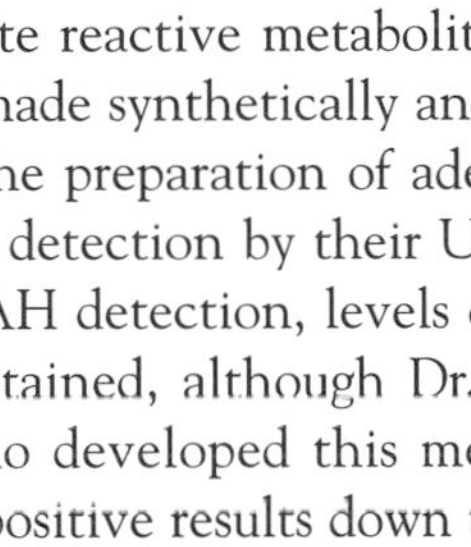

FIGURE 7 DNA adducts formed from acrolein (AC1 and 2) and crotonaldehyde (CA1).

the level of DNA damage, they are of considerable interest.

An alternative postlabeling technique, using t-butoxycarbonyl-L-[^{35}S]methionine N-hydroxysuccinimidyl ester, has been introduced for labeling 4-aminobiphenyl adducts and has been used on *in vitro* and *in vivo* samples from rats but not yet on human samples.

B. Immunological Methods

These approaches rely on the preparation of antisera which recognize specifically the modified bases in DNA. Such antibodies were prepared initially against methylated bases, but are becoming increasingly available for more complex modifications. Many variations exist on the method by which the antisera may be used, but one simple approach is described below. In the enzyme-linked immunosorbent assay (ELISA), DNA to be tested is coated onto the surface of a suitable plate. Antiserum, specific for the adduct of interest, is added and after incubation any noncomplexed antibody is removed. If this antiserum was prepared, for example, in a rabbit, a second goat antirabbit antibody, which was previously linked to a suitable marker enzyme, e.g., alkaline phosphatase, is now added. This will bind to the plate only if there was an interaction between the modified DNA and the primary antibody. The plate is again washed and the enzyme substrate, typically p-nitrophenylphosphate, is added. As hydrolysis proceeds, which will be proportional to the extent of modification originally present on the DNA, the color formed from the released nitrophenyl anion can be measured. By using specifically designed plates, 96 samples can be assayed at one time and the plates automatically washed and the color development measured. This assay is clearly attractive because of its ease of automation once established and is applicable equally to a wide variety of DNA adducts. The sensitivity of the assay can be further increased by using competitive versions of the assay, substrates which yield fluorescent products, by biotin–avidin enzyme complexes, or following the hydrolysis of ^{32}P-labeled substrates. The main restrictions relate to the preparation of DNA adequately modified to act as immunogen and the relative affinity constants of those antibodies produced for very low levels of modified bases compared to the normal sequences of DNA present in large excess. The former may be solved by

further development of *in vitro* immunization of spleen cells. The latter has both probable and theoretical limits which we may already be approaching. Current limits of detection are about 0.1 fmol/μg DNA or one adduct/10^8 bases.

The antibodies prepared to date have shown varying specificity toward different adducts. For example, it may be possible to distinguish between different alkyl substitutions at a particular site or to use the antibodies to detect adducts released into the urine by repair enzymes or spontaneous depurination. Such specific probes also allow for the location of adducts within cells and tissue or along the DNA chain. Image-enhanced immunofluorescence microscopic approaches have allowed the detection of as few as 700 O^6-ethylguanine residues per diploid genome. Although such experiments are still in a very early stage, these antibodies clearly provide tools for investigating not only the presence but also the location at which a particular adduct exists. Rapid improvements in image detection and analysis are occurring. Increased automation in the preparation and analysis of samples is helping to increase the sensitivity and reproducibility of the assays. However, the critical importance of the primary antibody cannot be avoided.

Recent developments in combinatorial chemistry have shown the possibilities of making molecules based on nucleic acids, proteins, and other synthetic polymers with very high ligand recognition capabilities, including purine and pyrimidine bases. Application of these molecules to carcinogen–DNA adduct detection is probably only a question of time.

C. Fluorescence Techniques

Guanosine shows significant fluorescence and this often increases with alkylation. Similarly, some highly fluorescent adenosine adducts have been prepared. However, the short wavelengths at which they absorb generally preclude the use of this technique to study such adducts unless the DNA is digested and the adducts are first separated, normally by HPLC. In contrast, studies on the PAHs and aflatoxins (Fig. 8) have made great use of fluorescence since these compounds absorb beyond 310 nm, where DNA gives little interference. In addition, the quantum yields of adducts may be increased by cooling to liquid nitrogen temperatures, and the sensitivity of the instru-

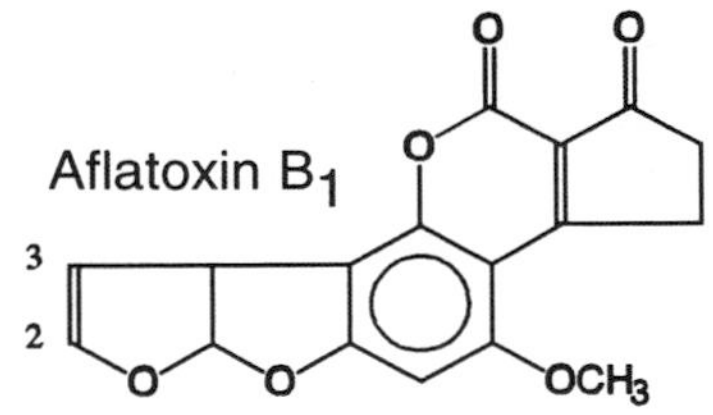

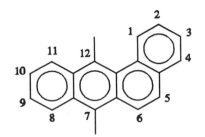

FIGURE 8 Aflatoxin B$_1$, an extremely potent carcinogen from *Aspergillus flavus*, is metabolically activated by epoxidation at the 2,3 positions.

ments can be increased by photon counting or laser excitation of the sample. The advantage of fluorescence analysis is that it requires no prior knowledge or preparation of the DNA adduct, only the knowledge that it is adequately fluorescent. Success depends, however, considerably on the type of metabolic activation which occurs. For example, in the case of 7,12-dimethylbenz[a]anthracene (Fig. 9), several groups have reported fluorescence spectra for DNA isolated from a variety of sources after exposure to the hydrocarbon. All describe metabolic activation as having occurred in the 1–4 positions. Dimethylanthracene absorbs strongly at long wavelengths to give a very characteristic spectrum. However, had metabolism occurred in the 8–11 positions, the residual phenanthrene chromophore would have been much harder to detect. Only after more thorough HPLC purification of the DNA adducts was it possible to be certain that the majority of adducts resulted from "Bay Region" activation.

Another limitation of this approach is that because of the relatively broad excitation and emission spectra, it is severely limited when attempts are made to analyze exposures to complex mixtures of PAHs. If a specific PAH adduct is to be detected and its excitation and emission spectra are known, then by determining the difference in wavelength between suitable maxima and scanning both the excitation and the emission monochromaters synchronously at the difference in wavelength, greater sensitivity and selectivity have been obtained.

In the case of PAHs themselves, significant improvements in the quality of spectra have been obtained by matrix isolation techniques, working at liquid helium temperatures to remove the effects of thermal broadening of the spectral lines. Under such conditions, it has been possible to analyze directly quite complex mixtures of hydrocarbons. However, the materials generally used for the matrix, such as nitrogen or hexane, are quite unsuited to PAH-modified DNA samples. Mixtures of water, ethylene glycol, and ethanol do, however, form suitable glasses in which DNA samples can be embedded. In such glasses the bound hydrocarbon moieties will be in any one of a large variety of microenvironments and, while the individual molecules may themselves have sharp excitation and emission spectra, the summation of these overlapping spectra is again a broad fluorescent spectrum. These subpopulations, or isochromats, may be individually excited with very narrow band pass light produced by a laser. This approach, called "fluorescence line narrowing," has been applied to a study of B[a]P bound to DNA. The spectra are much more characteristic than the broad band spectra of equivalent samples, and subtle differences in structure can be detected including resolution of complex mixtures containing up to nine PAH metabolites.

Numerous adducts, from PAHs to simple alkylating agents, are released from isolated DNA by acid hydrolysis. Free alkylated bases are released but, in the case of PAH diol epoxide–DNA adducts, they are acid labile and decompose to tetraols. These are not only more fluorescent than the adducts themselves, but are also more easily extracted from the large excess of unmodified bases. Detection levels of <1 adduct/10^5 bases using 40 μg of DNA have been obtained. The method does, however, require the certainty that hydrolysis of the adducts will occur and that the products will be stable or, if degradation occurs, that the products can still be recognized. In the case of aflatoxin, the major N^7 adduct undergoes, in addition to stabilization by ring opening, depurination. It was this adduct which, after extensive purification, was identified by its fluorescence in the urine of individuals who had high exposures to aflatoxins.

FIGURE 9 7,12-Dimethylbenz[a]anthracene.

Differences in fluorescence lifetimes of adducts can give clues to their conformation. Typically these measurements have been made in solution and provide information in distinguishing between internal and external binding on the DNA. Extensions of this approach using low-temperature laser-induced fluorescence in combination with polyacrylamide gel electrophoresis have been used to probe the sequence dependence of conformation of adducts. These studies, while having some limitations based on possible effects of the matrix, require far less material than NMR approaches. Similarly, information has been obtained regarding the environment of flourescent adduct by the hybridization of modified oligonucleotides to either complementary or mismatched sequences. Fluorescence detectors for HPLC, when optimized with high quantum yield compounds, can compete well in terms of sensitivity with radiochemicals in sensitivity.

D. Electrochemical Detection

Some DNA adducts which easily undergo reduction or oxidation reactions can be detected very well electrochemically: 8-hydroxyguanine (Fig. 10) is the most commonly measured by this HPLC detector. The other oxidized bases must be measured by gas chromatography/mass spectrometry (gc/ms) or by ELISA. One of the major challenges when studying oxidized bases is to ensure that no further oxidation occurs during sample preparation.

E. Mass Spectrometry

An alternative approach, applicable to both BP tetraols and related less fluorescent derivatives, has been developed in which, after adding an internal standard, the tetraols are oxidized with potassium dioxide to the corresponding dicarboxylic acids. These are derivatized with pentafluorobenzylbromide, purified by silica gel chromatography, and separated by gc/ms with selected ion monitoring (SIM) in the negative chemical ionization (NCI) mode. This provides specificity, based on the high resolving capacity of the capillary gc columns, discrimination, based on mass, and high sensitivity, based on the use of NCI/SIM. Identification of the PAH dicarboxylic acid is theoretically easier than the chiral and more difficult to prepare tetraols. This approach may be helpful in providing clues to the identification of adducts formed as a result of exposure to complex mixtures of PAHs.

Improvements in the sensitivity of mass spectrometry have enabled the detection of adducts formed in biological systems. Enhancements have been obtained by a number of approaches. These vary from relatively simple approaches such as the use of halogenated derivatizing agents which improve the sensitivity of detection to the use of high resolution or tandem (ms/ms) mass spectrometry systems in which the background of interfering ions can be minimized. SIM provides the highest sensitivity, when ionization conditions are used to minimize fragmentation, but little structural information. Because of the limited sample size available from biological systems, array detectors have advantages when the pattern of fragment ions is needed. Some of the first adducts to be analyzed by this approach were oxidation products of DNA. Questions have been raised regarding whether the levels measured reflect *in vivo* levels or, at least in part, additional oxidation occurring during the preparation of the samples. Recent studies have focused on DNA damage by ozone. While some adducts, detected by ^{32}P-postlabeling, are those typically seen in oxidized DNA, others may represent modifications characteristic of ozone. Their role in biological samples has yet to be investigated.

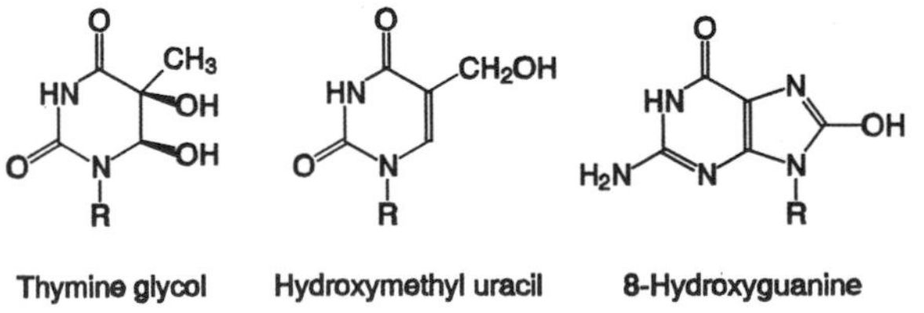

IV. ISOLATION AND STRUCTURE DETERMINATION OF DNA ADDUCTS

A major challenge still exists in the structural elucidation of adducts formed *in vivo*. Their presence is often known, but since the levels of modification of

FIGURE 10 Three of the major oxidized bases found in DNA. 8-Hydroxyguanine undergoes keto-enol tautomerism (enol form shown).

DNA are typically less than one adduct in 10^6 nucleotides and are often three or four orders of magnitude less, the quantities of these adducts which can be isolated are, therefore, extremely small. In general, clues as to possible structures of an adduct have been obtained by knowing the chemical responsible for adduct formation, its metabolism, and the possible structure of the ultimate carcinogenic metabolite. This can then be prepared synthetically or biosynthetically, at least in a transient state, which can be reacted directly with DNA or homopolymers *in vitro*. Digestion of the DNA to the modified nucleotides will often provide sufficient material for comparison with adducts formed *in vivo* and subsequent chemical analysis. Only a few adducts have been prepared by direct chemical synthesis. Structure identification is normally by nuclear magnetic resonance (NMR) and MS analysis. However, if isolated at the deoxyribonu-cleotide level, adducts with chiral centers will frequently separate as diastereomeric pairs with often approximately mirror image circular dichroism spectra. Such pairing of spectra often simplifies the identification of multiple adducts.

The most detailed structural information regarding the DNA adducts comes from NMR data involving NOESY and COSY experiments which have provided very detailed three-dimensional information regarding the solution conformation of numerous DNA adducts. These experiments complement and provide proof for molecular modeling studies (Fig. 11). It is, however, often difficult to prepare sufficient material for analysis and the sequences of oligonucleotides into which the adduct can be incorporated may also be limited if the reactive ultimate carcinogen is used to modify the oligonucleotides.

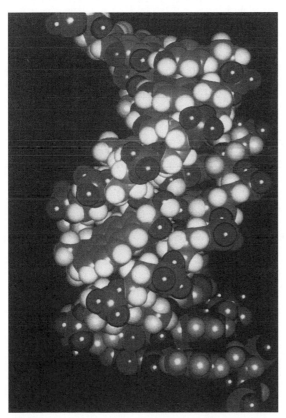

FIGURE 11 Molecular modeling of l-*t*-butylB[*a*]P diol epoxide guanine adduct in the minor groove of DNA. Despite the bulk of the *t*-butyl group, it appears to fit in the groove in a similar fashion to BPDE itself.

V. APPLICATIONS OF DNA ADDUCT ANALYSIS

A major goal of adduct analysis is to improve our ability to extrapolate data on carcinogen exposure to human risk. It is reassuring to find that good correlations have been obtained between carcinogenicity of genotoxic compounds and their ability to bind to DNA, especially when closely related series of compounds are investigated. Exceptions have, however, been noted. This is perhaps not unreasonable to expect based on the chemical diversity of carcinogens, their ability to bind to different bases, and the efficiencies with which an adduct can avoid repair or induce mutations. Nonlinearity of the dose–response curve can also contribute to these discrepancies.

As sensitivity of detection improves, more I compounds, a series of unidentified adducts intrinsically present in samples of DNA, will be detected. In some cases, as investigators analyzed samples for specific adducts, background levels have been detected in individuals for whom no specific exposure to the compound of interest was known. This may be particularly helpful in risk assessment: if there is a normal background present in all populations of a specific adduct, then attempts to regulate exposure to the progenitor compound to below a level which makes no significant impact on DNA adduct levels may be of little value. Caveats of course exist. For example, inhaled ethylene oxide may differ significantly in its carcinogenicity from that formed by metabolic activation of ethylene generated in and absorbed through the gastrointestinal tract.

Patients with familial adenomatous polyposis (FAP) have a high risk of developing duodenal adenomas and carcinomas. DNA adducts detected by ^{32}P-postlabeling as an index of genotoxicity are significantly higher in the duodenum of FAP patients than in controls. Bile obtained from the gallbladder of FAP patients immediately before colectomy, when incubated with DNA *in vitro*, produced significantly higher adduct levels than control bile samples, although the pattern of adducts were similar between the two groups. Incubation of bile with free radical scavengers and deconjugating enzymes did not influence adduct formation. The identification of the reactive compounds will be of considerable interest. Caution will be needed in adduct characterization since, in common with a few other non-3'-nucleotide derivatives, some bile acids can be phosphorylated by the kinase, although inefficiently.

Numerous studies have been conducted on the role of exposure to aflatoxins in conjunction with the he-

patitis B/C virus in the induction of hepatomas. Measurable adduct levels, both by synchronous fluorescence and immunohistochemistry, have been found in several populations and efforts to reduce exposure to both agents is clearly an important goal in reducing the incidence of liver cancer. 4-Aminobiphenyl-C-8-deoxyguanosine adducts have been detected in human bladder epithelium in smokers.

7-Alkylguanines are potentially useful markers of recent past exposure to environmental alkylating agents. Ethyl and higher homologs may be detected directly in urine. However, 7-MeG analysis in urine is complicated by the contribution from the breakdown of RNA in which it naturally occurs. Analysis of DNA circumvents this problem. 7-MeG is preferentially released from DNA rather than from RNA by hydrolysis at pH 9 at 70°C for 8 hr. After immuno-purification, quantitation by HPLC with electrochemical detection enables the detection of 0.5 pmol 7-MeG/DNA sample. 3-Methyl and ethyladenine have been shown to increase in cigarette smokers, but the alkylating agent is unknown, although NNK is a possible contender (Fig. 12).

As progress is made in improving the sensitivity of detection, we should be able to move away from study-

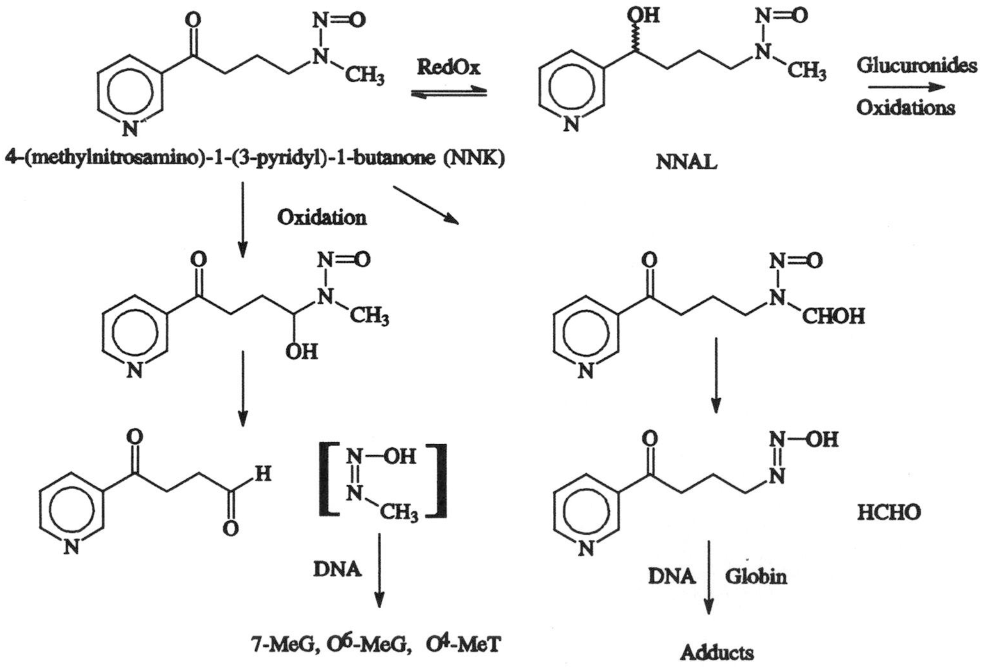

FIGURE 12 Metabolism of a tobacco-specific nitrosoamine NNK to DNA-alkylating derivatives. Metabolism to NNAL and glucuronides is considered detoxification.

ing only the most highly exposed cohorts. These include cigarette smokers, those occupationally exposed, and those being treated with genotoxic antineoplastic agents. The last group is particularly valuable since the doses given are close to the maximum tolerated dose and the most accurately known. These studies are especially valuable in children who, beyond their cancers, are often otherwise healthy and often tolerate higher doses/m^2 than older patients. These groups of patients provide valuable reference points for correlations with animal exposures to the same agent. Studies of adducts can also demonstrate the importance of different types of exposure. Forest fire fighters are exposed to a wide range of carcinogenic PAHs in smoke. Investigations of the association between occupational and dietary PAH exposures and the formation of white blood cell PAH–DNA adducts by ELISA found that adduct levels were not associated with cumulative hours of recent fire fighting activity. However, adduct levels were related to the frequency of charbroiled food intake within the previous week. These findings did not address the relative hazards of these two routes of PAH entry, oral and inhalation, which is critical to risk assessment analysis. The list of type of adducts and the cohorts in which they are found is growing rapidly.

VI. SUMMARY

Future studies of DNA adducts will probably move in three main directions. One will involve improvement in sensitivity and specificity of detection. The more often background levels of an adduct can be quantitated, the easier it will be to determine whether specific exposures or diets can modulate those levels. There will come a point, however, when detecting single adducts per cell will begin to dictate the minimum sample size needed for statistical significance.

However, a number of studies show levels of adducts with no clear distinction between exposed and control cohorts. Distinction between the background levels of adducts seen in all individuals and the specific changes which occur in the exposed cohort will be very helpful. A second direction, beyond detection-specific adducts, will include the identification of adducts found in DNA samples when individuals are exposed to no known specific agent (I compounds) or to complex mixtures when the specific chemical responsible for adduct formation is unknown. The third direction is in the area of molecular biology. Cloning the enzymes and regulatory elements responsible for adduct formation and repair and the construction of transgenic or knockout animals will help elucidate the molecular mechanisms of adduct formation, an aspect of increasing importance in risk assessment.

See Also the Following Articles

CARCINOGENESIS: ROLE OF ACTIVE OXYGEN SPECIES • CHEMICAL MUTAGENESIS AND CARCINOGENESIS • HORMONAL CARCINOGENESIS • MOLECULAR EPIDEMIOLOGY AND CANCER RISK • TOBACCO CARCINOGENESIS

Bibliography

Garner, R. C., Farmer, P. B., Steel, G. T., and Wright, A. S. (1991). "Biomonitoring and Carcinogen Risk Assessment." Oxford Univ. Press, Oxford.

IARC Scientific Publications No. 125 (1994). "DNA Adducts: Identification and Biological Significance."

Poirier, M. C. (1994). Human exposure monitoring, dosimetry, and cancer risk assessment. *Drug Metab. Rev.* **26,** 87–109.

Randerath, K., and Randerath, E. (1994). ^{32}P-postlabeling methods for DNA adduct detection. *Drug Metab. Rev.* **26,** 67–85.

Searle, C. E. (1984). Chemical carcinogenesis A. *Chem. Soc. Monogr.* **182.**

Strickland, P. T., Routledge, M. N., and Dipple, A. (1993). Methodologies for measuring carcinogen adducts in humans. *Cancer Epi Biomark. Prevent.* **2,** 607–619.

Carcinogenesis: Role of Reactive Oxygen and Nitrogen Species

Krystyna Frenkel
New York University School of Medicine

GLOSSARY

autoantibodies Antibodies recognizing antigen present in the same organism.

bioavailable Form that is not sequestered and is available for biochemical or chemical reactions within cells.

complete carcinogen A carcinogen that causes cell initiation and promotes cell transformation and growth to benign tumors, as well as mediates progression to malignancy.

chemokines Agents that even in minute amounts cause directed migration of cells.

cytokines Proteins produced by cells in response to inflammatory stimuli that affect the same or other cells in their growth, activation, priming, and death. Cytokines are an important part of the intercellular communication network.

growth factors Low molecular weight substances produced by cells that induce growth of the same (autocrine response) or other (paracrine response) cells.

inflammation A very complex process that is initiated by a release of cytokines and chemokines leading to the infiltration of phagocytic cells. Upon stimulation, phagocytes generate copious amounts of reactive oxygen and nitrogen species, proteases, as well as other enzymes and proteins. It can be manifested by fever, edema, hyperplasia, phagocytic infiltration, and oxidative stress.

oxidative stress Excessive production of and/or impaired removal of oxidants with a concomitant decrease in reducing capacity of cells.

oxidative modification of DNA bases Direct oxidation is characterized by a decrease in electron density. Such a modification can occur by oxidation of a double bond in a normal DNA base, of a methyl group, or by the addition of oxygen to a free pair of electrons. Indirect oxidative modification occurs when another molecule or macromolecule is oxidized and the product or by-product of that oxidation binds to DNA.

reactive oxygen species (ROS) and reactive nitrogen species (RNS) These are important players in normal physiology and signal transduction. They also participate in a plethora of damaging reactions, which lead to the disregulation of normal cell controls, thus contributing to various pathologies, including cancer.

transcription factors Factors needed for the transcription of genes into mRNA by binding to the specific recognition sequences in the promoter or enhancer regions of DNA.

tumor promoters Agents that support the development of initiated cells into transformed cells and tumors.

tumor suppressor genes Genes that prevent cell transformation and growth of tumors. Mutation of such genes usually abrogates their normal functioning and facilitates tumor development.

Carcinogenesis is a complex multistage process often taking decades until malignancy appears. Conventionally, the carcinogenic process has been divided into three main stages: initiation, promotion, and progression. Initiation requires an irreversible genetic damage causing mutations in transcribed genes. Promotion consists of a potentially reversible oxidant-mediated conversion step followed by a clonal expansion of the initiated cells into benign tumors, which can progress to malignancy when they acquire many additional genetic changes. Those genetic changes include modification of DNA bases, insertions and deletions, genetic instability consisting of loss of heterozygosity, chromosomal translocations, and sister chromatid exchanges, activation of oncogenes, and suppression of tumor suppressor genes. Although cell initiation is a frequent occurrence, tumor promotion and progression usually require a long time because of all of the genetic changes that have to accumulate within the same few cells.

It has been known for many years that antioxidants inhibit formation of tumors, even though they might not decrease DNA adducts, thought to be the initiating lesions. Hence, antioxidants are likely to interfere with the oxidant formation during promotion and/or progression stages of tumor development. Since then, numerous publications have shown that various types of reactive oxygen species (ROS) are generated during all stages of carcinogenesis, but especially during

that long time required to take an initiated cell to a fully disseminated cancer. This long period between the initiation stage and cancer development provides a wide-open window of opportunity to interfere with and suppress the carcinogenic process. This can be accomplished more readily when processes of tumor promotion/progression and factors responsible for them are known. Some of those factors are discussed in this article.

I. INTRODUCTION

The importance of oxidative stress to human cancer is underscored by the existence of cancer-prone syndromes characterized by the formation of high levels of oxidants and/or impairment(s) in their degradation or repair of the DNA damage they evoke. Those human congenital syndromes include Fanconi's anemia, xeroderma pigmentosum, Bloom's syndrome, ataxia telangectasia, Wilson's disease, and hemochromatosis, among others. The last two conditions also point to the contribution of an excess of bioavailable transition metal ions, such as copper and iron, to an overload of oxygen radicals in the liver and to the progression and outcome of those diseases. Hussain and colleagues clearly showed that livers of patients with Wilson's disease and hemochromatosis contain increased levels of inducible nitric oxide synthase (iNOS), as well as mutations in the p53 tumor suppressor gene, especially G:C to T:A transversions at codon 249. This finding is particularly important because hydrogen peroxide (H_2O_2)/iron treatment, as well as lipid peroxide-derived mutagenic aldehydes, such as 4-hydroxynonenal (HNE), cause the same type of mutations at codon 249. High levels of etheno compounds are present in liver DNA from patients having these two diseases. Interestingly, HNE causes formation of etheno derivatives in DNA and induces mutations at the 249 codon of the *p53* gene in HNE-treated lymphoblastoid cells. Notably, not only congenital syndromes exhibit mutations in the p53 gene, but also noncancerous colon tissues from ulcerative colitis patients, a colorectal cancer-prone chronic inflammatory disease. Frequencies of p53 mutations at codons 247 and 248 were strongly correlated with the progression of the disease being appreciably higher in inflamed than in noninflamed tissues. These studies strengthen the idea that chronic inflammation contributes to cancer, and the results are consistent with the hypothesis that p53 mutations at 247–249 codons are due to chronic inflammation-associated oxidative stress.

Oxidants are continuously formed and degraded during various normal cellular processes. ROS are required for the normal functioning of an organism and for the protection from invading bacteria. They are produced or utilized during mitochondrial respiration, metabolism of fats and xenobiotics, melanogenesis, and other peroxidatic reactions. Many types of cellular defenses keep these oxidants under control, but when they fail, extensive repair systems remove the damage from DNA and try to restore its integrity. ROS produced in small amounts can serve as second messengers in signal transduction. However, when ROS are formed at a time when they are not needed and/or in amounts exceeding antioxidant defenses and DNA repair capacity, then ROS can contribute to various diseases, with cancer being prominent among them. Tumor promoters and complete carcinogens induce chronic inflammation, ROS production, and oxidative DNA damage. Some of the oxidized DNA base derivatives are mutagenic, cytotoxic, and cross-linking agents. They can also cause hypomethylation, known to induce accelerated expression of some genes. This process might perhaps account for the ROS-mediated enhanced levels of various growth and transcription factors, and genes involved in antioxidant defenses.

II. OXIDANTS: REACTIVE OXYGEN SPECIES (ROS) AND REACTIVE NITROGEN SPECIES (RNS)

Extensive amounts of reactive oxygen and nitrogen species (ROS and RNS) are produced during inflammation, a normal bactericidal and tumoricidal process. However, *chronic* inflammation contributes to the long-lasting pathologic effects of the carcinogenic course of action, regardless of the type of cancer. ROS and RNS are generated by the activated "professional" phagocytic cells polymorphonuclear leukocytes (PMNs, neutrophils, granulocytes) and both circulating and resident macrophages. Target cells (i.e., epidermal keratinocytes or hepatocytes) can also form them in response to treatment with appropriate stimuli, such as tumor promoters or allergens. Although absolute amounts of ROS and RNS are much lower than those produced by stimulated phagocytes, these oxidants can set off a release and a synthesis of a cascade of various cytokines and chemotactic factors, which are instrumental to the initiation of inflammatory responses by phagocytic cells. ROS and RNS also mediate increased formation of growth and transcription factors needed for the accelerated growth of initiated cells.

Major ROS include superoxide anion radicals ($O_2^{\cdot-}$), their dismutation product hydrogen peroxide (H_2O_2), hypochlorous acid/hypochlorite (HOCl/OCl^-), singlet oxygen ($^1O_2$), and hydroxyl radicals ($\cdot OH$) (Table I). RNS are also produced during inflammation and contribute to its pathologic effects, with nitric oxide ($\cdot NO$), a product of iNOS, being a major player. The distinction between ROS and RNS is further blurred because of an avid interaction between $O_2^{\cdot-}$ and $\cdot NO$, which produces peroxynitrite ($ONOO^-$, a potent oxidant) at a near diffusion rate.

One of the most potent oxidants is $\cdot OH$. This can be generated by ionizing radiation and by iron autooxidation, as well as through the reduction of H_2O_2 by transition metal ions, such as iron or copper, in the well-known Fenton or Haber–Weiss reactions. Although to a lesser extent, $\cdot OH$ can also be formed in the absence of transition metal ions, when there is an opportunity for a homolytic scission. Because $\cdot OH$ are the most potent oxidizing species, they cause damage

TABLE I

Major ROS and RNS Produced during Inflammation

ROS or RNS $\longrightarrow$	Secondary ROS, RNS, and other reactive species
$O_2^{\cdot-}$	H_2O_2, $\cdot OH$, $ONOO^-$
H_2O_2	$\cdot OH$, HOCl/OCl^-
HOCl/OCl^-	$^1O_2$, RNHCl, RNCl$_2$, Cl$_2$, NO$_2$Cl
$\cdot OH$	Lipid peroxides
Lipid peroxides	Lipid hydroperoxides, aldehydes
$\cdot NO$	$ONOO^-$, N$_2$O$_3$, NO$_x$
$ONOO^-$	$^1O_2$, NO$_2^-$, NO$_3^-$, NO$_x$

only within a short distance from their generation. For this reason, H_2O_2, a neutral and not very reactive oxidant, is most likely responsible for reaching nuclear DNA and forming ·OH-like species at sites harboring transition metal ions. Even H_2O_2 generated outside of the target cells (i.e., by PMNs or macrophages) can pass through membranes of the target cells and cause damage in the neighboring or distant cells. Other ROS cannot cross cell membranes because they are charged (i.e., $O_2{}^{·-}$), lipophilic ($^1O_2$) reacting with membrane lipids, or react too rapidly ($HOCl/OCl^-$) with amino groups within membranes forming much longer acting chloramines. Of the RNS, ·NO can cross membranes. Although very reactive, $ONOO^-$ can diffuse within cells and might cross membranes of certain cells via anion transporters.

III. DIRECT OXIDATION OF DNA BASES

Both ROS and RNS can induce a plethora of genetic changes. Much is already known about the formation of oxidatively modified bases in cellular DNA. Figure 1 shows structures of oxidized DNA bases selected from well over 30 that are produced. The most extensively studied DNA base derivatives are thymidine glycol (dTG), 5-hydroxymethyl-2'-deoxyuridine (HMdU), and 5-hydroxy-2'-deoxyuridine (5-HdU), 5-hydroxy-

2'-deoxycytidine (5-HdC), and 5-hydroxymethyl-2'-deoxycytidine (HMdC), 8-hydroxy-2'-deoxyguanosine (8-OHdG), 8-hydroxy-2'-deoxyadenosine (8-OHdA), and their open-ring pyrimidine derivatives FaPy G and FaPy A. Many of these oxidized base derivatives are mutagenic (i.e., HMdU, 5-HdC, and 8-OHdG), whereas others block DNA replication (i.e., dTG). These oxidized bases can be formed directly by ROS, such as a site-specific attack by ·OH (or ·OH-like species), $^1O_2$ (i.e., 8-OHdG), or peroxyl radicals (HMdU). $HOCl/OCl^-$ can oxidize DNA bases through the evolution of $^1O_2$ in the presence of excess H_2O_2 and chlorinate cytosine and adenine residues in DNA and tyrosines in proteins. $ONOO^-$ oxidizes the guanine moiety in DNA to 8-OHdG but it reacts even more readily with 8-OHdG, which results in oxazolone derivative, cyanuric acid, and oxaluric acid as the end products. Hence, 8-OHdG might not be the best marker of oxidative stress and oxidative DNA damage if there is a possibility for $ONOO^-$ formation.

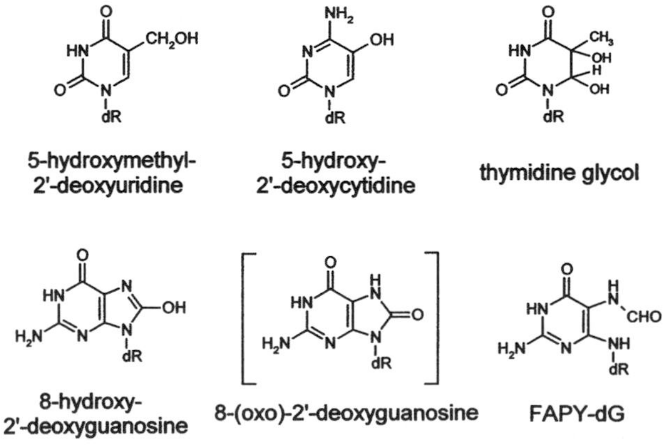

IV. INDIRECT ROS-MEDIATED MODIFICATION OF DNA BASES

In addition to the direct attack of oxidants on DNA bases, they can also be indirectly modified through interactions with electrophilic species produced by a ROS attack on other molecules or during ROS formation by such molecules.

A. Etheno-Base Derivatives Formed in DNA due to Lipid Peroxidation

ROS attacking unsaturated lipids cause the formation of lipid peroxides, which upon decomposition release aldehydes, such as malondialdehyde (MDA) and HNE. Both MDA and HNE are mutagenic and capable of binding to the amino group-containing dG, dA, and/or dC to form etheno derivatives, which contribute an additional ring to purines and pyrimidines (Fig. 2). Etheno compounds are present in DNA isolated from various types of tumors or from nontumorous sections of tumor-bearing animals and humans attesting to the existence of ROS and lipid peroxides in those tumors or tissues.

FIGURE 1 Selection of oxidized DNA nucleosides formed in DNA of humans, animals, and/or mammalian cells grown in culture. FAPY-dG, formamido-aminopyrimidine product of opening of the imidazol ring of dG.

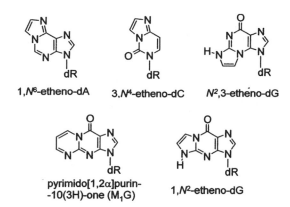

FIGURE 2 Selected products of interactions between aldehydes derived from lipid hydroperoxides (i.e., malondialdehyde or 4-hydroxynonenal) and amino group-containing 2′-deoxyribonucleosides in DNA of humans and animals.

B. Quinone–DNA Adducts Formed Due to ROS

An important example of processes leading to reactions of quinones with DNA is the redox cycling of the quinone–semiquinone couple derived from catecholestrogens. These evolve during estrogen metabolism by cytochrome P450 1A1 (CYP 1A1). Interestingly, lipid hydroperoxides acting as cofactors for peroxidatic oxidation also contribute to the formation of catecholestrogens (Fig. 3). Oxidation of semiquinone to quinone by molecular oxygen produces $O_2^{\cdot-}$ and H_2O_2 and, in the presence of iron or copper, forms $\cdot OH$, which can oxidize unsaturated lipids to lipid peroxides or, if formed *in situ*, cause oxidation of DNA bases. Thus, during metabolic estrogen transformation, several types of DNA modification should be anticipated: oxidized bases, etheno products derived from aldehydes released by lipid hydroperoxides, and quinone adducts. It is no wonder that estrogens have been implicated as contributors to hormonal cancers in humans.

Another example of the importance of quinones in carcinogenesis and ROS generated during metabolism is benzo[*a*]pyrene (BP), a polycyclic aromatic hydrocarbon (PAH) and a major pollutant. Long and co-workers showed that up to 50% of female knockout mice lacking NAD(P)H:quinone oxidoreductase (NQO1, enzyme reducing quinones by two electrons to the nonredox-cycling hydroquinones) develop tu-

mors when initiated with BP and promoted with phorbol ester 12-O-tetradecanoylphorbol-13-acetate (TPA) by the end of the experiment at 31 weeks, whereas the wild-type mice had none. Some (25%) of these tumors in NQO1($-/-$) mice progressed to malignancy. BP is metabolically activated by CYP 1A1 and related enzymes to a variety of oxygenated derivatives, including three BP quinines (Fig. 4), which in the presence of P450 reductase form semiquinones. Hence, again quinone–semiquinone couples can redox cycle and generate ROS. These results also underscore the important role that antioxidant enzymes, such as NQO1, play in carcinogenesis.

C. Effects of Inflammation-Derived ROS on Metabolism of Exogenous Carcinogens

Stansbury and colleagues showed that HOCl/OCl$^-$ (a powerful oxidant generated during inflammation by H_2O_2-mediated oxidation of chloride ions catalyzed by myeloperoxidase, an enzyme released by PMNs during activation) oxidizes BP 7,8-dihydrodiol to pyrene dialdehyde (Fig. 4), a novel BP-derived product that binds to DNA. These results point to ROS generated during inflammation as having a potential to change PAH metabolism and form DNA-binding species different from diol epoxides or quinones (Fig. 4). Oxidation and activation of polyaromatic amines by HOCl/OCl$^-$ have been known for many years. These could be some of the reasons why chronic inflammation contributes to carcinogenesis.

D. Oxidative Deamination and Nitration of DNA Bases

Although $\cdot NO$ has many physiological functions, when it is generated during chronic inflammation, it can oxidatively deaminate 5-methylcytosine, cytosine, guanine, and adenine, leading to the formation of thymine, uracil, xanthine, and hypoxanthine moieties in DNA. If not repaired, deaminated bases can mispair during DNA replication and cause mutations. Moreover, the nitrosating potential of $\cdot NO$ contributes to the formation of carcinogenic nitrosamines. In the presence of $O_2^{\cdot-}$, $\cdot NO$ produces a powerful oxidant, $ONOO^-$, which oxidizes dG and

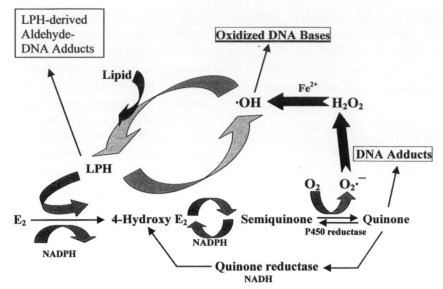

FIGURE 3 Redox cycling of quinone–semiquinone couples leading to the formation of three general types of modified bases in DNA: quinone–DNA adducts, oxidized bases, and etheno compounds, which are products of lipid hydroperoxide (LPH)-derived aldehydes' reactions with amino group-containing DNA bases. This redox cycling is illustrated by the metabolism of estradiol, a physiological hormone, which is suspected as a contributor to human cancers, such as those of breast, endometrium, and prostate. It also applies to other carcinogens, which are metabolized to quinones and semiquinones that can redox cycle. Adapted from JNCI Monograph No. 27, p. 86, 2000, published by the Oxford Univ. Press, with permission from the publisher.

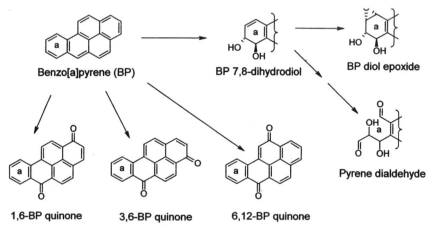

FIGURE 4 Metabolism of benzo[*a*]pyrene (BP, a carcinogenic polycyclic aromatic hydrocarbon) to metabolites that can form adducts with DNA bases and depurinating adducts, as well as contribute to the oxidation of bases in DNA through the redox cycling of quinone–semiquinone couples. The newly described pyrene dialdehyde potentially can form mono-adducts with DNA bases, as well as form intra- and interstrand DNA cross-links and DNA–protein cross-links. Pyrene dialdehyde is produced by oxidation of BP 7,8-dihydrodiol with HOCl/OCl$^-$ generated by activated PMNs during inflammation.

8-OHdG and also has nitrating properties evident from the formation of 8-nitroguanine in DNA and 3-nitrotyrosine in proteins. Upregulated iNOS and 3-nitrotyrosine have been found in tumor tissues and, in some cases, such as in metastatic melanoma, were correlated with poor survival of the patients, according to Ekmekcioglu and co-workers.

V. CARCINOGEN-MEDIATED INFLAMMATORY AND OXIDATIVE RESPONSES

As already mentioned, carcinogens, such as PAHs, can be metabolized by ROS-mediated pathways and they also contribute to ROS formation. Virtually all types of complete carcinogens and tumor promoters tested cause oxidative DNA base damage *in vivo* and, when analyzed, H_2O_2 is also evident in the target tissues. Carcinogens have been known to evoke inflammation thought to be necessary for tumorigenesis. An important question arises as to the mechanism(s) by which inflammatory responses are induced. Tumor promoters, such as TPA, induce inflammation very rapidly through protein kinase C, which provides a signal for a plethora of responses. A prominent response among them is a rapid release of interleukin (IL)-1α from suprabasal keratinocytes, which initiates a cascade of other cytokines and chemotactic factors synthesis, including IL-1α, tumor necrosis factor (TNF)-α, IL-8, granulocyte/macrophage-colony stimulating factor, and others. Frenkel and colleagues and Li and co-workers showed that similar to TPA, 7,12-dimethylbenz[a]anthracene (DMBA, a carcinogenic PAH) also induces IL-1α and TNF-α release and causes mRNA upregulation, which leads to further cytokine production in mouse skin. DMBA-induced IL-1α was responsible for PMN infiltration into mouse skin, as >65% of that infiltration was inhibited by preinjection of mice with anti-IL-1α antibody (Ab). Interestingly, anti-IL-1α Ab did not have appreciable effects on the incidence of DMBA-induced papillomas or carcinomas, but very potently inhibited the carcinoma volume, whereas anti-TNF-α Ab suppressed the incidence and volume of benign tumors but not carcinomas. DMBA mediated a substantial increase in HMdU and 8-OHdG in mouse skin, lev-

els of which declined over time but remained elevated after tumors appeared. It will be important to establish whether DMBA-induced oxidative DNA base damage is modulated by anti-IL-1α and/or anti-TNF-α Ab and whether these two Abs have comparable or different effects on that DNA base damage.

Upregulation of proinflammatory cytokines causes infiltration of phagocytic cells into the affected area. Circulating phagocytes are primed by IL-1α, whereas infiltrating cells may be further primed by TNF-α, which increases ROS production when those cells are activated by an appropriate stimulus. It is not yet known which of the DMBA metabolites is responsible for the start of this inflammatory process and whether the same or a different metabolite is needed for PMN activation. However, H_2O_2, HMdU, and 8-OHdG formation in DMBA-treated mouse skin attests to that activation. It appears then that immune responses to carcinogen treatment are very important in the determination of which pathway predominates and culminates in a preferential formation of benign and/or malignant tumors. Elevated levels of inflammatory cytokines have been found in many types of human cancer, including ovarian, lung, skin, and liver, as well as in many chronic inflammatory conditions, which are known cancer risk factors.

VI. FACTORS CONTRIBUTING TO CYTOKINE UPREGULATION

Upregulation of inflammatory cytokines' mRNAs requires binding of transcription factors, such as activator protein (AP)-1 and/or nuclear factor (NF)-κB, to the specific sites in the promoter or enhancer regions of the cytokine genes. Formation and activation of transcription factors required for cytokine upregulation depend on the redox status of the cell and its effect on those factors. Increased H_2O_2 production causes rapid phosphorylation of the inhibitor (IκB) and its dissociation from the NF-κB complex, which allows for NF-κB translocation from cytosol into the nucleus. Before binding to the appropriate consensus sequence giving a signal for the initiation of the transcription process, NF-κB must be reduced by the thioredoxin system, which itself depends on glutathione (GSH), a major cellular reductant in the nucleus. Often, more than one binding site is needed for the transcription to occur or more than one type of a transcription factor is required. AP-1, another transcription factor, is formed from c-*fos* and c-*jun*, two immediate early genes produced under conditions of oxidative stress. Interestingly, AP-1 binding also requires reduced sulfhydryl groups in the cysteine residues, which is accomplished under conditions of increased reductive power of GSH, NAD(P)H, and antioxidant enzymes. For this reason, the AP-1 pathway is often referred to as an antioxidant-regulated pathway. Interestingly, recent results show that the presence of oxidized bases at the recognition sequence can modulate binding of the transcription factors and, thus, interfere with gene expression, including those of cytokines. This is a very exciting area of investigation, which might show how oxidation of bases at specific sites of DNA could interfere directly with or enhance the carcinogenic process.

VII. OXIDIZED DNA BASES IN HUMAN CANCER

Elevated levels of oxidized purines were found in DNA isolated from human breast tumors, whereas increased levels of oxidized pyrimidines (HMdU) were present in white blood cell (WBC) DNA of women at high risk for breast cancer, as well as those diagnosed with breast cancer. Changes in the diet to lower the consumption of fat and increase that of fruits and vegetables caused a statistically significant decline in HMdU present in WBC DNA of the dieting high-risk subjects. The formation of oxidized bases in the DNA of breast cancer patients is due to extensive oxidative stress that is evident in breast cancer patients, whose phagocytes produce more $O_2^{\cdot-}$ and H_2O_2 than those of healthy controls (Ray *et al.*). At the same time, antioxidant enzymes superoxide dismutase (SOD) and GSH peroxidase are appreciably increased, whereas catalase is decreased. The high SOD content could rapidly dismutate $O_2^{\cdot-}$ to H_2O_2, which cannot be completely degraded to water because of the decreased catalase activity. Thus, the accumulated H_2O_2 can migrate into other cells and their nuclei, where it generates $\cdot$OH-like species in a site-specific manner that oxidize DNA bases. Results obtained by Gowen and colleagues further underscore the importance of oxidative DNA base damage to breast cancer. The authors discovered that the BRCA1 gene product is required for the transcription-coupled repair of oxidative DNA base damage. BRCA1 mutations confer susceptibility to human breast cancer, which provides strong evidence that oxidative DNA base damage contributes to breast cancer, at least in women carrying the mutated BRCA1 gene.

In comparison to healthy controls, autoantibodies (aAb) that recognize HMdU were increased in sera of women diagnosed with breast cancer, thus providing another proof of oxidative stress and a biologic response to the consequences of that stress in cancer. More importantly, sera of apparently healthy women, who 1 to 6 years *after* that blood donation, were diagnosed with breast, colon, or rectal cancers, and sera of those at high risk for cancer contained elevated anti-HMdU aAbs. Thus, the enhanced presence of oxidized bases (i.e., HMdU) in WBC DNA, anti-HMdU aAb in serum, and possibly other antioxidized DNA base aAb can potentially serve as biomarkers of susceptibility to cancer. These biomarkers may allow preventive measures to be undertaken before an overt malignancy develops and, therefore, may also serve as efficacy markers of cancer-preventive agents.

VIII. CONCLUSIONS

Studies of factors contributing to the carcinogenic process, especially those modulated by oxidative stress, are by necessity correlative in nature. However, a discovery of more specific inhibitors and an increased use of molecular biology techniques have started to yield more direct proof of the involvement of oxidative stress and oxidative DNA base damage in carcinogenesis. Oxidative stress is characterized by increased ROS production, decreased antioxidant defenses, and impaired DNA repair capacity. All are evident during chronic inflammation evoked by a variety of agents or health conditions, many of which are known risk factors for different types of cancer. In summary, there is ever increasing scientific evidence that changes occurring during chronic inflammation, which include increased expression of inflammatory cytokines and downregulation of protective cytokines leading to further exacerbation of oxidative stress, play a direct role in the process of carcinogenesis. Oxidative modification of DNA bases present at specific sites of tumor suppressor genes, such as p53, which plays a pivotal role in cell cycling and apoptosis, causes a decline in their expression. Oxidized bases are also capable of changing binding patterns of transcription factors, and thus affect gene expression of many genes, which can lead to the disregulation of genetic machinery responsible for normal cell functioning.

Acknowledgments

Support by NCI (CA37858), NIA (AG14587), and NIEHS (ES00260) is gratefully acknowledged.

See Also the Following Articles

CHEMICAL MUTAGENESIS AND CARCINOGENESIS • HORMONAL CARCINOGENESIS • HYPOXIA AND DRUG RESISTANCE • TOBACCO CARCINOGENESIS

Bibliography

Ardestani, S. K., Inserra, P., Solkoff, D., and Watson, R. R. (1999). The role of cytokines and chemokines on tumor progression: A review. *Cancer Detect. Prev.* **23**, 215–225.

Arrigo, A. P. (1999). Gene expression and the thiol redox state. *Free Radic. Biol. Med.* **27**, 936–944.

Bartsch, H. (2000). Studies on biomarkers in cancer etiology and prevention: A summary and challenge of 20 years of interdisciplinary research. *Mutat. Res.* **462**, 255–279.

Bolton, J. L., Trush, M. A., Penning, T. M., Dryhurst, G., and Monks, T. J. (2000). Role of quinones in toxicology. *Chem. Res. Toxicol.* **13**, 135–160.

Cavalieri, E., Frenkel, K., Rogan, E., Roy, D., and Liehr, J. G. (2000). Estrogens as endogenous genotoxic agents: DNA adducts and mutations. *J. Natl. Cancer Inst. Monogr.* **27**, 75–93.

Ekmekcioglu, S., Ellerhorst, J., Smid, C. M., Prieto, V. G., Munsell, M., Buzaid, A. C., Grimm, E. A. (2000). Inducible nitric oxide synthase and nitrotyrosine in human metastatic melanoma tumors correlate with poor survival. *Clin. Cancer Res.* **6**, 4768–4775.

Frenkel, K. (1997). Carcinogenesis: Role of active oxygen species. *In* "Encyclopedia of Cancer" (J. R. Bertino, ed.), pp. 233–245. Academic Press, San Diego.

Frenkel, K. (1992). Carcinogen-mediated oxidant formation and oxidative DNA damage. *Pharmacol. Ther.* **53**, 127–166.

Frenkel, K., Karkoszka, J., Glassman, T., Dubin, N., Toniolo, P., Taioli, E., Mooney, L., and Kato, I. (1998). Serum autoantibodies recognizing 5-hydroxymethyl-2-deoxyuridine, an oxidized DNA base, as biomarkers of cancer risk in women. *Cancer Epidemiol. Biomark. Prevent.* **7**, 49–57.

Frenkel, K., Wei, L., and Wei, H. (1995). 7,12-Dimethyl-benz[a]anthracene induces oxidative DNA modification in vivo. *Free Radic. Biol. Med.* **19**, 373–380.

Ghosh, R., and Mitchell, D. L. (1999). Effect of oxidative DNA damage in promoter elements on transcription factor binding. *Nucleic Acids Res.* **27**, 3213–3218.

Gowen, L. C., Avrutskaya, A. V., Latour, A. M., Koller, B. H., and Leadon, S. A. (1998). BRCA1 required for transcription-coupled repair of oxidative DNA damage. *Science* **281**, 1009–1012.

Hussain, S. P., Raja, K., Amstad, P. A., Sawyer, M., Trudel, L. J., Wogan, G. N., Hofseth, L. J., Shields, P. G., Billiar, T. R., Trautwein, C., Hohler, T., Galle, P. R., Phillips, D. H., Markin, R. Marrogi, A. J. and Harris, C. C. (2000). Increased p53 mutation load in nontumorous human liver of wilson disease and hemochromatosis: oxyradical overload diseases. *Proc. Natl. Acad. Sci. USA* **97**, 12770–12775.

Klein, C. B., Snow, E. T., and Frenkel, K. (1998). Molecular mechanisms in metal carcinogenesis: Role of oxidative stress. *In* "Molecular Biology of Free Radicals in Human Diseases" (O. I. Aruoma and B. Halliwell, eds.), pp. 79–137. OICA International, London.

Li, X., Li, C. and Frenkel, K. (2001). Differences in the effects of inflammatory cytokines interleukin (IL)-1α and tumor necrosis factor (TNF)-α on 7,12-dimethylbenz(a)anthracene (DMBA)-induced carcinogenesis. *Proc. Am. Assoc Cancer Res.* **42**, 806.

Li, X., Eckard, J., Shah, R., Malluck, C. and Frenkel, K. (2002). Interleukin-1α up-regulation *in vivo* by a potent carcinogen 7,12-dimethylbenz(a)anthracene (DMBA) and control of DMBA-induced inflammatory responses. *Cancer Res.* **62**, 417–423.

Long, D. J., Waikel, R. L., Wang, X. J., Perlaky, L., Roop, D. R., and Jaiswal, A. K. (2000). NAD(P)H:quinone oxidoreductase 1 deficiency increases susceptibility to benzo(a)-pyrene-induced mouse skin carcinogenesis. *Cancer Res.* **60**, 5913–5915.

Lyons, C. R. (1995). The role of nitric oxide in inflammation. *Adv. Immunol.* **60**, 323–371.

Marnett, L. J. (2000). Oxyradicals and DNA damage. *Carcinogenesis* **21**, 361–370.

Neurath, M. F., Becker, C., and Barbulescu, K. (1998). Role of NF-kappaB in immune and inflammatory responses in the gut. *Gut* **43**, 856–860.

Qian, S., and Buettner, G. (1999). Iron and dioxygen chemistry is an important route to initiation of biological free radical oxidations: An electron paramagnetic resonance spin trapping study. *Free Radic. Biol. Med.* **26**, 1447–1456.

Ray, G., Batra, S., Shukla, N. K., Deo, S., Raina, V., Ashok, S. and Husain, S. A. (2000). Lipid peroxidation, free radical production and antioxidant status in breast cancer. *Breast Cancer Res. Treat.* **59**, 163–170.

Stansbury, K. H., Noll, D. M., Groopman, J. D., and Trush, M. A. (2000). Enzyme-mediated dialdehyde formation: An alternative pathway for benzo[a]pyrene 7,8-dihydrodiol bioactivation. *Chem. Res. Toxicol.* **13**, 1174–1180.

Caspases in Programmed Cell Death

J. Marie Hardwick
Johns Hopkins School of Public Health

I. Discovery
II. Structure of Caspases
III. Activation of Caspases
IV. Regulation of Caspase Activation
V. Role in Caspases in Development and Disease

GLOSSARY

apoptosis A type of "programmed cell death" or "cell suicide" (genetically controlled process of self-destruction) in which the cell undergoes DNA condensation, membrane blebbing, and other specific characteristics that are usually the result of activation of intracellular proteases called caspases.

protease Enzyme that cleaves polypeptide chains.

Caspases (Cys active site; Asp cleavage site specificity; -ase conventional for proteases) are a family of cysteine proteases that facilitate apoptotic cell death in metazoans. These proteases are expressed inside cells and cleave a subset of intracellular proteins to facilitate the biochemical and morphological changes that occur during cell suicide. Caspases and granzyme B are the only mammalian proteases known to cleave after aspartate residues, aiding in the study of these proteases and their substrates. Over 80 cellular substrates have been identified and there may be as many as 200 in total (Table I). Cleavage of these substrates can inactivate, activate, or alter their functions, and many, if not all, of these cleavage events contribute to cell death. Thus, caspase activation leads to the activation of nucleases, condensation of chromatin, changes in the cytoskeleton, and other events characteristic of apoptotic cells. Cells also encode many proteins that positively and negatively regulate the activation and function of these potentially deadly proteases. Caspases are essential for embryonic development, and the dysregulation of caspases has been implicated in a number of human disease states.

I. DISCOVERY

Genetic studies in the nematode *Caenorhabditis elegans* demonstrated that a gene encoding CED-3 mediates programmed cell death of all 131 somatic cells that are destined to die by programmed cell death. That is, in

TABLE I
Caspase Substrates (Partial List)

Substrate	Function
Poly(ADP)-ribose polymerase	DNA repair, other?
β-actin	Cell structure
Nuclear lamin proteins	Nuclear envelope structure
α/β-fodrin	Cell structure
Gelsolin	Cell structure
Caspases	Activated by proteolysis to kill cells
Rb	Tumor suppressor, sequesters E2F, blocks cell cycle
DNA-PK (protein kinase)	DNA repair? Recombination?
Protein kinase C	Activated by cleavage, signal transduction
MEKK1	Ser/Thr kinase (induces/inhibits apoptosis)
Huntington's disease protein	Unknown function, contains trinucleotide repeat
SRE/BP	Transcription factor
rho-GDI	Signaling
hnRNPs C1 and C2	Splicing
ICAD	Inhibitor bound to apoptosis endonuclease CAD
IkB	Inhibitor bound to NF-κB
p21Waf1	Cdk inhibitor induced by p53
Bcl-2	Antiapoptotic becomes proapoptotic with cleavage
Bcl-xL	Antiapoptotic becomes proapoptotic with cleavage
Bid	C-terminal cleavage fragment kills cells
Presenilin	Regulates neuronal death/survival
Acinus	Chromatin condensation during apoptosis
ROCK	Rho GTPase involved in actomyosin-based contractility, activated by caspases

the absence of CED-3 function, this 959 cell organism has an extra 131 cells that normally die by programmed cell death during development. However, the biochemical function for CED-3 was not uncovered until the cloning of the human protease ICE (IL-1β converting enzyme, renamed caspase-1), which is responsible for cleaving the precursor form of pro-IL-1β to release the active proinflammatory IL-1β cytokine.

Subsequently, a dozen additional human caspases have been cloned and partially characterized. Caspase-1 clearly has a role in inflammation *in vivo*, and the role of caspases-1, -4, and -5 in apoptosis is still debated. However, most caspases appear to have a direct role in promoting cell death, although some caspases are likely to have additional functions as well.

II. STRUCTURE OF CASPASES

Caspases are synthesized as zymogens (inactive enzyme precursors) that must be cleaved into large (17–21 kDa) and small (10–13 kDa) subunits that form the active tetrameric enzyme ($p20_2$:$p10_2$) (Fig. 1). An additional cleavage event can remove the N-terminal prodomain (3–24 kDa) of caspases. The long prodomains of some caspases contain protein–protein interaction motifs (called CARD, caspase recruitment domains; or DED, death effector domains) that target these zymogens to protein complexes within the cell to facilitate caspase activation. Other caspases have short prodomains with unknown function. The three-dimensional structure of some caspases has been solved. The active site Cys and His residues are in the large subunit, but both subunits together form the substrate-binding cleft. The two heterodimers, each folded into a cylinder consisting of a central six-stranded β sheet and five α helices, are in a head-to-tail orientation, producing an enzyme with two active sites on opposite ends of the tetramer (Fig. 1). The active site cleft recognizes a four amino acid sequence. Other than the required Asp present at the P1 position, the amino acid present at the P4 position (fourth amino acid N-terminal of the cleavage site) confers the greatest speci-

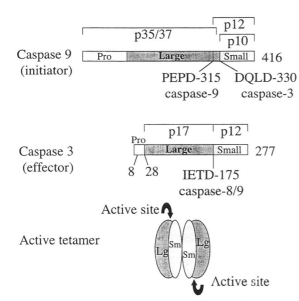

FIGURE 1 Caspases contain three segments: prodomain (Pro), large subunit (Lg), and small subunit (Sm). Caspases are activated when cleaved by other caspases (except caspase 9, which can be active prior to cleavage). The resulting fragments (indicated as p with their approximate size in kilodaltons) form the tetrameric enzyme containing two active sites. The amino acid sequence (single letter code) of the cleavage sites in caspase-9 and caspase-3 are indicated by position (amino acid number) and the name of the caspase that cleaves at that site. Initiator (upstream, long prodomain) caspases can self-cleave and can cleave effector (downstream, short prodomain) caspases.

ficity. Caspases have been classified into three groups based on their peptide substrate specificities (Table II). However, substrate specificity determined by the analysis of tetrapeptide substrates often differs from the sequences recognized within intact protein substrates.

III. ACTIVATION OF CASPASES

Some caspases are constitutively present in cells as inactive zymogens, but increasing evidence suggests that some caspases are synthesized *de novo* following a death stimulus. Once activated, caspases cleave and activate other caspases to produce a loosely defined caspase cascade during cell death. In general, the long prodomain caspases, also called initiators (caspase-8, -9, -10), cleave and activate the short prodomain caspases, also called effectors (caspase-2, -3, -7). This is consistent with the observation that the cleavage site specificity of caspases 8, 9, and 10 (Leu-X-X-Asp) is similar to the "activating" cleavage site separating the large and small subunits of caspases 3 and 7 (Ile-X-X-Asp). The effector caspases cleave most of the 80 or

so substrates identified to date that facilitate apoptosis. Many of these substrates (Table I) contain cleavage sites with the sequence Asp-X-X-Asp, consistent with the substrate specificity of the effector caspases-2, -3, and -7 (Table II). Of these, caspase-3 is the best studied and is capable of cleaving most of the identified cellular substrates. Despite the fact that caspases-3 and -7 have identical peptide substrate specificities *in vitro* (Asp-Glu-Val-Asp), they are likely to have only partially overlapping lists of intracellular substrates, but the determinants for this additional specificity are currently unknown. Some caspases may also be activated via autoactivation through conformational changes, but this area is less well understood.

The proximity model probably explains how most long prodomain caspases are activated to initiate the caspase cascade. In this model, caspases are recruited via their prodomains to protein complexes. While in close proximity, they become activated, probably by cross-catalytic cleavage of the zymogens. The two best-understood kinds of protein complexes that facilitate caspase activation are the "apoptosome" found in the cytosol and the "disc" located on the cytoplasmic tails of several members of the tumor necrosis factor (TNF) receptor family expressed on the plasma membrane. Receptor-mediated cell death is referred to as the extrinsic pathway (type I cells). When bound by their extracellular ligands, a protein–protein interaction motif called the "death domain" (DD) located in the cytoplasmic tail of the death receptors TNFR, Fas/CD95 and TRAIL, bind to a similar DD present in an adapter protein called FADD. (In the case of TNFR, TNFR binds directly to TRADD, which binds to FADD.) The CARD/DED domain present in FADD in turn binds to the CARD/DED in the prodomain of caspases such as caspase-8. This complex of proteins is known as a "disc" and may contain other components as well. Clustering of caspase-8 leads to its cross-catalytic activation. Other prodomain-binding factors have also been identified (Table II). Defects in receptor-mediated cell death are associated with autoimmune disorders in mice and humans.

Activation of cell death from within a cell (intrinsic pathway/type II cells) leads to mitochondrial damage through the action of activated proapoptotic Bcl-2 family members. Damaged mitochondria release a number of components from their intermembrane space into the cytosol. One of these factors is cytochrome *c*, which

TABLE II
Human Caspase Family

Caspase class/ caspase No.	LAP No./alternate names	Prodomain (binding partner)	Activation site at p20/p10	Cleavage site preference
Class I (ICE-like)				
Caspase-1	ICE	Long (CARDIAK)	WFKD↓	WEHD↓
Caspase-4	LAP1/Tx, Ich2, ICE rel II	Long	WVRD↓	(W/L)EHD↓
Caspase-5	TY, ICE rel III	Long	WVRD↓	(W/L)EHD↓
			P4 P3 P2 P1↓P1'	
Class II (CED-3-like)				
CED-3	(from C. elegans)	Long (CED-4)	DSVD↓	DETD↓
Caspase-3	LAP4/CPP32, YAMA	Short	IETD↓	DEVD↓
Caspase-7	LAP3/Mch3, CMH-1	Short	IQAD↓	DEVD↓
Caspase-2	LAP2/Ich1	Long (RAIDD)	DQQD↓	DEHD↓
Class III				
Caspase-6	LAP5/Mch2	Short	TEVD↓	VEHD↓
Caspase-8	LAP7/FLICE, Mch5, MACH	Long (FADD)	VETD↓	LETD↓
Caspase-9	LAP6/Mch6	Long (Apaf1)	PEPD↓	LEHD↓
Caspase-10	Mch4	Long	IEAD↓	LENIeD↓

serves not only in the electron transport chain in mitochondria, but also functions as a cofactor for Apaf-1 in the cytosol. Binding of cytochrome c and ATP induce oligomerization of Apaf-1 and caspase-9 into a 700- to 1400-kDa apoptosome that activates caspase-9. Caspase-3 is recruited to the apoptosome and is activated by caspase-9. Other factors released from mitochondria during cell death include SMAC/DIABLO, AIF, some caspases, and others. The extrinsic and intrinsic pathways appear to have cross-talk mechanisms. Cleavage of the Bcl-2 family member BID by TNFR-activated caspase-8 leads to BID-induced release of cytochrome c from mitochondria.

IV. REGULATION OF CASPASE ACTIVATION

Caspase activation has potentially severe consequences and must be tightly regulated. FLICE inhibitory proteins (FLIPs) bind to the cytoplasmic protein complex (disc) of death receptors to modulate/inhibit the recruitment/activation of caspases. FLIPs are either inactive caspase-like proteins (lacking enzyme active sites) or small bridging molecules that mimic the prodomains of caspases.

Cells also encode a direct inhibitor of caspases, XIAP. XIAP is found on the X chromosome and is a member of the IAP (inhibitor of apoptosis) family. XIAP contains three BIR (baculovirus IAP repeat) motifs in its N terminus that bind to and inhibit caspases. The linker region between BIR1 and BIR2 of XIAP binds the catalytic cleft of caspases-3 and -7 and inhibits their activities. In addition, the N-terminus of the small subunit of caspase-3 binds in a pocket in BIR2. Similarly, a pocket in the BIR3 domain of XIAP binds the N-terminus of the small subunit of caspase-9 (that is generated upon cleavage between the large and small subunits by caspase-9, but not caspase-3). SMAC/DIABLO is released from mitochondria during cell death and binds to the pocket in the BIR domain of XIAP, preventing XIAP from inhibiting caspases. Antiapoptotic Bcl-2 (b-cell lymphoma/leukemia gene 2) proteins prevent release of cytochrome c, SMAC, AIF, and other factors from mitochondria, therefore preventing caspase activation. IAP proteins may regulate other cellular functions as well. The C-terminal RING fingers of IAP proteins have E3 ubiquitin ligase activity that likely targets other binding partners to ubiquitin-dependent degradation.

V. ROLE OF CASPASES IN DEVELOPMENT AND DISEASE

Knockout mice lacking caspase-1, -2, -6 or, -11 all exhibit normal embryonic development but have defects in the adult. However, deletion of caspase-7, -8, or -9 results in embryonic lethality, whereas caspase-3 knockouts have perinatal lethality. Thus, some caspases are required for normal development whereas others are required for postnatal functions. Mice lacking caspase-8 or FADD have almost identical cardiac defects, supporting the argument that these factors work in the same pathway. Similarly, deletion of Apaf-1, caspase-9, or caspase-3 results in excessive numbers of neurons, particularly in the brain cortex, but other brain regions as well. The activation of caspases has been implicated in a number of disease states, including ischemia and Alzheimer's and Huntington's diseases. Mutation of caspase-10 was found in some autoimmune lymphoproliferative disease syndrome patients, and caspase-8 is deleted or silenced in some childhood neuroblastomas. Similarly, factors that regulate caspase activation are also defective in some cancers such as follicular lymphoma (Bcl-2) and MALT lymphoma (cIAP2).

See Also the Following Articles

Bcl-2 Family Proteins and the Dysregulation of Programmed Cell Death • P-Glycoprotein as a General Anti-Apoptotic Protein • Tumor Necrosis Factors

Bibliography

Adams, J. M., and Cory, S. (1998). The Bcl-2 protein family: Arbiters of cell survival. *Science* **281**, 1322–1326.

Baens, M., Maes, B., Steyls, A., Geboes, K., Marynen, P., and De Wolf-Peeters, C. (2000). The product of the t(11;18), an API2-MLT fusion, marks nearly half of gastric MALT type lymphomas without large cell proliferation. *Am. J. Pathol.* **156**, 1433–1439.

Chinnaiyan, A. M., Tepper, C. G., Seldin, M. F., O'Rouke, K., Kischkel, F. C., Hellbardt, S., Krammer, P. H., Peter, M. E., and Dixit, V. M. (1996). FADD/MORT1 is a common mediator of CD95 (Fas/APO-1)-and TNF-receptor-induced apoptosis. *J. Biol. Chem.* **271**, 4961–4965.

Clem, R. J., Cheng, E. H. Y., Karp, C. L., Kirsch, D. G., Ueno, K., Takahashi, A., Kastan, M. B., Griffin, D. E., Earnshaw, W. C., Veliuona, M. A., and Hardwick, J. M. (1998). Modulation of cell death by Bcl-x_L through caspase interaction. *Proc. Natl. Acad. Sci. USA* **95**, 554–559.

Deveraux, Q. L., and Reed, J. C. (1999). IAP family proteins—suppressors of apoptosis. *Genes Dev.* **13**, 239–252.

Du, C., Fang, M., Li, Y., Li, L., and Wang, X. (2000). Smac, a mitochondrial protein that promotes cytochrome c-dependent caspase activation by eliminating IAP inhibition. *Cell* **102**, 33–42.

Hengartner, M. O., and Horvitz, H. R. (1998). Programmed cell death in C. elegans. *Curr. Opin. Genet. Dev.* **4**, 581–586.

Irmler, M., Thome, M., Hahne, M., Schneider, P., Hofmann, K., Steiner, V., Bodmer, J.-L., Schroter, M., Burns, K., Mattmann, C., Rimoldi, D., French, L. E., and Tschopp, J. (1997). Inhibition or death receptor signals by cellular FLIP. *Nature (Lond.)* **399**, 190–195.

Kroemer, G., and Reed, J. C. (2000). Mitochondrial control of cell death. *Nature Med.* **6**, 513–519.

Li, H., Zhu, H., Xu, C., and Yuan, J. (1998). Cleavage of BID by caspase 8 mediates the mitochondrial damage in the Fas pathway of apoptosis. *Cell* **94**, 491–501.

Luo, X., Budihardjo, I., Zou, H., Slaughter, C., and Wang, X. (1998). Bid, a Bcl-2 interacting protein, mediates cytochrome c release from mitochondria in response to activation of cell surface death receptors. *Cell* **94**, 481–490.

Nicholson, D. W. (1999). Caspase structure, proteolytic substrates, and function during apoptotic cell death. *Cell Death Differen.* **6**, 1028–1042.

Ray, C. A., Black, R. A., Kronheim, S. R., Greenstreet, T. A., Sleath, P. R., Salvesen, G. S., and Pickup, D. J. (1992). Viral inhibition of inflammation:cowpox virus encodes an inhibitor of the interleukin-1-beta converting enzyme. *Cell* **69**, 597–604.

Teitz, T., Wei, T., Valentine, M. B., Vanin, E. F., Grenet, J., Valentine, V. A., Behm, F. G., Look, A. T., Lahti, J. M., and Kidd, V. J. (2000). Caspase 8 is deleted or silenced preferentially in childhood neuroblastomas with amplification of MYCN. *Nature Med.* **6**, 529–535.

Thornberry, N.A., Rano, T. A., Peterson, E. P., Rasper, D. M., Timkey, T., Garcia-Calvo, M., Houtzager, V. M., Nordstrom, P. A., Roy, S., Vaillancourt, J. P., Chapman, K. T., and Nicholson, D. W. (1997). A combinatorial approach defines specificities of members of the caspase family and granzyme B. Functional relationships established for key mediators of apoptosis. *J. Biol. Chem.* **272**, 17907–17911.

Tsujimoto, Y., Cossman, J., Jaffe, E., and Croce, C. M. (1985). Involvement of the bcl-2 gene in human follicular lymphoma. *Science* **228**, 1440–1443.

Wang, J., Zheng, L., Lobito, A., Chan, F. K., Sneller, M., Yao, X., Puck, J. M., Straus, S. E., and Lenardo, M. J. (1999). Inherited human caspase 10 mutations underlie defective lymphocyte and dendritic cell apoptosis in autoimmune lymphoproliferative syndrome type II. *Cell* **98**, 47–58.

Yang, X., Chang, H. Y., and Baltimore, D. (1998). Autoproteolytic activation of procaspases by oligomerization. *Mol. Cell* **1**, 319–325.

Zheng, T. S., Hunot, S., Kuida, K., and Flavell, R. A. (1999). Caspase knockouts: Matters of life and death. *Cell Death Differen.* **6**, 1043–1053.

Zou, H., Li, Y., and Wang, X. (1999). An APAF-1 cytochrome c multimeric complex is a functional apoptosome that activates procaspase-9. *J. Biol. Chem.* **274**, 11549–11556.

Cationic Lipid-Mediated Gene Therapy

William M. Siders

Genzyme Molecular Oncology and Genzyme Corporation, Framingham, Massachusetts

Seng H. Cheng
Johanne M. Kaplan

Genzyme Corporation, Framingham, Massachusetts

GLOSSARY

alloantigens A foreign cellular protein recognized by the immune system.

cationic lipid A positively charged lipid used to condense plasmid DNA.

CpG motif An immunostimulatory sequence found within bacterial DNA that consists of an unmethylated cytidine–guanosine dinucleotide sequence surrounded by specific flanking nucleotides.

cytokine One of a group of molecules involved in cell-to-cell signaling during inflammation or an immune response.

liposomes An enclosed lipid layer used to encapsulate plasmid DNA.

naked DNA Plasmid DNA that has not been complexed to lipid.

suicide gene A gene encoding an enzyme that converts an otherwise nontoxic drug into a toxic metabolite.

transfection The introduction of foreign DNA into a cell.

transgene A gene found within plasmid DNA that encodes a specific protein.

xenograft The introduction of tissue from one species into another species.

Although the field of gene therapy initially concentrated on treating monogenic disorders, the concept of treating cancer by modifying the tumor cells or enhancing a specific immune response soon emerged. Within the field of gene therapy, there are two primary approaches: viral-mediated gene transfer and nonviral-mediated gene transfer. Both of these strategies have several potential benefits as well as disadvantages. For instance, in viral-mediated gene

Encyclopedia of Cancer, Second Edition
Volume 1

transfer, the use of recombinant adenoviruses to deliver therapeutic genes is widely being explored. This virus has a broad tissue tropism and has been shown to infect a wide variety of both dividing and nondividing cells. In addition, advances in the area of adenovirus biology have led to the ability to rapidly generate recombinant viruses that are capable of packaging the full-length genomic sequence of most genes. However, despite the overall utility of recombinant adenoviruses, issues involving their safety and efficacy in clinical trials have generated some concern regarding their use. In addition, the use of currently available adenoviral vectors *in vivo* has been shown to result in an inflammatory response as well as the generation of an immune response to adenoviral proteins that may prevent readministration of the vector. Due to these potential limiting issues, the field of nonviral-mediated gene transfer is being reexamined. For years, several areas of research have utilized cationic lipids complexed to plasmid DNA (pDNA) as a means to transfect cells. More recently, advances within this field have made transfection and gene expression in target cells more effective, and efforts are underway to apply these to *in vivo* cancer models. The efficiency of transfection of a tumor cell or antigen-presenting cell is dependent both on the efficacy of DNA delivery to the nucleus and on the effectiveness of DNA expression. Although significant progress has been made in the field of optimizing gene expression cassettes, this article primarily examines the use of lipid-mediated gene transfer as a means to treat cancer *in vivo*.

I. FORMULATION AND STABILITY OF LIPID/PLASMID DNA COMPLEXES

The transfection of pDNA into cells using cationic lipids is a multistep process that involves (1) binding of the lipid/pDNA complex to the cell, (2) cell entry that is generally thought to be through endocytosis, and (3) trafficking of the pDNA to the nucleus. Once inside the nucleus, expression is dependent on the transcriptional expression cassette used to encode the transgene. Although the exact mechanisms of entry and transport have not been fully characterized, it is clear that there are several steps along this pathway where the lipid must protect the pDNA from degra-

dation. Indeed, it has been suggested that for every 100 copies of pDNA that enter into a cell, only 1 copy will reach the nucleus and express its transgene. Therefore the choice of lipids, as well as the lipid-to-pDNA ratio used in formulating the lipid and pDNA complex, is extremely important. The formation of lipid/pDNA particles typically involves the condensation of negatively charged pDNA with positively charged cationic lipids. Altering the proportion of lipid and pDNA in the complex can modify the overall stability of this complex as well as its size and charge. Neutral lipids, such as dioleyl phosphatidylethanolamine (DOPE), are generally required to help cationic lipids generate maximal transfection efficiencies. Thus, high transfection efficiencies could be obtained *in vitro* with these lipids, in some cases approaching 90%. However, as reported in the literature, the ability to transfect cells *in vitro* rarely translated to a high level of transfection of target cells *in vivo* due to considerations such as the instability of the lipid/pDNA complexes in blood. Because good correlations between *in vitro* and *in vivo* transfection efficiency in general do not exist, it is now recognized that for *in vivo* use, the best way to compare various lipid/pDNA formulations is *in vivo*, using the expression of a reporter transgene as an end point. Great efforts have been expended to develop lipids capable of achieving a high level of *in vivo* transfection efficiency, including novel multivalent cationic lipids, as well as many structural analogs of first-generation lipids, such as DMRIE and DOTAP. DC-chol, a cholesterol-based lipid, in conjunction with DOPE, was the first lipid formulation to be used in human cancer clinical trials and is discussed in a later section.

II. PRECLINICAL STUDIES

Even though no direct correlation can be made as to whether a particular cationic lipid might yield a high level of transfection efficiency *in vivo*, in retrospect, the labor-intensive work of trial and error *in vivo* screening has led to the discovery of several lipids that exhibit good clinical potential. However, prior to testing in human clinical trials, these lipid/pDNA formulations must undergo rigorous testing for efficacy and safety in animal cancer models, which adds another level of complexity. Investigators must decide what type of transgene to express and the route of administration, as well as the lipid/pDNA formulation to use. It is clear from several studies that the choice of formulation will depend on the route of administration. Formulations that are optimal for route of administration, for example, may not necessarily result in high levels of transgene expression following a different route of administration.

A. Route of Administration

The two standard routes of administration utilized for lipid/pDNA complexes in cancer applications are intravenous (iv) and intratumoral (it). Although lipid/pDNA complexes can be injected intramuscularly, direct administration of pDNA alone (naked DNA) in this instance results in similar if not more sustained transgene expression levels by this route. Thus it is unclear what benefit, if any, the use of cationic lipids in conjunction with pDNA would be for the intramuscular route. Successful transfer of pDNA to the lung via the iv route has been achieved using several different formulations. The primary cell type transfected in these studies has been shown to be endothelial cells, although gene expression was also detected from some monocytes. These data suggest the possibility of loco-regional treatment of pulmonary metastases with cytokine or immunomodulating gene therapy. Delivery of tumor suppressor genes, such as retinoblastoma (RB) or p53, in this manner has already been shown to significantly decrease the number of pulmonary metastases in several animal models. Despite successful demonstrations of gene transfer by systemic administration, dose-dependent toxicity can be associated with the iv delivery of some lipid/pDNA complexes in animal models. Some researchers have suggested that the toxicity that accompanies iv administration of complexes is in large part thought to be associated with the high level of unmethylated CpG motifs within the pDNA. The interaction of these motifs (discussed in more detail later) with components of the immune system elicits high levels of cytokines, including IFN-γ, TNF-α, and IL-12. Indeed, it has been demonstrated that a 50% reduction in the level of these CpG motifs leads

to a significant decrease in proinflammatory cytokines, without affecting transgene expression. In preparation for human clinical trials, several safety and biodistribution studies have been conducted examining the systemic administration of selected lipid, including DMRIE:DOPE, and pDNA formulations. Results from these studies indicated that at the doses tested, iv injection of these particular lipid/pDNA complexes did not result in high levels of toxicity and that statistical differences were observed in only a few clinical parameters. Biodistribution analysis indicated that although the presence of pDNA could be detected within the heart, liver, kidney, lung, and spleen following iv administration, no organ toxicity was associated with the presence of the plasmid. It is also important to note that no gonadal transmission of pDNA was found, suggesting that the potential for transfer of pDNA to germ cells by systemic administration at these doses is extremely low.

Direct intratumoral administration is the preferred method for injecting lipid/pDNA complexes to treat cancer as it targets gene delivery directly to the tumor cells. This method relies upon the accessibility of the tumor or the ability to insert a catheter into the tumor at distal locations for delivery of the complexes. Several murine solid tumors have been successfully transfected *in vivo* with pDNA expressing several types of genes, including those coding for cytokines, suicide genes, and alloantigens. Although a large body of evidence indicates that the combination of lipid and pDNA is superior to naked pDNA, some investigators have proposed that cationic lipids may reduce the transfection efficiency of the tumor cells. To address this issue, pharmacokinetic studies have been performed to examine both the transfection efficiency and the level of gene expression following it injection of either naked pDNA or lipid/pDNA complexes. Following the injection of naked DNA, approximately 50% was cleared from the injected tumors within 2 h, whereas 94% of lipid complexed pDNA remained within the tumor for the same time period. Even though the addition of cationic lipids resulted in a higher level of retention at the tumor site, the transgene expression levels were similar for both naked pDNA and lipid-complexed pDNA. It is interesting to note that in both cases expression of the transgene was limited to the injection site, suggesting little to no diffusion of the pDNA throughout the tumor. Upon further examination, estimates of the transfection efficiency of lipid/pDNA complexes following it injections have revealed that from 0.05 to 1.0% of the tumor cells actually expressed the transgene. However, by varying the choice of lipid used, increases in transfection efficiency and transgene expression could be observed. Despite these low levels of transgene expression, encouraging results have been seen in several tumor models, including the Renca renal cell carcinoma and the aggressively growing B16 melanoma model.

B. Immunomodulatory versus Suicide Genes

The initial screening of immunomodulating cytokines as cancer therapeutics by lipid-mediated gene transfer involved *ex vivo* transfection of the tumor cells followed by drug selection for cells with high levels of transgene expression. This method resulted in the generation of a clonal population of cells expressing high levels of the cytokine being analyzed. Eventually these cells were injected into mice and were found to have a reduced tumorigenic potential. As a result of advances in lipid formulations, the possibility of achieving loco-regional expression of cytokines was considered. For instance, considering that high levels of recombinant IL-2 protein are required for enhancing immune responses by systemic treatment and that these doses are associated with several toxic side effects, localized expression of the gene at the tumor site would help circumvent this toxicity. In addition, due to the short half-life of several cytokines in circulation, transfection of tumor cells with a pDNA expressing the cytokine gene would result in a continuous expression of the cytokine at the tumor site for a defined period of time. In support of this, the administration of recombinant IL-2 protein at the tumor site has been demonstrated to be more effective in initiating an immune response than systemic administration of the protein. Following multiple it injections of lipid and pDNA complexes encoding IL-2, inhibition of tumor growth and eventually tumor regression in the Renca model were observed due to the induction of a specific CD8$^+$ T-cell response. This immune response, generated with as little as 10 μg of pDNA, was capable of inhibiting the formation of a tumor injected 4 days following treatment. Similar experiments performed in the B16 melanoma tumor model demonstrated that although circulating levels of IL-2 could not be detected, a delay in tumor growth could be observed. However, a specific IL-2 effect was observed only when B16 cells were transfected *in vitro* prior to implantation *in vivo*. Interestingly, antitumor effects were also observed when tumors were injected with complexes containing pDNA that did not express a transgene.

In addition to trying to modulate the immune system by cytokines, another form of therapy is being examined that involves the introduction of alloantigens into tumor cells, such as foreign MHC class I molecules. Expression of these genes results in proteins within the tumor cells that are recognized as foreign and elicit a cellular immune response. Direct intratumoral injections using lipid and plasmid DNA coding for the foreign MHC class I molecule elicited a potent immune response characterized by both CD8$^+$ T-cell and NK-cell activation. An important outcome from these studies was that during the development of the cellular immune response generated against the alloantigen, a tumor-specific cytotoxic response also developed. This observation demonstrates that although intratumoral injections using current lipid formulations can result in low transfection efficiencies, a robust antitumor response can be generated. Findings from these preclinical studies eventually resulted in a human clinical trial in which DC-Chol was used to transfer a plasmid encoding an alloantigen directly to tumor cells of patients.

The use of suicide genes, such as HSV-thymidine kinase (HSV-tk) or *Escherichia coli* purine nucleoside phosphorylase (PnP) genes, requires the addition of a prodrug, which generally is relatively nontoxic at very high levels unless specifically activated by cellular enzymes into a toxic metabolite. In the case of HSV-tk, expression of this enzyme will convert the inactive gancyclovir prodrug into its phosphorylated toxic form that can become incorporated into DNA and cause chain termination, thus killing the cell expressing the tk protein. One of the added benefits of this type of prodrug therapy is the so-called "bystander" effect.

Nearby cells that contact the transfected cell via gap junctions are also susceptible to the effects of the activated prodrug. Therefore, in treatments such as these, not all tumor cells need to be transfected in order to generate a robust anti-tumor response. Because gene expression from intratumoral injections is typically limited to the vicinity of the injection site, the bystander effect of suicide gene expression makes this a very attractive therapy. To limit expression of the suicide gene, tumor-specific promoters are typically used to drive gene expression. For instance, promoters for both the α-fetoprotein gene, abnormally expressed in hepatocellular carcinoma, and the tyrosinase gene, overexpressed in several cases of malignant melanoma, have been used to drive expression of the HSV-tk gene in a tumor-specific manner. It is clear that with this type of therapy, multiple injections will be required due to the localized expression of the transgene within the tumor following lipid/pDNA complex administration. Unlike viral-mediated gene therapy, the benefit of using lipids to mediate the transfer of pDNA is that delivery of successive injections of complex is possible. Using this treatment regimen, the delivery of suicide genes using lipid/pDNA complexes has been shown to be efficacious in numerous tumor models, including several human xenograft models.

C. Adjuvancy Effect of Lipid/pDNA Complexes

Many of the results from *in vivo* studies involving lipid-mediated gene transfer have attributed the antitumor efficacy to expression of the transgene. However, it is becoming increasingly evident that the pDNA itself, irrespective of any transgene, can induce immunostimulatory effects. Treatment of tumor cells *in vitro* with lipid/pDNA complexes results in significant phenotypic changes in the tumor cell, including increases in the surface level of MHC class I molecules, as well as increased expression of heat shock proteins. In addition to these effects, a large body of evidence now exists that implicates unmethylated CpG residues within the pDNA as being immunostimulatory. Bacterial DNA contains a high level of unmethylated CpG dinucleotides that are rarely found in eukaryotic cells. Approximately 80% of these motifs are methylated in eukaryotes. The high frequency of unmethylated CpG residues in pDNA appears to be recognized by the immune system as a danger signal. Consequently, the immune system becomes activated and an inflammatory response ensues. However, the motifs present in pDNA are highly contextual, sometimes inhibitory and sometimes stimulatory, depending on the nucleotides flanking the CpG residues. Several studies have reported nonspecific effects associated with the treatment of tumors with noncoding plasmids. Treatment of tumors with noncoding vectors in some cases led to an antitumor immune response and activation of the innate immune system. This was characterized by the release of IL-12 and IFN-γ and an influx of NK cells. Studies are now being performed to specifically examine the immune response generated by such treatments, which includes the induction of tumor-specific cytotoxic T-cell responses. Methylation of the pDNA has been shown to inhibit or reduce this immunostimulatory effect, suggesting that it is in fact mediated by the presence of CpG motifs. Given these effects, the choice of transgene, as well as the consequence of noncoding pDNA, becomes extremely important to consider.

The Krieg laboratory has pioneered research in this area by demonstrating that CpG oligonucleotides can substitute for the activity initially ascribed to empty or null vector effects. Treatment with immunostimulatory CpG oligonucleotides *in vivo* induces high levels of IFN-γ, IL-12, and IL-6, leading to activation of NK cells and an innate immune response. In addition, CpG oligonucleotides can directly activate specific populations of dendritic cells (DCs). These oligonucleotides have exhibited therapeutic efficacy in several tumor mouse models. Although CpG motifs have typically been regarded as being immunostimulatory, it has been shown that treatment with CpG oligonucleotides may inhibit some immune responses by decreasing the level of MHC class II expression from macrophages. Although work with CpG oligonucleotides reinforces the concept that these motifs can have wide-ranging immunostimulatory effects, whether all of these effects can be observed using noncoding pDNA remains to be determined.

Therefore, a balance must be achieved between the desired immunostimulatory properties and the levels of CpG motifs present.

III. CLINICAL TRIALS

One of the eventual goals of optimizing both lipid/pDNA formulations and gene expression cassettes is to initiate human clinical trials to examine both the safety and the efficacy of the lipid and pDNA complexes. Through recent enhancements in these fields, a few lipids, such as DC-chol, have yielded positive results in several animal models leading to their use in a small number of human clinical trials. Although it is not yet possible for lipid-mediated gene transfer to compete with the efficiency with which an adenovirus can infect a cell and express its transgene, several benefits exist as to why lipid/pDNA complexes would be the preferred delivery vehicle. For example, unlike lipid/pDNA complex, viral vectors have been shown to induce a cellular immune response to viral proteins that are still expressed by the virus. In addition, a humoral immune response develops that is strong enough to inhibit repeat administration. Repetitive administration protocols likely will be required to induce and maintain cytotoxic T-cell responses against tumor cells. However, although lipid/pDNA complexes do not appear to elicit an immune response, there does appear to be a window or refractory period during which readministration of lipid/pDNA complexes is not effective. In particular,

it has been suggested that readministration of the lipid and plasmid DNA complex too soon after the initial injection did not result in transgene expression. As the time period between injections increased, so did transgene expression. Lipid and plasmid DNA complexes are also attractive because they are non-replicating and will not integrate into the host genome.

Early cancer clinical trials involving lipid-mediated gene transfer consisted of *ex vivo* modification of autologous tumor cells with pDNA encoding immunomodulatory genes. It was thought that reintroduction of these tumor cells (following inactivation) would elicit a tumor-specific immune response that would cross-react with tumor cells in the host. However, the technical challenges associated with modifying and establishing human tumor cell lines has prompted investigators to examine the *in vivo* transfer of pDNA-encoded genes by lipid-mediated gene transfer for the treatment of cancer. In this regard, results from only a handful of studies have been reported in the literature. A majority of these studies, as shown in Table I, examine the potential of transferring plasmids encoding allogeneic MHC class I molecules by intratumoral injections. The first trial of this type was performed by Gary Nabel and involved the transfer of the HLA-B7 gene into 5 HLA-B7-negative patients with advanced melanoma. Although this study largely examined safety parameters, evidence of an immune response was observed. Following intratumoral injections of complex, expression of the HLA-B7 protein could be detected in tumor biop-

TABLE I
Clinical Trials Involving Lipid-Mediated Gene Transfer for Cancer Therapy

Trial	Gene	Cancer	Lipid	Route of administration
Phase I	HLA B7-1	Melanoma	DC-chol/DOPE	Intratumoral
Phase I	HLA B7-1	Renal cell carcinoma	DMRIE/DOPE	Intratumoral
Phase II	HLA B7-1	Metastatic cancer	DMRIE/DOPE	Intratumoral
Phase I/II	IL-2	Melanoma, renal cell carcinoma and sarcoma	DMRIE/DOPE	Intratumoral
Phase I	E1A	Metastatic solid tumors	Not specified	Intratumoral and peritumoral
Phase I	E1A	Ovarian	Not specified	Intraperitoneal
Phase I	IL-2 and SEB[a]	Melanoma	Not specified	Intratumoral
Phase I	IL-2	Melanoma	Not specified	Intradermal

[a]SEB, staphlococcal enterotoxin B.

sies of all five patients. Similar to results from preclinical studies, the pDNA remained localized to the site of injection and was not detected within the serum of patients. Analysis of several serum biochemical markers indicated that no toxicity occurred as a result of the intratumoral injection of lipid/pDNA complex. An increase in the cellular immune response to the autologous tumor was also detected in two patients, eventually leading to regression of the injected tumor nodule in one patient. Taken together, these data indicate that intratumoral injections of lipid/pDNA complexes can be both safe and efficacious. Results from ongoing clinical trials are eagerly being awaited and typically involve similar intratumoral injection regimens utilizing various pDNA-encoding cytokines such as IL-2.

IV. CONCLUSION

It is clear that lipid/pDNA complexes can achieve a good transfection rate and express an encoded transgene for a short-term period. However, several factors remain to be addressed, including new lipid formulations to increase transfection efficiency and the immunostimulatory properties of the vector DNA. The most successful cancer gene therapy will more than likely include a balance between immunostimulatory properties of the pDNA and the ability to efficiently express the desired transgene. Studies have suggested that both the cationic lipid alone and the plasmid DNA (containing no transgene) alone possess immunostimulatory properties. For treating cancer, a high level of CpG motifs may be desirable to activate an innate immune response. However, studies have also shown that high levels of TNF-α or IFN-γ can inhibit gene transcription or decrease the stability of the mRNA transcript. Thus a balance must be struck between these two components when trying to induce a specific immune response with a plasmid encoding a transgene. Ultimately, as researchers, we need to ask ourselves what we are looking for in a cancer therapy. Are we looking for a nonspecific activation of the innate immune response, ultimately leading to an adaptive cellular response, or the generation of a specific response based on the expression of a particular transgene, such as IL-2 or IL-12?

See Also the Following Articles

CYTOKINE GENE THERAPY • GENE THERAPY VECTORS, SAFETY CONSIDERATIONS • SUICIDE GENES • TARGETED VECTORS FOR CANCER GENE THERAPY

Bibliography

Clark, P. R., Stopeck, A. T., Ferrari, M., Parker, S. E., and Hersh, E. M. (2000). Studies of direct intratumoral gene transfer using cationic lipid-complexed plasmid DNA. *Cancer Gene Ther.* **7,** 853–860.

Gallucci, S., Lolkema, M., and Matzinger, P. (1999). Natural adjuvants: Endogenous activators of dendritic cells. *Nature Med.* **5**(11), 1249–1255.

Gao, X., and Huang, L. (1995). Cationic liposome-mediated gene transfer. *Gene Ther.* **2,** 710–722.

Lanuti, M., Rudginsky, S., Force, S. D., Lambright, E. S., Siders, W. M., Chang, M. Y., Amin, K. M., Kaiser, L. R., Scheule, R. K. and Albelda, S. M. (2000). Cationic lipid:bacterial DNA complexes elicit adaptive cellular immunity in murine intraperitoneal tumor models. *Cancer Res.* **60,** 2955–2963.

Mahato, R. I., Anwer, K., Tagliaferri, F., Meaney, C., Leonard, P., Wadhwa, M. S., Logan, M., French, M., and Rolland, A. (1998). Biodistribution and gene expression of lipid/plasmid complexes after systemic administration. *Hum. Gene Ther.* **9,** 2083–2099.

Nabel, G. J., Nabel, E. G., Yang, Z., Fox, B. A., Plautz, G. E., Gao, X., Huang, L., Shu, S., Gordon, D., and Chang, A. E. (1993). Direct gene transfer with DNA-liposome complexes in melanoma: Expression, biologic activity, and lack of toxicity in humans. *Proc. Natl. Acad. Sci. USA* **90,** 11307–11311.

Nomura, T., Nakajima, S., Kawabata, K., Yamashita, F., Takakura, Y., and Hashida, M. (1997). Intratumoral pharmacokinetics and *in vivo* gene expression of naked plasmid DNA and its cationic liposome complexes after direct gene transfer. *Cancer Res.* **57,** 2681–2686.

Parker, S. E., Vahlsing, H. L., Serfilippi, L. M., Franklin, C. L., Doh, S. G., Gromkowski, S. H., Lew, D., Manthorpe, M., and Norman, J. (1995). Cancer gene therapy using plasmid DNA: Safety evaluation in rodents and non-human primates. *Hum. Gene Ther.* **6,** 575–590.

Weiner, G. J., Liu, H., Wooldridge, J. E., Dahle, C. E., and Krieg, A. M. (1997). Immunostimulatory oligonucleotides containing the CpG motif are effective as immune adjuvants in tumor antigen immunization. *Proc. Natl. Acad. Sci. USA* **94,** 10833–10837.

Yew, N. S., Zhao, H., Wu, I., Song, A., Tousignant, J. D., Przybylska, M., and Cheng, S. H. (2000). Reduced inflammatory response to plasmid DNA vectors by elimination and inhibition of inflamatory CpG motifs. *Mol. Ther.* **1,** 255–262.

Zabner, J., Fasbender, A. J., Moninger, T., Poellinger, K. A., and Welsh, M. J. (1995). Cellular and molecular barriers to gene transfer by a cationic lipid. *J. Biol. Chem.* **270,** 18997–19007.

Cell Cycle Checkpoints

Clare H. McGowan

The Scripps Research Institute

GLOSSARY

centrosomes Organizing centers for the two arrays of microtubules that form the mitotic spindle.

chromatids Two equal components of a replicated chromosome that are segregated into daughter cells by the processes of mitosis.

cyclin-dependent kinases (Cdks) A family of protein kinases that drive cell cycle progression. Cyclins are essential cofactors of Cdks. The periodic synthesis and destruction of cyclins contribute to the temporal regulation of Cdks; they probably also contribute to substrate specificity.

kinetochore A specialized region of chromatids that serve as the attachment site for microtubules of the mitotic spindle.

At its simplest, the cell cycle is a process in which cellular components are first duplicated and then distributed equally between two daughter cells. Complexity within the cell cycle arises because of the need to coordinate a number of physically independent pathways that allow duplication and segregation of all cellular components and because of the requirement for a high level of fidelity in these processes. The human somatic cell cycle has evolved with many checkpoint systems that ensure the levels of coordination and fidelity required for survival, both of individual cells and of the body as a whole. Cytotoxic anticancer therapy makes use of a wide variety of agents that activate a small number of cell cycle checkpoint pathways.

I. INTRODUCTION

The cell cycle is a process by which all the components of one cell are duplicated and equally distributed between two daughter cells. Checkpoints are regulatory pathways that ensure that the biochemically independent processes of the cell cycle are coupled. The eukaryotic cell cycle is defined as consisting of four phases. G1 is a gap phase in which cellular growth occurs. S phase is the synthetic period in which DNA is replicated and is followed by another gap, G2, in which more growth may occur, and the integrity of the DNA may be checked. G2 is followed by mitosis (M phase) during which the nuclear and cytoplasmic contents are divided. Complexity within the cell cycle arises because a large number of macromolecular components and organelles need to be exactly replicated and equally segregated. To ensure a high rate of success and to maintain genetic constancy, the replication and duplication of the cytoplasmic components and the nuclear components of the cell must be entrained. Soluble cytoplasmic components and multicopy organelles such as mitochondria increase in abundance, being evenly distributed throughout the cytoplasm, they are equally segregated by chance when cytokinesis occurs. Single copy organelles, such as the Golgi, are fragmented into numerous pieces that disperse throughout the cytoplasm so that each daughter cell receives enough components to rebuild a viable Golgi apparatus after division. The replication and segregation of chromosomal DNA perhaps represent the cells greatest challenge in producing two equivalent daughters. Chromosomal DNA must be replicated with complete fidelity, once and only once in each cycle, and the two daughter cells must receive an exact copy of parental DNA.

Defects in replication or in segregation will cause daughters to differ from their parents.

To achieve equal distribution of the genetic material, DNA is replicated and condensed; the centrosomes are duplicated and each half migrates to opposite sides of the cell where they act as foci for the separation of replicated chromatids. The sister chromatids all have to be attached to the centrosomes so that one full complement of chromosomal DNA is pulled into each of the two forming daughter cells. In metazoans, the nuclear membrane is disassembled to allow segregation of the replicated DNA; following division, it is reassembled to allow chromosomal decondensation and replication in the subsequent cycle. The concept of checkpoint control arose from the comprehension that replication and distribution of all the macromolecular structures of the cell have to be coupled with the replication and distribution of all the others. Moreover, it came from an understanding that extracellular or intrinsic cellular events that delay the completion of a specific cell cycle process must inhibit the progression all other processes until the problem that delayed the first pathway has been fixed (see Fig. 1).

A detailed explanation of the functioning of the human cell cycle is provided in an accompanying article. A brief description is given here. The human cell cycle is driven by the sequential activation of a number of kinases known as cyclin-dependent kinases (Cdks). The cell cycle stage is determined by sequential changes in the spectrum of proteins that are phos-

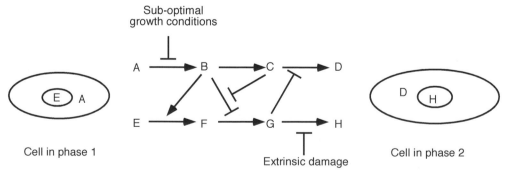

FIGURE 1 Theoretical checkpoint interactions. Horizontal arrows represent physically dependent steps of two independent processes. One process converts A to B. A second process converts C to D. Extracellular conditions, such as suboptimal growth factors or damage, delay the conversion of A to B. A inhibits the conversion of C to D. Thus, if progress in the pathway A to B is inhibited, the conversion of C to D is also slowed. The vertical arrow represents elements of the checkpoints that coordinate the two pathways.

phorylated and functionally altered by the activation and inactivation of distinct Cdk species. As its name implies, each kinase is composed of a catalytic subunit and a cyclin subunit. The regulated accumulation and destruction of the cyclin subunit is one mechanism by which coordination of cell cycle progression is achieved. The activity of Cdks is also controlled by a number of posttranslational mechanisms, including inhibitor phosphorylation, and by association with inhibitory proteins. Any or all of these regulatory mechanisms can theoretically be used by the checkpoint machinery to delay cell cycle progression.

II. CHECKPOINTS

A. Definition

Checkpoints were defined by Hartwell and Wienert as control mechanisms that enforce dependency between processes that are not physically dependent. An example of a checkpoint is the prevention of nuclear envelope breakdown that occurs when DNA synthesis is stopped by the addition of drugs such as hydroxyurea. Hydroxyurea inhibits an enzyme needed to generate the nucleotides required for DNA replication. It is not physically possible for cells to synthesis DNA in the presence of hydroxyurea; therefore, the accumulation of cells with an S-phase content of DNA is the result of a chemical block and not a checkpoint. However, hydroxyurea does not directly block the enzymes required for nuclear envelope breakdown. The block in nuclear envelope breakdown is actively imposed by a cell, it is the result of a checkpoint that is activated in cells that cannot complete DNA replication (see Fig. 2).

One line of evidence that cells actively block nuclear envelope breakdown came from the experiments of Schlegel and Pardee who observed that addition of caffeine to hydroxyurea-treated cells leads to nuclear envelope breakdown. Caffeine cannot bypass the requirement for nucleotide synthesis. Thus, DNA remains unreplicated. However, caffeine does uncouple the block in nuclear envelope breakdown from completion of DNA replication. Early evidence that mammalian cells use active processes to couple biochemically independent cell cycle processes came from a

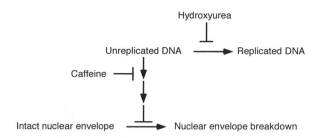

FIGURE 2 Caffeine inhibits a checkpoint that couples nuclear envelope breakdown to the replication of DNA. Hydroxyurea physically prevents the replication of DNA but does not directly affect the process of nuclear envelope breakdown. Caffeine does not affect DNA replication. Caffeine inhibits the checkpoint pathway that is activated in cells that are unable to complete DNA replication.

variety of experimental observations. Cell fusion experiments, in which S-phase cells were fused with G2 cells, showed that the G2 nucleus delayed mitotic entry until S-phase nuclei completed DNA replication. This experiment suggested that ongoing DNA replication in the S-phase nucleus generates a signal that inhibits the onset of mitosis in the G2 nucleus. When replication is complete, both nuclei progress into mitosis. Evidence also came from analysis of genetic human disorders. Normal human cells reduce the rate of DNA synthesis and delay mitosis in response to irradiation. Cells from patients with the recessive trait ataxia telangiectasia (AT) fail to show this reduction in the rate of DNA synthesis and fail to delay mitotic onset following DNA damage. This was taken to mean that AT cells lack a function required to delay cell cycle progression when DNA is damaged. However, it was not until studies of the radiation response of budding yeast formalized the concept of checkpoint that the full significance of these and many other mammalian cell cycle experiments was appreciated.

The concept of cell cycle checkpoint was proposed by studies of Hartwell and Weinert based on the radiation response of the budding yeast *Saccharomyces cerevisiae*. They found that when wild-type yeast are irradiated, they delay cell cycle progression for a period of time that is proportional to the dose of irradiation. After the delay, cells resume cell cycle progression and proliferate. In mutants, such as Rad9, cells do not delay cell cycle progression following irradiation, instead they progress to the next stage of the cell cycle and die. Hartwell and Weinert found that if cells lacking Rad9 function were extraneously prevented from progressing through the cell cycle for a time, following release of the block, the cells resume progression and proliferate normally. This experiment was interpreted to mean that when wild-type cells are irradiated, they require Rad9 function to block cell cycle progression until damage is repaired. Cells that lack Rad9 proceed through the cell cycle and die because the daughter cells inherit damaged DNA. Extraneously blocking progression provided the time needed to repair damage and complete the division cycle successfully. This experiment led to the hypothesis that an important function of the checkpoint was to provide time for DNA repair prior to cell cycle progression.

In the last two decades, genetic analysis of S. pombe and S. cerevisiae and of a number of human cancer-prone disorders, notably AT, has revealed a complex system of checkpoints that prevent cell cycle progression in response to both extrinsic and intrinsic events. The DNA damage checkpoint, the DNA replication

checkpoint, and the spindle checkpoint have been extensively studied, and as they have proven relevance to cancer, they are discussed to illustrate the principles of checkpoint control.

B. Anatomy of a Checkpoint

Checkpoint pathways are signal transduction pathways, as such they are composed of a sensor component that detects the defective process, a transducer that transmits the signal from the sensor, and a target that is a regulator of cell cycle machinery. A generic checkpoint pathway is shown in Fig. 3. Sensors that monitor the completion of DNA synthesis, unattached chromatids, or damaged DNA trigger the checkpoints that preserve genetic integrity. In principle, sensors can detect perturbation of any cellular process. For example, cells have mechanisms for ensuring that they have attained sufficient cellular mass to execute successful cell division. Although the exact mechanisms by which cells measure cellular mass

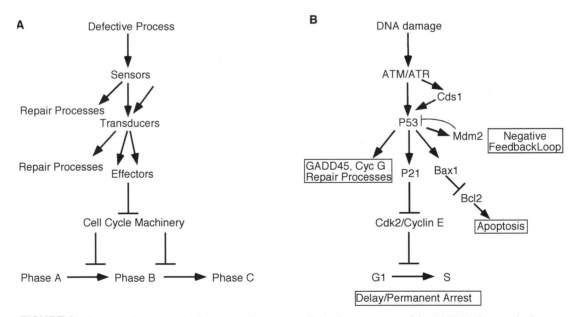

FIGURE 3 Elements of a generic checkpoint are shown in parallel with components of the G1 DNA damage checkpoint. (A) Multiple sensors might input to the same transduction element. Effectors could act to inhibit the cell cycle machinery at more than one point. The repair process may be initiated by activation of the sensor or by the transducer. (B) ATM is activated in response to DNA damage, which in turn activates the transcriptional activity of the transducer p53. p53 induces expression of effector molecule p21. p21 binds to and inhibits Cdks, thus cells are held in G1. Activation of p53 may occur as a direct consequence of interaction with ATM or indirectly through Chk1 or Cds1. Activation of p53 stimulates expression of a number of proteins that enhance repair. It also stimulates expression of Mdm2, a protein that facilitates the degradation of p53 and hence contributes to the downregulation of p53. Activation of p53 also increases the expression of apoptosis-promoting factor Bax. Prolonged stimulation of the pathway by irreparable damage leads to permanent arrest or apoptosis.

are not known, it is clear that cells growing under suboptimal conditions spend extended time in the gap phases, primarily in G1, acquiring increased mass. In many checkpoint responses, the exact signals that initiate the pathway are not clear. In the case of damaged DNA, the primary lesion is often processed, in preparation for repair, and it may be the processed site of damage, not the original damage product that initiates the checkpoint response. Regardless of how it monitors a defect, the sensor is expected to transmit a signal to an effector molecule that is capable of influencing the activity of the cell cycle engine. Theoretically, the detection and transmission of a checkpoint signal could be carried out by a single enzyme; however, multiprotein cascades may have the advantage that they facilitate signal amplification and allow integration of signals from several sources. The effector molecule may block cell cycle progression by altering the activity of one or more of the regulators of cell cycle machinery. Experimental evidence suggests that a variety of strategies are used to inhibit cell cycle progression. Increased inhibitory phosphorylation, transcriptional upregulation of tight binding inhibitors, decreased transcription of the cyclin subunit, regulated destruction of inhibitors, and sequestration of enzymes from their essential substrates are all mechanisms that have been implicated in the enforcement of checkpoint control.

C. Purpose

The immediate purpose of a checkpoint is to halt the progression of physically independent cell cycle activities until a defective process is repaired. If a cell already has the components necessary to repair the defective process, all that is required is time. Consider what happens if a single chromatid fails to attach to the spindle. The unattached kinetochore generates a signal that halts mitosis and microtubules are maintained in the dynamic state that typifies M phase. They remain in this state until the kinetochore attaches to the spindle. Repair of the defective process only requires that the cell remain in the M-phase state long enough for the kinetochore and spindle to contact each other. However, many extracellular challenges that provoke checkpoint responses also induce a complex program of transcriptional induction that provides enzymes needed to repair the defective process. For example, if progression is slowed due to lack of nucleotides, enzymes in the nucleotide biosynthetic pathways may be up regulated or, if DNA is damaged, repair enzymes may be upregulated. By inducing the expression of repair proteins, the process can be sped up, and the length of time cells remain delayed can be reduced. Thus, the ultimate purpose of a checkpoint, to increase survival, is probably best served by providing the maximum amount of repair capacity, as well as allowing the extra time needed for repair. The induction of repair enzymes may be directly under the control of the checkpoint sensor/transducer or it may be initiated by a distinct pathway.

D. Adaptation

Much of the time, damage inflicted on a cell can be repaired, and, after a delay for repair, cell cycle progression continues. However, the question of what happens if a cell suffers irreparable damage is of profound importance for the treatment of cancer. Several currently used therapies rely on genotoxic agents that severely damage DNA. Selectivity for tumor cells relies on the fact that cancerous cells are rapidly dividing, and thus are more sensitive to genotoxic agents. A compromise between inflicting sufficient damage to kill the tumor cells while preserving as many normal cells as possible has to be made. This difficult task is made more difficult by the fact that cells from many cancers have enhanced survival rates following genotoxic treatment. Such cancers are highly unyielding to therapy. Understanding how normal and tumor cells react to irreparable damage is a fundamental requisite for rationally designed therapy.

How a cell responds to irreparable damage depends on the nature of the damage, the species, and, within mammalians, even on the cell type. If unicellular eukaryotes, such as yeast, suffer irreparable damage, they undergo a prolonged arrest. Eventually, cells may adapt to the checkpoint and resume cell cycle progression even though damage remains unrepaired. If the damage is in an essential gene, the daughter cells will not be viable. However, if the damage does not cause loss of an essential function, the daughter cells may well be altered but they will be viable. Considering how much DNA encodes nonessential functions and how many mutations might not adversely affect the capacity to survive, it is perhaps advantageous to a microorganism to adapt the checkpoint response and resume proliferation, even in the presence of irreparable damage. In multicellular organisms the goal is survival of the organism as a whole. Thus, adaptation by individual cells may have been selected against. Mammalian cells that have suffered irreparable damage can either execute a pathway of self-destruction known as apoptosis or become permanently arrested. This permanent arrest is a form of senescence termed premature senescence. Premature senescence is a state in which cells remain metabolically alive, actively contributing to the good of the organism, but barred from further division. Thus, damaged senescent cells cannot compromise the well-being of the whole organism by giving rise to progeny containing altered genetic material. The fate of an irremediably damaged cell is determined in part by cell type. For instance, in lymphoid cells that suffer irreparable DNA damage, the apoptopic pathway is readily activated. However, damaged fibroblasts rarely undergo apoptosis, instead they remain alive, but permanently refrain from further division following irreparable damage. The processes of both damage-induced apoptosis and permanent arrest are under the control of the tumor suppressor gene p53 (see later). Many cancer cells lack p53 function and behave more like unicellular organisms than the disciplined members of a multicellular organism. Chromosomal losses, rearrangements, and amplifications are found in cells that lack p53 function. These things are rarely, or never, seen in cells that retain wild-type p53 function. It is therefore thought that normal cells with irreparable damage are restrained from proliferation by the presence of functional p53. When p53 is lost, the restraint on progressing in the presence of damaged DNA is also lost. The odds of successful proliferation with damaged DNA are quite high. The odds of successful proliferation when cells are permanently arrested or suicidal (apoptosis) are zero. It is not surprising that the damage survival rates of cancer cells, lacking the machinery to strictly enforce the genetic integrity checkpoint, are higher than wild-type cells. The continued proliferation of tumor cells in the presence of damaged DNA could be the result of a failure to detect the initial damage and thus a failure to initiate the checkpoint response. Alternatively, it can also occur if damage is detected and processed, but that the checkpoint signal it initiates is not effectively transmitted to the cell cycle machinery. The failure of cancer cells to enforce strict checkpoint during genotoxic therapy is of profound importance for the treatment of the disease.

III. p53 AND THE G1 DNA DAMAGE CHECKPOINT

Normal human cells have remarkably sensitive systems for responding to DNA damage in G1. This checkpoint may be essential to ensure that repair occurs before replication. If the replication fork encounters a fault and collapses, the act of replication could convert a minor repair problem on one strand of DNA into a more serious problem, such as a break that affects both strands. The G1 checkpoint is thought to operate as shown in Fig. 3. A family of protein kinases represented by ATM (ataxia telan-giectasia mutated) acts as sensors that are activated by damaged, and perhaps by unreplicated DNA. The mechanism of activation is not clear. ATM is structurally related to DNA-PK (DNA-dependent protein kinase), a kinase that is dramatically stimulated by free DNA ends. ATM is stimulated by DNA damage, but it is not known if stimulation of the kinase activity is the consequence of direct binding to damaged DNA or if other proteins sense the damage and activate the kinase. The G1 DNA damage checkpoint is largely dependent on the function of the tumor suppressor protein p53. The p53 gene is the tumor suppressor most frequently mutated in human cancer. It encodes a transcription factor that is activated in response to DNA damage and to a lack of nucleotide precursors. Cells defective for p53 are unable to arrest in G1 following DNA damage and show reduced rates of apoptosis following irreparable damage. Activation of p53 results from increased protein stability and increased transcriptional activity following DNA damage. The ATM gene product is required for the full activation of p53 in response to γ-irradiation. Other ATM-like kinases, such as ATR (ATM and Rad3 related), may contribute in response to other forms of damage. ATM can phosphorylate p53 directly *in vitro*. However, kinases that operate downstream of ATM, such as Chk1 and Cds1, can also phosphorylate p53 at relevant sites. Thus, although it is apparent that the activation of p53 is dependent on ATM, the exact contribution of direct and mediated phosphorylation is not currently clear. One of the transcriptional targets of p53, p21, an inhibitor of Cdk activity, binds preferentially to Cdk2-containing complexes and delays the G1–S phase transition. A pulse of p53 activation and of p21 synthesis is the mechanism by which cells delay the G1–S transition while damage repair is in progress. It is thought that the long-term arrest seen following irreparable damage is mediated through prolonged expression of p21. In many cell types, increased expression of the p53-regulated protein Bax initiates apoptosis by titrating out the antiapoptosis activity of Bcl2. p21 and other p53-regulated gene products may also play a direct role in the repair of damaged DNA.

IV. REPLICATION AND DNA DAMAGE CHECKPOINTS THAT DELAY MITOSIS

In mammalian cells, inhibitory phosphorylation of Cdc2 is necessary for proper mitotic delay in response to blocked replication and following DNA damage. The inactivation of Cdc2 by phosphorylation of the inhibitory sites may not account fully for the checkpoint response; however, the nature of the secondary mechanism is not known. The current model, shown in Fig. 4, is largely based on studies in the model organism *S. pombe*. Regulation of the G2/M transition has also been studied in a number of cancer cell lines that lack p53 and thus lack the G1 damage checkpoint.

Inhibitory phosphorylation is required to prevent premature mitosis in the presence of unreplicated or damaged DNA. Thus, it is thought that regulation of the kinases that inhibit, or of the phosphatases that activate Cdc2, is likely to be an important mechanism by which cells are held in G2 following DNA damage. Indeed, it is known that phosphatase Cdc25 is inactivated in response to DNA damage.

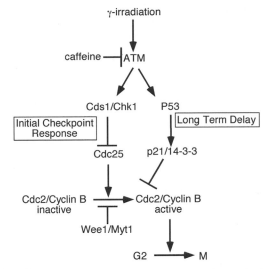

FIGURE 4 The G2 DNA damage checkpoint. The G2 checkpoint involves a protein kinase cascade in which activated ATM phosphorylates and activates Cds1. (The placement of Chk1 downstream of ATM is an assumption based on data from yeast.) Cds1/Chk1 in turn phosphorylate and inactivate phosphatase Cdc25. The mitotic kinase Cdc2/Cyclin B is thus maintained in its phosphorylated and inactive state. Theoretically, upregulation of the kinases Wee1/Myt1 could also delay the G2–M transition, but experimental evidence for this is lacking. The long-term arrest of cells in G2 requires p53-induced expression of CDK inhibitor p21 and members of a family of 14-3-3 proteins which bind to specific phosphoproteins, including Cdc25.

Two human checkpoint kinases are known that can phosphorylate and inactivate Cdc25 *in vitro*, and it is thought that one or both of these kinases inactivate Cdc25 in the presence of incompletely replicated or damaged DNA. ATM is required for the G2 delay response seen following ionizing irradiation of human cells. However, ATM is not required to respond to UV-induced damage and is not required for the block on entry into mitosis that occurs when DNA replication is delayed. Caffeine can override both ATM-dependent and -independent checkpoint responses. Although caffeine has many biological targets, its effects on cell cycle and checkpoint control are most probably mediated through inhibition of ATM and its homologues. Thus, a caffeine-sensitive, ATM-like kinase probably regulates these ATM-independent checkpoint responses. A likely candidate for some of these roles is ATR. However, unidentified relatives may also exist. The activation of Chk1/Cds1 and the inhibition of Cdc25 are likely to be the mechanism by which delay at the G2–M transition is initiated following DNA damage. In the presence of irreparable damage, p53-induced expression of p21 and a 14-3-3 protein are required for long-term maintenance of the arrest. Genotoxic agents are widely used in therapy, and because more than 50% of tumor cancer are defective for p53, cancerous cells are largely dependent on the initial G2 damage checkpoint to maintain viability. A full understanding of the G2 damage checkpoint may facilitate the design of agents that render cancer cells more susceptible to death by genotoxic agents.

V. CHROMOSOME SEGREGATION CHECKPOINT

The use of agents that act on the mitotic spindle is also common in anticancer therapy. Like many drugs, they were discovered serendipitously and their use is empirically defined. As details of the relationship between the mitotic spindle and the chromosome segregation checkpoint improve, it is likely that this information may lead to rational improvements in the use of agents that interfere with mitotic spindle function. The generation of cells with extra chromosomes, amplifications of large chromosomal regions, translocations, or loss of certain chromosomes is a common characteristic of cancer cells that is not seen in normal human cells. This chromosomal instability or aneuploidy (variability in chromosomal number) is thought to result from defects in the checkpoints that ensure perfect segregation of chromosomes in mitosis. Thus, a better understanding of the chromosome segregation checkpoint is likely to contribute not only to the development of better treatment but also to a better understanding of the etiology of the disease.

Cell cycle progression is halted if a single chromatid fails to attach correctly to the mitotic spindle. The signal to halt is generated by unattached kinetochores (see Fig. 5). The exact pathway is not clearly defined, but it is thought that phosphorylation of specific kinetochore proteins recruits a component of the spindle checkpoint machinery, Mad2. In animal cells, Mad1, Mad2, Mad3, Bub1, and Bub2 are all found at the kinetochores of unattached chromosomes and, by

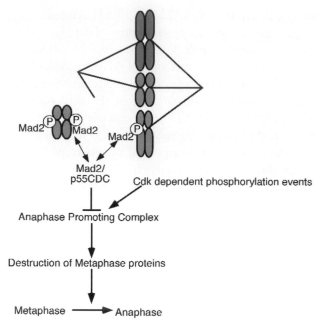

FIGURE 5 The chromosome segregation checkpoint. Specific phosphoproteins are located on the kinetochores of unattached chromosomes. Mad2 associates with the phosphorylated kinetochores and with p55Cdc. The Mad2/p55Cdc complex, which is not restricted to the kinetochore region, inhibits APC function. The binding of microtubules and/or the generation of tension on the kinetochore results in loss of kinetochore phosphorylation, loss of Mad2 binding, and loss of the Mad2/p55Cdc inhibitory function. Thus, correct attachment of all kinetochores relieves inhibition of the APC. The Cdk-dependent phosphorylation of substrates and of recognition factors within the APC allows for differentially regulation of proteins that are tagged for destruction by a common mechanism.

analogy with *S. cerevisiae*, are thought to play an essential role in generating the spindle checkpoint signal. When a kinetochore is attached to the two opposing sets of microtubules that form the mitotic spindle, the kinetochore is maintained under tension and loss of phosphorylation is seen. Mad2 dissociates from the kinetochore region, and inhibition of the Anaphase promoting complex (APC) is relieved. As its name implies, the APC is a complex that allows entry into anaphase. It is a multiprotein complex that catalyzes the ubiquitination of specific proteins that maintain cells in metaphase. Ubiquitination renders the proteins susceptible to proteolytic destruction. Release of Mad2 allows activation of the APC and destruction of the signal that prevents progression into anaphase. Activation of the APC is controlled by the temporally restricted phosphorylation of its regulatory components and of its substrates.

VI. CONCLUSIONS

The past few years have seen a rapid increase in our knowledge of the regulation of cell cycle checkpoints. Knowledge of the mechanisms that maintain dependency between the many biochemically independent processes of the cell cycle is improving our understanding and treatment of the variety of diseases that comprise cancer. The concept of checkpoints as defined by Hartwell is proving an excellent intellectual framework on which to base the more complex models that must be constantly rebuilt in the light of increased knowledge and understanding.

See Also the Following Articles

BCL-2 FAMILY PROTEINS AND THE DYSREGULATION OF PROGRAMMED CELL DEATH • CELL CYCLE CONTROL • CELL–MATRIX INTERACTIONS • CELLULAR RESPONSES TO DNA DAMAGE • DNA METHYLATION AND CANCER • P53 GENE THERAPY

Bibliography

Elledge, S. (1997). Cell cycle checkpoints; preventing an identity crisis. *Science* **274,** 1664–1671.

Hartwell, L., and Weinert, T. (1989). Checkpoints: Controls that ensure the order of cell cycle events. *Science* **246,** 629–634.

Hartwell, L. H., and Kastan, M. B. (1994). Cell cycle control and cancer. *Science* **266,** 1821–1828.

Morgan, S. E., and Kastan, M. B. (1997). p53 and ATM: Cell cycle, cell death, and cancer. *Adv. Cancer Res.* **71,** 1–25.

Cell Cycle Control

Randy Y. C. Poon

Hong Kong University of Science and Technology

GLOSSARY

anaphase-promoting complex/cyclosome A multiprotein complex that promotes the entry into anaphase by targeting proteins for ubiquitin-mediated degradation.

checkpoints Mechanisms that ensure that each stage of the cell cycle is completed before the next stage is initiated.

cyclin-dependent kinases A family of serine/threonine protein kinases that require cyclin binding for activity.

cyclins A family of proteins first identified as proteins that oscillate in amount in synchrony with the cell cycle.

maturation-promoting factor Activity that drives M phase of the cell cycle and that is composed of cyclin B and CDC2. Also known as M phase-promoting factor.

restriction point A point in late G_1 phase of the cell cycle, after passing which the cell is committed to another round of the cell cycle. Known as START in yeast.

ubiquitin-mediated degradation A mechanism by which many proteins in the cell are tagged for selective proteolysis by the proteasome first modified with covalent attachment of polyubiquitins.

The cell cycle is the sequence of events through which a cell duplicates its genome, grows, and divides into two daughter cells. The ability of a cell to duplicate into two daughter cells is one of the most fundamental properties that define life. Most cancers are in essence caused by deregulation of the cell cycle,

Encyclopedia of Cancer, Second Edition
Volume 1

and many oncogenes and tumor suppressor genes are intrinsic components of the cell cycle or can influence its progression.

I. INTRODUCTION

The cell cycle is divided into four phases. After cell division, daughter cells undergo a period of growth (G_1) when most cellular proteins, RNA, membranes, and other macromolecules are synthesized. G_1 is followed by a period of DNA synthesis (S) and then by another period of growth (G_2). G_2 is followed by mitosis (M), within which chromosome condensation, nuclear envelope breakdown, formation of mitotic spindles, attachment of chromosomes to the mitotic spindles, and separation of sister chromatids occur. The stages outside M phase are collectively known as interphase. The cell cycle is completed with separation of the two daughter cells (cytokinesis). Most nondividing mammalian cells exit the cell cycle at G_1 into a G_0 quiescent state, or they can also exit the cell cycle during differentiation and senescence.

Since the 1970s, cell cycle research has moved from merely descriptive studies for events such as chromosome condensation and spindle organization to a fairly comprehensive molecular comprehension through a combination of biochemical and genetical studies. These studies show that the molecular components and the mechanisms that control the cell cycle are conserved throughout evolution from yeast to human. It has also become apparent that many oncogenes and tumor suppressor genes are intrinsic components of the cell cycle or can influence its progression.

The cell cycle is driven by an evolutionarily conserved engine composed of a family of protein kinases called cyclin-dependent kinases (CDKs). The orderly events of the cell cycle depend on many factors, but the turning on and off of different CDKs to drive different phases of the cell cycle remains a good approximation. The activities of CDKs are highly regulated by protein–protein interaction and phosphorylation. The ubiquitin-mediated proteolysis of CDK regulators and other proteins is also critical for cell cycle transitions. It was an important revelation that like so many other processes in the cell, the cell cycle is regulated by phosphorylation and proteolysis.

II. CYCLIN AND CDC2 ARE COMPONENTS OF MPF, A FACTOR THAT REGULATES ENTRY INTO M PHASE

Early cell fusion experiments with mammalian cells and microinjection experiments with amphibian oocytes demonstrated the existence of an M-phase dominant factor. Fusion of cells in G_1, S, or G_2 to cells in M phase induced nuclear envelope breakdown and chromosome condensation of the interphase nuclei, suggesting that M phase is dominant over other cell cycle phases. When the cytoplasm from frog eggs (arrested in second meiotic M phase) is microinjected into oocytes (arrested in second meiotic G_2), the oocytes are induced to enter M phase. This activity, termed maturation-promoting factor or M phase-promoting factor (MPF), can also be found in mitotic cells in all eukaryotes ranging from yeast to human. MPF can drive cells into mitosis and is interchangeable between different organisms, indicating that MPF is not only able to induce certain special meiotic G_2-arrested cells into M phase, but represents a universal M-phase activator in all eukaryotic cells.

Biochemical purification of MPF revealed that it contains two subunits: a serine/threonine protein kinase Cdc28p/Cdc2p first identified in yeast and a regulatory subunit called cyclin first identified in murine invertebrates.

Cell division cycle (CDC) mutants were identified in the yeast *Saccharomyces cerevisiae* and *Schizosaccharomyces pombe* as mutants that arrest cells at a unique stage of the cell cycle when shifted from the permissive temperature to the restrictive temperature. Among the 70 or so CDC genes that have been identified, one CDC gene, the *CDC28/cdc2* (in *S. cerevisiae* and in *S. pombe*, respectively), encodes a related and functionally interchangeable 34-kDa serine/threonine protein kinase that is essential for cells to progress through mitosis and a point in late G_1 called START. START is similar to the restriction point (R) in higher eukaryotic cells; after passing START or the restriction point, the cell is committed to another round of cell cycle.

The importance of cell cycle control is underlined by the fact that its components have been conserved

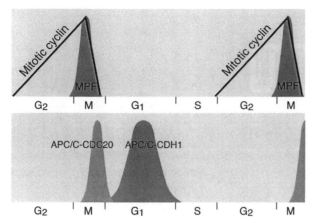

FIGURE 1 Schematic diagram of the relationship between the levels of mitotic cyclin, MPF, and APC/C in successive cell cycles.

phase. The behavior of cyclins suggests that they may be components of the cell cycle engine.

These important early works established that cell cycle transitions can be driven by complexes containing CDC2 and cyclin. The presence of CDC2 in MPF accounts for the protein kinase activity associated with MPF. Moreover, the cell cycle oscillation of the cyclin immediately suggests a mechanism for producing high MPF activity in M phase and low MPF activity in interphase (Fig. 1).

down to details in different eukaryotes. Homologues of *CDC28/cdc2* have been found in other eukaryotes and can functionally complement yeast *CDC28/cdc2* mutations. Indeed, human CDC2 was isolated by looking for human cDNA that can complement a *S. pombe cdc2* temperature sensitive mutation.

The other component of MPF, cyclin, was first discovered as proteins that varied in abundance during the embryonic cell cycles of marine invertebrates. The level of cyclins oscillates in synchrony with the cell cycle, accumulates progressively throughout interphase, and disappears abruptly at the end of M

III. CYCLINS AND CYCLIN-DEPENDENT KINASES DRIVE DIFFERENT PARTS OF THE MAMMALIAN CELL CYCLE

Cell cycle regulation in multicellular higher eukaryotes are necessarily more complex than unicellular lower eukaryotes. In yeast, Cdc28p/Cdc2p is involved in the regulation of both G_1–S (START) and G_2–M transitions. In contrast, mammalian cells contain a family of CDC28p/Cdc2p-like kinases that are regulated by a family of cyclin subunits.

Cyclins are defined as proteins that are related in sequence to the originally isolated mitotic A- and B-type cyclins. The region that shares the highest homology in the cyclin family is a ~100 residue region

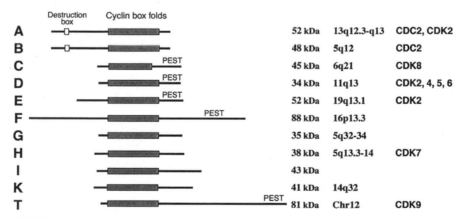

FIGURE 2 The human cyclin family. The cyclin proteins are aligned schematically in relation to the cyclin box region. The position of the destruction box in mitotic cyclins and the PEST region in other cyclins are indicated. The predicted size of the cyclins, their chromosomal localization, and their CDK partners are shown. For cyclins that have more than one subtype, the diagram represents that of cyclin A2, B1, D1, E1, G1, and T1.

known as the cyclin box (Fig. 2). Following the cyclin box, a region with low sequence conservation with the cyclin box can nevertheless fold into the same three-dimensional structure to form a second cyclin box fold. A similar cyclin box fold can be found in diverse proteins like the transcriptional factor TFIIB and the A pocket region of the retinoblastoma protein pRb.

Cyclin-dependent kinases are defined as protein kinases whose kinase activities are depended on binding to a cyclin subunit. All CDKs are related in sequence to the archetypal member CDC2 (also called CDK1) (Fig. 3). The levels of most CDKs are relatively constant in the cell cycle, but their activities are highly regulated due to the fluctuation of the levels and activities of their cyclin partners and other regulators.

Cyclin B–CDC2 is the principal mitotic cyclin–CDK complex that regulates the G_2–M transition (MPF). Identification of physiological substrates for cyclin–CDK is difficult, partly because CDKs have a loose substrate specificity of a serine/threonine followed by a proline (similar to that of the MAP kinase family). One cyclin B–CDC2 substrate involved in M phase is nuclear lamin. Nuclear lamins form dimers that make up the intermediate filaments; intermediate filaments in turn make up the nuclear lamina that lines the inside of the nuclear envelope. Breakdown of the nuclear envelope is essential for M-phase progression and separation of the chromosome into the two daughter cells. It was found that cyclin B–CDC2 phosphorylates a serine residue in lamins, which lead

to the depolymerization of the intermediate filaments and, in turn, nuclear envelope breakdown. If lamins with the regulatory serine changed to a nonphosphorylatable alanine are introduced into the cell, the mutant lamins no longer depolymerize during mitosis.

Cyclin A is synthesized and destroyed slightly earlier than cyclin B during G_2 and can also associate with CDC2. It is unclear whether cyclin B–CDC2 and cyclin A–CDC2 complexes have distinct roles in G_2–M transition, but it is likely that in addition to being an activating subunit, different cyclins also act as different targeting subunits for the recognition of substrates. One example is the ZRXL motif (basic/Cys-Arg-basic-Leu) found in many proteins, such as E2F, p107, p130, and the p21 family of CDK inhibitors that bind to a conserved hydrophobic docking site on the surface of cyclin A.

The second member of the CDK family, CDK2, is an important regulator for G_1 phase and S phase. CDK2 associates mainly with cyclin A and cyclin E, although it can also associate with cyclin D in human normal fibroblasts. The levels of cyclin E–CDK2 and cyclin A–CDK2 peak during G_1–S transition and in S phase, respectively. Introduction of a dominant-negative mutant of CDK2 into the cell arrests the cell in G_1 phase. CDK3 is very similar in sequence to CDK2, but its precise function is not known.

CDK4 and CDK6 are partners of D-type cyclins (D1, D2, and D3) that function in G_1 before cyclin E–CDK2. The main target of cyclin D–CDK4/6 is the retinoblastoma gene product pRb. Phosphorylation of

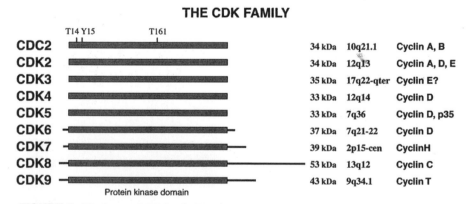

THE CDK FAMILY

		size	localization	cyclin partners
CDC2	T14 Y15 T161	34 kDa	10q21.1	Cyclin A, B
CDK2		34 kDa	12q13	Cyclin A, D, E
CDK3		35 kDa	17q22-qter	Cyclin E?
CDK4		33 kDa	12q14	Cyclin D
CDK5		33 kDa	7q36	Cyclin D, p35
CDK6		37 kDa	7q21-22	Cyclin D
CDK7		39 kDa	2p15-cen	CyclinH
CDK8		53 kDa	13q12	Cyclin C
CDK9		43 kDa	9q34.1	Cyclin T

Protein kinase domain

FIGURE 3 The human CDK family. Boxed regions represent protein kinase homologous regions between different CDK proteins. Major phosphorylation sites in CDC2 are indicated. The predicted size of each CDK, chromosomal localization, and cyclin partners are shown.

pRb by cyclin D–CDK4/6 (and by cyclin E–CDK2) releases the transcription factor E2F and histone deacetylase from pRb. E2F is needed for the transcription of genes important for entry into S phase (including cyclin A), but is usually inactivated by sequester through binding to hypophosphorylated pRb. The adenoviral protein E1A is able to bind to pRb and displaces E2F, therefore disrupting the normal control of the G_1–S by cyclin D–CDK4/6 and pRb. Hypophosphorylated pRb also acts as a transcriptional repressor of genes important for entry into S phase by binding to histone deacetylase (HDAC), in turn leading to the remodeling of chromatin.

It has become apparent that several cyclins and CDKs have non-cell cycle regulatory functions. Apart from binding to CDK4/6, cyclin D can also bind and activate the estrogen receptor. CDK7, which is a component of CDK-activating kinase (CAK) (see later), is also a component of the basal transcription factor TFIIH and can phosphorylate the carboxy-terminal repeat domain (CTD) of the large subunit of RNA polymerase II. Phosphorylation of the CTD is believed to be important for transcription initiation. Other cyclins and CDKs (cyclin C-CDK8, cyclin T-CDK9, and cyclin K) also associate with RNA polymerase II and can phosphorylate CTD. Cyclin T–CDK9 also interacts directly with the human immunodeficiency virus type-1 Tat protein. Interaction of Tat with cyclin T–CDK9 enhances Tat binding to the viral TAR RNA stem–loop structure, which is important in promoting transcription elongation and overcoming transcriptional pausing induced by the TAR element. CDK5 was identified as one of the CDK partners of cyclin D in human normal fibroblasts. However, there is no other indication that CDK5 has a function in normal cell cycle control, but instead CDK5 was found to have essential functions in neuronal development. CDK5 is activated in postmitotic neurons by binding to a protein called p35, which shares no sequence homology to cyclin.

IV. REGULATION OF CDK BY CYCLINS

The activity of CDK is, by definition, dependent on binding to a cyclin subunit. The crystal structure of CDK2 shows that it has an overall bilobed structure typical of serine/threonine protein kinases, but there are several deviations that explain why CDK2 is not active in the absence of cyclin. ATP in the catalytic core of monomeric CDK2 is incorrectly aligned for phosphotransfer. A large structural change is seen in CDK2 following cyclin A binding, with CDK2 adopting a structure more closely resembling that of other active protein kinases and the ATP now becomes correctly aligned for phosphotransfer.

The abundance of cyclin is controlled both at transcriptional and at posttranslational levels. Posttranslational regulation of cyclin mainly occurred through ubiquitin-dependent proteolysis, which will be discussed later. Transcription of cyclin D increases when quiescent G_0 cells are stimulated to enter the cell cycle by growth factors through the integration of multiple signal transduction pathways. In yeast, transcription of the cyclin genes is controlled by a series of feedback loops. G_1 cyclin (Cln)–Cdc28p complexes stimulate *CLN1* and *CLN2* transcription in a positive feedback loop. After G_1, mitotic cyclin (Clb)–Cdc28p complexes repress *CLN* transcription and induce *CLB* transcription in another positive feedback loop. The regulation of cyclin transcription in mammalian cells may also involve feedback controls, with the role of E2F being the better characterized. Phosphorylation of pRb (and the related proteins p107 and p130) by D- and E-type cyclin–CDK complexes leads to the release and activation of E2F. E2F is then able to act as a transcriptional activator for genes involved in S-phase progression, including that of cyclin A. E2F can in turn interact with cyclin A, and the transcriptional activity of E2F is turned off by cyclin A–CDK2 phosphorylation.

Subcellular localization of CDKs and their regulators involves a variety of mechanisms, including the use of nuclear localization sequence, nuclear exporting sequence, phosphorylation, and anchoring to other proteins by direct interaction. One example highlighted here is cyclin B1, which is localized in the cytoplasm during G_2 and translocated into the nucleus at prophase. Cyclin B1 degradation begins as soon as the last chromosome aligns on the metaphase plate. Nuclear import of cyclin B1 involves binding of cyclin B1 to importin-β. The cytoplasmic localization of cyclin B1 during G_2 is mediated by the binding of the nuclear-exporting sequence (NES) in cyclin B1 to the export mediator

CRM1. Phosphorylation of serine residues (by CDC2) in the NES of cyclin B1 is important for its nuclear translocation, possibly through disruption of the CRM1–cyclin B1 interaction. Hence, this mechanism allows the localization of cyclin B1–CDC2 to the nucleus when the complexes are active.

V. REGULATION OF CDK BY PHOSPHORYLATION

Given that the kinase activity of CDK is dependent on binding to cyclin, one question that arises is how the progressive synthesis of cyclin induces the abrupt activation of CDK (Fig. 1). It is clear that apart from binding to cyclin, other regulators are involved in controlling the activity of CDK.

The phosphorylation control of CDC2 is the best understood. Monomeric CDC2 is inactive and unphosphorylated. On binding to cyclin, CDC2 is phosphorylated at three sites: Thr14, Tyr15, and Thr161. Thr161 is located on an activating T loop that blocks the catalytic site of CDK, and its phosphorylation is required for full activation of the protein kinase. Thr14 and Tyr15 are located near the catalytic core of CDC2, and their phosphorylation inhibits CDC2 activity. During G_2, cyclin B–CDC2 complexes are held in the Thr161- and Thr14/Tyr15-phosphorylated inactive state until a threshold of the complexes is reached and then the Thr14 and Tyr15 residues are dephosphorylated for an abrupt activation of MPF.

Thr161 is phosphorylated by the CDK-activating kinase (CAK) and dephosphorylated by the CDK-interacting phosphatase KAP. The activity of CAK is constant in the cell cycle, and KAP only dephosphorylates Thr161 when cyclin is degraded. Hence Thr161 phosphorylation may not be an important regulation for CDKs. It is intriguing that in higher eukaryotes, CAK itself is composed of a cyclin–CDK pair (cyclin H and CDK7) with a third subunit called MAT1. However, CAK in yeast is entirely unlike its higher eukaryote counterpart. Whether cyclin H-CDK7-MAT1 is the real CAK in higher eukaryotes is still a contentious issue. MAT1 activates cyclin H-CDK7 by acting as an assembly factor, as well as substituting for the phosphorylation of Thr170 in CDK7 (equivalent site to Thr161 in CDC2). Interestingly,

CDK7 Thr170 can be phosphorylated by targets of CAK, such as cyclin A–CDK2, in an autocatalytic loop. Phosphorylation of the Thr170 and another residue in the activating loop (Ser164) promotes cyclin H binding even in the absence of MAT1. Hence there appears to be interplay between phosphorylation and MAT1 binding on the activation of CAK.

The Thr14 and Tyr15 residues of CDC2 can be phosphorylated by the protein kinases MYT1 and WEE1, respectively. Both Thr14 and Tyr15 can be dephosphorylated by members of the CDC25 phosphatase family (A, B, and C). Significantly, active CDC2 can inactivate WEE1 and activate more CDC25 by directly phosphorylating these proteins or indirectly phosphorylating upstream components. Hence, a small amount of active cyclin–CDC2 can lead to a rapid and complete activation of all cyclin–CDC2 by this autocatalytic loop.

VI. REGULATION OF CDK BY CDK INHIBITORS

In addition to regulation by cyclin and phosphorylation, CDKs are also negatively regulated by CDK inhibitors. These inhibitors are highly relevant to tumorigenesis. CDK inhibitors fall into two families based on sequence homology (Fig. 4). One family includes p16, p15, p18, and p19 (also called INK4A-D or CDKN2A-D, respectively), and the other family includes p21 (CIP1/WAF1), p27 (KIP1), and p57 (KIP2). The p16 family of inhibitors contains ankyrin repeats and is specific for cyclin D–CDK4/6 complexes. Intriguingly, an alternative reading frame of *INK4A* encodes a protein called ARF that shares no sequence homology to p16. ARF does not interact with CDKs, but can regulate the cell cycle by inhibition of the p53 regulator MDM2 (see later). In contrast to the p16 family, the p21 family can bind and inhibit a broader spectrum of CDKs, including CDK2, CDK4 (weaker), and CDC2 (weakest). Furthermore, the mechanism through which the p21 family and the p16 family inhibit CDKs appears to be different: p21 forms a stable complex with cyclin–CDK, whereas p16 dissociates cyclin from CDK.

The putative functions of different CDK inhibitors are best seen by disruption of these genes in mice. Mice with targeted deletion of the *INK4A* gene that

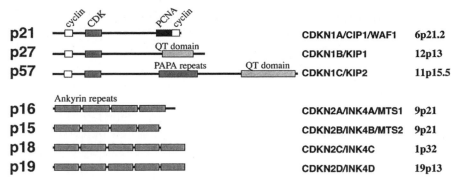

FIGURE 4 The human CDK inhibitor family. The p21 family and the p16 family are shown. CDK- and cyclin-binding regions in p21, p27, and p57 are indicated. The PCNA-binding domain of p21 is at the C-terminal region and is not found in p27 and p57. The precise function of the conserved QT domain and PAPA repeats is unknown. Boxed regions in p16, p15, p18, and p19 indicate ankyrin repeats. Common alternative names and the chromosomal localization of the CDK inhibitors are shown.

eliminates both p16 and ARF are viable, but develop spontaneous tumors at an early age and are highly sensitive to carcinogenic treatments. Significantly, a very similar phenotype was obtained when only ARF was knocked out without disrupting p16, suggesting that ARF could be as important, if not more so, as p16 as a tumor suppressor. The expression is also known to be increased during senescence.

One putative function of p15 is for arresting the cell cycle in response to TGFβ. TGFβ induces the synthesis of p15, which inhibits cyclin D–CDK4/6 and displaces p21/p27 that normally associates with cyclin D–CDK4/6 to redistribute to other cyclin–CDK complexes. This may be a general mechanism of how the p16 family of inhibitors arrests the cell cycle. Mice with the disrupted *INK4C* gene are larger in size and frequently develop pituitary tumors (similar to disruption of p27). Mice with the disrupted *INK4D* gene, however, have no increase in tumor but instead have some defects in spermatogenesis.

One major function of p21 is the inhibition of cell cycle progression following DNA damage because DNA damage induces p53, which in turn activate the transcription of p21. A role for p21 in various cell cycle-arresting states, such as senescence and differentiation independent of p53, has also been suggested. Furthermore, p21 (but not p27 and p57) can inhibit DNA replication by binding to the proliferating cell nuclear antigen (PCNA) and may regulate methylation of newly replicated DNA by disrupting the association between PCNA and DNA (cytosine-5)

methyltransferase. In marked contrast to mice that lack p53 (which develop tumors spontaneously), mice that lack p21 develop normally. Nonetheless, p21-/- embryonic fibroblasts are significantly impaired in their ability to arrest in G_1 following DNA damage by ionizing irradiation, indicating that p21 is important, but not sufficient for the DNA damage checkpoint.

The level of p27 is elevated or has been implicated in a number of cell-resting states, such as quiescence, contact inhibition, and anchorage-dependent arrest. Mice with disrupted p27 gene are larger in size due to a general increase in cell number. These mice are also defective in ovarian follicular development and frequently develop pituitary tumors.

Mice lacking p57 have altered cell proliferation and differentiation, resembling some features of the human hereditary disorder Beckwith–Wiedemann syndrome, which is characterized by a variety of overgrowth and predisposition to cancer. Indeed, both the Beckwith–Wiedemann syndrome and the gene encoding p57 were mapped to 11p15 and are imprinted, and some Beckwith–Wiedemann syndrome patients have mutations in the p57 gene.

VII. REGULATION OF CDK BY ASSEMBLY FACTORS AND CHAPERONES

The role of MAT1 as an assembly factor in formation of the cyclin H–CDK7 complex (see earlier discussion) indicates that the assembly of cyclin–CDK complexes can be a regulated event. Aside from their roles as inhibitors of CDK kinase activity, it is now appreciated that the p21 class of CDK inhibitors actually promotes the formation of cyclin D1–CDK4/6 complexes and targets them to the nucleus. In this connection, control of the subcellular localization of cyclin–CDK, their regulators, and their substrates in general is clearly an important topic that needs to be further investigated.

Proper folding of CDK4 and CDK6 involves binding to CDC37 and the heat shock protein HSP90. HSP90 is a ubiquitous and highly conserved chaperone that supports protein folding. CDC37 and HSP90 also bind and promote the activity of diverse protein kinases such as v-Src and RAF, suggesting that CDC37-HSP90 may be a general chaperone for protein kinases.

VIII. REGULATION OF THE CELL CYCLE BY UBIQUITIN-MEDIATED PROTEOLYSIS

Mitotic cyclins (cyclin A and cyclin B) contain a sequence motif known as the destruction box that is required for their destruction at the end of mitosis. Inactivation of mitotic cyclin–CDC2 complexes is important for events during exit from mitosis, including spindle disassembly, chromosome decondensation, cytokinesis, and reformation of the nuclear envelope.

Cyclin destruction involves a nonspecific ubiquitin-activating enzyme (E1), which activates and transfers ubiquitin to an ubiquitin carrier protein (E2). Ubiquitin is then transferred to cyclin by a cyclin-specific ubiquitin ligase (E3) known as the anaphase-promoting complex/cyclosome (APC/C). The ubiquitinated cyclins are then degraded rapidly by a constitutively active proteasome complex. The importance of APC/C lies in its ability to drive metaphase–anaphase transition by triggering the destruction of the mitotic cyclins, as well as proteins involving sister chromatid cohesion and formation of the prereplication complex. Furthermore, the spindle assembly checkpoint (see later) is executed by inhibition of the APC/C.

APC/C is a large complex containing more than 10 subunits. APC/C-dependent proteolysis depends on binding to activators: the WD40 repeat-containing proteins CDC20 and CDH1. CDC20 and hence APC/C-CDC20 complexes are present only during mitosis. In contrast, the level of CDH1 remains constant during the cell cycle, but it only associates with APC/C during G_1 (Fig. 1).

The activity of APC/C–CDC20 appears to be regulated by phosphorylation. The APC/C core particle is phosphorylated by cyclin B–CDC2 in a CKS1-dependent manner before the APC/C is activated by CDC20. Other protein kinases, such as the polo kinase and protein kinase A, have been shown to stimulate and inhibit, respectively, the APC/C core particle. Degradation of CDC20 itself at the end of anaphase is dependent on APC/C. After anaphase, CDC20 is replaced by CDH1 until cells enter S phase, at which time APC/C–CDH1 interaction is blocked by cyclin–CDK2 phosphorylation of CDH1. While APC/C–CDC20 targets destruction box-containing proteins for ubiquitination, the APC/C–CDH1 recognizes a distinct KEN box motif, which is also present in CDC20. After CDH1 dissociates from APC/C at S phase, the mitotic cyclins are able to accumulate and drive cells into mitosis. At the end of anaphase, a phosphatase CDC14 is released from CFI1, which usually sequesters CDC14 in the nucleolus. This process again involves APC/C–CDC20. CDC14 is then able to dephosphorylate CDH1 and promotes APC/C–CDH1 formation.

Sister chromatids are held together by a multisubunit complex called cohesin. During anaphase, sister chromatid separation is triggered by the cleavage of the cohesin subunit SCC1 by separin (ESP1/CUT1). Before anaphase, separin is inhibited by binding to the protein securin (PDS1/CUT2/PTTG). Separin is allowed to cleave cohesin only after securin is degraded by APC/C–CDC20-mediated proteolysis.

Inappropriate firing of DNA replication origins during G_2 is suppressed by CDK activities and the protein geminin. Geminin interacts tightly with CDT1, a replication initiation factor necessary for loading of MCM proteins into the prereplication complex at origins. Geminin is degraded by APC/C–CDC20, which allows the formation of prereplication complex and later DNA replication in S phase.

Hence APC/C–CDC20 appears to be at the center of several important processes during M to G_1 transition. By simutaneously destroying the mitotic cyclins, securin, and geminin, APC/C–CDC20 triggers sister chromatid separation, exit from mitosis, cytokinesis, and formation of prereplication complex (Fig. 5).

Unlike mitotic cyclins, G_1 cyclins do not have a destruction box, but contain PEST sequences at the C-terminal portion of the protein that are partly responsible for their relatively short half-life. Phosphorylation of human cyclin E (on Thr380) and cyclin D1 (on Thr286) is important for their ubiquitin-dependent degradation. Interestingly, the CDK2 partner of cyclin E can be phosphorylated by CDK2, but cyclin D1 is apparently not phosphorylated by CDK4, but instead by GSK-3β, possibly linking cyclin D1 turnover to mitogen signal transduction pathways. Ubiquitin-dependent proteolysis of G_1 cyclins and some CDK inhibitors involves their phosphorylation-dependent association with SCF complexes. SCF complexes are ubiquitin ligases composed of SKP1, cullin-1, and an F box-containing protein. Additional components of SCF complexes also include RBX1/ROC1 and SGT1. SCF complexes containing different F box-containing proteins target diverse proteins for ubiquitination. Targets of SCF complexes include cell cycle regulators (cyclins, CDK inhibitors, CDK regulators), transcription factors (E2F), I-κB

(inhibitor of the transcription factor NF-κB), and kinetochore proteins.

IX. CHECKPOINTS

The intricate mechanisms that regulate the activity of CDKs and APC/C ensure that they are turned on and off at the correct time in the cell cycle. It is essential to regulate the cell cycle to ensure that each stage of the cell cycle is completed before the next stage is initiated. Deregulation of this kind of checkpoint control may allow cell cycle progression to become insensitive to external signals, spindle assembly, or DNA damage, giving rise to mutagenesis of the genome. Important checkpoints in mammalian cells include the inhibition of entry into mitosis when DNA replication is not completed, inhibition of the exit from mitosis when the mitotic spindles are improperly formed, and inhibition of S phase and mitosis when the DNA is damaged.

The DNA damage checkpoint provides a good example of how checkpoints are linked to the cell cycle (Fig. 6). When cellular DNA is damaged, continued progression through the cell cycle and DNA replication are undesirable because this would lead to

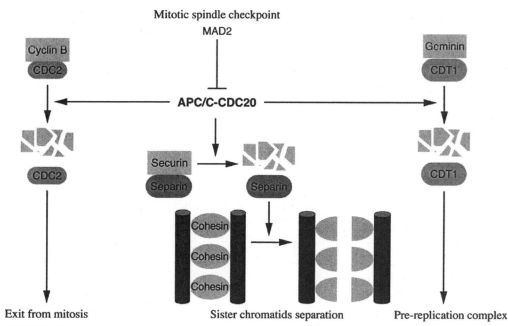

FIGURE 5 APC/C targets degradation of the mitotic cyclins and securin, leading to sister chromatid separation and exit from mitosis.

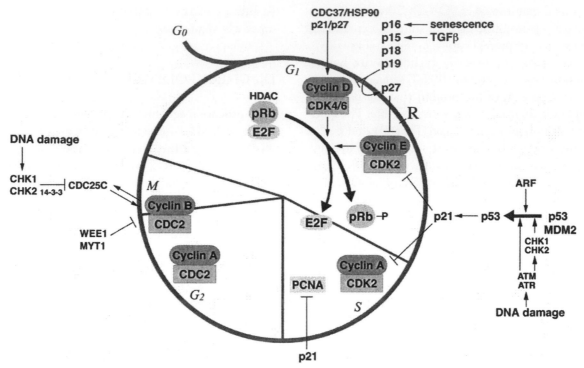

FIGURE 6 Summary of the regulation of the cell cycle by different cyclin–CDK complexes. Selective regulatory pathways for different cyclin–CDK complexes are also shown (see text).

increased DNA mutagenesis and contribute to tumorigenesis. Two options adopted by damaged cells are either to stop the cell cycle, thus allowing time for DNA repair, or to eliminate the damaged cells by apoptosis. Tumor suppressor p53 is critical for both cell cycle checkpoint and apoptosis following DNA damage. A number of the transcriptional activated targets of p53 have been identified, including the CDK inhibitor p21 (which inhibits cyclin–CDK complexes and causes cell cycle arrest) and MDM2. Control of p53 is provided, at least in part, by MDM2 on both the transcriptional activity and the half-life of p53 in a negative feedback loop. MDM2 can bind to the N-terminal transactivation domain of p53 and inhibit p53-mediated transcription, shuttle p53 out of the nucleus, and promote p53 for ubiquitin-mediated degradation. After DNA damage, protein kinases such as ATM, CHK2, or related kinases are activated and phosphorylate residues at the N-terminal region of p53. These phosphorylations inhibit the binding of MDM2 to p53, therefore leading to an increase in p53 level, nuclear localization, and transcriptional ac-

tivity. ARF binds to MDM2 and sequesters it into the nucleolus, hence inhibiting the degradation of p53. Moreover, ARF can be induced by mitogenic stimuli, including the adnoviral E1A, RAS, E2F, and MYC. Therefore, ARF appears to function as a p53-dependent fail-safe mechanism to counter uncontrolled proliferation. In a variety of cancers, the p53-mediated DNA damage checkpoint is commonly eliminated because of mutation of p53, overexpression of MDM2, or disruption of the ARF gene *INK4A*.

The DNA damage checkpoint involving the p53–p21 pathway arrests cells mainly in G_1. The G_2 DNA damage checkpoint involves activation of the protein kinases CHK1 and CHK2. These protein kinases can phosphorylate CDC25C, and in turn create a binding site for 14-3-3. Binding of 14-3-3 to CDC25C inhibits the dephosphorylation of CDC2 Thr14/Tyr15 by CDC25C. This increases the phosphorylation of Thr14/Tyr15 and leads to the inactivation of CDC2 kinase activity.

Chromosomes that are not attached to spindles from the two spindle poles send signals to block the inactivation of cyclin B–CDC2 and sister chromatid separation. This mitotic spindle checkpoint is essential to ensure the proper segregation of the chromosomes at mitosis. Several proteins important for this checkpoint are localized selectively to unattached kinetochores and disappear from them after the attachment of mitotic spindle. One of these proteins, MAD2, can associate with the APC/C–CDC20 complex and inhibit its ubiquitin ligase activity (Fig. 5). The mutation of mitotic spindle checkpoint genes has been implicated to play a role in chromosomal instability in cancers.

X. CELL CYCLE CONTROL AND CANCER

Cancer is in essence caused by cells with deregulated cell cycle control and proliferation. Conceptually, an unchecked cell cycle can be caused by increases in positive regulators of the cell cycle, such as cyclins; decreases in negative regulators of the cell cycle, such as CDK inhibitors; or loss of functions of proteins involved in checkpoint controls. Hence, many positive regulators of the cell cycle are proto-oncogene products, and many negative regulators of the cell cycle and checkpoint proteins are tumor suppressors.

One good example is the cyclin D–CDK4/6-p16-pRb pathway, which is frequently targeted during tumorigenesis. Overexpression of cyclin D1 (also identified as the PRAD1 proto-oncogene) is common in tumors. CDK4 is mutated (an Arg24-to-Cys24 substitution) in some sporadic and familial melanomas, which renders the CDK4 insensitive to p16 inhibition. As discussed earlier, cyclin D–CDK4/6 phosphorylates pRb at the G_1–S transition. Many transformed cells do not have functional pRb, and these cells inevitably have a downregulated level of cyclin D1–CDK. This and other evidence suggest that hypophosphorylated Rb stimulates cyclin D1 expression, and cyclin D1 then turns off its own expression in a negative feedback loop by activating CDK4/6 and phosphorylating pRb. In contrast, the level of the cyclin D–CDK inhibitor p16 is elevated in pRb-negative tumor cells, suggesting that pRb may suppress p16 expression, allowing cyclin D–CDK to phosphorylate pRb. Inactivation of the *INK4A* gene (*MTS1*) (affecting both p16 and ARF) through gene deletions, point mutations, or transcriptional silencing by promoter methylation is prevalent in many types of cancers. Inactivation of the *INK4A* gene has the serious effect of disrupting the cell cycle regulation of cyclin D–CDK4/6 as well as that of p53–MDM2. Moreover, cyclins encoded by the two transforming herpesviruses, herpesvirus saimiri and human herpesvirus 8 (or Kaposi-sarcoma-associated herpesvirus), can form active kinase complexes with CDK6. More importantly, viral cyclin–CDK6 complexes are resistant to inhibition by p16 and p21. It is likely that one or more components of the cyclin D–CDK4/6-p16-pRb pathway are deleted, amplified, rearranged, or mutated in the majority of tumors.

See Also the Following Articles

Bcl-2 Family Proteins and the Dysregulation of Programmed Cell Death • Caspases in Programmed Cell Death • Cell Cycle Checkpoints • Cell–Matrix Interactions • Cell-Mediated Immunity to Cancer • Cellular Responses to DNA Damage

Bibliography

Hartwell, L. H., and Kastan, M. B. (1994). Cell cycle control and cancer. *Science* **266**, 1821–1828.
Hunter, T., and Pines, J. (1994). Cyclins and cancer II: Cyclin D and CDK inhibitors come of age. *Cell* **79**, 573–582.
Morgan, D. O. (1997). Cyclin-dependent kinases: Engines, clocks, and microprocessors. *Annu. Rev. Cell Dev. Biol.* **13**, 261–291.
Murray, A., and Hunt, J. (1993). "The Cell Cycle." Oxford Univ. Press, Oxford.
Nurse, P. (2000). A long twentieth century of the cell cycle and beyond. *Cell* **100**, 71–78.
Sherr, C. J., and Roberts, J. M. (1999). CDK inhibitors: Positive and negative regulators of G_1-phase progression. *Genes Dev.* **13**, 1501–1512.
Zachariae, W., and Nasmyth, K. (1999). Whose end is destruction: Cell division and the anaphase-promoting complex. *Genes Dev.* **13**, 2039–2058.

Cell–Matrix Interactions

Roger Chammas
Ricardo R. Brentani
Ludwig Institute for Cancer Research, and
USP Medical School, São Paulo, Brazil

GLOSSARY

extracellular matrix glycoproteins Large proteins modified by the addition of carbohydrate residues.

glycosaminoglycans Linear heteropolymers consisting of alternating units of uronic acids and hexosamines, which can be extensively sulfated.

growth factors Proteic components that trigger cell proliferation and/or differentiation upon interaction with specific cell surface receptors.

integrins Cell surface receptors that integrate both extracellular and intracellular compartments; composed by two distinct subunits also modified by glycosylation.

proteoglycans Large macromolecules in which the core protein is modified by glycosaminoglycans.

For quite some time it has been well established that interactions between cells and the surrounding extracellular matrix (ECM) are crucial in order to determine basic cellular behavioral patterns such as cell growth and cell death, differentiation, and motility. Such patterns are involved in diverse biological mechanisms such as embryonal morphogenesis, inflammation, immune response, parasitic invasion, cellular transformation, and metastasis. This article considers the role of cell–matrix interactions in the acquisition of aspects of the transformed phenotype and in tumor progression. Attention will be given to those cell–matrix interactions that are concerned with the control of cell growth, cell survival, and cell death leading to increased cell proliferation. Furthermore, the role of cell–matrix interactions in cell motility and invasiveness is examined, as metastatic dissemination of cancer cells is ultimately the cause of death of the vast majority of cancer patients.

I. INTRODUCTION

From a mechanistical point of view, it is clear that in cell proliferation, differentiation, and motility, both expression of hitherto silent genes and activation of already expressed gene products take place. This means that upon docking of extracellular matrix components to their corresponding cell surface receptors, signals must be generated and subsequently transduced in order to unleash the desired biological response. Thus, the extracellular matrix plays an instructive role in the cellular processes mentioned previously. In addition to being instructive, the ECM is also selective. Increasing evidence shows that the ECM is a reservoir for a variety of peptide growth factors, which reside in a latent form in the matrix. Either release of these growth factors from or their presentation by ECM molecules may influence cell survival in different microenvironments.

In the case of *de novo* gene expression, it thus becomes obvious that the response of the genome to signals generated outside the cell is the consequence of a long and complex chain of events that can easily be perturbed. Receptors for ECM proteins are not always randomly distributed in the plasma membrane. Engaged receptors are rather segregated into defined domains within the plasma membrane, providing a supramolecular structure, which allows for the concentration and activation of cytoplasmic proteins involved in signal transduction. These cytoplasmic proteins may be common transducers to different signaling pathways, accounting for biologically relevant cross talks between different cellular communication systems (e.g., peptide growth factors and ECM). In order to better understand how this chain of events is initiated, we have to turn our attention to the matrix components and their cellular receptors. ECM major components include collagens, elastin, noncollagenous glycoproteins, and proteoglycans. More recently, different investigators included a new group of proteins in the ECM, the matricellular proteins. Matricellular proteins bind both to extracellular matrix proteins and to cells and they are apparently devoid of a structural role as most ECM proteins, acting as modulators of cell–matrix proteins. Osteonectin (SPARC, secreted protein acidic and rich in cysteine), thrombospondin, and members of the galectin family may be considered examples of matricellular proteins. This article focuses on noncollagenous glycoproteins, their receptors, and proteoglycans, emphasizing their involvement in tumor progression.

II. NONCOLLAGENOUS MATRIX GLYCOPROTEINS

Whereas noncollagenous matrix glycoproteins do not belong to a single proteic family, they nevertheless display several interesting common features. Extracellular matrix glycoproteins are large extended molecules (some molecules may reach 0.1 μm), organized in distinct subfamilies. Fibronectins (FN) are organized as dimers of two ~200-kDa peptide chains. Variability among members of the fibronectin family is due to alternative splicing, at least 20 different variants have been described so far. Laminins are heterotrimers, the three laminin polipeptide chains α, β, and γ associate forming either a cross- or a Ψ-shaped structure consisting of a long arm and two or three short arms. There are at least five genes coding for the α chain, three for the β chain, and two for the γ chain. Two splice variants exist for one of the α chains (α3A and α3B). So far at least 11 laminin molecules have been identified. The long arm rod is formed through the interaction of the carboxy termini of the three polypeptide chains, which form a coiled-coil α helix, via typical heptad repeats. Each of the short arms is composed of only one peptide chain. Tenascin-C, also called hexabrachion, is the prototype of the tenascin family. Tenascin-C is formed by six polypeptides bound by one of their ends. All of these assemblies are held together by disulfide bonding. Their secretion and deposition at the extracellular matrix depend on the correct assembly and posttranslational modifications in the endoplasmic reticulum and Golgi apparatus. All these proteins display globular domains. At least in the case of laminins, one such domain binds to an identical one displayed by another laminin molecule. This allows for oligomerization of assembled laminins in the extracellular space. ECM molecules not only self-aggregate, but also interact with each other, thus forming a complex extracellular supramolecular structure. One of the biological implications of this complex arrangement is that not all ECM domains are readily available for cellular interactions at a given time. These hidden domains may be uncovered by limited proteolysis or by differential turnover of ECM molecules. Upon exposure these domains may turn on different cellular processes, as cell migration in wound repair, for example. A second biological implication of self-aggregation is the generation of an interesting binding mechanism in which cells displaying occupied ECM (e.g., laminin) receptors bind one another through their respectively bound laminin molecules. Examples of such an interacting mechanism are provided by the attachment of *Staphylococcus aureus* to mouse melanoma cells and mouse and human monocytes, *Trychomonas vaginalis* to canine kidney cells, *Trypanosoma cruzi* to monkey kidney cells and thymic epithelial nurse cells, and immature T lymphocytes.

Extracellular matrix protein families share other interesting similarities. They are usually coded by a large number of short exons. Furthermore, the exons are often repeated and shared by different ECM molecules. It is likely that a combinatorial assembly of different modules through exon shuffling mechanisms gave rise to the diversity of ECM molecules. Fibronectins, for example, are composed of only three kinds of repeats (type I, II, and III FN repeats), which are also found in different ECM subfamilies. All of the other glycoproteins described earlier display several epidermal growth factor (EGF) repeats shown to modulate cell proliferation. It was tempting to speculate that such an effect was determined by EGF repeats. In the case of soluble laminin, the mitogenic activity has been ascribed to a laminin fragment displaying multiple EGF repeats. Cells devoid of EGF receptors were not responsive to the mitogenic activity of soluble laminin. Although there is no evidence for interaction between laminin fragments and the EGF receptor, it seems clear that EGF receptors are necessary for the efficient mitogenic activity of soluble laminin. EGF-like sequences have been also identified in the human core protein of the large cartilage-specific proteoglycan. Polymerase chain reaction (PCR) analysis has indicated distinct mRNA species in human cartilage cells, generated by alternative splicing. It has been speculated that such splicing might provide a mechanism of feedback regulation for the proliferation of cartilage cells. As was the case for soluble laminin, the matrix molecule neither binds the EGF receptor directly nor competes with EGF in its proliferative activity.

Laminins display another domain with mitogenic activity, determined by the peptide IKVAV localized near the carboxy terminus of the α chain devoid of EGF repeats. Furthermore, EGF repeats have been described in a large number of proteins devoid of a proliferation-inducive capacity. One possible role for these repeats could be the interaction with similar repeats. This has been shown to be the case for interactions between the products of the genes *notch* and *delta*, active in the neurogenesis of *Drosophila* and stem cell proliferation in avian and mammal systems or the genes *lin 12* and *gln-1* in the worm *Caenorhabditis elegans*. Indeed, a mutation in one of the EGF repeats of the *notch* gene or the experimental generation of deletion mutants abrogates its interactive capacity. Of course, albeit unattractive, the possibility that such repeats fulfill a structural role only cannot be excluded.

If one cannot predict a function through a structural motif, as illustrated earlier, this very same example may be useful for illustrating another emerging concept in cancer biology. In the absence of direct binding to growth factor receptors, the mitogenic activity of ECM molecules may suggest a further level of complexity involving ECM receptors. A possible explanation is that ECM molecules may sensitize cells so that they may respond to suboptimal amounts of growth factors. Cross talking between both engaged ECM and growth factor receptors has been demonstrated in different experimental systems, determining cell survival and proliferation. The biological implications for such mechanisms are plenty. Cells in different environments, defined by the composition of extracellular matrices, might respond differently to the same (quantities of) growth factors. There is increasing evidence that cell adhesion to an appropriate extracellular matrix is necessary for cell survival. When normal cells are dislodged from their matrices they undergo apoptosis. The term anoikis has been coined to define the death of the homeless cell (from greek, *an*, no; *oikis*, home). Upon malignant transformation, the neoplastic cell acquires resistance to anoikis. Experimental evidence indicates that many protooncogenes are involved in ECM-dependent signal transduction via integrin receptors, leading to cell proliferation and survival.

Other common domains found in the ECM glycoproteins are (1) the extracellular calcium-binding domain and (2) fibronectin type I, II, and III domains. Because many ECM glycoproteins share fibronectin domains, it is tempting to speculate that fibronectin was coded for by an ancestral gene(s), part of which was utilized for the construction of genes coding for the remaining glycoproteins. The cell-binding domain in fibronectin contains a specific tripeptide sequence in one of the fibronectin type III domains, the tripeptide Arg-Gly-Asp (RGD), which is shared by other glycoproteins also involved in cell adhesion, such as vitronectin, nidogen (entactin), fibrillin, epiligrin (a member of the laminin family), fibrinogen, and von Willebrand factor. Abundant experimental evidence employing competing peptides, monoclonal antibodies, or site-directed mutagenesis has clearly established the fact that the cellular receptors recognize their respective ligand via the latter's RGD domain, yet preserving absolute ligand specificity. For example, fibronectins are able to compete with vitronectin for receptor binding only when reduced by proteolysis to a 11-kDa RGD-containing fragment. Two non-mutually exclusive explanations can account for this ligand specificity: (1) the flanking amino acid sequences create different conformations, which modulate the affinities of the receptor for RGD, and (2) further specific interactins are required in order to stabilize each ligand–receptor pair. For example, distinct sequences (so-called synergy sequences) located upstream of the RGD domain enhance its cell-binding activity. RGD sequences are also found in a variety of different venoms (e.g., plant, snake, and scorpion venom peptides), which disrupt cellular interactions, and are involved in the pathophysiology of envenomation. Mammalian glycoproteins also display these so-called disintegrin domains (e.g., members of the growing ADAMs family, proteins bearing both a disintegrin and a metalloproteinase domains). For most of these proteins it is not yet known if they act as adhesion or deadhesion molecules.

Diversity among matrix glycoproteins is not reached only through differential gene usage or alternative splicing, as mentioned previously. Posttranslational modifications, as glycosylation, glycation, and sulfation (e.g., in tyrosine residues), account for the generation of glycoprotein variants, which may be expressed in specific tissues, in distinct developmental stages, or in the course of chronic diseases (e.g., diabetes). Gly-

cosylation of laminin has been shown to be rather critical for cell adhesion and for cell spreading. A number of laminin-binding proteins are indeed carbohydrate-binding proteins, as cell surface galactosyltransferase, calreticulin, calnexin, and members of the galectin family (β-galactoside-binding proteins). The functional role of these molecules in the supramolecular organization of matrices is yet unknown.

III. INTEGRINS

Most, if not all, RGD receptors belong to the integrin family. The term integrin was used for the first time to define an ECM receptor with a dual function: (1) its extracellular domain had affinity for ECM glycoproteins (e.g., fibronectin) and (2) its cytoplasmic domain was associated with cytoskeletal proteins. Thus, integrins integrate both extracellular and intracellular environments. Integrins are constituted by two distinct polypeptide chains noncovalently bound, called generically α and β chains. Sixteen different α and 8 β chains have thus far been reported, forming at least 22 distinct functional heterodimers. Splice variants of both α and β chains (usually in their cytoplasmic domains) increase integrin diversity even further. It becomes clear that there is high promiscuity among members of the integrin family, i.e., not only can several α chains bind to the same β chain or vice versa, but different integrin heterodimers can also bind to the same ligand; conversely, the same ligand can bind to distinct integrins. Integrins not only mediate cell–matrix interactions but may also participate in cell–cell interactions. There are 10 known $\beta1$ integrins, composed by $\alpha1$ to $\alpha9$ and the α_V subunits. All of them bind to extracellular matrix proteins, as collagens, fibronectins, laminins, tenascins, and plasma proteins as vitronectin and fibrinogen. The leukocyte $\alpha4\beta1$ integrin binds to the vascular cell adhesion molecule (a member of the Ig superfamily), egg $\alpha6\beta1$ integrin binds to sperm cell fertilin, a disintegrin. Members of the $\beta2$ integrin subfamily (four distinct heterodimers) mediate cell–cell interactions, mediating the firm adhesion of leukocytes to the inflamed endothelium, and in the formation of the immunologic synapse, enhancing lymphocyte–target cell interactions. There are two $\beta3$ integrins:

$\alpha_{IIb}\beta3$ and $\alpha_V\beta3$. $\alpha_{IIb}\beta3$ is found in platelets and mediates platelet binding to fibronectin, fibrinogen, von Willebrand factor, and vitronectin. $\alpha_V\beta3$ has a broader distribution than $\alpha_{IIb}\beta3$, but a similar distribution. There is only a $\beta4$ integrin so far ($\alpha6\beta4$ integrin), which is found in epithelial cell hemidesmosomes, thus mediating a cell–matrix interaction. α_V chains also associate with $\beta5$, $\beta6$, and $\beta8$ subunits forming extracellular matrix receptors. There are two $\beta7$ integrins ($\alpha4\beta7$ and $\alpha_E\beta7$), mainly associated with intercellular interactions, e.g., lymphocyte homing to lymph nodes/ Peyer's patch and skin, respectively.

Integrin functions are illustrated in different diseases. For example, a severe disease called leukocyte adhesion deficiency (LAD I), which is characterized by recurrent life-threatening infections, is a natural knockout of the $\beta2$ integrin gene. Normal levels of the corresponding α chains are synthesized but not targeted to the cell surface. Heterologous expression of the murine $\beta2$ subunit gene in LAD I cells restored cell surface expression of the integrin. LFA-1, a $\beta2$ integrin, is also expressed in lymphocytes. LFA-1 recognizes and binds to ICAM-1 expressed at the surface of target cells, leading to a closer contact between effector and target cell membranes. This allows for scanning of peptides presented in the context of target cell MHC molecules through the lymphocyte T-cell receptor and subsequent lysis of the target cell. It is believed that downregulation of ICAM-1 expression by the myc oncogene in Epstein–Barr-positive Burkitt lymphoma cells is associated with the latter's ability to evade T cell surveillance.

Integrin chains display short cytoplasmic domains. Furthermore, it has become well established that some integrin β chains may undergo tyrosine phosphorylation upon docking of the corresponding ligands. This was shown for the interaction of $\alpha_{IIb}\beta3$ and fibrinogen in platelets. This effect could be reversed by RGD peptides and was not observed in platelets from Glanzman's patients, which lack this receptor (another natural knockout). Tyrosine phosphorylation could also be induced by plating cells on fibronectin. The question was how integrins transduce signals from the extracellular environment.

Integrins are found in clusters in specialized membrane domains of adherent cells. These domains are called point contacts, focal contacts, and adhesion plaques. On the cytoplasmic side, $\beta1$ integrin chains nucleate the organization of a variety of cytoskeleton-associated anchor proteins, such as talin, vinculin, paxillin, zyxin, and α-actininin. This complex finally binds to actin fibers. Thus, integrins mediate tight contacts between extracellular matrix components and the cytoskeleton. Recruitment of cytoskeleton anchor proteins to these specialized membrane domains depends in part on the activity of a tyrosine kinase called focal adhesion kinase (FAK). FAK was initially described as a substrate for v-SRC and was subsequently shown to be likewise phosphorylated upon docking on fibronectin. In addition to FAK, docking onto ECM components leads to tyrosine phosphorylation of tensin and paxillin. FAK is involved in PI-3K and PKB (Akt) activation, associated with cell survival. Some integrins are also found in other specialized membrane domains and may signal through FAK-independent pathways. $\alpha1\beta1$, $\alpha5\beta1$, and $\alpha_V\beta3$ integrins are found in caveolae, where they may recruit Shc, which in turn triggers the ras/raf/MAPkinase cascade, associated with cell proliferation.

Further consequences of adhesion to ECM consist of a fluctuation in intracellular Ca^{2+} concentration, an increase in cytoplasmic pH, and a higher turnover of phosphatidylinositol polyphosphates. These effects can be also triggered by growth factors, as platelet-derived growth factor. It is clear therefore that cell adhesion to ECM components may elicit cellular responses through well-known second messenger pathways. It is thus also not surprising that profound alterations in cell–matrix adhesions occur when cells are transformed by activated oncogenes. To exemplify, c-erbB2, an oncogene that is amplified and/or overexpressed in a significant proportion of human breast cancers, downregulates the expression of the $\alpha2$ integrin and thus inhibits collagen-induced morphogenesis of an immortalized human mammary epithelial cell line.

Oncogenic transformation of cells also leads to downregulation of $\alpha5\beta1$ expression. However, transfection of transformed Chinese hamster ovary cells with $\alpha5\beta1$ genes led to the suppression of the transformed phenotype, concomitant of course, with greater adhesiveness toward fibronectin. These results would support the notion that $\alpha5\beta1$ acts as a tumor supressor gene. The hypothesis was tested in chimeric mice containing high proportions of α5 null cells. Tumorigenesis and tumor progression in these animals were essentially the same as in wild-type mice. Experimental and clinical evidence point to a role for integrins in invasion and metastasis. For example, uncloned murine melanoma cells could be separated into high- and low-metastasizing subpopulations by adhesion to laminin and fibronectin, respectively. One of the members of the β3 family, $\alpha_V\beta3$, is also expressed in melanocytes and melanoma cells. It is interesting to note that vertical growth phase human melanomas accumulate large amounts of this integrin, as compared to its expression on normal melanocytes. $\alpha_V\beta3$ is not only a receptor for extracellular matrix proteins, it also serves as a local coactivator for the urokinase plasminogen activator in the invadopodia (membrane protrusion of invading cells). The latter is a serine proteinase that activates plasminogen, which in turn activates ECM-degrading metalloproteinases.

Concerning the mechanism of ligand binding, it was well established that effective extracellular matrix recognition depends on an integrin-binding site composed by both integrin subunits. Ligand–receptor interactions are usually divalent cation dependent. However, studies employing either cross-linking strategies or exploiting the molecular recognition theory/principle of complementary hydropathy have shown that fibronectin binds to the β subunit of both $\alpha5\beta1$ and $\alpha_{IIb}\beta3$ integrins. Integrin glycosylation also affects its function. Studies on the interaction of laminin-1 with the $\alpha6\beta1$ integrin receptor have shown that underglycosylated integrins are less efficient as mediators of cell spreading than fully mature integrins. Interestingly, cells do not spread efficiently on underglycosylated laminin. Laminin may act as a lectin-like molecule recognizing specific glycans, as those found in α-dystroglycan and those found in β1 integrins (e.g., the HNK-1 epitope, found in different glycoconjugates, including β1 integrins). β1 integrins are substrates for specific glycosyltransferases as *N*-acetylglucosaminyltransferase V (GnT V, MGAT V), which is upregulated upon malignant transformation. Heterologous expression of GnT V in cultured "normal" epithelial cells led to malignant transformation accompanied by altered adhesion to laminin and fibronectin. It is still not clear how altered glycosylation leads to transformation. It is tempting to speculate that altered cell adhesion is a primary event leading to genetic instability that renders cells transformed. GnT V is also upregulated in *ras*-transformed cells. *ras*-transformed fibroblasts accumulate a galactoside-binding protein (galectin-3), which recognizes GnT V-dependent N-glycans as those present in β1 integrins. As mentioned earlier, galectin-3 is also a laminin-binding protein. Exogenous galectin-3 mediates cell spreading on laminin surfaces. Glycosylation of integrins may define binding sites for endogenous lectins that may act as functional modulators of integrin-containing supramolecular structures. More recently, it has been shown that $\alpha5\beta1$ integrins are covalently modified by chondroitin-sulfate chains, i.e., they are facultative proteoglycans. The physiological significance of this posttranslational modification is still unknown.

The close interconnection between ECM components and the cytoskeleton mediated, for example, by integrins, as discussed earlier, raises the interesting possibility that the complex may also be employed as a mechanoreceptor in order to elicit cellular responses to mechanical stimuli. In fact, cells grown on deformable substrata have been shown to affect specific gene activation; stimulation of cell growth has been obtained by stretching fibroblasts or myocytes. When cells are cultured on tension-resisting collagen gels, they secrete ECM proteins, organize long actin bundles, and grow. When gels are released and tension dissipates, these effects are abolished. Similar results have been obtained when mammary epithelial cells are grown on deformable basement membrane substrata. More recently, evidence has been provided demonstrating that the cellular responses to mechanical stresses (mechanotaxis) are indeed mediated by β1 integrins, and mechanotactic signals are transduced through the activation of tyrosine phosphorylation.

IV. PROTEOGLYCANS

Proteoglycans are ubiquitous glycoproteins found in the extracellular matrix, on cell membranes, and in secretory vesicles (e.g., in mast cells). The glycan chains of these glycoconjugates are long, unbranched carbohydrate heteropolymers, called glycosaminoglycans (GAG).

GAG chains bind specific serine residues in the protein core via a reducing xylosyl residue. Proteoglycans may have up to a hundred GAG chains. Initial studies led researchers to group the proteoglycans according to the nature of their GAG chains. GAG chains can be divided into four distinct groups: (1) heparin and heparan sulfate glycosaminoglycans, (2) chondroitin and dermatan sulfate glycosaminoglycans, (3) keratan sulfate glycosaminoglycan, and (4) hyaluronic acid. Proper proteoglycans are modified by either heparan sulfate or chondroitin/dermatan sulfate. Keratan sulfates are indeed long sulfated polylactosamines, which can be either O linked to serine (as in proper proteoglycans) or N linked to asparagine residues. Hyaluronic acid is not synthesized attached to an aglycone (e.g., a core protein) and it is not further modified as the other GAG chains are. Heparin and heparan sulfate are polymers of [glucuronic acid $\beta(1\text{-}4)N$-acetylglucosamine $\alpha(1\text{-}4)$]. Hyaluronic acid is a polymer of [glucuronic acid $\beta(1\text{-}3)N$-acetylglucosamine $\beta(1\text{-}4)$]. Chondroitin sulfate is a polimer of [glucuronic acid $\beta(1\text{-}3)N$-acetylgalactosamine $\beta(1\text{-}4)$] and can be converted into dermatan sulfate by an epimerase that converts glucuronic acid in iduronic acid, thus dermatan sulfate is a polimer of iduronic acid $\beta(1\text{-}3)N$-acetylgalactosamine $\beta(1\text{-}4)$. The parent polymer is further modified by sulfate groups added either to the hydroxyl groups of the carbohydrate residues (O sulfation) or to the hexosamine after de-N-acetylation (N-sulfation). Details of GAG biosynthesis and its control are still in debate. It is clear though that these polymers are highly diverse and that the patterns of these modifications vary during development, aging, and diseases. It is tempting to speculate that diversity among GAG chains may serve as an extracellular code, which needs to be deciphered.

Many proteoglycan core proteins have been cloned. We now realize that diversity among proteoglycans is not only dependent on GAG chain diversity. Among heparan sulfate proteoglycans, there are those that are matrix associated, such as perlecan and agrin, and there are those that are cell membrane associated as members of the syndecan and glypican families. Among chondroitin sulfate proteoglycans, there are the small, interstitial leucine-rich matrix proteoglycans, such as decorin, biglycan, and fibromodulin, which may interfere with collagen fibrillogenesis, and there are the large matrix chondroitin sulfate proteoglycans, such as aggrecan and versican. There are also cell-associated chondroitin sulfate proteoglycans, such as CD44. The list would go on and on. It is clear that proteoglycan functions depend not only on the GAG chain, but also on the core protein, as discussed later.

A. Matrix-Associated Proteoglycans

Proteoglycans are very versatile molecules, capable of binding to cell surface, to other extracellular matrix components, and to a variety of growth factors. This latter capacity, which is discussed further, determines a means of concentrating such growth factors (through immobilization) near the cells that will be stimulated. These growth factors may be kept in an inactive or latent form. Many proteoglycan interactions occur through their glycosaminoglycan moieties. These interactions seem to be charge dependent or rather a function of the degree of sulfation. Glycosaminoglycan binding takes place at consensus sequences found in many proteins. Indeed many of the extracellular matrix proteins do bind proteoglycans. Such binding allows for matrix assembly and organization of its supramolecular structure. These binding sites are rich in basic amino acids and two motifs have been proposed: BBXB and BBBXXB, where B is a basic amino acid and X may be any amino acid.

Binding of glycosaminoglycans is also dependent on the size and/or the number of glycosaminoglycan side chains. It was speculated that larger molecules can engage in multiple interactions. Thus, the presence of chondroitin sulfate chains helps stabilize the interactions of this glycosaminoglycan with fibronectin and collagen. The large cartilage proteoglycan aggrecan contains a hyaluronic acid-binding domain, which also binds the hyaluronic acid link protein. These interactions create a stable aggregate among these three molecules found in cartilages. The small fibroblast proteoglycan decorin also binds both collagen and fibronectin through its core protein. It has been shown that soluble proteoglycans can inhibit cell adhesion to fibronectin or collagen, presumably by steric hindrance or by occupying glycosaminoglycan-binding sites.

Perlecan, the low-density heparan sulfate proteoglycan, is found in basement membranes and is involved in endothelial/epithelial cell attachment to these specialized extracellular matrices. Its core protein is a multidomain structure with regions of homology with laminin, LDL receptor, and N-CAM. The murine perlecan core protein displays an RGD sequence in a globular region within domain III, which is homologous to domain IVb of the laminin α1 chain. Adhesion of aortic endothelial cells to mouse perlecan core protein was inhibitable by anti-integrin antibodies. Heparan sulfate GAG chains present in perlecan interfere with the RGD–integrin interaction. A similar binding is observed in *C. elegans* and seems essential to body wall muscle cell differentiation. It is interesting to note that human perlecan has no RGD sequences. Perlecan also binds laminin and is essential in basement membrane assembly.

B. Membrane-Bound Proteoglycans

Membrane-bound proteoglycans may be substituted predominantly by either heparan sulfate or chondroitin sulfate chains. Syndecans are transmembrane heparan sulfate proteoglycans (that may also present chondroitin sulfate chains) found in almost all cells. Syndecans may serve as growth factor coreceptors, integrin coreceptors, and lipoprotein lipase-binding proteins. For example, syndecan-1 binds mammary epithelial cells to fibronectin and fibrillar collagens through its heparan sulfate GAG chains. Glypicans are also heparan sulfate proteoglycans, which are linked to the cell surface via glycosyl-phosphatidylinositol (GPI) anchors that are believed to act as growth factors coreceptors. Glypican-3 binds FGF and is also able to induce cell death in a GAG-independent way. Mutations in glypican-3 are associated with the Simpson–Golabi Behmel overgrowth syndrome (SGBS). SGBS patients are at a higher risk for developing Wilm's tumor and neuroblastomas.

CD44 is a membrane-bound chondroitin sulfate proteoglycan, which also displays a hyaluronic acid-binding domain, as aggrecan. CD44 has been shown to mediate lymphocyte binding to the high endothelial venules of lymphoid organs and is thus responsible for the homing of lymphocytes. CD44 also binds extracellular matrix glycoproteins, such as collagens and fibronectin. It has been shown that its short cytoplasmic domain can be phosphorylated at two out of six serine residues. Mutagenesis of either of the two serines precludes phosphorylation of the other one. The amino acids that surround Ser^{333} and Ser^{325} make them poor substrates for both protein kinases A and C, but suitable substrates for casein-kinase 2.

CD44 is actually a group of glycoproteins ranging from 85 to more than 200 kDa in size. Part of this heterogeneity is due to posttranslational modifications, but cloning and sequencing have shown that many isoforms also vary in their primary structure. All of them share a very conserved cytoplasmic domain, a transmembrane domain, and the N-terminal 150 residues. Studies on metastatic cancer cells have led to the production of antibodies specific for surface antigens present in metastatic cells only. Using this antibody, it was possible to isolate cDNAs that code for splice variants of CD44. The metastatic epitope was found in an enlarged extracellular region absent from "standard" CD44. Transfection and overexpression of this variant into one of various nonmetasta-sizing cells rendered them highly metastatic. However, intravenous injection of a metastasis-specific monoclonal antibody directed against the enlarged extracellular region epitope prevents metastasis formation associated with the variant CD44.

PCR analysis of human tumor cell lines has shown that human tumor homologues contain up to five additional domains in the extracellular region of standard (epithelial) CD44. Cell lines studied were lung, breast, and colon. Examination of material from breast or colon cancer patients has also revealed the overproduction of several alternatively spliced CD44 variants whereas only the standard protein was found in control samples. Interestingly, with the aid of the just-described monoclonal antibody, it was possible to show that the CD44 variant, sharing sequences with those variants involved in metastasis formation, is also transiently expressed on activated T and B lymphoyctes. The fact that the same CD44 variant seems involved in lymphocyte activation and recirculation and in the spread of cancer cells indicates that both processes resemble each other at the molecular level. There is experimental evidence for a role of CD44, as a hyaluronan-binding protein, in dynamic interactions (as adhesion under flow) between lymphocytes and endothelial cells/subendothelial matrices. The role of CD44 in carcinoma metastasis is still elusive.

Another hyaladherin (hyaluronic acid-binding protein) is called RHAMM (receptor for hyaluronic acid-mediated motility). RHAMM promotes the disassembly of focal adhesion plaques, leading to the locomotion of fibroblasts and transformed cells. This seems not to be a CD44 function.

C. Selected GAG/Proteoglycan Binding Proteins

Several proteins cited throughout this text bind either glycosaminoglycans or proteoglycans under physiological conditions. It has been more and more appreciated that glycosaminoglycans play a role as modulators of different protein functions. Glycosaminoglycan chains provide an anionic surface for intermolecular interactions. Due to a variable degree of sulfation, gradients of local pH may be formed along GAG chains, favoring a number of reactions/interactions we would not assume possible under physiological conditions. We have already discussed the role of GAG chains/proteoglycans in the assembly of extracellular matrices through their coordinate binding to laminins, fibronectins, and collagens. Enzymes as cathepsins bind to GAG chains and have their function modulated by the acidic microenvironment provided by them. Heparan sulfate GAG chains may resemble the overall charge distribution of selectin-binding sialomucins. Indeed, low molecular weight heparins are efficient ligands to P-selectin.

Among peptide growth factors, it has been long recognized that extracellular matrices are true reservoirs for FGFs, PDGF, vascular endothelial growth factor (VEGF), TGF-βs, chemokines (as IL-8 and MIP-1β), hemopoietic growth factors (as GM-CSF and IL-3), scatter factor, and EGF-related growth factors, among others. It has been assumed that release of these immobilized growth factors would depend on matrix remodelling. Studies on FGFs consolidated the notion that GAG chains are indeed growth factor coreceptors.

FGF-2 promotes the proliferation of cells of both ectodermic and neural origin. It is also a very potent angiogenic factor. Measurements of FGF-2 binding have evidenced the existence of both high- and low-affinity receptors at the cell surface level. Further studies have shown that low-affinity receptors, which

are more abundant, are heparan sulfate proteoglycans (HSPG; perlecan, glypican, syndecan). These HSPG can be effectively competed out by heparin. The association of FGF-2 to heparin has proven beneficial because it protects the growth factor from degradation. The biological response, however, depends on the interaction with high-affinity receptors, which display tyrosine kinase activity and are phosphorylated upon docking of FGF-2. Mutant CHO cells that do not express heparan sulfate proteoglycans are unable to bind FGF-2 unless heparin or heparan sulfate is added to the medium. These results, coupled to the observation that FGF-2 dissociates rapidly from heparan sulfates but slowly from high-affinity receptors, led to the suggestion that prior binding to heparan sulfate proteoglycans is obligatory for proper presentation of the growth factor to its high affinity receptor. An octasaccharide from heparin was found sufficient to promote the effects of the intact proteoglycan. It was also shown that heparin facilitates FGF dimerization. This observation is of physiological significance, as effective signaling through FGF receptors depends on their dimerization.

Interestingly enough, this effect of heparin was also observed for a number of other growth factors. For example, it also potentiates the mitogenic activity of FGF-1 on endothelial cells. Another angiogenic factor that promotes the proliferation of endothelial cells is vascular endothelial growth factor. The binding of VEGF to its specific cell surface receptors is likewise modulated by interaction with heparin, albeit at a 10-fold lower affinity. Again, interaction with heparin promotes dimerization of the growth factor. It is clear, however, that the binding site for heparin on the VEGF molecule is distinct from that which recognizes its specific receptor.

While the structural diversity of proteoglycans has been long appreciated, we are just now learning about the genes involved in their biosynthesis. Biosynthesis of heparan sulfate glycosaminoglycans depends on the activity of a heparan sulfate copolymerase, which adds alternating units of both glucuronic acid and *N*-acetylglucosamine to a nascent GAG chain. There are at least two human genes coding for such activity, *EXT1* and *EXT2*, which were initially described as putative tumor suppressor genes associated with growth plate tumors (hereditary multiple exostoses).

It is interesting to note that in the absence of heparan sulfate GAG chains, which are necessary for the adequate function of different growth factors, tumors may arise more frequently.

In the case of platelet-derived growth factor, another mesenchymal growth modulator, binding to proteoglycans seems to be more complex. Enzymatic proteoglycan digestion indicates that at least part of the attachment of PDGF B and LA (one of the splice variants of the PDGF A chain) is mediated by either chondroitin or dermatan sulfates. However, the carboxy-terminal part of PDGF LA seems to attach to cells via a heparin sulfate proteoglycan. Contrary to the results on other growth factors, proteoglycan interactions of PDGF are not involved in receptor-triggered cellular responses.

Other chondroitin sulfate proteoglycans, such as decorin, biglycan, and betaglycan, bind TGF-β. As FGFs, TGF-β is another morphogenetic growth factor, which has at least three cell surface receptors. Two of them are high affinity receptors. The low-affinity receptor is the proteoglycan betaglycan. Betaglycan has two isoforms: a membrane-bound and a soluble isoform. The soluble form may represent a matrix reservoir for TGF-β.

Thus, proteoglycans can act as versatile deposits of growth factors, at times able even to improve the effects of the latter by conformational modifications such as dimerization or by presenting them in a favorable conformation to their physiological receptors.

See Also the Following Articles

Bibliography

Brentani, R. R. (1989) The molecular basis of the metastatic phenotype. *Crit. Rev. Oncogen.* **1,** 51–59.

Chammas, R., Veiga, S. S., Travassos, L. R., and Brentani, R. R. (1993). Functionally distinct roles for glycosylation of alpha and beta integrin chains in cell-matrix interactions. *Proc. Natl. Acad. Sci. USA* **90,** 1795–1799.

Engel, J., and Bozic, D. (1999). Modules in ECM and adhesion molecules. *In* "Guidebook to the Extracellular Matrix: Anchor and Adhesion Proteins (T. Kreis and R. Vale, eds), 2nd Ed., pp. 344–351. Oxford Univ. Press, New York.

Frisch, S. M., and Ruoslahti, E. (1997). Integrins and anoikis. *Curr. Opin. Cell Biol.* **9,** 701–706.

Giancotti, F. G., and Ruoslahti, E. (1999). Integrin signaling. *Science* **285,** 1028–1032.

Jasiulionis, M. G., Chammas, R., Ventura, A. M., Travassos, L. R., and Brentani, R. R. (1996). alpha6beta1 integrin, a major cell surface carrier of beta1-6 branched oligosaccharides, mediates migration of EJ-ras transformed fibroblasts on laminin-1 independently of its glycosylation state. *Cancer Res.* **56,** 1682–1689.

Koenig, A., Norgard-Sumnicht, K., Linhardt, R., and Varki, A. (1998). Differential interactions of heparin and heparan sulfate glycosaminoglycans with the selectins: Implications for the use of unfractionated and low molecular weight heparins as therapeutic agents. *J. Clin. Invest.* **101,** 877–889.

Lander, A. D., and Selleck, S. B. (2000). The elusive functions of proteoglycans: In vivo veritas. *J. Cell Biol.* **148,** 227–232.

Lind. T., Tufaro, F., McCormick, C., Lindahl, U., and Lidholt, K. (1998). The putative tumor suppressors EXT1 and EXT2 are glycosyltransferases required for biosynthesis of heparan sulfate. *J. Biol. Chem.* **273,** 26265–26268.

McCormick, C., Leduc, Y., Martindale, D., Mattison, K., Esford, L. E., Dyer, A. P., and Tufaro, F. (1998). The putative tumor suppressor EXT1 alters the expression of cell surface heparan sulfate. *Nature Genet.* **19,** 158–161.

Pilia, G., Hughes-Benzie, R. M., Mackenzie, A., Baybayan, P., Chen, E. Y., Huber, R., Neri, G., Cao, A., Forabosco, A., and Schlessinger, D. (1996). Mutations in GPC3, a glypican gene cause the Simpson-Golabi-Behmel syndrome. *Nature Genet.* **12,** 241–247.

Taverna, D., Ullman-Cullere, M., Rayburn, H., Bronson, R. T., and Hynes, R. O. (1998). A test of the role of alpha5/fibronectin interactions in tumorigenesis. *Cancer Res.* **58,** 848–8553.

Tlsty, T. D. (1998). Cell-adhesion-dependent influences on genomic instability and carcinogenesis. *Curr. Opin. Cell Biol.* **10,** 647–653.

Veiga, S. S., Elias, M. C. Q. B., Gremski, W., Porcionatto, M. A., da Silva, R., Nader, H. B., and Brentani, R. R. (1997). Post-translational modifications of alpha5beta1 integrin by glycosaminoglycan chains: The alpha5beta1 integrin is a facultative proteoglycan. *J. Biol. Chem.* **272,** 12529–12535.

Cell-Mediated Immunity to Cancer

Jason S. Gold
Alan N. Houghton

Memorial Sloan-Kettering Cancer Center and
Weill Medical School of Cornell University

GLOSSARY

adoptive immunotherapy The strategy of passively immunizing against a tumor by infusing T cells specific to the tumor or natural killer cells activated with cytokines.

antigen-presenting cell A cell that is specialized in activating a T-cell-mediated immune response by presenting antigen in the context of sufficient costimulation to naive T cells.

cancer-testis antigens Tumor antigens that are only expressed on cancer cells and immune privileged germ cell tissue.

cell-mediated immunity Immunity that can be transferred by the cellular fraction of blood but not serum. The specificity of a cell-mediated immune response is determined by the T-cell receptor of T cells.

costimulation Signals that allow activation of a naive T cell upon encountering antigen. Costimulation can be transmitted by the interaction of molecules on the cell surface of the antigen-presenting cell with molecules on the cell surface of the T cell or by cytokines in the local milieu.

differentiation antigen Tumor antigens shared by tumors and similarly differentiated normal tissue. The best described differentiation antigens are melanosomal differentiation antigens, which are shared between melanoma and normal melanocytes.

immune surveillance The concept that the immune system recognizes and destroys incipient neoplasms. Thus hosts with impaired immunity may be more susceptible to cancer, and cancers in immunocompetent hosts must evolve to evade the natural immune response.

MHC molecules Molecules on the surface of cells that present antigen in the form of peptide epitopes so that it can be recognized by T cells. MHC class I molecules typically present cytoplasmic proteins. MHC class II molecules present antigens present in endosomal and lysosomal compartments.

tumor antigens Antigens on tumors that the immune system is capable of recognizing and responding to. Tumor antigens may be present exclusively on cancer cells or may be shared with normal tissue.

T-cell receptors Molecules on the surface of T cells capable of recognizing antigen complexed to MHC. Each T cell has one specificity of T-cell receptors.

vaccination The strategy of actively inducing immunity by giving the host an antigenic substance. Vaccination against cancer can involve administration of whole tumor cells or tumor cell preparations, as well as recombinant or synthetic tumor antigens. In contrast to vaccination against infectious diseases, in the clinical setting, vaccination against cancer usually implies vaccinating against a disease after it has occurred rather than prophylactically.

Cell-mediated immunity to cancer principally relies on the specificity of the interaction between T cells and tumor antigens presented by tumors and antigen-presenting cells (APC), although other types of cells may be the ultimate effectors. Many tumor antigens have been discovered in recent years. The immune system has been shown to recognize antigens that are shared between cancer and normal tissue, as well as those that are created by genetic alterations in the tumor. In immunocompetent hosts, many tumors may be recognized and destroyed at an early stage, and those that progress may be forced to evolve mechanisms to evade an immune response. Much effort has been directed toward developing strategies of immunizing individuals so that their immune systems can recognize and respond to established malignancies.

I. INTRODUCTION

It has long been accepted that the immune system evolved to protect the host from microbial invasions. It is harder to explain how the immune system might evolve to fight cancers. In fact, as recently as this past decade, immunologists questioned whether the immune system could recognize cancer cells and whether the immune system was capable of mounting a response that could reject tumors.

In the setting of a microbial invasion, the immune system must only differentiate "self" from "foreign" in order to direct its attack. Cancers, however, arise from the host's own tissues, and thus almost all the genes expressed by tumors are also expressed by normal tissues. Can the immune system attack "altered self" while sparing "self"? Another question is why the immune system would evolve to fight tumors. Although microbial invasion can affect an individual of any age, malignancy is more common after childbearing, and thus the ability to protect against cancer might not exert the same sort of evolutionary pressure as the ability to protect against infection.

Nevertheless, immune recognition of cancers has now been well documented in humans. Also, it has been shown that the immune system is capable of rejecting cancer in experimental systems. Further, evidence shows that the immune system may have a role in protecting the host from developing tumors (the concept of immune surveillance), and that in order for cancer to progress beyond microscopic loci, it must acquire mechanisms to evade an immune response.

Historically, the immune system has been said to have two arms. Humoral immunity was originally described as immunity that could be transferred from one individual to another through the transfer of the serum fraction of blood and is mediated by antibodies. Cellular immunity was thus defined as immunity that could be transferred through the cells of blood. An antitumor immune response can involve either or both arms of the immune system. This article focuses on cellular immunity to cancer.

II. CELLS OF THE IMMUNE SYSTEM

Specific immunity resides in B lymphocytes and T lymphocytes. The ability to react and respond to specific antigens is called adaptive immunity. B lymphocytes are responsible for the secretion of immunoglobulin, or antibodies. Antibodies directly bind to antigen and usually are directed at extracellular or cell surface antigens, such as bacteria, toxins, or viral proteins expressed on the surface of cells. T lymphocytes can only recognize antigens that are presented to the T cell by another host cell (called an antigen-presenting cell) that is genetically identical. The

T-cell receptor is expressed on the surface of T cells and has a similar structure to immunoglobulins. However, T-cell receptors do not directly bind to antigens. Rather, T-cell receptors bind to peptides (between 8 and 16 amino acids in length) presented on the surface of APCs; these peptides are processed from longer proteins inside APC to form the antigens recognized by T cells. Peptides (or in some cases lipids or carbohydrates) are presented to T-cell receptors by major histocompatibility (MHC) molecules on APCs. MHC molecules in humans are called HLA and are extremely polymorphic, distinguishing one individual from another (except for identical twins). A T cell activated by recognizing antigen can either destroy the host cell presenting the antigen or secrete immune substances known as cytokines that stimulate inflammation and recruit other immune cells. T lymphocytes are responsible for recognizing intracellular pathogens (because the antigens recognized by T cells must be processed inside the cell). B cells develop in the bone marrow and T cells develop in the thymus. Each B or T cell can recognize a single antigen. B or T cells capable of broadly recognizing host tissues are normally deleted from the immune repertoire during development or paralyzed (a process called anergy), but B or T cells capable of recognizing "nonself" are allowed to fully develop. However, B cells or T cells that do not strongly recognize self but can bind to specific types of tissues in the body may be allowed to develop.

T lymphocytes can be further divided into CD4$^+$, or helper, T cells and CD8$^+$, or cytotoxic, T cells. CD4$^+$ T cells recognize antigens presented by MHC class II (class II MHC) molecules. Class II MHC molecules present antigens derived from proteins broken down in lysosomal/endosomal compartments within cells. The cellular compartments sample molecules from the cell surface and outside the cell. Class II MHC is expressed by only specialized APCs that are capable of activating T cells. CD4$^+$ T cells have been called helper T cells because their primary response when activated is to secrete cytokines that enhance the response of CD8$^+$ T cells, B cells, inflammatory cells (especially macrophages), and other immune/inflammatory cells. In contrast, CD8$^+$ T cells, recognize antigens in the context of class I MHC molecules. Class I MHC molecules, which are present on all cells, present primarily cytoplasmic and nuclear antigens. The primary response of activated CD8$^+$ cells is to lyse cells presenting the specific antigens, and thus they are known as cytotoxic T cells (CTLs). A third type of lymphocyte is neither a B cell nor a T cell and is known as a natural killer (NK) cell. These cells can directly lyse a host cell without recognizing a specific antigen and can also produce cytokines. Although the exact mechanism by which NK cells recognize cells is not entirely understood, there are signals for both activating and inhibiting NK cells. One of the best understood inhibitory signals is self class I MHC molecules. NK cells have been described as cells that recognize "missing self." Thus virus-infected cells or tumor cells that lose MHC expression in an effort to evade a T-cell response are susceptible to lysis by NK cells. NK T cells form another set of lymphocytes that can mediate tumor immunity. These cells express both NK and T-cell markers and are able to kill target cells like CTLs and also produce cytokines.

Adaptive immunity, driven by B cells and T cells, develops in response to antigens. The frontline defense of the immune system does not require prior recognition of antigen, which is called innate immunity. NK cells are part of the innate immune system. Macrophages, eosinophils, basophils, and mast cells are other cells involved in innate immunity, participating in inflammatory responses, and will not be further discussed here.

A critical step of the adaptive immune response by T cells is presentation of antigen. The initial response of T cells to antigens that leads to activation is called priming. Although any APC can present antigenic peptides, only "professional" APCs can activate T-cell responses. Once T cells are primed, they can recognize nonprofessional APCs. Professional APCs are specifically designated to activate T lymphocytes. Thus antigen presented on an APC can license a T cell to respond to subsequent exposures to antigen presented on other host cells. In contrast, antigen presented to a naive T cell by a host cell that is not a professional APC can potentially tolerize that T cell such that it is rendered anergic to subsequent exposures to that antigen (one of the mechanisms for peripheral tolerance). The dendritic cell is the most potent and best described professional antigen-presenting cell. Dendritic cells are derived from the bone marrow and reside in epithelial surfaces, lymph nodes, and the spleen. They can capture and process antigens from a variety of sources, including bacterial and viral infections and tumors.

III. ANTIGEN PROCESSING AND PRESENTATION

T cells can only recognize antigen presented to them by MHC molecules. MHC molecules have been divided into two classes. Almost all cells express class I MHC, with red blood cells and spermatozoa being exceptions. The class I MHC molecule is translated into the endoplasmic reticulum where it associates with peptide fragments of cytoplasmic and nuclear proteins. The class I MHC/peptide complex is then transported to the cell surface, where it is accessible to T cells.

Specialized cells, including B cells, macrophages, and dendritic cells, express class II MHC. The class II MHC molecule is routed to specialized lysosomal/endosomal compartments after translation. There it associates with fragments of proteins that are also routed to that compartment for degradation or arrive in that compartment from outside the cell through phagocytosis. The class II MHC/peptide complex is also transported to the cell surface.

Humans have three sets of genes for class I MHC molecules, known as HLA-A, HLA-B, and HLA-C. There are also three sets of genes for class II MHC molecules, known as HLA-DR, HLA-DP, and HLA-DQ. Because each of these genes is highly polymorphic and each individual has two alleles for each of the class I MHC molecules and two alleles for each of the two chains of the class II MHC molecules, the number of possible combinations of MHC molecules is enormous. Because each polymorphic MHC molecule has a different affinity for peptide, a peptide that can bind to the HLA-A1 molecule may not bind to the HLA-A2 molecule. Thus the sets of peptides that can be seen by the immune systems of two genetically different individuals are distinct.

In order for an antigen to be presented by an MHC molecule, it must first be processed. For class II MHC, this is accomplished mainly by the proteolytic degradation of proteins in the endosomal/lysosomal compartment by resident proteolytic enzymes. For class I

MHC, this is slightly more complex, as a full-length protein present in the cytoplasm or nucleus must be converted into peptide fragments before transport into the endoplasmic reticulum for binding to MHC molecules. The proteasome is a complex of enzymatic proteins responsible for degrading intracellular proteins. Proteins destined for the proteasome are cleaved into peptides that then can be transported into the endoplasmic reticulum by the transporter associated with antigen processing (TAP). It should be noted that cleavage of a protein by the proteasome into certain peptide fragments and transportation of certain peptide fragments by TAP into the endoplasmic reticulum are also responsible for the repertoire of peptides that can be seen by $CD8^+$ T cells.

In order to activate a T-cell response, antigen must be presented in the context of costimulatory signals, only present on professional APCs. How do tumor antigens then activate an immune response if cancer cells are not professional APCs? Tumor antigens from necrotic or apoptotic cancer cells can be taken up and presented by APCs. This process is called crosspresentation. By the process of phagocytosis or other fluid uptake, tumor antigen can access the class II MHC compartment of an APC, but it is not obvious how exogenous tumor antigens might be presented by the class I MHC processing pathway (which typically involves cytoplasmic and nuclear proteins). One possibility is that exogenous peptides can bind to heat shock proteins, which are stress proteins produced in abundance by many cancer cells. Heat shock proteins bind to receptors on professional APCs and can efficiently deliver peptides into the class I MHC pathway. This process may be one mechanism for crosspresentation. In addition, heat shock proteins can activate professional APCs, leading to more efficient stimulation of T cells. Thus tumor antigens released from damaged or dying cells can be presented to the immune system by professional APCs.

IV. T-CELL RESPONSE

T cells recognize antigen on the surface of APCs in the context of self-MHC molecules. The T-cell receptor confers the specificity of this response. Each T cell has a unique T-cell receptor that interacts with the antigenic peptide bound to an MHC molecule. CD8 or CD4 molecules on the surface of the T cell served as coreceptors. CD8 interacts with class I MHC molecules and CD4 interacts with class II MHC independently of peptide binding; thus CD8$^+$ T cells recognize peptides presented by class I MHC and CD4$^+$ T cells recognize peptides presented by class II MHC. When a T cell encounters its cognate peptide/MHC complex, the T-cell receptor binds, leading to signals through the T-cell receptor that activate the T cell.

A naive T cell, one that has never encountered its cognate peptide/MHC complex, needs costimulation in order to be fully activated. If it does not receive costimulatory signals, it can be rendered tolerant to subsequent exposures to antigen (a form of peripheral tolerance). Molecules such as B7-1/B7-2 and ICAM-1 on the surface of professional APCs typically provide costimulation. Costimulation may also be provided by cytokines secreted by the APC or by other cells nearby (see Fig. 1). Once a T cell has experienced antigen in the setting of sufficient costimulation, it may proliferate. Thus a clone of T cells with identical T-cell receptors is generated. They may become effector or helper T cells, and if the signal is sufficient a small subset may become memory T cells. Effector and helper T cells respond to antigen without the need for further costimulation, but are themselves destroyed in the ensuing immune response in a process called activation-induced cell death. Memory T cells can also respond to antigen without the need for costimulation, but these remain quiescent during the initial immune response and are only activated upon repeat exposure to antigen.

CD4$^+$ and CD8$^+$ T cells classically have different effector responses. CD4$^+$, or helper, T cells secrete soluble cytokines that act locally and at a distance to enhance the function of other immune cells, such as B cells, CD8$^+$ T cells, or macrophages. Activated

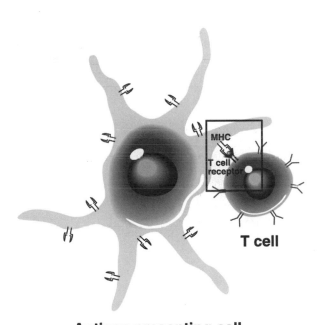

Antigen presenting cell

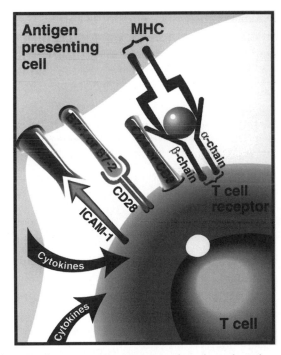

FIGURE 1 Activation of a naive T cell by an antigen-presenting cell (APC). A T cell recognizes antigen presented on the surface of an APC. The T-cell receptor binds to a peptide fragment, known as an epitope, complexed to an antigen-presenting MHC molecule. The coreceptors for MHC, CD4, and CD8 on the surface of the T-cell facilitate this interaction. CD4$^+$ T cells recognize epitopes complexed with class II MHC molecules, and CD8$^+$ T cells recognize epitopes complexed with class I MHC molecules. Each T cell has T-cell receptors of one specificity that bind a particular peptide epitope and MHC complex. In order to activate a naive T cell (one that has never before experienced antigen), the antigen/MHC complex must be present within the context of sufficient costimulation. Costimulation can be provided by B7-1 or B7-2 on the APC binding to CD28 on the T cell, and by LFA-1 on the APC binding to ICAM-1 on the T cell. Costimulation can also be provided by cytokines in the local environment. Mature dendritic cells are professional APCs and thus are able to provide sufficient costimulation.

CD4$^+$ T cells can be categorized by the profile of cytokines they secrete and the types of cells they stimulate when activated. Th$_1$ helper T cells enhance the function of macrophages and CD8$^+$ T cells through the cytokines they produce, most classically IFN-γ but also TNF-β. Thus Th$_1$ cells are central players in cell-mediated immunity. In contrast, Th$_2$ cells produce a humoral immune response through a set of cytokines, IL-4, IL-5, and IL-10, that enhance B cells and may inhibit T-cell-mediated immune responses.

CD8$^+$ T cells are typically cytotoxic T lymphocytes because their classic effector function is to lyse cells. However, it should be noted that secretion of cytokines, mainly IFN-γ, by CD8$^+$ T cells is also a function of activation. CD8$^+$ T cells lyse their targets through two main mechanisms: one involves the release of cytotoxic proteins known as perforin and granzymes from specialized vesicles, and the second involves induction of programmed cell death through the stimulation of fas on the target cell. Effector CD8+ T cells are armed with lytic granules, and upon activation they can release the contents of these granules. One of these is the protein perforin, which can destroy the integrity of the cell membrane through the formation of pores. These pores allow entry of proteolytic enzymes, including granzymes, which are also released from the lytic granules. Another way cytotoxic T cells arm themselves is through the expression of fas ligand on their cell surface. The interaction of fas ligand on the CD8$^+$ T cell with fas on the target cell induces apoptosis of the target. Some cancer cells expressed fas, although the degree of actual expression of fas *in vivo* by cancers remains controversial.

V. TUMOR ANTIGENS

T cells can recognize antigens presented by cancer cells, although cancer cells are not typically professional APCs and do not easily elicit T-cell immunity. The greatest advance in cancer immunology has come from the molecular identification of antigens recognized by the immune system. Several competing classification schemes have been proposed to categorize tumor antigens. No one scheme has been widely accepted. The classification used here encompasses most of the tumor antigens identified and is based on the presence or expression of antigens recognized on tumors in normal host tissue (see Table I).

TABLE I
Tumor Antigens

Class	Type	Example
Alterations or atypical gene products	New epitope by mutation	p16/INK4A
		β-Catenin
	Altered trafficking by stability	CDC27
	Psuedogene	HPX42B
	Antisense DNA	RU2
	Translocation	GDP-L-fucose:β-D-galactoside-2-α-L-fucosyltransferase
Cancer-testis antigens		MAGE family
		BAGE family
		GAGE family
		NY-ESO-1
Differentiation antigens	Melanosomal differentiation antigens	Tyrosinase
		TRP-1/gp75
		TRP2
		gp100
		MelanA/MART-1
Signal transduction molecules		HER2/neu
		EphA3
Viral antigens		Epstein–Barr virus
		Human T-cell leukemia virus

A. Alterations or Atypical Gene Products

Cancer results from the accumulation of genetic mutations, so it may seem obvious that at least some of these mutations could be recognized by the immune system. However, the manner in which the immune system detects genetic change would not be easy to predict.

In some cases, a mutation can create a new epitope or increase the immunogenicity of an existing epitope. In the case of genes encoding p16/INK4A, p53, and β-catenin, the immune system can recognize the products of point mutations that are implicated in the pathogenesis of malignancy. In these cases, T cells potentially strike at the heart of genetic lesions that drive the cancer. In addition to recognizing point mutations, T cells have also been shown to recognize new epitopes created by genetic translocations joining two distinct genes in a fusion protein.

In addition to creating a new epitope, a mutation can alter trafficking and stability by its gene product, thus allowing for MHC presentation of an unaltered epitope that is not seen in normal cells. Cancer cells can also present antigens from alternative transcripts, including those from cryptic start sites and alternative reading frames, and even from parts of the genome that are normally invisible, such as pseudogenes and antisense products from the minus strand of DNA.

B. Cancer Testis Antigens

Another class of tumor antigens are not unique to cancer but are only shared with germline cells, which do not express classical MHC molecules and thus do not present these antigens to the immune system. These antigens are operationally tumor specific. Expression of these normally silent antigens is sometimes introduced in cancer cells, perhaps due to changes in the transcriptional regulation such as methylation of DNA.

The prototype of this family is the MAGE-1 protein, which was the first human gene product recognized by CD8$^+$ T cells from cancer patients. The list of cancer-testes antigens includes the MAGE family and related GAGE and BAGE families, along with the NY-ESO-1 antigen.

C. Differentiation Antigens

Antigens shared by cancer cells and their normal cell counterparts are known as differentiation antigens. Prototypical differentiation antigens are the melanosomal differentiation antigens shared by melanoma and normal melanocytes. In fact, antigens characteristic of melanocytic differentiation were determined, in part, from the recognition of melanoma cells by autologous serum. Most melanosomal differentiation antigens are proteins involved in the synthesis of melanin, such as tyrosinase, TRP-1/gp75, TRP2, and gp100/pmel17. MelanA/MART-1 is another melanoma differentiation antigen of unknown function. Immunity against melanosomal differentiation antigens is, in fact, autoimmunity and destruction of melanocytes as well as tumor cells can ensue. It is thought that immunity against differentiation antigens can develop because these antigens are not expressed in the thymus, so reactive T cells are not deleted and peripheral tolerance is incomplete. In melanoma, which is the best studied cancer type in humans in the field of cancer immunology, differentiation antigens are the most frequent antigens recognized by T cells.

D. Signal Transduction Molecules

Another group of antigens includes the signal transduction molecules, which do not fit in any of the categories just described. These molecules are present in normal tissue but can be overexpressed by cancers. In cancer patients, T cells reactive to HER2/neu, a receptor tyrosine kinase that is overexpressed in several types of cancer, including breast, ovarian, and lung, have been identified. Another tyrosine kinase, EphA3, is recognized by autologous T cells in a human patient.

E. Viral Antigens

Viruses are implicated in the pathogenesis of some types of cancers, including hepatoma (hepatitis virus), lymphomas and nasopharyngeal cancer (Epstein–Barr virus), and leukemias (HTLV). Viral-infected cells can express strong antigens that are recognized by T cells.

VI. IMMUNE SURVEILLANCE AND IMMUNE EVASION

Lewis Thomas originally proposed the concept that the immune system protects the organism against the development of malignancies, known as immune surveillance. This idea fell out of favor in the 1970s, but has reemerged. Experiments with animals having specific deficiencies in their immune systems have shown a higher rate of tumor formation. If it is true that the immune system identifies many tumors at an early stage before they become clinically apparent, then it follows that tumors escaping surveillance can develop mechanisms to evade the immune system. Mechanisms by which the tumors can escape immune attack include loss of MHC molecules, loss of immunogenic antigens, and loss of antigen-processing machinery. It appears that the most common of these mechanisms is the loss of MHC molecules. In fact, many tumors have been shown to have lost expression of some or all of their MHC I genes.

VII. INDUCTION OF CELL-MEDIATED IMMUNITY TO CANCER

The roots of cancer immunology are in the therapy of cancer. Treatment of "tumors" by injection of infected purulent materials is documented in both Eastern and Western ancient medical writings and dates back at least several millennia. It can be argued that the birth of modern tumor immunology began with the treatment of cancer with bacterial extracts by William B. Coley around the end of the 19th century. With a better understanding of the molecular basis of immunity, the field of immunotherapy is rapidly growing. Approaches to the induction of cell-mediated immunity against cancer can be grouped into three broad categories: (1) immune modulation, (2) passive/adoptive immunotherapy, and (3) active immunotherapy/vaccination (see Table II). Most efforts using these strategies are in clinical trials, so our discussion is brief.

A. Immune Modulation

The strategy of immune modulation involves attempting to activate the immune system against the cancer through the administration of immunostimulatory substances. In particular, approaches involve systemic treatment with the cytokines IL-2, IL-12, IFN-α, and IFN-β. IL-2 is a primary growth factor for T cells and thus can potentially expand existing T cells that recognize the tumor. IL-12 is a cytokine known to bias the immune system toward a Th_1, or cell-mediated, immune response. Recombinant human IL-2 is routinely used in the treatment of melanoma and renal carcinoma. Experimental evidence suggests that cell-mediated immune responses

---

TABLE II
Strategies for Immunotherapy of Cancer Using Cell-Mediated Immunity

Strategy	Type	Example
Immune modulation	Cytokines	IL-2
		IL-12
		IFN-α
		IFN-β
Passive/adoptive immunotherapy		Transfer of T cells
		Transfer of NK/LAK cells
Active immunotherapy/vaccination	Whole tumor cell/tumor cell preparation vaccines	Tumor cells transduced with cytokine
		Dendritic cells pulsed with tumor preparations
		Dendritic cells pulsed with RNA from tumors
		Heat shock protein preparations
	Antigen-specific vaccines	Recombinant protein
		Synthetic peptide
		Naked plasmid DNA
		Recombinant viruses

are more potent than humoral immune responses against cancer and that IL-12 can induce tumor regression. However, IL-12 is still being tested in early clinical trials. The interferons IFN-α and IFN-β bind to the same receptor and have similar effects that can enhance cell-mediated immunity. IFN-α and IFN-β both increase expression of the antigen-processing and -presenting machinery, as well as activating NK cells. The interferons are widely used for cancer therapy, including treatment of melanoma, renal cancer, and leukemias.

B. Passive/Adoptive Immunotherapy

Adoptive immunotherapy involves the *ex vivo* activation and expansion of T cells or NK cells and passive transfer of these cells into the cancer patient. This is an experimental approach with some risks and needs to be explored more intensively. Cells for adoptive therapy can be obtained either from the patient or from a separate individual. In the case of adoptive transfer between different individuals, the goal here is for T cells from the donor to attack the recipient's cancer in a process called graft versus tumor. The MHC haplotype of the transferred T cells, of course, must match the patient to be treated.

Adoptive transfer of T cells against viral antigens expressed by the Epstein–Barr virus has been successfully used to treat lymphomas induced by the Epstein–Barr virus following bone marrow transplantation. Other experimental approaches use T cells expanded from tumor lesions (called tumor-infiltrating lymphocytes by some) and T cells expanded by exposure to specific tumor peptides plus APCs. In addition to T cells, NK cells may be used for adoptive therapy. The entity originally called lymphocyte-activated killer (LAK) cells used in some of the earliest adoptive therapy trials has been shown to consist mostly of activated NK cells.

C. Active Immunotherapy/Vaccination

Investigation into active immunotherapy or vaccination of cancer patients is the most active area of cancer immunotherapy. It should be noted that in tumor immunology, the word "vaccination" is used to mean the deliberate induction of specific immunity to treat

a cancer and does not typically indicate that the vaccine is given prophylactically to prevent disease, as is the case in infectious disease. Similar to vaccines against infectious diseases, vaccines against cancer have been developed both where the vaccine does not target any specific antigens and where the vaccine is based on a specific antigen (whole tumor cell/tumor cell preparation vaccines versus antigen-specific vaccines).

1. Whole Tumor Cell/Tumor Cell Preparation Vaccines

The first cancer vaccines were based on cancer cells given with adjuvant. Newer approaches using whole cell vaccines involve tumor cells transfected to express cytokines, costimulatory molecules, or allogeneic molecules. In particular, GM-CSF, which is a central growth factor for professional antigen-presenting cells, is receiving attention. Another strategy involves extracting heat shock proteins from autologous tumor cells and administering that preparation as a vaccine. Heat shock proteins have bound peptides from the tumor cell and, when extracted, can chaperone these antigens into the class I MHC pathway of an APC. Dendritic cells have also been used as an adjuvant with tumor cell preparations. Dendritic cells taken from the host can be pulsed with autologous tumor cell lysate or apoptotic bodies from autologous tumor cells and administered back to the patient.

2. Antigen-Specific Vaccines

The last two decades have been characterized by a search for cancer antigens that can be recognized by the immune system. Vaccines based on these defined tumor antigens are being studied in clinical trials. In some approaches, the whole antigen has been delivered to the patient as a recombinant protein, as DNA (either naked DNA are expressed by recombinant virus), or loaded onto dendritic cells and then administered as a vaccine. Naked DNA and recombinant viruses are particularly attractive strategies because of the ease of making and administering the vaccine. Xenogeneic vaccination, which is immunization with the homologous antigen from another species, has in some cases proven more potent in inducing an immune response than vaccination with syngeneic antigen.

Increased understanding of MHC molecules is allowing better determination of potentially immunogenic epitopes of many tumor antigens. Epitopes for class I MHC molecules are being identified at an increasing rate, and class II MHC epitopes have begun to be discovered. Vaccination with these minimal peptide epitopes with or without adjuvant has followed. These peptides can also be loaded on dendritic cells and administered as a vaccine. Epitopes for some tumor antigens, particularly differentiation antigens, are poorly immunogenic. It is thought that T cells against self-antigens have low or intermediate affinity for these antigens because more potent T cells were deleted during thymic T-cell development. Modifying these epitopes at the amino acid level to make them stronger binders to MHC or to the T-cell receptor has increased the efficacy of peptide-based vaccines in experimental models. These enhanced peptides are called heteroclitic vaccines. Although motifs for epitopes have thus far only been identified for some of the more common human MHC alleles, efforts to identify epitopes for other alleles are ongoing.

VIII. CONCLUSION

The immune system is capable of recognizing and rejecting tumors. Both humoral and cell-mediated immune responses are potentially important for tumor immunity. The cell-mediated immune response is particularly effective in experimental models. Nevertheless, the fact that some tumors grow progressively despite evidence of immune recognition demonstrates the difficulty of controlling large or metastatic tumors with the immune system. Immunotherapy strategies have encountered these obstacles, but ongoing research is aimed at better understanding the principles and more effective manipulation of the cell-mediated immune response against cancer.

See Also the Following Articles

ANTIBODIES IN THE GENE THERAPY OF CANCER • DIFFERENTIATION AND THE ROLE OF DIFFERENTIATION-INDUCERS IN CANCER TREATMENT • IMMUNE DEFICIENCY: OPPORTUNISTIC TUMORS • MOLECULAR BASIS OF TUMOR IMMUNITY • T CELLS AGAINST TUMORS • T CELLS, FUNCTION OF • TUMOR ANTIGENS

Bibliography

Banchereau, J., and Steinman, R. M. (1998). Dendritic cells and the control of immunity. *Nature* **392**(6673), 245.

Boon, T., Coulie, P. G., and Van den Eynde, B. (1997). Tumor antigens recognized by T cells. *Immunol. Today* **18**(6), 267.

Bremers, A. J., and Parmiani, G. (2000). Immunology and immunotherapy of human cancer: Present concepts and clinical developments. *Crit. Rev. Oncol. Hematol.* **34**(1), 1.

Delon, J., and Germain, R. N. (2000). Information transfer at the immunological synapse. *Curr. Biol.* **10**(24), R923.

Houghton, A. N. (1994). Cancer antigens: Immune recognition of self and altered self. *J. Exp. Med.* **180,** 1.

Houghton, A. N., Gold, J. S., and Blachere, N. E. (2001). Immunity against cancer: Lessons learned from melanoma. *Curr. Opin. Immunol.* **13,** 134.

Marincola, F. M., Jaffee, E. M., Hicklin, D. J., and Ferrone, S. (2000). Escape of human solid tumors from T-cell recognition: Molecular mechanisms and functional significance. *Adv. Immunol.* **74,** 181.

Pardoll, D. M. (1998). Cancer vaccines. *Nature Med.* **4**(5 Suppl.), 525.

Rosenberg, S. A. (1999). A new era for cancer immunotherapy based on the genes that encode cancer antigens. *Immunity* **10**(3), 281.

Cellular Responses to DNA Damage

Jean Y. J. Wang
Se Won Ki

University of California, San Diego

GLOSSARY

apoptosis Programmed cell death.

ataxia telangiectasia mutated (ATM) This gene is recessively mutated in the human disease ataxia telangiectasia (AT). Cells derived from AT patients exhibit the characteristics of radiation sensitivity and cell cycle checkpoint defects, in particular, following the exposure to ionizing radiation. ATM encodes a protein kinase.

ATM- and Rad3-related gene (ATR) Also encodes a protein kinase.

Bcl-2 homology domain Conserved regions of Bcl-2 family proteins, which can either inhibit or promote apoptosis.

cell division cycle 25 of fisson yeast, *Schizosaccharoyces pombe* (Cdc25) Cdc25 encodes a dual speci-ficity protein, which dephosphorylates Cdc2. Cdc25 is conserved through evolution; mammalian cells have three Cdc25: Cdc25A, B, and C.

cyclin dependent protein kinase (Cdk) In mammalian cells, Cdk2-cyclin A or -cyclin E promotes S phase entry and progression. Cdc2 (also known as Cdk1)–cyclin B promotes M phase entry.

checking DNA synthesis 1 (Cds1) Cloned in fission yeast, *S. pombe*, as a multicopy suppressor of temperature-sensitive DNA polymerase-α mutant. A mammalian homologue of Cds1 has been cloned and is referred to as hCds1 (human Cds1) or Chk2. The hCds1 encodes a protein kinase that is activated by ATM and ATR.

checkpoint Mechanisms that monitor cell cycle events and can stop cell cycle progression until conditions are favorable.

checkpoint kinase 1 (Chk1) Identified in fission yeast, *S. pombe*, as a kinase required for the DNA damage checkpoint. A mammalian homologue of Chk1 has been cloned and is referred to as hChk1. The hChk1 encodes a protein kinase that is activated by ATM and ATR.

direct IAP-binding protein with low pI/second mitochondria-derived activator of caspases (Diablo/Smac) A mammalian protein that promotes apoptosis by binding to and antagonizing inhibitor of apoptosis proteins (IAPs), which inhibit caspases.

DNA damage Alterations in the physical and the chemical structure of DNA resulting from endogenous cellular process or exposure to exogenous agents.

DNA repair Mechanisms that recognize and remove DNA lesions from the genome. These mechanisms include enzymes that directly undo the lesions (e.g., photolyase for the cleavage of cyclobutane ring), excision repairs (nucleotide excision repair, base excision repair and mismatch repair), recombination repair (homologous recombination and nonhomologous end joining), postreplication repair, and SOS repair.

p21^{cip1} A heat-stable inhibitor of Cdk.

retinoblastoma tumor suppressor protein RB is a repressor of transcription. RB inhibits cell proliferation and apoptosis.

14-3-3 Adaptor protein conserved through evolution with a higher affinity for phosphoserine-containing proteins. In yeast and mammalian cell, 14-3-3 is involved in DNA damage response.

Cellular DNA can be damaged by physiological and environmental agents, which cause a variety of lesions, including base modifications, crosslinkings, and strand breaks. If not repaired, these DNA lesions can interfere with transcription, DNA replication, and chromosome segregation to cause mutations or cell death. To protect the genome, a number of DNA repair mechanisms have evolved and are highly conserved through evolution. DNA repair is continuously required in living cells to prevent the accumulation of mutations. DNA repair is further activated when cells are exposed to environmental agents that induce lesions in DNA. Under conditions of genotoxic stress, which causes the formation of nonphysiological DNA lesions, the activation of DNA repair is coupled with an inhibition of cell proliferation. The mechanism that coordinates DNA repair with cell proliferation is commonly known as cell cycle checkpoints. The inhibition of cell cycle progression is critical to prevent the replication or the segregation of damaged DNA. Therefore, DNA repair and the inhibition of cell cycle progression are two important cellular responses to DNA damage.

Insights into how cells respond to DNA damage have come from the characterization of the yeast RAD genes, isolated from yeast mutants that were hypersensitive to UV or X ray. The majority of the RAD genes encode proteins and enzymes that are involved in DNA repair. Some of the RAD gene products function in the DNA damage checkpoints to coordinate cell cycle inhibition with DNA repair. Irradiation of yeast mutants with defects in the RAD genes causes a passive cell death, resulting from genome damage that is incompatible with life.

The mammalian homologues of many of the yeast RAD genes have been identified, supporting conservation of the DNA repair and cell cycle checkpoint mechanisms. Interestingly, however, DNA damage can activate in mammalian cells additional cellular responses that are not found in yeast. For example, human fibroblasts can undergo a terminal growth arrest that resembles senescence following ionizing radiation. Moreover, mammalian cells can undergo apoptosis in response to DNA damage. Apoptosis is an active form of cell death that is programmed in the genome of multicellular organisms. Terminal growth arrest and apoptosis are irreversible cell fates that cannot be adopted by unicellular organisms. Therefore, the mechanisms that are common to unicellular and multicellular life, i.e., DNA repair and cell cycle checkpoints, are those that help promote the survival of damaged cells. In contrast, terminal growth arrest and apoptosis are mechanisms that suppress damaged cells and help protect a multicellular organism against cells with DNA damage.

The cellular responses to DNA damage are important to the study of cancer for two reasons. First, defects in DNA damage responses can contribute to the development and progression of cancer. This is because defects in DNA damage responses can lead to the accumulation of mutations as well as the accumulation of mutated cells. Second, defects in DNA damage responses can contribute to the development of drug resistance in cancer. This is because a majority of the cancer therapeutics cause lesions in DNA and exert their antiproliferative effects through the induction of growth arrest or apoptosis.

It has been well established that defects in the conserved mechanisms of DNA repair and cell cycle checkpoints can promote the development of cancer. For example, mismatch repair defects are associated with the hereditary human nonpolyposis colon carcinoma. Mutation of the conserved cell cycle checkpoint gene (Cds1) is associated with a fraction of the hereditary Li–Fraumeni syndrome. However, because DNA repair and cell cycle checkpoints promote cell survival, cancer cells must maintain some checkpoint activity and a reasonable repair capacity to sustain proliferation. In contrast, terminal growth arrest and apoptosis are safeguard mechanisms used to suppress damaged cells. Thus, these mechanisms are preferentially inactivated during cancer development.

Given the importance of the DNA damage response to the development, progression, and treatment of cancer, understanding how cells respond to DNA damage has been an active area of cancer research. This article provides an overview on the cellular responses to DNA damage, particularly, cell cycle checkpoints, terminal growth arrest, and apoptosis.

I. CELL CYCLE CHECKPOINTS

The inhibition of cell cycle progression has the important role of allowing time for DNA repair when a proliferating cell suffers from nonphysiological levels of DNA damage. Mechanistically, cell cycle checkpoints are signaling pathways composed of protein kinases. Because protein phosphorylation is rapid and reversible, checkpoint kinases provide a swift response that can be easily reversed to allow the resumption of cell proliferation. The checkpoint kinases are conserved through evolution. Among them, the protein kinase encoded by the fission yeast Rad3, the budding yeast MEC1, and the mammalian ATR and ATM genes appear to play a central role in the overall coordination of the DNA damage responses.

A. The Conserved G2 Checkpoint Pathway

A proliferating cell can become arrested in the G2 phase of the cell cycle in response to DNA damage. The arrest in G2 is mediated by the inhibition of M-phase promoting factor (MPF). The DNA damage-activated signaling pathway that inhibits the entry into mitosis is commonly known as the G2 checkpoint (Fig. 1). In mammalian cells, MPF is the cyclin B/Cdc2 kinase complex. During S and G2 phases, the

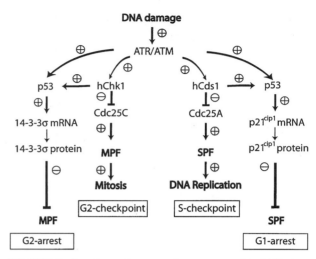

FIGURE 1 Signal transduction pathways activated by DNA damage. Checkpoint kinases (ATR, ATM, hChk1, and hCds1) activate G2 and S checkpoints rapidly upon DNA damage. DNA damage also activates p53 through checkpoint kinases to cause G1 and G2 arrests, which require *de novo* gene expression. +, activation; −, inhibition.

cyclin B/Cdc2 complex is formed and kept in the inactive state through the phosphorylation of Cdc2. The activation of MPF depends on the phosphatase encoded by the cdc25C gene in mammalian cells. The Cdc25C phosphatase dephosphorylates Cdc2 to activate MPF. In the G2 checkpoint pathway, Cdc25C is the target of inhibition by the checkpoint kinases. Inhibition of Cdc25C prevents the activation of MPF, thus causing a damaged cell to arrest in G2.

The G2 checkpoint pathway is elucidated through genetic studies in the fission yeast *S. pombe*. In *S. pombe*, activation of the G2 checkpoint requires the function of Rad3 and Chk1. Rad3 is required for DNA damage to activate Chk1, and Chk1 is required for DNA damage to inhibit Cdc25. The fission yeast G2 checkpoint mechanism is conserved in mammalian cells. The human homologue of Rad3 is ATR, and the human homologue of Chk1 is hChk1. Current evidence supports a pathway in which DNA damage activates the protein kinase activity of hChk1, most likely through ATR and possibly also through ATM (Fig. 1). The activated hChk1 phosphorylates Cdc25C to inhibit its function (Fig. 1). Interestingly, mouse ATR and Chk1 genes are essential for survival. The knockout of either gene causes lethality of mice in early embryogenesis. These observations suggest that this conserved G2 checkpoint pathway may be required during normal cell cycle progression, possibly to block the premature entry into mitosis.

B. The S-Phase Checkpoint Pathway

DNA damage also activates checkpoints to inhibit DNA synthesis. The inhibition of DNA synthesis can be achieved at two levels, either to prevent the entry into S phase or to block the progression of ongoing DNA replication in S-phase cells. In mammalian cells, DNA damage activates p53 to prevent G1 cells from entering S phase. This p53-dependent G1 arrest mechanism is very well understood (Fig. 1). The inhibition of ongoing DNA replication by DNA damage, also referred to as the S-phase checkpoint, is still under investigation.

In mammalian cells, "S-phase checkpoint" is commonly used to describe the rapid and transient inhibition of DNA replication in response to DNA damage. In the yeast literature, S-phase checkpoint (or replication checkpoint) is used to describe a mechanism that causes the inhibition of mitosis when replication is not completed. The mammalian S-phase checkpoint that targets DNA replication is biochemically distinct from the replication checkpoint that targets mitosis. Because the replication checkpoint causes the inhibition of MPF, it has the same target as the G2 checkpoint (Fig. 1). However, the mammalian S-phase checkpoint is a mechanism that inhibits the DNA replication machinery.

The genomic DNA of mammalian cells is replicated as 50,000 to 100,000 replicons, which are sequentially activated through S phase. The origin of each replicon is activated once and only once in each round of DNA replication. Activation of the replication origins requires the activity of cyclin E–cdk2 and cyclin A–cdk2, which are collectively referred to in this article as the S-phase promoting factor (SPF). A signal transduction pathway has been described that can mediate the S-phase checkpoint activated by ionizing radiation. In this pathway, ionizing radiation activates the ATM kinase to phosphorylate and activate the hCds1 kinase (Fig. 1). The hCds1 kinase phosphorylates Cdc25A. The phosphorylated Cdc25A is targeted for degradation by the proteasome. The Cdc25A gene, similar to Cdc25C, encodes a protein phosphatase that dephosphorylates cdk2 to activate

the SPF. Degradation of Cdc25A, therefore, can cause an inhibition of DNA replication. This S-phase checkpoint pathway can explain the phenotype of "radiation-resistant DNA synthesis" (RDS), which is characteristic of ATM-deficient cells. In the absence of ATM, ionizing radiation cannot activate hCds1. Hence, ionizing radiation cannot induce the degradation of Cdc25A and cannot inhibit DNA replication in ATM-deficient cells.

The conserved G2 checkpoint pathway and the recently identified mammalian S-phase checkpoint pathway are quite similar in design. Both pathways are activated by ATR/ATM kinases and both pathways target Cdc25 phosphatases (Fig. 1). Phosphorylation is a rapid and reversible mechanism to modify protein functions. Thus, these checkpoint mechanisms are designed to be deployed swiftly upon DNA damage and to be reversed after DNA repair. These checkpoint pathways are different from the p53-dependent cell cycle arrest, which is slower in onset and can result in terminal growth arrest.

II. p53-DEPENDENT CELL CYCLE ARREST

The p53 protein is a transcription factor that is frequently mutated in human cancer. Checkpoint kinases can phosphorylate and activate p53 to cause cell cycle arrest (Fig. 1). p53-dependent cell cycle arrest requires the *de novo* synthesis of mRNA and protein. While p53 itself can be rapidly activated by checkpoint kinases, the p53-dependent arrest is slower in onset than the cell cycle arrest caused by the inhibition of Cdc25 phosphatases.

A. G1 Arrest

p53-dependent G1 arrest is mediated by the transcription upregulation of p21Cip1. The heat-stable p21Cip1 protein is a stoichiometric inhibitor of the SPF. An increased expression of p21Cip1 can therefore inhibit S-phase entry, contributing to a cell cycle arrest in G1. The p21Cip1-dependent inhibition of SPF can cause the accumulation of unphosphorylated RB. In fact, RB is required for DNA damage to induce G1 arrest because RB-deficient cells cannot be arrested in G1 by DNA damage. RB functions as a transcription corepressor to inhibit the expression of cyclin E and cyclin A, thus leading to the inhibition of DNA synthesis.

Taken together, current evidence suggests that checkpoint kinases can activate p53-dependent G1 arrest through transcription regulation. The p53-dependent upregulation of p21Cip1 causes the activation of RB. The activation of RB causes the downregulation of cyclins E and A. This p53-dependent G1 arrest can be reversed by mechanisms that reduce the levels of p21Cip1 and inactivate RB. However, this G1 arrest can become permanent if the repression of cyclin E and A transcription becomes irreversible.

B. G2 Arrest

p53-dependent G2 arrest is mediated by the transcription upregulation of 14-3-3σ. The 14-3-3σ protein belongs to a family of adaptor proteins that are conserved through evolution. Yeast 14-3-3 proteins play an essential role in the G2 checkpoint response by sequestering the inactive Cdc25 phosphatase in the cytoplasm. The mammalian 14-3-3β protein can bind to and sequester Cdc25C in the cytoplasm. The 14-3-3σ protein binds to and retains the cyclin B–Cdc2 complex (MPF) in the cytoplasm. The cyclin B–cdc2 kinase complex must function in the nucleus to initiate mitosis. Thus, the cytoplasmic retention of cyclin B–Cdc2 can inhibit M-phase entry, contributing to a cell cycle arrest in G2 (Fig. 1). The p53-dependent G2 arrest response is distinct from the hChk1-dependent inhibition of Cdc25C. Again, the transcription upregulation of 14-3-3σ by p53 occurs slower than the phosphorylation of Cdc25C by hChk1 (Fig. 1). Thus, p53-dependent G2 arrest may be a secondary mechanism to maintain the G2 checkpoint.

The induction of p21Cip1 by DNA damage also contributes to the maintenance of G2 arrest. Similar to the arrest in G1, this p21Cip1-mediated G2 arrest again requires RB. The mechanism of RB-dependent G2 arrest is likely due to the repression of gene expression. The promoter of the cdc2 gene contains binding sites for E2F. Therefore, RB can inhibit the expression of cdc2, which will enforce the inhibition of mitosis.

III. p53-DEPENDENT APOPTOSIS

DNA damage can also activate p53 to cause apoptosis. The induction of apoptosis by DNA damage is unique to higher eukaryotes, and the dependence of this response on p53 is conserved through evolution. In *Drosophila*, DNA damage can activate the fly p53 protein to upregulate the expression of Reaper. The fly Reaper gene encodes a small protein that can activate apoptosis. The Reaper gene itself does not appear to be conserved. However, a functional homologue of Reaper has been identified in the mammalian genome, and this gene is known as Diablo/Smac. At present, it is not known if Diablo/Smac is a transcriptional target of p53. Mammalian p53 does upregulate the expression of several proapoptotic Bcl2 homology (BH) domain proteins, such as Bax and Noxa, which can activate apoptosis by causing the release of cytochrome C from the mitochondria.

IV. TERMINAL GROWTH ARREST

DNA damage can cause a terminal growth arrest in some mammalian cells. The phenotype of the arrested cells is similar to that of senescent cells and has been described in the literature as premature senescence. Senescence differs from arrest in that it is irreversible. In a recent study, mouse fibroblasts were found to undergo an irreversible arrest that was induced by a high dose of cisplatin, mitomycin D, or epotoside. This arrest occurred to cells in G1, S, or G2 phase of the cell cycle. Interestingly, this irreversible G1, S, and G2 arrest did not occur in cells derived from RB-deficient mice. Indeed, RB became dephosphorylated in S-phase cells that are exposed to a high dose of cisplatin, mitomycin C, or epotoside. The dephosphorylation of RB caused an inhibition of DNA replication, and this inhibition was not observed in Rb-deficient cells.

Because RB can repress genes that are required for DNA replication, it is perhaps not surprising to find that RB can inhibit S-phase progression if it is dephosphorylated in S-phase cells. The fact that RB can cause an irreversible growth arrest in response to heavy damage suggests that the RB-dependent transcription repression may also contribute to DNA damage-induced terminal growth arrest. Indeed, RB and RB-related p107 and p130 proteins play essential roles in developmentally regulated terminal growth arrest. Current results have demonstrated that RB is necessary to enforce p53/p21Cip1-mediated cell cycle arrest. In addition, RB is required for the irreversible arrest of heavily damaged cells. These observations suggest that the reversibility of DNA damage-induced growth arrest may be dependent on the reversibility of RB-mediated transcription repression.

V. CHOICE BETWEEN GROWTH ARREST AND APOPTOSIS

It is clear that p53 can activate cell cycle arrest or apoptosis in response to DNA damage. Despite the understanding on how p53 activates growth arrest and apoptosis, the rules that govern these two mutually exclusive functions of p53 are not known. The choice between growth arrest and apoptosis appears to be determined by the extent of damage and by the developmental lineage of a cell. For example, neuroblasts readily undergo apoptosis when exposed to a relatively low dose of ionizing radiation that does not cause the death of mature neurons. This differential apoptosis response to DNA damage could be due to two possible reasons. First, neuroblasts may have a lower repair capacity so that they are more sensitive to damage-induced apoptosis. Alternatively, DNA damage-induced apoptosis may be dependent on the differentiation program but not the extent of damage. Taken together, current observations suggest that a multitude of factors may impinge on p53 to determine whether a damage cells will choose to arrest or to die.

There are two possible ways to regulate p53-dependent growth arrest versus apoptosis. The first is to modify p53 itself, i.e., the p53 protein that activates the transcription of p21Cip1 may be modified differently from the p53 that activates the transcription of Bax. This mechanism would predict that the enzymes that modify p53 are in control of the cell fates. Alternatively, the choice between growth arrest and apoptosis may not be determined by p53 alone, but are determined by other factors that can restrict the function of p53. For example, activation of apoptosis inhibitors parallel to the activation of p53 may promote growth arrest. However, p53-independent

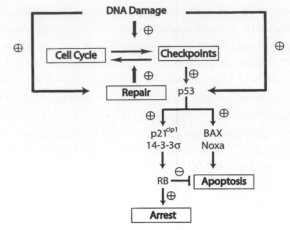

FIGURE 2 Cellular responses to DNA damage. DNA repair and cell cycle checkpoints are activated upon DNA damage in yeast and mammalian cells. Checkpoints can be reversed after DNA is repaired. Additionally, in mammalian cells, p53-dependent growth arrest and apoptosis can be activated upon DNA damage. The RB protein plays a role in p53-mediated growth arrest, which can be irreversible. Moreover, RB also inhibits apoptosis.

apoptosis factors may be activated by DNA damage and these additional factors may corporate with p53 to kill cells.

Supporting the idea that the function of p53 is determined by cofactors is the finding that growth arrest in the DNA damage response is dependent on the retinoblastoma tumor suppressor protein (RB) (Fig. 2). The RB protein, in addition to the inhibition of proliferation, can also inhibit apoptosis (Fig. 2). Dephosphorylation and the maintenance of RB in damaged cells may restrict the p53 function to the induction of growth arrest. Phosphorylation and inactivation of RB, however, may be required for p53 to induce apoptosis.

VI. SUMMARY AND FUTURE PROSPECTS

The cellular responses to DNA damage can be summarized in a simple outline that is depicted in Fig. 2. DNA damage activates DNA repair and cell cycle checkpoints. The checkpoints are reversed after the damage is repaired. These responses are designed to protect the genome and to promote the survival of damaged cells. DNA damage also activates p53, which can cause cell cycle arrest or apoptosis. These p53-

dependent responses are slower in onset due to the requirement for gene expression. p53-dependent cell cycle arrest can help maintain cell cycle checkpoints. p53-dependent arrest can also be prolonged to cause the onset of premature senescence. The retinoblastoma tumor suppressor protein RB is required for DNA damage to induce growth arrest. RB also contributes to the inhibition of apoptosis in DNA-damaged cells.

Several important components of this simple outline are not understood. First, we do not understand the nature of the "DNA damage" signal. This signal can be in the form of a specific lesion in DNA, e.g., a modified base or single-stranded DNA. Alternatively, this signal may be a DNA/protein complex that is formed because of the processing of the primary lesions. Understanding the nature of this signal will provide insights on the overall design of the DNA damage responses. Second, we do not understand how cells recover from the checkpoints. The widely accepted notion that checkpoints are reversed when DNA is properly repaired is based on rationalization rather than experimental data. At present, we cannot rule out the possibility that each checkpoint pathway has an intrinsic half-life that is independent of the status of DNA repair. This might explain the requirement for the p53-mediated and transcription-dependent mechanisms to maintain the cell cycle arrest in G1 and G2. Third, we do not understand how cells choose between p53-dependent growth arrest and apoptosis. The widely accepted notion that these two choices are determined by the extent of DNA damage may be correct, but does not illuminate the molecular basis for the choice. Finally, there has not been a systematic study on the functional status of these DNA damage-regulated events during cancer development, except for p53. Malignant cancer cells must inactivate some of these responses to allow the accumulation of genetic alternation, but the complete elimination of these responses is not likely to be tolerated, as this would compromise cancer cell survival. The study of DNA damage response pathways in cancer might therefore provide clues to the interrelationship among DNA repair, cell proliferation, and apoptosis.

See Also the Following Articles

Bibliography

Brown, E. J., and Baltimore, D. (2000). ATR disruption leads to chromosomal fragmentation and early embryonic lethality. *Genes Dev.* **14,** 397–402.

Diffley, J. F. (1996). Once and only once upon a time: Specifying and regulating origins of DNA replication in eukaryotic cells. *Genes Dev.* **10,** 2819–2830.

Du, C., Fang, M., Li, Y., Li, L., and Wang, X. (2000). Smac, a mitochondrial protein that promotes cytochrome c-dependent caspase activation by eliminating IAP inhibition. *Cell* **102,** 33–42.

Falck, J., Mailand, N., Syljuasen, R. G., Bartek, J., and Lukas, J. (2001). The ATM-Chk2-Cdc25A checkpoint pathway guards against radioresistant DNA synthesis. *Nature* **410,** 842–847.

Flatt, P. M., Tang, L. J., Scatena, C. D., Szak, S. T., and Pietenpol, J. A. (2000). p53 regulation of G(2) checkpoint is retinoblastoma protein dependent. *Mol. Cell Biol.* **20,** 4210–4223.

Friedberg, E. C., and Siede, W. (1995). "DNA Repair and Mutagenesis." ASM Press, Washington, DC.

Harbour, J. W., and Dean, D. C. (2000). Rb function in cell-cycle regulation and apoptosis. *Nature Cell Biol.* **2,** E65–E67.

Harrington, E. A., Bruce, J. L., Harlow, E., and Dyson, N. (1998). pRB plays an essential role in cell cycle arrest induced by DNA damage. *Proc. Natl. Acad. Sci. USA* **95,** 11945–11950.

Knudsen, K. E., Booth, D., Naderi, S., Sever-Chroneos, Z., Fribourg, A. F., Hunton, I. C., Feramisco, J. R., Wang, J. Y., and Knudsen, E. S. (2000). RB-dependent S-phase response to DNA damage. *Mol. Cell Biol.* **20,** 7751–7763.

Liu, Q., Guntuku, S., Cui, X. S., Matsuoka, S., Cortez, D., Tamai, K., Luo, G., Carattini-Rivera, S., DeMayo, F., Bradley, A., Donehower, L. A., and Elledge, S. J. (2000). Chk1 is an essential kinase that is regulated by Atr and required for the G(2)/M DNA damage checkpoint. *Genes Dev.* **14,** 1448–1459.

Norbury, C. J., and Hickson, I. D. (2001). Cellular responses to DNA damage. *Annu. Rev. Pharmacol. Toxicol.* **41,** 367–401.

Verhagen, A. M., Ekert, P. G., Pakusch, M., Silke, J., Connolly, L. M., Reid, G. E., Moritz, R. L., Simpson, R. J., and Vaux, D. L. (2000). Identification of DIABLO, a mammalian protein that promotes apoptosis by binding to and antagonizing IAP proteins. *Cell* **102,** 43–53.

Vousden, K. H. (2000). p53: Death star. *Cell* **103,** 691–694.

Zhou, B. B., and Elledge, S. J. (2000). The DNA damage response: Putting checkpoints in perspective. *Nature* **408,** 433–439.

Chemical Mutagenesis and Carcinogenesis

Joshua W. Hamilton
Dartmouth Medical School

GLOSSARY

carcinogen Any chemical or physical agent that increases cancer burden by increasing the incidence, altering the tissue distribution, increasing the malignant or metastatic potential, or decreasing the latency period of cancers in an individual or a population.

genotoxin Any chemical or physical agent that directly or indirectly causes DNA damage, i.e., a covalent chemical modification to a DNA molecule.

mutagen Any chemical or physical agent that directly or indirectly leads to a heritable alteration in the genetic sequence of bases in DNA.

Experimental carcinogenesis and human epidemiology studies have clearly identified specific chemicals that can act as human carcinogens. Certain chemicals have been associated with increased human cancer incidence in both occupational and environmental exposure settings.

I. INTRODUCTION

It is now widely recognized that exposure to chemicals in the workplace and the environment can contribute to human cancer risk. This was first postulated in 1775 by Dr. Percival Pott, who recognized an association between occupational exposure to chemicals in soot and an increased incidence of scrotal cancer in London chimney sweeps. Other sporadic clinical observations of this type throughout the 19th century also suggested an association between certain occupational exposures to specific chemical agents and increased human cancer. However, it was not until the 20th century that science and medicine actively investigated this aspect of cancer etiology. Boveri first hypothesized that cancer was a genetic disease in 1921, prior to the discovery of the genetic material. In 1915, Yamagawa and co-workers demonstrated that application of coal tar could induce tumors in animals. In the 1930s Kenneway and co-workers demonstrated that pure chemicals isolated from coal tar could also induce animal tumors. Parallel discoveries in the 1950s of the structure of the DNA double helix and its establishment as the hereditary material on the one hand and mutagenic potential of ionizing radiation and certain chemical carcinogens in humans and experimental systems on the other set the stage for extensive investigations into the relationship between chemically induced mutations and human cancer.

Public perceptions, and the regulatory policies resulting from them, have had a strong influence on the direction of chemical carcinogenesis studies and their interpretation. The infamous Delaney Clause of the 1950s led to an intensive focus on the potential carcinogenicity of food additives and other contaminants, and also established the paradigm of the animal tumor model as a test system for predicting carcinogenicity of chemicals in humans. Similarly, the environmental movement of the 1960s and 1970s, which began with the publication of Rachel Carson's *Silent Spring* and the subsequent discovery of Love Canal, led to the establishment of the Federal Environmental Protection Agency and "Superfund," clean air, and clean water legislation. This movement was accompanied by a growing public concern that the widespread use of pesticides and exposure to chemicals from toxic waste sites could cause cancer, and more generally to the belief that chemicals in the environment, particularly man-made chemicals, were responsible for a major fraction, perhaps the majority, of human cancers. The 1980s saw the elucidation of the first oncogenes, genes that appeared to be responsible for the initiation of cancer as first predicted by Boveri. This era also saw the development of the Ames *Salmonella* bacterial mutagenesis assay and hundreds of similar genetic toxicology assays. These developments firmly established the basic paradigm for the field of chemical carcinogenesis; that chemicals that can cause mutations are presumed to be carcinogens. By extension, it was predicted that any chemical or physical agent that could covalently damage DNA could also cause mutations through its DNA-damaging mechanism, and hence could also be a carcinogen. The data that followed over the next decade appeared to strongly support this central tenet, as the

vast majority of chemicals that were initially tested for DNA damage or mutations were also shown experimentally to be animal carcinogens. However, most of the chemicals that were initially tested were either known or suspected carcinogens, were agents of concern, or were closely related structurally to these known and suspected carcinogens.

Over the most recent decade, our understanding of the molecular basis of cancer has substantially improved. In addition, investigations into the molecular basis of chemical carcinogenesis, as well as more extensive human cancer epidemiology studies using modern molecular tools, have greatly expanded our knowledge in this area. This has led to a reevaluation of the overall role of chemicals in human cancer, as well as a modification of the basic paradigms that form the initial foundations of the field. In contrast to earlier predictions, estimates suggest that perhaps only 4–8% of human cancers can be directly attributed to specific chemical exposures. Moreover, these exposures are primarily occupationally related or involve specific environmental contaminants, and it is therefore unlikely that environmental exposures to most chemicals contribute significantly to the overall burden of human cancer. The reasons for this are severalfold. First, while many chemicals have the potential to be genotoxic (DNA damaging), mutagenic, or carcinogenic in various test systems, the levels of most environmental human exposures are usually too low, or are too transient, to have an appreciable impact on cancer relative to other risks. Second, it is also now clear that humans have many protective mechanisms that can act as practical threshold barriers to most minor chemical exposures. These include physiological barriers to chemicals, xenobiotic metabolism and other pharmacokinetic mechanisms of detoxification, a highly efficient DNA repair system, various active apoptotic mechanisms, and various immune and other active surveillance mechanisms. These thresholds are often not present, or are exceeded or bypassed, in many test systems, including rodent bioassays. For example, some agents are only carcinogenic in animals when administered by large bolus intraperitoneal or intramuscular injections that bypass the normal dose, time course, and route of exposure that would otherwise have resulted in detoxification. Chemicals are also usually given to test animals at or near their maximum tolerated dose (MTD), whereas people are usually exposed to these same chemicals at levels that are thousands or even millions of times lower. About half of all chemicals that have been tested in rodents, whether natural or man-made, have been shown to increase tumor formation. However, the list of chemicals that have been tested to date is highly biased.

Third, based on a growing database, it is now also clear that while there are considerable overlaps among groups of chemicals that are genotoxic, mutagenic, or carcinogenic, these properties are not equivalent. For example, not all chemicals that are genotoxic are mutagenic. This is likely to be due to both the ability of the cell to recognize certain kinds of damage with extremely high efficiency at low levels and the observation that not all types of damage are equally mutagenic to the cell during DNA replication. Similarly, there are many chemicals that are mutagenic but not genotoxic. For example, certain metal ions that do not cause DNA damage can interact with and directly alter the fidelity of DNA polymerase, at least *in vitro*, and thereby lead to mutations due to replication errors. Moreover, DNA-intercalating agents such as ethidium bromide, which can transiently stack between the base pairs of the DNA, can also cause mutations in the form of frameshifts (additions or losses of DNA base pairs), without any covalent modification of DNA.

Most importantly, there is a large list of chemicals of concern that are carcinogenic, based on evidence in experimental animals or as demonstrated directly in human epidemiology studies, but that have not been found as overtly genotoxic or mutagenic in experimental test systems. Approximately one-third of chemical mutagens are negative as chemical carcinogens in animals, and vice versa. Examples of carcinogenic agents that are not genotoxic or mutagenic include the so-called solid-state carcinogens (e.g., smooth plastic implants) and the carcinogenic metals, arsenic and cadmium. In fact, in the case of cadmium and arsenic, it has been difficult to demonstrate that they are carcinogenic as single agents in animal models, despite strong epidemiological evidence that they are carcinogenic in humans. Moreover, many chemicals that were initially thought to act by genotoxic and mutagenic mechanisms may, in fact, act primarily through other as yet unclear mechanisms that do not involve DNA damage or mutations per se. For example, although the human lung toxin and carcinogen chromium(VI) is moderately positive for DNA damage and mutations in certain experimental test systems, there is growing evidence that it may act as a human carcinogen primarily through cell signaling and tumor promoter-associated mechanisms rather than or in addition to its genotoxic or mutagenic effects. It is therefore important, in assessing the overall carcinogenic potential of a chemical, to consider whether it is a genotoxin, mutagen, or animal or human carcinogen separately and to also classify the type of mechanism involved. Thus, chemically induced DNA damage, chemical mutagenesis, and chemical carcinogenesis are considered separately.

II. CHEMICALLY INDUCED DNA DAMAGE

A. Types of Chemical Interactions with DNA

Two basic types of chemical interaction with DNA are noncovalent and covalent binding. Examples of the primary types of noncovalent interactions include (a) ionic interactions, such as when Mg^{+2} and other cations interact with the negative phosphate groups on the outside of the DNA helix; (b) minor groove-binding chemicals, such as the dye Hoechst 33258; and (c) intercalating agents, such as ethidium bromide and bleomycin, which are planar aromatic compounds capable of stacking between the parallel base pairs inside the DNA helix. These various noncovalent interactions can each have toxicological consequences. For example, such interactions can affect the structure of the DNA helix or disrupt DNA–protein interactions within chromatin, leading to changes in DNA replication and RNA expression. They can also alter the fidelity of DNA and RNA polymerases, in the former case increasing the probability of mutations. Noncovalent chemical–DNA interactions are not considered damage per se; however, the noncovalent interactions of some chemicals can subsequently lead to the generation of covalent DNA damage. For example, intercalation of bleomycin into DNA and subsequent binding of iron to the drug can lead to the generation of reactive oxygen species that can damage the DNA at sites adjacent to the drug intercalation site. At high levels, this damage will kill the cell, which is the basis for the use of bleomycin as an anticancer drug, but at lower levels this damage can also result in mutations. Covalent interactions occur when the chemical, or a portion of the chemical, is covalently adducted to the DNA helix or when it causes other types of covalent modifications, such as oxidative damage. Chemicals that can directly adduct to DNA are often referred to generically as "DNA-alkylating agents." The various types of DNA damage are discussed in further detail.

B. Types of DNA Damage

1. Spontaneous DNA Damage

In the context of this topic there are two basic classes of DNA damage to consider, i.e., so-called "spontaneous" or background damage and chemically induced damage. Spontaneous DNA damage includes deamination, loss of bases to form abasic sites, and oxidative damage. Deamination, i.e., chemical loss of amino groups on bases, occurs frequently and spontaneously. It has been estimated that approximately 10,000 deamination events occur per cell per day, on average, in humans and other mammals. Deamination usually leads to the formation of unusual bases, e.g., cytosine deamination forms uracil (which is the thymine analog in RNA but not a normal DNA base) and adenine deamination forms hypoxanthine. These deaminated bases are potentially mutagenic. If left unrepaired, some abnormal bases can form an alternative base pair with the wrong partner during replication, leading to a mutation at that site. For example, uracil can base pair with adenine because it is a structural analog of thymine so that deamination of cytosine to uracil can result in a transition from a C–G base pair to a T–A base pair if undetected. However, the common deamination products are detected by specific enzymes called DNA glycosylases, each of which recognizes a specific inappropriate base in DNA (e.g., uracil glycosylase). Some deamination events do not have a mutagenic consequence, e.g., deamination of guanine leads to the formation of xanthine, which, if unrepaired, normally will still be base paired

preferentially with cytosine during replication. From the standpoint of mutations, the most important deamination is of 5-methylcytosine, as this leads to formation of thymine, which is a normal DNA base. If this mismatch is left unresolved, it can lead to a transition mutation to a T–A base pair during replication. In fact, it has been observed that sites of 5-methylcytosine are typically "hot spots" for mutation, with a much higher mutation frequency than other sites. Repair of these mismatches requires a complex repair process that queries each strand to identify the parental and daughter strands of the helix. This allows it to determine whether the site should be methylated to determine which base is incorrect.

Abasic sites occur when a glycosidic bond in DNA weakens and the helix releases the base at that site. This also occurs at a high spontaneous level, with approximately 20,000 purines and 1000 pyrimidines lost per cell per day on average. These abasic sites are also recognized and repaired by the cellular repair machinery. Background oxidative DNA damage and radiation-induced DNA damage are often classified as "spontaneous" damage because they are part of the normal background. A low level of reactive oxygen species (primarily hydroxyl radical and superoxide) is generated chemically or enzymatically in cells on a continuous basis, and some of these reactive byproducts will attack DNA to cause oxidative base damages such as 8-oxodeoxyguanosine. Similarly, background levels of ultraviolet (UV) and ionizing radiation are encountered by virtually all organisms. Low levels of background DNA damage (pyrimidine dimers and 6-4 photoproducts from UV; oxidized bases, and single and double strand breaks from ionizing radiation) can occur from this radiation. However, these lesions are also normally recognized and repaired by the cellular machinery.

It is important to consider spontaneous or background levels of DNA damage in considering chemically induced DNA damage for several reasons. First, it is clear that all the cells in our bodies are continuously challenged by these background levels of DNA damage, which, if left unrepaired, are potentially mutagenic and therefore possibly carcinogenic. Thus, normal individuals will have low background levels of DNA damage and mutations even in the absence of chemical exposure, which must be taken into account when assessing the added impact of chemical exposures that might contribute to these levels. One obvious way that this might occur is that chemicals can directly damage DNA and thereby induce mutations. However, additional mechanisms might include altering important cellular processes, such as DNA damage recognition and repair, replication fidelity, cell cycle checkpoints, apoptotic mechanisms, or overall cell proliferation rates, each of which might strongly influence the mutation rate from these background forms of DNA damage. Alternatively, one must consider very low levels of chemically induced DNA damage in the context of the background damage and repair that is always present. This additional damage may be inconsequential with respect to increasing the overall rate of mutation until a specific threshold of damage is attained such that the probability of mutation is increased to a measurable level. Understanding the relationship between background and chemically induced DNA damage and mutations has important implications for risk assessment, particularly for determining the appropriate model for extrapolating from measurable effects at high-dose human or animal exposures to possible risks from very low-dose exposures.

2. Chemically Induced DNA Damage

Chemically induced DNA damage includes oxidative damage, simple alkylation, bulky monoadducts, and DNA cross-links. Chemically induced oxidative DNA damage can result from the generation of hydrogen peroxide in the cell or from redox reactions generated by chemicals such as menadione, bleomycin, and certain metals inside the cell. Simple alkylation typically occurs when a reactive parent compound has a reactive methyl or ethyl group that can covalently interact a DNA base, leaving the alkyl group behind. Examples of alkylation agents include direct-acting compounds, such as methyl- or ethyl-methanesulfonate, and indirect-acting agents, such as methyl- or ethyl-nitrosourea, which require activation to a reactive intermediate metabolite by the phase I cytochrome P450 system. Simple alkylation normally involves the addition of a methyl or ethyl group to the N^2, N^7, and O^6 of guanine but also occurs at other nucleophilic sites of DNA. The O^6-methylguanine adduct in particular is highly mutagenic if unrepaired. Many organic mutagen–carcinogens form bulky monoadducts with DNA, typically following metabolism of the parent compound to a reactive intermediate by the phase I cytochrome P450 system. Examples of chemical carcinogens that do this are mycotoxin, aflatoxin B1 (AFB1), and the polycyclic aromatic hydrocarbon, benzo[a]pyrene (BaP), each of which has been shown to induce bulky monoadducts that cause specific mutations at the site of adduction.

With the advent of modern molecular biology techniques, it has been possible to determine the precise mutations that result from each type of chemical adduct and to compare this mutational pattern with the mutations found in oncogenes and tumor suppressor genes of tumors produced by that chemical in experimental animals. For example, BaP is metabolized to the reactive intermediate benzo[a]prene-7,8,-diol-9,10-epoxide (BPDE), which forms an adduct at the N^2 of guanine and results in a G–C to T–A mutation. Use of site-specific adducts of BPDE in shuttle vectors has shown that this lesion almost exclusively results in G–C to T–A mutations at the site of the lesion. Cells in culture or tumors from animals treated with BaP or BPDE have certain activated oncogenes, and the mutations that occur in these oncogenes are G–C to T–A mutations. Oncogenes that have been synthesized to contain specific G–C to T–A mutations have been shown to be sufficient to transform cells to tumorigenic cells in culture, indicating that this type of mutation in and of itself can contribute to the carcinogenic process. Thus, these empirical observations, at least in the example of BaP, match the predictions of the basic paradigm linking chemical genotoxicity to mutagenesis and carcinogenesis, i.e., that certain chemicals can cause cancer by attacking and damaging DNA, generating DNA adducts that cause specific mutations in critical cancer genes that, in turn, can contribute to a cancer cell genotype and phenotype.

DNA cross-links are another category of DNA damage induced by chemicals and some forms of radiation. The three basic types are interstrand (covalent linkage of two bases on opposite DNA strands), intrastrand (linkage of bases on the same strand), and DNA–protein cross-links. Different bifunctional agents can induce one, two, or all three types of cross-links, in addition to other types of DNA lesions, with varying efficiencies. For example, the human lung carcinogen chromium(VI) induces both DNA inter-strand and DNA–protein cross-links, in addition to the formation of Cr–DNA monoadducts and the generation of reactive oxygen species that can also damage DNA. Similarly, the cancer chemotherapy agents mitomycin C and cisplatin can each induce a spectrum of monoadducts, DNA interstrand cross-links, and DNA intrastrand cross-links. DNA interstrand cross-links, in particular, are very difficult for the cell to repair because both strands of DNA are involved, and if left unrepaired these lesions can be lethal to the cell. This is believed to be the principal basis for the ability of mitomycin, cisplatin, and similar cross-linking agents to kill cancer cells. However, at lower doses it is not clear whether DNA interstrand cross-links are mutagenic. Similarly, DNA–protein cross-links do not appear to be strongly associated with an increase in mutations. These lesions are generally well recognized and repaired by the cellular machinery. Most chemically induced DNA intrastrand cross-links are also easily recognized and repaired, as they usually cause severe distortions of the DNA helix. UV light can cause thymine dimers and 6-4 photoproducts, two specific forms of interstrand cross-links. Thymine dimers are also recognized and repaired in cells, whereas the 6-4 photoproduct appears to be poorly recognized and is very mutagenic if left unrepaired. Formation of this adduct is probably the primary basis for the increased risk of skin cancer in heavily sun-exposed people and in xeroderma pigmentosum (XP) patients who are deficient in specific repair enzymes (discussed in further detail later). Ionizing radiation and some chemicals can cause single and double strand breaks in the DNA helix. Single strand breaks are usually repaired by the cellular machinery and are a normal intermediate in many DNA replication and maintenance processes. Double strand breaks can be repaired, although poorly and with slow kinetics, as this involves a more complex repair process, and so these are considered lethal to a dividing cell. This is one of the primary cellular lesions induced by therapeutic ionizing radiation that leads to tumor cell cytotoxicity.

Assays for DNA damage are generally of two types: they are either very specific for a particular type of damage or they detect overall levels of DNA damage without information about the type of damage. For example, carcinogen-binding assays with radiolabeled compounds provide information about covalent adduction but not other types of DNA damage (e.g., oxidative damage or strand breaks). Oxidative damage can be assessed by HPLC analysis of altered bases or use of lesion-specific antibodies. DNA alkaline elution is a technique that can be used to measure DNA interstrand and DNA–protein cross-links, as well as frank strand breaks and so-called "alkali labile sites," i.e., regions of weakness in the DNA helix, presumably as a result of damage, that are elaborated in the presence of strongly alkaline conditions. Assays using ^{32}P postlabeling for altered bases can be used to assess a spectrum of adducts from a given agent, but the technique must be customized to each agent and its DNA damage products, and many agents are not amenable to this analysis for technical reasons. Similarly, HPLC and antibody-based detection of adducts can be developed, but these methods are agent specific. Sister chromatid exchanges occur at a low level in all dividing cells but are increased by many different chemical and physical agents that damage DNA. These events can be detected by differential staining or antibody techniques. However, it is not clear whether chemically induced exchanges between identical chromatids represent DNA damage, successful or unsuccessful repair of damage, or whether there are mutations associated with these events (e.g., by unequal exchange of sequences). Light microscopy can be used to measure increases in chromosomal aberrations, and formation of micronuclei and "unscheduled DNA synthesis" (i.e., DNA synthesis not associated with replication, which is presumed to be DNA repair in response to induced DNA damage) in treated cells can also be used to assess the effects of genotoxic agents, but these techniques also do not distinguish individual lesions. It is therefore often useful to use several complementary assays when assessing DNA damage from a particular chemical.

C. Repair of DNA Damage

Eukaryotic DNA repair is a highly efficient and coordinated process that normally protects cells and organisms from chemical or genetic alterations to the genetic material. This is a continuous process in the cell that counteracts the background levels of DNA damage that occur in each cell every day. That DNA repair is critical both for suppressing the cancer process and for maintaining life itself can be illustrated by two related observations. First, as mentioned earlier, it has been estimated that in the absence of any other chemical or physical agent, each cell of the body loses or experiences damage to several thousand DNA bases per day through spontaneous chemical degeneration of the DNA helix, which would be potentially mutagenic or lethal were it not repaired on an ongoing basis. These tens of thousands of potentially mutagenic lesions are occurring in each of the trillions of cells in our body on a daily basis. However, the average life span of U.S. citizens is now expected to extend well into the eighth decade, and cancer is not a significant risk for most of us until the sixth or seventh decade of life. Second, among the hereditary mutations described to date that are known to predispose humans to cancer, the majority involve defects in genes whose proteins mediate specific steps of DNA repair. For example, individual mutations in eight different genes all result in the clinical disease xeroderma pigmentosum. XP patients have a high rate of skin cancer from even low levels of sun exposure, and all of the XP mutations occur in genes involved in DNA excision repair. Studies of the different "complementation groups" of these XP mutations have given us major insights into the specific genes and proteins involved in DNA excision repair in mammals. Mutations in various other DNA repair genes are also associated with an increased risk of cancer and other diseases, including a gene involved in mismatch repair that predisposes to colorectal cancer (hereditary nonpolyposis colon cancer, HNPCC) and genes associated with Bloom's syndrome, Fanconi's anemia, and trichithiodystrophy.

There are four basic types of repair, i.e., direct repair, base excision repair (BER), (poly)nucleotide excision repair (NER), and postreplication repair (recombination and mismatch repair). Sexual reproduction has been described as a fifth form of DNA repair, and the ultimate form of genomic DNA repair, as the pairing of alleles from two different individuals provides an opportunity for the genome of the offspring to contain at least one intact copy of each critical gene. Direct repair involves chemically restoring a damaged base to its original structure, e.g.,

by reversal of a UV light-induced lesion by the photoreactivation enzyme, photolyasem, or removal of a methyl or ethyl group from guanine by O^6-methylguanine methyltransferase. BER involves removal of a damaged base from the DNA helix and subsequent replacement by the repair machinery. Different lesions are recognized by specific enzymes, e.g., uracil glycosylase. Nucleotide excision repair (more properly polynucleotide excision repair) involves recognition of a wide variety of DNA damages, excision of a patch of DNA surrounding the lesion by an enzyme complex, and repair of the gap by the replication machinery. Mismatch repair is a process that is linked to DNA replication, whereby mismatches created by DNA polymerase infidelity are corrected as part of the replication process. HNPCC genes are involved in mismatch repair. Why HNPCC mutations would specifically predispose people to colon cancer rather than a general increase in overall cancer risk is not clear. These examples of genetic predispositions to cancer illustrate how important DNA repair is for suppressing carcinogenesis from background and chemically induced DNA damage.

III. CHEMICALLY INDUCED MUTATIONS

A. Types of Mutations

The three basic classes of genetic mutations are point mutations, clastogenic mutations, and aneuploidy events. Point mutations are arbitrarily defined as changes in the DNA sequence of 10 bp or less. These can include single base pair changes (purine-to-purine and pyrimidine-to-pyrimidine transitions and purine–pyrimidine transversions) and small insertions or deletions of 1–10 bp. Transitions and transversions can result in changes in the coding of an individual amino acid if it occurs in the first or second codon position, but can be silent mutations if in the "wobble" position of many amino acid codons. These mutations can also result in creation of stop codons that result in mRNA and protein truncation. These can also cause changes in other types of genetic information, such as alterations in binding sites for transcription factors and other regulatory proteins within promoter regions, methylation sites within promoter regions, and mRNA splice sites that define the final mRNA structure and sequence. Insertions or deletions that are not divisible by three and that occur within coding regions of base pairs will result in frameshifting, such that the remainder of the coding sequence will have a dramatically altered amino acid information. This often results in the creation of premature termination signals and truncated gene products.

Clastogenic mutations include insertions or deletions of greater than 10 bp, inversion of a sequence of DNA within the same chromosome, duplication of DNA sequence (which can include entire gene segments or gene clusters), and gene amplification. Amplification events can result in homogeneously staining regions (HSRs) that are visible in chromosome karyotypic analysis, or extrachromosomal "minichromosomes" that contain high copy numbers of an amplified gene or genetic cluster. Amplification events are inducible even in normal cells, at least in cell culture, and also reversible, suggesting that they represent a survival strategy for upregulating certain important genes during times of severe stress. Translocation events can occur, where regions of different chromosomes swap locations. This is a common event in cancer and appears to be important in the etiology of certain cancers. The classic example of this is the "Philadelphia chromosome," which is a translocation of the short "p" arms of chromosomes 9 and 22 +(9;22) and a hallmark of chronic myelogenous leukemia. Many translocations in cancer result in the juxtapositioning of an oncogene with a strong promoter region, resulting in substantial upregulation of oncogene expression (e.g., BCL-2/IG). Other translocations result in either truncation of a gene product, which can be an activation event for certain oncogenes (e.g., MYB), or creation of a chimeric gene product (e.g., PML-RARα in acute promyelocytic leukemia or BRC-ABL in chronic myelogenous leukemia).

Aneuploidy involves gain or loss of one or more entire chromosomes. Only two human aneuploidy events are compatible with life if they are germline or occur somatically in the early embryo, namely, trisomy 21 (Down's syndrome) and XO (Turner's syndrome). However, most malignant cancers arising from somatic mutations exhibit extensive genetic rearrangement and aneuploidy events, resulting in what is called "loss of heterozygosity" (LOH) or, more properly, loss of dizygosity as the genes that remain are haploid (single copy). This genetic instability and increasing haploidy is considered to provide a selective advantage to the tumor, but whether these events are primarily causal in development of a fully malignant phenotype, and/or are a result of processes that occur in a more advanced cancer phenotype, is still not fully understood.

B. Chemically Induced Mutations

As described earlier, certain chemicals are genotoxic, i.e., they can directly or indirectly cause covalent DNA damage. Certain forms of damage potentially result in mutations if unrepaired. The biochemical mechanism for this, at least for the handful of chemicals that have been investigated at this level of mechanistic detail, is primarily by causing DNA polymerase to misread a template base (usually containing, or immediately adjacent to a site of covalent DNA damage) and causing polymerase to insert the incorrect base into the daughter strand when forming a base pair. Lesions that are most mutagenic appear to not only cause DNA polymerase to make this mistake, but also form an alternative base pair that is poorly recognized as being incorrect by the DNA replication machinery, thereby eluding postreplication mismatch repair as well. For example, the BPDE lesion bound to the N^2 of guanine can cause the damaged base to rotate about its glycosidic bond, flipping the base over. This results in polymerase adding an adenine at the site to form a base pair with the "Hoogsteen" face of the flipped guanine, ultimately resulting in the G–C to T–A transversion that is characteristic of BPDE mutations. Similarly, the O^6-methylguanine lesion, which is caused by many simple alkylating agents, can continue to base pair with a protonated cytosine, such that the site appears normal to the machinery, but O^6-methylguanine can also be inappropriately base paired with thymine, resulting in a G–C to A–T transition. Moreover, the cellular machinery appears to poorly recognize the alternative thymine-containing base pair as well. Thus, the O^6-methylguanine adduct can persist without detection, and this lesion can cause mutations during replication that are poorly detected. The prevalence of this adduct in background levels of oxidative DNA damage and its high mutagenic potential are probably why evolution has developed a specific repair pathway (O^6-methylguanine methyltransferase) that recognizes and removes this lesion from DNA.

As mentioned previously, chemicals can influence mutations in the absence of inducing overt DNA damage. One class of agents that can do this are chemicals that noncovalently interact with DNA. DNA-intercalating agents such as ethidium bromide, acridine orange, bleomycin, actinomycin, and the various anthracyclines (e.g., daunorubicin, doxorubicin) can insert between the base pairs of DNA, forming stable interactions by virtue of their planar multiring structure and the formation of favorable electronic interactions with the ring systems of the purine and pyrimidine DNA bases. However, this intercalation has the effect of "stretching" the DNA helix along its long axis, and also altering DNA–protein interactions along the face of the helix. Intercalating agents can cause frameshift mutations, especially in sequential runs of the same base, e.g., a run of four or more adenines. Adjacent bases in these runs can share electronic pairing of the opposite bases, such that if DNA polymerase adds or omits a base on the opposite strand, the error can be difficult to detect. Intercalating agents appear to be able to increase the probability of these frameshift events occurring, as one typically sees insertion or deletion of single bases in these contiguous runs. Minor groove-binding drugs can also influence the rate of mutation, although the mechanism for this is not clear. Other agents, especially certain metal ions, can influence the fidelity of DNA polymerase itself, at least in *in vitro* and cell culture systems. Agents that block or suppress specific steps in DNA repair can increase mutations, presumably resulting from background and spontaneous DNA damage events.

Another class of nongenotoxic chemicals that can increase mutagenesis in the presence of other agents are called "comutagens." An example of this is 2,3,7,8-dibenzo-*p*-dioxin (TCDD, dioxin) and similar polyhalogenated hydrocarbons, which are strong inducers of specific isozymes of cytochrome P450. This can lead to increased activation of other agents such as BaP, resulting in much greater mutagenesis following a low-level exposure than would otherwise occur. An-

other example is agents that can influence DNA damage recognition and/or repair of DNA lesions. Arsenic, which is not genotoxic or mutagenic per se, is a strong comutagen when present with other genotoxic agents such as BaP or AFB1. The precise mechanism for this is not clear, but arsenic has been shown to influence the expression of DNA repair genes and to affect the fidelity of DNA replication and repair. Thus, one might predict that arsenic is most carcinogenic in combination with other agents, such as cigarette smoke or UV irradiation, and animal data and human epidemiology studies support this prediction.

As mentioned earlier, although the vast majority of mutations seen in human tumors are large insertions, deletions, rearrangements, and aneuploidy events, the vast majority of tests for genotoxicity and mutagenesis, and therefore the vast majority of our information about chemical carcinogens, have focused on their ability to cause point mutations, especially single base pair transitions and transversions. The development of the *Salmonella* reversion assay by Bruce Ames and colleagues in the early 1980s (the "Ames test") led to an ability to rapidly screen chemicals for their potential to cause simple point mutations in this bacterial system. While this provided a high throughput and rapid and inexpensive screening system, there are two apparent drawbacks of this assay. First, it is a prokaryotic system, which differs in important respects from human cells in its uptake, metabolism, and DNA machinery. Second, it focuses on reversion mutations (i.e., reverting from a mutant to a wild-type sequence) under strong selective pressure for specific phenotypes. Thus, there is a strong bias to only observing certain mutations in this system. Similar assays have also been developed in yeast and other lower eukaryotes, utilizing both reverse and forward (wild-type to mutant) mutation screening, and in mammalian cells with screens for both forward and reverse mutations. Use of mammalian forward mutation systems addresses some concerns about the bacterial and yeast systems, but these systems still have limitations with respect to metabolism of most promutagens. This latter issue has been partially addressed by the development of cell lines that have been transfected with specific P450 isozymes to provide key metabolic activation steps.

Most of these assay systems also use immortalized cell lines, either derived from tumors or transformed to an immortalized phenotype by a viral or other genetic change. These cellular systems, being simple, uniform monolayers, also lack the multicellular, three-dimensional aspects of whole animal tissues, and also lack other pharmacokinetic and pharmacodynamic properties of intact animals. Nonetheless, these various assays have provided a great deal of information about the mutagenic potential of hundreds of chemicals to establish a growing database of information. Recent development of transgenic mice and rats (e.g., the "Big Blue" mice and rats) has allowed the screening of mutations in shuttle vectors following *in vivo* exposure, which largely alleviates the problems of cell culture systems. However, these systems still focus predominantly on single point mutations and selectable markers. *In vivo* systems that can look at other mutational events *in vivo* are limited but include dominant lethal, heritable translocation, and mouse spot test and specific locus assays. However, these systems are time-consuming, expensive, and have low throughput.

The use of diverse genetic toxicology assays over the past two decades has provided a database of several hundred chemicals that are positive for DNA damage and/or point mutations. However, we still have little mechanistic insight into how chemicals might cause or influence the larger mutations that are the hallmark of human clinical tumors, and this remains an important goal. Vogelstein and co-workers have described a genetic model for colon cancer that is likely to be a relevant genetic paradigm for most cancers. According to this model, it requires four to seven distinct genetic changes in separate genes to progress from a normal colonic epithelium to a malignant and metastatic colon cancer. Although there appears to be a favored order to this process, these events do not strictly require a specific order of occurrence, but rather it is an accumulation of these genetic changes that results in cancer. Interestingly, the majority of these genetic events, and some of the key steps in the process, involve the inactivation of tumor suppressor genes rather than the activation of oncogenes. The precise mechanism for this inactivation is not well understood but is clearly critical to elucidate. It will be important in future studies to examine the genetic mechanisms underlying this process, e.g., focusing on how genotoxic and nongenotoxic chemicals can lead to genetic and phenotypic changes in cells that promote the carcinogenic process in addition to or in the absence of point mutations. In particular, a critical need remains for the development of moderate to high throughput molecular *in vivo* assays that can provide information on large mutations and other genetic events important in human cancers.

IV. CHEMICAL CARCINOGENESIS

A. Chemical Carcinogenesis in Animals

Kenneway first demonstrated in the 1930s that a pure chemical could cause cancer in animals. Experimental evidence of tumorigenicity in animals has remained the gold standard for determining whether something is considered a potential human chemical carcinogen, particularly in the absence of strong human epidemiology data. The mouse or rat 2-year tumorigenicity study is currently the primary assay for experimentally assessing chemical carcinogenesis in animals for the purposes of human risk assessment. Generally, chemicals are administered at the maximum tolerated dose (MTD), and one-half the MTD for the lifetime of the animals, typically by gavage or in the diet, and tumor incidence is assessed in comparison to control animals. It is important to note that the background incidence of tumors in the control animals of these studies can be substantial. For example, in the two most widely used strains, B6C3F1 mice and F344 rats, the overall incidence of tumors can be as high as 50–60% and individual tissues can have a tumor incidence of 10–50%. Thus, a chemical must increase the tumor burden above this spontaneous background. Agents are considered positive that increase overall incidence, shift the overall tissue distribution or specific sites of tumors, or decrease the time to tumors.

It is important to note that these long-term rodent tumor assays do not usually provide information about involved mechanisms. However, other short- and long-term experimental animal tumor assays can provide such information. The mouse two-stage skin cancer assay and similar assays developed in mouse lung and rat liver have provided a paradigm for assessing the basic mode of action of different chemicals. In the mouse two-stage skin cancer assay, four basic phases of carcinogenesis have been defined, initiation, early promotion (promotion I), late promotion (promotion II), and progression. Different chemicals can act during one or more of these phases and can be operationally defined by their mode of action in this model. For example, most genotoxic mutagens act as classic "initiating agents" in this assay, as a single application of one of these chemicals will usually result in increased skin tumors in the absence of any other treatment. A classic "tumor promoter," such as the phorbol ester, tetradecanoyl phorbol acetate (TPA), will usually not cause skin tumors by itself, but will substantially increase the tumor incidence of another agent if applied daily for several weeks or months following application of an initiating agent. Tumor promotion can experimentally be divided into an early and late phase in this system, the first of which appears to be reversible (tumor incidence decreases if chemical promotion is terminated) and the second of which is usually irreversible. The final phase of tumor progression is a period of time in which existing tumors progress from a nonmalignant to a fully malignant and metastatic phenotype. "Progressors" are chemicals that enhance this last phase of the process. "Complete carcinogens" are initiating agents that cause a substantial increase in fully malignant tumors in virtually all treatment animals, and therefore appear to be able to push cells through the entire process, without any additional help during the promotion or progression phases. A "cocarcinogen" in this assay is one that is not an initiating agent by itself, but enhances tumorigenesis when applied simultaneously with or prior to an initiating agent. Conversely, an "anticarcinogen" is one that can suppress the potency of another initiating chemical when given in combination. Likewise, other chemicals can be identified in this system that act as "chemopreventive agents" by being able to suppress the promotion and/or progression phases following initiation by another chemical. Much of our experimental evidence for the mechanism of action of chemicals as carcinogens is derived from these multistage tumor models.

Another mechanism of action that has been described for some chemicals that induce tumors in long-term rodent assays appears to involve the induction of cell proliferation. Many agents that are only tumorigenic in animals at their MTD may be directly inducing cell proliferation or causing tissue damage leading to compensatory cell proliferation. In the case of chemicals that only act by this mode of action, it seems unlikely that this will also occur at the lower doses that humans are typically exposed to (often at thousands or millions of times lower than the MTD). Thus, there is some concern about determining the carcinogenic potential of some chemicals only at or near their MTD in these rodent assays. It is well known that cell proliferation is a strongly cocarcinogenic process. For example, in the rat liver, tumor induction by an initiator such as AFB1 can be substantially increased by giving the AFB1 in conjunction with a partial hepatectomy in which a large portion of the liver is surgically removed, leading to rapid proliferation of the liver to its fully restored size over the subsequent 72 h. Similarly, hepatitis B is strongly synergistic with AFB1 as a risk factor in human liver cancer, which is likely due to the continual proliferative response induced by this chronic viral infection. Conversely, it has been shown that mutagenesis from chemical and physical genotoxins can be strongly suppressed in mammalian cell culture by inhibiting cell division, presumably by providing an opportunity for cells to repair DNA damage before DNA replication, whereas the same treatment in cells that are rapidly dividing induces high levels of mutagenesis. Thus proliferation alone can be a strongly cocarcinogenic process, and agents or conditions that involve continual cell proliferation, such as chronic viral infections, other inflammatory responses, or chronic tissue injury, may strongly influence both background and chemically induced carcinogenesis. An additional mechanism of carcinogenesis that can be influenced by chemicals may involve disruption of cell–cell communication, which may be most important during the later phases of carcinogenesis when cells are acquiring a malignant and metastatic phenotype.

Because of the large expense of long-term rodent tumor bioassays, many of the chemicals that have been screened to date were already strongly suspected of being carcinogenic in humans, based on human epidemiology studies or short-term assays such as those described in the preceding sections. The majority of these chemicals are genotoxic mutagen–carcinogens, as this class of agents is of considerable concern. However, more than a third of the chemicals that have been shown to be positive in long-term tumor assays are not overtly genotoxic or mutagenic. These nongenotoxic chemicals likely are acting through other epigenetic mechanisms as described earlier. There is concern about both false-positive and false-negative results in these assays. For example, there are agents that are positive in these long-term rodent assays but do not appear to be carcinogens in humans who are exposed to lower doses and different exposure conditions. Conversely, many chemicals that are known to be human carcinogens based on strong epidemiology evidence have been negative or equivocal in long-term rodent tumor assays (e.g., the carcinogenic metals arsenic and cadmium) or require nonphysiological exposures (e.g., intraperitoneal, intratracheal or implantation) to be positive (e.g., nickel and chromium). Thus, while animal tumorigenicity data are useful in assessing the carcinogenic potential and mechanism of action of many chemicals, there are limitations to these systems both for screening and for human risk assessment that are important to consider when evaluating individual agents.

One of the more controversial uses of animal tumorigenicity data is in quantitative human risk assessment. This involves a mathematical extrapolation from the tumor incidence that is observed at high doses in rodents (often at only one or two doses at or near the MTD) to the potential cancer risk that might occur at the very low doses encountered by humans. This risk extrapolation from high to low doses may be required to extend over a dose range of three to six orders of magnitude. The conservative assumptions used by the U.S. Environmental Protection Agency and most other state and federal regulatory agencies that perform these risk assessments is that the dose–response will be linear over this range. This linear, low-dose extrapolation model was initially based on the so-called "one-hit" hypothesis, i.e., that one molecule of a chemical mutagen–carcinogen can theoretically interact with one critical target (i.e., DNA base) within a cell, thereby causing a change (mutation) that produces a cancer cell that can give rise to a tumor. We have little or no empirical data to support or reject this or other alternative models regarding the shape of the dose–response curve. However, as discussed earlier, it is likely that there are practical

thresholds to the carcinogenic response to chemicals *in vivo*, and our current model of the multihit, multistage nature of the cancer process in humans suggests that the one-hit model is not a valid risk assessment model. Thus, it is likely that these risk assessments substantially overestimate risk at low doses. There has been a move toward the use of mechanistic information, when available, to do risk assessments of specific chemicals. For example, it appears that virtually all of the biological effects of TCDD can be attributed to its interaction with a cellular receptor, the Ah receptor, leading to activation of the receptor as a transcription factor. The K_d of TCDD for the Ah receptor in humans is known, and we would predict, based on basic receptor pharmacology principles, that there would be little or no biological effect of TCDD in humans at doses well below those that would be required to bind half or more of the available receptors. As additional mechanistic information such as this becomes available for individual chemicals, it will be increasingly possible to do meaningful, mechanistically based risk assessments that more accurately predict actual cancer risk to the human population in occupational and environmental exposure settings.

B. Evidence for Chemically Induced Cancers in Humans

There is substantial evidence from human epidemiology studies that chemicals can increase cancer in humans. Cigarette smoking alone is estimated to be responsible for approximately 30% of all cancer deaths, and this is clearly related to the hundreds of toxic chemicals in cigarette smoke, which collectively and individually have been shown to cause cancer in animals. Many of these chemicals are genotoxic mutagens, such as BaP, and others act as classic tumor promoters, comutagens, and cocarcinogens in the assays described earlier. Other major causes of cancer deaths include diet (35%), infection (10%), reproductive and sexual behavior (7%), and alcohol (3%) and, therefore, like tobacco use, are presumed to be largely preventable by identifying and instituting appropriate lifestyle changes. Human exposure to chemicals has been associated with cancer risk in environmental and occupational settings, but these exposures overall are estimated to contribute to only a small fraction of total cancer deaths. Approximately 4% of all cancer deaths have been attributed to occupational exposures, presumably involving exposures to individual chemicals and chemical mixtures in most cases. Similarly, exposure to pollution, industrial products, medicines or medical procedures, and food additives has been estimated to only account for an additional 2–4% of total cancer deaths. This is evident by examining data for death rates from major individual cancers over the past century. If occupational and environmental chemical exposures were responsible for a large and growing number of cancers, one might predict that cancer death rates should have increased from the 1950s onward, when there was a concomitant increase in manufacturing, use, and environmental release of industrial chemicals. However, with the exception of increases in male and female lung cancer from cigarette smoking, and a few other exceptions, most individual cancer death rates have been relevantly constant or have declined over the past century. Thus, the vast majority of cancers appear to be attributable to other causes. In particular, it is unlikely that exposure to trace levels of chemicals in the environment—in air, water, soil, as pesticide residues on food, and similar background exposures—contribute significantly to individual cancer risk, despite a public perception that this is the case.

However, certain chemicals have been linked to human cancer in specific occupational or environmental settings. Hill first described an association between tobacco snuff and nasal polyps in 1761. Pott was the first to describe an occupational exposure of chimney sweeps to soot and their increased incidence of scrotal cancer. In the 1920s, the Germans described a strong association between occupational exposure to chromium dusts and an increase in lung and other respiratory tract cancers. This led to the development of industrial hygiene practices to reduce exposure as well as alterations in the manufacturing processes. Workers who began their employment in the chromium ore industries after the institution of these practices have demonstrated cancer risks similar to the general population. Occupational exposure to several other metals, particularly nickel, arsenic, and cadmium, has also been strongly associated with increased cancer risk, especially respiratory tract cancers. However, with the exception of arsenic (dis-

cussed later), there does not appear to be an increased cancer risk from exposure to the much lower environmental levels of these metals, particularly via non-inhalation routes of exposure.

Epidemiological studies of past occupational exposures have provided the best evidence for a link between individual chemicals and human cancer. Groups of workers in the late 19th and early 20th century who were exposed to 2-naphthylamine during its purification demonstrated a very high incidence of bladder cancer, some up to 100%. Similarly, occupational benzene exposure has been strongly associated with an increased incidence of acute myelogenous leukemia. Occupational exposure to vinyl chloride, an important chemical used in the manufacture of plastics, has been associated with an increased risk of liver angiosarcoma. This increased risk is fairly low even in exposed workers; however, the relative rarity of this particular cancer allowed its increased incidence to be detected. The relationship between increased human cancer risk and occupational exposure to other chemicals has been more controversial. This includes agents such as phenoxy herbicides and their contamination products (including TCDD), formaldehyde, and several organic solvents. The various conflicting studies published to date for some of these agents suggest that if there is an increased risk, it may be relatively low even in occupational settings.

Occupational exposure to asbestos has been clearly associated with an increased risk of lung carcinoma and mesothelioma. There appears to be a strong synergy between asbestos and cigarette smoking for the former neoplasm. In fact, asbestos alone appears to be a weak or nonsignificant risk factor for this cancer in the absence of smoking, whereas asbestos exposure alone is clearly associated with mesothelioma risk and smoking appears to play a smaller or inconsequential role in this disease. This illustrates a common issue in both occupational and environmental exposures, namely, that humans are exposed to many agents simultaneously. Moreover, these agents can act additively, synergistically, or even antagonistically in contributing to overall cancer risk. Wood dust exposure, especially in the furniture manufacturing industries, is associated with an increased risk of lung cancer and other lung diseases and exhibits an interaction with smoking. The mechanistic basis for increased cancer risk from wood dust is not known, but may involve both a physical component (small, respirable fibers) and one or more specific chemical components.

Use of certain drugs in medical therapies has also been associated with an increased risk of cancers. The most well-known example of this is the use of various DNA-damaging agents in cancer chemotherapy. By the nature of their mechanism of action, it is predicted that the majority of these drugs will have carcinogenic potential. The therapeutic goal when using these agents is to saturate the more rapidly dividing target tumor cells with sufficient DNA damage to arrest cell division and induce cell death. However, other normal dividing tissues are also receiving considerable DNA damage during systemic treatment with these agents, and surviving nontarget cells would be expected to have increased mutations that may contribute to carcinogenesis in these tissues, giving rise to so-called "second site" neoplasms. Ironically, because of the latency period of these tumors, this is usually only observed in long-term, disease-free survivors of the initial treatment. For example, in children with cancer, approximately 3–12 percent of survivors will develop second site cancers by 25 years after treatment. In adults, the risk of second site cancers is highly dependent on initial tumor type and mode of treatment. The greatest risk is for survivors of Hodgkin's disease, in which there is a 10–15% risk of second site tumors at 15 years after therapy. Not surprisingly, the risk of second site tumors is highest for those cancer patients receiving both radiation therapy and chemotherapy. A few other drugs in non-cancer therapeutic treatments have also been shown to increase cancer risk. Use of diethylstilbestrol (DES) is a well-known but unusual example of hormonally induced cancer, where the adult female offspring of DES-treated mothers have an increased risk of clear cell vaginal adenocarcinoma. Other hormone therapies have also been associated with increased cancer risk, especially liver cancer risk associated with the use of estrogens in premenopausal women. Phenacatin use has been associated with an increased risk of renal carcinoma, and use of the immunosuppressive drug azothioprine has been associated with an increased risk of lymphoma, skin cancer, and Kaposi's sarcoma.

Environmental exposure to certain chemicals is associated with an increased cancer risk. Exposure of certain populations to AFB1 through contaminated diet is clearly associated with an increased risk of liver cancer, although as mentioned earlier, the risk is synergistically greater with simultaneous infection by hepatitis B virus. AFB1 exposure is endemic in tropical areas of Africa, China, and South and Central America. Regulation of AFB1 levels in the food supply in the United States and the Western world has largely eliminated this risk to those populations. Environmental exposure to arsenic in drinking water in various regions throughout the world is also an important factor in the increased incidence of several cancers, as well as an increased risk of vascular disease and type 2 diabetes. Exposure to arsenic in drinking water occurs primarily as a result of leaching of arsenic from natural geological sources into well water. Arsenic is odorless, tasteless, and colorless and is therefore usually undetectable without chemical analysis. Certain areas of South America, southeast Asia, Europe, Asia, and North America contain appreciable arsenic levels in groundwater. Long-term exposure to arsenic through drinking water has been associated with elevated incidences of skin, lung, bladder, liver, kidney, and other cancers and can approach 10-fold above control levels in some areas.

Chemical carcinogens that are associated with lifestyle include those in tobacco products, Betel nut chewing, and consumption of alcoholic beverages. As mentioned previously, dietary factors have been associated with up to 35% of all cancers. Many of these "dietary factors" may involve specific chemicals in the diet, apart from contaminants such as AFB1 or arsenic. These may include certain components of fats or fatty acids; various specific chemical inducers or inhibitors of cytochrome P450s, such as some of the natural plant chemicals found in dark green vegetables; heterocyclic amines and other food mutagens, especially those produced by cooking; polycyclic aromatic hydrocarbons produced by charring of meat and other foods; and nitrosamines found in certain foods. Conversely, certain plant chemicals may act as chemopreventive agents, such as some of those identified in certain fruits, vegetables, and teas. However, while it may be possible to optimize our diets to achieve the best balance between factors that enhance and suppress carcinogenesis, we may be limited in the extent to which this is possible because virtually all foods appear to contain both types of agents. However, specific chemicals are being identified from the diet that may be useful pharmacologically in pure form as chemopreventive agents.

V. SUMMARY

Experimental carcinogenesis and human epidemiology studies have clearly identified specific chemicals that can act as human carcinogens. Certain chemicals have been associated with increased human cancer incidence in both occupational and environmental exposure settings. Experimental cell and animal systems have been useful in helping identify potential human carcinogens, as well as in determining their basic mechanisms of action. Many of the chemicals that are known carcinogens act by causing covalent DNA damage that can lead to mutations in critical oncogenes and tumor suppressor genes, which in turn can contribute to the carcinogenic process. However, many other chemicals initiate or promote carcinogenesis through non-genotoxic mechanisms that may also be important, including cell proliferation and disruption of cell–cell communication. Moreover, chemicals that are identified in experimental systems as being positive for a particular end point such as DNA damage, mutations, cell transformation, and animal tumor formation, while having the potential to be carcinogenic, may not represent a major cancer risk in humans due to differences between these end points and the actual cancer process or limitations in the assay systems that do not allow direct comparisons with human exposures. In this regard, it is difficult to do meaningful human risk assessment when one must extrapolate from high-dose animal exposures to the more typical low human exposures using theoretical models that are based on unproven hypotheses and assumptions. There is a clear need to understand better the mechanisms of action of nonovertly genotoxic carcinogens. It will be important to determine the mechanistic basis for the induction of large clastogenic mutations and aneuploidy events, which are a hallmark of human cancers, and to develop effective screening assays for assessing the potential of chemicals to induce these types of genetic events.

See Also the Following Articles

ANIMAL MODELS FOR COLON CANCER CHEMOPREVENTION • CARCINOGEN–DNA ADDUCTS • CARCINOGENESIS: ROLE OF ACTIVE OXYGEN SPECIES • CELLULAR RESPONSES TO DNA DAMAGE • HORMONAL CARCINOGENESIS • MOLECULAR EPIDEMIOLOGY AND CANCER RISK • MISMATCH REPAIR: BIOCHEMISTRY AND GENETICS • MULTISTAGE CARCINOGENESIS • TOBACCO CARCINOGENESIS

Bibliography

Ames, B. N., and Gold, L. S. (1998). The prevention of cancer. *Drug Metab. Rev.* **30,** 201–223.

EPA. (1996). "Proposed Guidelines for Carcinogen Risk Assessment." Office of Research and Development, U.S. Environmental Protection Agency, Washington, DC.

Garner, R. C. (1998). The role of DNA adducts in chemical carcinogenesis. *Mutat. Res.* **402,** 67–75.

Hoffmann, G. R. (1996). Genetic toxicology. *In* "Casarett and Doull's Toxicology, the Basic Science of Poisons" (C. D. Klaassen, ed.), 5th Ed., pp. 269–300. McGraw-Hill, New York.

Hussain, S. P., and Harris, C. C. (2000). Molecular epidemiology and carcinogenesis: Endogenous and exogenous carcinogens. *Mutat. Res.* **462,** 311–322.

Kinzler, K. W., and Vogelstein, B. (1996). Lessons from hereditary colorectal cancer. *Cell* **87,** 159–170.

Kirsch-Volders, M., Aardema, M., and Elhajouji, A. (2000). Concepts of threshold in mutagenesis and carcinogenesis. *Mutat. Res.* **464,** 3–11.

Klaunig, J. E., Kamendulis, L. M., and Xu, Y. (2000). Epigenetic mechanisms of chemical carcinogenesis. *Hum. Expt. Toxicol.* **19,** 543–555.

Nickoloff, J. A., and Hoekstra, M. F. (1998). "DNA Damage and Repair," Vol. II. Humana Press, Totowa, NJ.

Pitot, H. C., III, and Dragan, Y. P. (1996). Chemical carcinogenesis. *In* "Casarett and Doull's Toxicology, the Basic Science of Poisons" (C. D. Klaassen, ed.), 5th Ed., pp. 201–268. McGraw-Hill, New York.

Chemoprevention, Pharmacology of

Ethan Dmitrovsky
Michael B. Sporn
Dartmouth Medical School

I. Introduction
II. Pharmacology
III. Clinical Considerations
IV. Conclusions

GLOSSARY

biomarkers and intermediate end points Markers of the carcinogenesis process that highlight cells or tissues at risk for malignant conversion; these may serve as surrogates of response in clinical cancer chemoprevention trials.

cancer chemoprevention Use of dietary, nutritional, or pharmacological interventions to inhibit development of invasive cancer by blocking DNA damage that initiates carcinogenesis or by arresting or reversing the progression of premalignant cells that have already acquired genomic damage.

premalignancy Cells or tissues that are at an intermediate step in the carcinogenesis process and have acquired some, but not all, features of transformation; these cells are diagnosed based on histopathologic features and often exhibit genetic changes.

primary prevention Therapeutic interventions to prevent primary cancers from arising in high-risk individuals.

secondary prevention Therapeutic interventions to prevent second cancers from arising in patients cured of a primary cancer.

Carcinogenesis is a chronic and multistep process that results in malignancy. Malignant cells acquire the ability to invade or metastasize. Metastasis is often the first evidence of malignant disease. During the continuum of carcinogenesis, therapeutic interventions can be used to arrest or reverse this process. This is known as cancer chemoprevention. Effective cancer chemoprevention should suppress or block the clinical manifestation of malignancies by treating lesions before clinical signs or symptoms arise. A strong rationale for cancer chemoprevention as an attractive therapeutic strategy stems from considerable preclinical, clinical, and epidemiological findings. Cancer chemoprevention has been shown to be a valid clinical approach in the use of tamoxifen in a randomized phase III trial that demonstrated how this selective estrogen receptor modulator (SERM) reduced the risk of breast cancer in high-risk women. Other clinical trials have demonstrated favorable activity in the treatment of certain premalignant diseases, as will be discussed. Effective cancer chemoprevention should involve lifestyle, dietary, nutritional, pharmacological, and other interventions. This article focuses on the pharmacological basis for clinical cancer prevention by emphasizing candidate classes of agents that are promising for use in cancer chemoprevention.

I. INTRODUCTION

Cancers arise as a result of carcinogenesis, a chronic and multistep process. This stems from mutagenic damage to growth-regulating genes and their products that alters gene expression and ultimately confers changes that lead to the development of invasive or metastatic malignant disease. This process leads to progressive changes of cells that result in premalignancy and eventually overt malignancy. The steps defined in this process include (1) initiation, where DNA damage occurs; (2) promotion, where genetic or epigenetic alterations confer additional genomic damage; and (3) progression to invasive or metastatic disease. Conceivably, each of these steps would be attractive pharmacological targets for cancer chemoprevention.

It has been recognized that carcinogenic exposure leads to fields of altered cells that exist before malignancies are clinically evident. This concept was first proposed by Slaughter in 1953 and provided a basis for understanding how carcinogen-exposed cells that result from failure to repair genomic damage are of clonal origin. Some of these genetically altered cells may progress to a malignant phenotype. It is possible that markers of these carcinogenic changes at affected tissues will determine clones of genetically altered cells that are at especially high risk for malignant conversion. It is not known what precise cassette of carcinogenic or genetic changes are required for the maintenance or progression of premalignant lesions.

Distinct changes may be required for each affected tissue or carcinogenic agent. These alterations likely involve dominant genetic changes through the activation of oncogenes and recessive genetic events through the inactivation of tumor suppressor genes. The underlying genetic properties of a cell may promote susceptibility for malignant transformation such as in inherited cancer-prone syndromes. Tumor–matrix interactions and neoangiogenesis also have important roles in the maintenance or progression of premalignant cells. Because carcinogenesis is of a chronic nature, pharmacological interventions are attractive to arrest or reverse these progressive changes evident following genomic damage. The concept of cancer chemoprevention, coined by Sporn, stresses therapeutic interventions at the earliest steps of carcinogenesis, as this would avoid the clinical consequences of malignancies.

A clinical validation of the concept of cancer chemoprevention was shown through a randomized trial using the SERM tamoxifen to reduce breast cancer risk in high-risk women. Risk reduction was found only for hormone-sensitive breast cancers and provided a basis for Federal Drug Administration (FDA) approval. Undesirable estrogenic effects, such as those involving the endometrium, have resulted in an active search for a SERM that would preserve the chemopreventive effects of tamoxifen in the breast while retaining desirable estrogenic effects, such as those in preventing osteoporosis and promoting hypocholesterolemia. This clinical finding in reduction of hormone sensitive breast cancer risk has underscored the need to identify other pharmacological agents that would be effective in preventing hormone-resistant breast cancers.

Many interventions could reduce specific cancer risk, including lifestyle changes, dietary interventions, and effective screening of high-risk individuals, as will be discussed elsewhere in this encyclopedia. This article focuses on chemopreventive agents that exert their actions through specific pharmacological mechanisms. Representative classes of chemoprevention agents will be discussed, including specific agonists or antagonists for members of the steroid receptor superfamily of nuclear receptors, selective cyclooxygenase-2 (COX-2) or inducible nitric oxide synthase (iNOS) inhibitors, and other agents.

II. PHARMACOLOGY

Pharmacological cancer chemoprevention strategies could target multiple steps during carcinogenesis. Agents can act by blocking DNA damage that occurs as an initiating step in carcinogenesis or by blocking or reversing the progression of premalignant cells that have already acquired genomic damage. Agents may also act at the promotion or progression steps of carcinogenesis. In targeting these steps of carcinogenesis, cell–stromal interactions, as well as neoangiogenesis, would play important roles in the development of invasive malignancy. An empirical approach to cancer chemoprevention has been replaced by clinical strategies that emphasize the mechanisms of action of candidate chemopreventive agents in the design of clinical trials. These strategies build on basic scientific insights into pathways involved in cancer chemoprevention.

Several examples illustrate this point. Inducible COX-2 is involved in the synthesis of prostaglandins from arachidonic acid and is often activated during inflammation. Evidence exists for COX-2 as a therapeutic target for cancer chemoprevention. Genetic findings implicate a role for COX-2 in preventing colon carcinogenesis. Genetically modified mice have been engineered to harbor defects of the adenomatous polyposis coli (APC) gene, which results in intestinal adenomatous polyps as well as an increase in COX-2. The relevancy of this genetically modified mouse model to disease in humans is shown by the finding that COX-2 overexpression relative to adjacent normal tissues was found as frequent in clinical colon cancers. The role of COX-2 in colon carcinogenesis was examined further by engineering mice with defects in COX-2 and APC. In contrast to the increase in intestinal polyps observed in APC-deficient mice, a reduction in polyp formation occurred in mice deficient in COX-2. These and other studies provided a basis for clinical trials that target inducible COX-2 with pharmacological inhibitors in selected patients at risk for colon carcinogenesis. These findings were extended to the clinical setting. Beneficial clinical effects have been reported with selective COX-2 inhibitors in the treatment of patients with the familial adenomatous polyps (FAP) syndrome.

These clinical findings obtained in patients with an inherited risk for colon carcinogenesis set the stage for use of COX-2 inhibitors (Fig. 1) in other individuals with high risk for colon cancer. A further rationale for targeting COX-2 in colon carcinogenesis comes from epidemiological findings in individuals who chronically received nonsteroidal anti-inflammatory drugs (NSAIDs) and have reduced incidence of carcinogenesis. While NSAIDs do not selectively inhibit COX-2 rather than COX-1, these and other findings support the view that a selective COX-2 inhibitor would have a beneficial impact in colon cancer prevention. Selective COX-2 inhibitors would be expected to have reduced side effects than a nonselective inhibitor, as the constitutively expressed COX-1 is not targeted. This could favor chronic clinical administration as would be needed for the prevention of colonic or other tumors.

Another example of successful targeting of a pathway involved in the suppression of carcinogenesis is found in the use of SERMs to reduce breast cancer risk. Administration of the SERM tamoxifen (Fig. 1) has been shown to reduce breast cancer risk in women at high risk for hormone-sensitive breast cancer. A positive proof of a principle randomized trial has provided a basis for additional clinical breast cancer prevention trials that test other SERMs that would exert the desired tissue estrogenic actions, such as in preventing osteoporosis, while antagonizing undesirable estrogenic effects that promote carcinogenesis in breast, uterine, or ovarian tissues. This possibility is under clinical study with the SERM raloxifene. Distinct raloxifene response elements exist and could contribute to different pharmacological effects of this SERM relative to others. In the future, other SERMs will be examined in relevant clinical trials. These could exploit the fact that a second estrogen receptor (ERβ) has been identified that may exert distinct biological effects.

An analogous chemopreventive approach could target the androgen receptor in prostate cancer. Prostatic intraepithelial neoplasia (PIN) has been identified as a precursor lesion in prostatic carcinogenesis. Whether antiandrogen-based strategies will prevent the progression of PIN to prostate cancer is the subject of future work in this field. The development of transgenic prostate cancer models should be of assistance in evaluating the efficacy and activities of pharmacological agents that target the androgen receptor in prostate carcinogenesis.

Antiproliferative, differentiating-inducing as well as proapoptotic agents can target carcinogenesis. The retinoids, derivatives of vitamin A, are a class of prevention agents that could exert desired clinical chemoprevention effects by targeting these and other biological pathways. The retinoids are natural and synthetic derivatives of vitamin A that have diverse

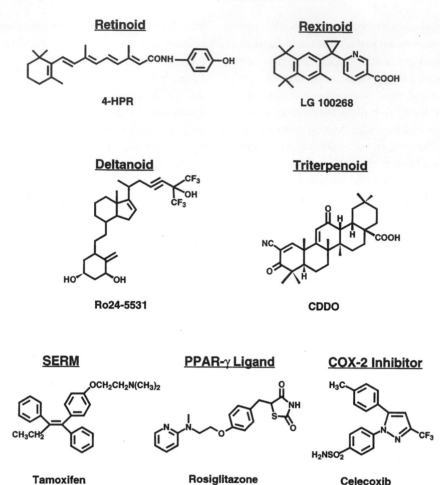

FIGURE 1 Structures of candidate cancer chemoprevention agents. These are representative pharmacological agents that target distinct pathways and exhibit specific mechanisms of action. Several interact with nuclear receptors, others affect enzymatic pathways, and some have mechanisms of actions that are currently under active investigation.

chemical structures, pharmacological properties, nuclear receptor affinities, and associated toxicity profiles. A strong rationale for a role of retinoids in cancer therapy or prevention stems from results obtained from experimental animal models, epidemiological studies, and clinical trials. Wolbach and Howe focused initial attention on vitamin A-dependent pathways as important in epithelial cell homeostasis in 1925. These investigators found that vitamin A deficiency in rodents caused squamous metaplasia in the trachea as well as at other epithelial sites. Notably, correction of this deficiency by vitamin A treatment reverses these metaplastic changes. These metaplastic changes are similar to those that arise in smokers, implicating a role for vitamin A-dependent signals in

suppressing lung carcinogenesis. Further evidence for an association between vitamin A and cancer incidence stems from epidemiological data demonstrating an inverse relationship between vitamin A levels and incidence of cancer at specific epithelial sites.

These and other findings provided a basis for use of retinoids in cancer prevention. Additional support for a retinoid role in cancer prevention derived from clinical trials conducted using retinoids that resulted in the successful treatment of certain premalignant conditions such as oral leukoplakia, cervical dysplasia, and xeroderma pigmentosum. Other clinical trials revealed retinoid activity in reducing some second primary cancers. These include independent retinoid trials that demonstrated a reduction in second aerodigestive tract cancers in patients having prior head and neck, lung, or hepatocellular carcinomas. In contrast to these promising trials, a randomized intergroup trial conducted in subjects treated with 13-*cis* retinoic acid following resection of stage I lung cancers did not show clinical benefit in smokers, although a reduction in second cancers was observed in subjects who never smoked. These findings, when coupled with those reported in large randomized trials using β-carotene in primary lung cancer prevention in high-risk individuals, indicate that a negative clinical interaction can exist when a chemopreventive agent is administered to active smokers. There is a need to combine lung cancer prevention agents with smoking cessation.

Mechanisms responsible for the reported reduction of second cancers by retinoid treatment of nonsmokers need to be determined. A better understanding of relevant mechanisms should prove useful in the selection of the optimal retinoid for use in cancer chemoprevention. Two classes of retinoid nuclear receptors exist. These are the retinoid acid receptors (RARs) and the retinoid X receptors (RXRs). These share homology with other members of the steroid receptor superfamily of nuclear receptors, which include the glucocorticoid receptor, vitamin D receptor, and estrogen receptor, among others. There are three subtypes of RARs (RARα, RARβ, and RARγ) and RXRs (RXRα, RXRβ, and RXRγ) and several isoforms exist. Orphan nuclear receptors have been identified where the physiological ligands remain to be discovered.

The ligand-binding domain of individual retinoid nuclear receptors is where specific retinoids bind. These nuclear receptors also contain DNA-binding domains that recognize defined responsive elements in genomic DNA. Following these ligand–receptor and receptor–DNA interactions, direct target genes that signal retinoid biological effects are activated or repressed. Retinoid nuclear receptors can heterodimerize or homodimerize and associate with two classes of coregulator proteins known as inhibitory corepressors and stimulating coactivators. Protein–protein interactions between retinoid receptors and their coregulators provide another level of regulation to the retinoid signaling pathway, as these can affect the basal transcriptional machinery through chromatin remodeling via changes in the state of acetylation. Coregulators represent additional pharmacological targets in cancer prevention.

Pharmacological agonists and antagonists have been engineered to affect specific components of the retinoid signaling pathway. For instance, all-*trans* retinoic acid is an agonist for the RAR but not the RXR pathway, whereas the ligand 9-*cis* retinoic acid is bifunctional, activating the RAR and RXR pathways. An RXR agonist, known as a rexinoid, has been approved for clinical use by the FDA. Other retinoids target the AP-1 transcription factor. Some retinoids, such as N-(4-hydroxyphenyl)retinamide (4HPR) act through receptor-independent mechanisms (Fig. 1) and preferentially signal apoptosis in responsive cells. Randomized cancer chemoprevention clinical trials have emphasized the use of classical retinoids that activate the RAR pathway. Because repressed expression of RARβ is frequent in several epithelial cancers, including lung cancers, this could contribute to the clinical chemopreventive effects observed in subjects entered into trials to reduce primary or second lung tumors. The mechanisms responsible for RARβ repression are under active study. Preclinical evidence points to a role for methylation-induced silencing of this nuclear receptor. Perhaps demethylation agents that target RARβ sequences could be used in conjunction with the optimal retinoid to overcome RARβ repression and elicit the desired clinical chemoprevention effects. Clinical cancer chemoprevention studies could consider the use of retinoids that do not activate the classical retinoid signaling pathway. This approach might bypass a common defect observed in aerodigestive tract tumors, the suppression of RARβ.

There is a need for additional candidate cancer chemoprevention agents that target specific cellular pathways. A partial list of candidate cancer chemoprevention agents appears in Fig. 1. In addition to pharmacological agents designated as retinoids, rexinoids, or SERMs, agents that act through other nuclear receptors include those affecting the vitamin D receptor (known as deltanoids) and those acting through PPAR-γ. One promising class of potential chemoprevention agents is synthetic triterpenoids, which are derivatives of natural products, known as cyclosqualenoids. Triterpenoids exhibit potent differentiation-inducing, antiproliferative, and anti-inflammatory activities. Pertinent to their potential role in cancer chemoprevention, one of the synthesized triterpenoids known as CDDO (Fig. 1) suppresses induction of the inflammatory enzymes iNOS and COX-2. Whether these findings will be extended into the setting of clinical cancer chemoprevention is the subject of ongoing work.

III. CLINICAL CONSIDERATIONS

Clinical cancer chemoprevention trials have features distinct from therapeutic trials. To exert the desired clinical effects, chemoprevention agents are often administered on a chronic basis and should have few, if any, associated clinical toxicities. For individuals who are at increased risk for cancer, primary cancer prevention with chemopreventive agents, when coupled with lifestyle or dietary changes, would be an attractive approach to reduce cancer risk. Even in individuals at high risk for a primary cancer, a cancer chemoprevention agent would not be clinically adopted when clinical side effects are evident when used in cancer chemoprevention. In contrast, subjects who have already had a cured primary cancer may accept some side effects of chemoprevention agents if this would reduce the risk of a second primary cancer. Because candidate cancer chemopreventive agents are often selected for use based on mechanisms of action, one way to limit clinical toxicities of cancer chemopreventive agents would be through combination therapy. Agents targeting different chemopreventive pathways would each be administered at dosages lower than when these are used as single agents. This could yield more than additive chemopreventive activities while retaining acceptable clinical toxicity profiles. Perhaps synergistic clinical actions would be exerted by pharmacological agents that affect distinct chemopreventive pathways.

Cancer chemoprevention trials are of a large size and require long clinical follow-up. If clinical outcome is the sole end point for the assessment of chemopreventive activity, then progress in this field will not be rapid. For this reason, biomarkers or intermediate end points have been proposed as ways to assess chemoprevention responses even before the

clinical outcome is known. Biomarkers and intermediate end points are indicative of changes that increase the risk of cancer development in affected cells or tissues. Examples could indicate genomic instability that leads to additional chromosomal abnormalities (such as aneuploidy or loss of heterozygosity), cell cycle deregulation that alters the proliferative state, or changes in transcription due to the basal methylation or acetylation status of the genome, among other changes. Specific genetic alterations that occur in carcinogenesis include those affecting oncogenes (*ras* family, *myc* family, epidermal growth factor receptors, and others) or tumor suppressor genes, such as p53. These changes might be targets for cancer chemoprevention or surrogate markers for response to cancer chemopreventive agents.

IV. CONCLUSIONS

Pharmacological interventions can be used to reverse or arrest the progression of carcinogenesis at specific cell or tissue sites. Cancer chemoprevention is an attractive approach to reduce the societal burden of cancer by treating carcinogenesis before lesions become clinically evident. Given the chronic nature of interventions for cancer chemoprevention, pharmacological agents should be administered with few, if any, associated clinical toxicities. Biomarkers or intermediate end points could prove useful to identify chemopreventive targets as well as highlight those changes that would place cells or tissues at high risk for malignant transformation. Changes in these markers represent potential surrogate end points for clinical cancer chemoprevention trials. In the near term, as the clinical cancer chemoprevention field advances, it will be important to understand how preventive agents act and when they should be administered for primary or secondary cancer chemoprevention.

Acknowledgments

This work was supported in part by NIH RO-1-CA8756 (E.D.), RO1-CA62275 (E.D.), RO1-CA78814 (M.B.S.), the Department of Defense Grants DAMD17-99-1-9168 and DAMD17-98-1-8604, the American Cancer Society Grant RPG-90-019-10-DDC (E.D.), the National Foundation for Cancer Research (M.B.S.), and the Oliver and Jennie Donaldson Trust. M.B.S.

is the Oscar M. Cohn Professor. We thank Dr. Nanjoo Suh, Dartmouth Medical School, for helpful consultation and Ms. Ann Frost for expert editorial assistance.

See Also the Following Articles

CELLULAR RESPONSES TO DNA DAMAGE • CHEMOPREVENTION TRIALS • ESTROGENS AND ANTIESTROGENS • MOLECULAR EPIDEMIOLOGY AND CANCER RISK • MOLECULAR MECHANISMS OF CANCER INVASION • MULTISTAGE CARCINOGENESIS • NUTRITIONAL SUPPLEMENTS AND DIET AS CHEMOPREVENTIVE AGENTS • TUMOR CELL MOTILITY AND INVASION

Bibliography

Alpha-Tocopherol, Beta-Carotene Cancer Prevention Study Group. (1994). The effect of vitamin E and beta carotene on the incidence of lung cancer and other cancers in male smokers. *N. Engl. J. Med.* **330,** 1029–1035.

Fisher, B., Costantino, J. P., Wickerham, D. L., Redmond, C. K., Kavanah, M., Cronin, W. M., Vogel, V., Robidoux, A., Dimitrov, N., Atkins, J., Daly, M., Wieand, S., Tan-Chiu, E., Ford, L., and Wolmark, N. (1998). Tamoxifen for prevention of breast cancer: report of the National Surgical Adjuvant Breast and Bowel Project P-1 Study. *J. Natl. Cancer Inst.* **90,** 1371–1388.

Hennekens, C. H., Buring, J. E., Manson, J. E., Stampfer, M., Rosner, B., Cook, N. R., Belanger, C., LaMotte, F., Gaziano, J. M., Ridker, P. M., Willett, W., and Peto, R. (1996). Lack of effect of long-term supplementation with beta carotene on the incidence of malignant neoplasms and cardiovascular disease. *N. Engl. J. Med.* **334,** 1145–1149.

Hong, W. K., Endicott, J., Itri, L. M., Doos, W., Batsakis, J. G., Bell, R., Fofonoff, S., Byers, R., Atkinson, E. N., Vaughan, C., Toth, B. B., Kramer, A., Dimery, I. W., Skipper, P., and Strong, S. (1986). 13-cis-retinoic acid in the treatment of oral leukoplakia. *N. Engl. J. Med.* **315,** 1501–1505.

Hong, W. K., Lippman, S. M., Itri, L. M., Karp, D. D., Lee, J. S., Byers, R. M., Schantz, S. P., Kramer, A. M., Lotan, R., Peters, L. J., Dimery, I. W., Brown, B. W., and Goepfert, H. (1990). Prevention of second primary tumors with isotretinoin in squamous-cell carcinoma of the head and neck. *N. Engl. J. Med.* **323,** 795–801.

Kraemer, K. H., DiGiovanna, J. J., Moshell, A. N., Tarone, R. E., and Peck, G. L. (1988). Prevention of skin cancer in xeroderma pigmentosum with the use of oral isotretinoin. *N. Engl. J. Med.* **318,** 1633–1637.

Lippman, S. M., Lee, J. J., Karp, D. D., Vokes, E. E., Brenner, S. E., Goodman, G. E., Khuri, F. R., Marks, R., Winn, R. J., Fry, W., Graziano, S. L., Gandara, D. R., Okawara, G., Woodhouse, C. L., Williams, B., Perez, C., Kim, H. W., Lotan, R., Roth, J. A., and Hong, W. K. (2001). Random-

ized phase III intergroup trial of isotretinoin to prevent second primary tumors in stage I non-small-cell lung cancer. *J. Natl. Cancer Inst.* **93,** 605–618.

Meyskens, F. L., Jr., Surwit, E., Moon, T. E., Childers, J. M., Davis, J. R., Dorr, R. T., Johnson, C. S., and Alberts, D. S. (1994). Enhancement of regression of cervical intraepithelial neoplasia II (moderate dysplasia) with topically applied all-trans-retinoic acid: A randomized trial. *J. Natl. Cancer Inst.* **86,** 539–543.

Muto, Y., Moriwaki, H., Ninomiya, M., Adachi, S., Saito, A., Takasaki, K. T., Tanaka, T., Tsurumi, K., Okuno, M., Tomita, E., Nakamura, T., and Kojima, T. (1996). Prevention of second primary tumors by an acyclic retinoid, polyprenoic acid, in patients with hepatocellular carcinoma. Hepatoma Prevention Study Group. *N. Engl. J. Med.* **334,** 1561–1567.

Nason-Burchenal, K., and Dmitrovsky, E. (1999). The retinoids: Cancer therapy and prevention mechanisms. *In* "Handbook of Experimental Pharmacology" (H. Nau and W. Blaner, eds.), Vol. 139. pp. 301–322. Springer, Berlin.

Omenn, G. S., Goodman, G. E., Thornquist, M. D., Balmes, J., Cullen, M. R., Glass, A., Keogh, J. P., Meyskens, F. L., Valanis, B., Williams, J. H., Barnhart, S., and Hammar, S. (1996). Effects of a combination of beta carotene and vitamin A on lung cancer and cardiovascular disease. *N. Engl. J. Med.* **334,** 1150–1155.

Pastorino, U., Infante, M., Maioli, M., Chiesa, G., Buyse, M., Firket, P., Rosmentz, N., Clerici, M., Soresi, E., Valente, M., Belloni, P. A., and Ravasi, G. (1993). Adjuvant treatment of stage I lung cancer with high-dose vitamin A. *J. Clin. Oncol.* **11,** 1216–1222.

Slaughter, D. P., Southwick, H. W., and Smejkal, W. P. (1953). "Field cancerization" in oral stratified squamous epithelium: clinical implications for multicentric origin. *Cancer* **6,** 963–968.

Sporn, M. B., Dunlop, N. M., Newton, D. L., and Smith, J. M. (1976). Prevention of chemical carcinogenesis by vitamin A and its synthetic analogs (retinoids). *Fed. Proc.* **35,** 1332–1338.

Steinbach, G., Lynch, P. M., Phillips, R. K. S., Wallace, M. H., Hawk, E., Gordon, G. B., Wakabayashi, N., Saunders, B., Shen, Y., Fujimura, T., Su, L.-K., and Levin, B. (2000). The effect of celecoxib, a cyclooxygenase-2 inhibitor, in familial adenomatous polyposis. *N. Engl. J. Med.* **342,** 1946–1952.

Suh, N., Wang, Y., Honda, T., Gribble, G. W., Dmitrovsky, E., Hickey, W. F., Maue, R. A., Place, A. E., Porter, D. M., Spinella, M. J., Williams, C. R., Wu, G., Dannenberg, A. J., Flanders, K. C., Letterio, J. J., Mangelsdorf, D. J., Nathan, C. F., Nguyen, L., Porter, W. W., Ren, R. F., Roberts, A. B., Roche, N. S., Subbaramaiah, K., and Sporn, M. B. (1999). A novel synthetic oleanane triterpenoid, 2-cyano-3,12-dioxoolean-1,9-dien-28-oic acid, with potent differentiating, antiproliferative, and anti-inflammatory activity. *Cancer Res.* **59,** 336–341.

Wolbach, S. B., and Howe, P. R. (1925). Tissue changes following deprivation of fat-soluble vitamin A. *J. Exp. Med.* **42,** 753–777.

Chemoprevention Trials

Edward S. Kim
Fadlo R. Khuri
Waun Ki Hong

University of Texas M. D. Anderson Cancer Center, Houston

GLOSSARY

chemoprevention Treatment with natural or synthetic agents that prevent the development of cancer in cancer-naive patients (primary chemoprevention) or in patients who have been cured of a prior cancer (secondary chemoprevention)

DNA damage Genomic damage resulting from carcinogen exposure that leads to abnormalities in coding sequence (point mutations, amplifications, deletions, additions) or in chromosomal content (aneuploidy).

epithelial cancer Cancer that originates in the epithelial lining of any organ.

field cancerization Hypothesis in which diffuse epithelial injury results from chronic carcinogen exposure; genetic changes and the presence of premalignant and malignant lesions in one region of the field are associated with an increased risk of cancer developing throughout the entire field.

intermediate end point Any biological or genetic variable that changes during chemopreventive treatment and that can be used as a marker to predict a reduction in cancer incidence in chemoprevention trials.

multistep carcinogenesis Hypothesis stating that a cancer cell evolves from a normal cell as a result of a sequence of genomic injuries, which leads to a progressively dysplastic appearance and abnormal biological behavior.

oncogene A gene that, when expressed at abnormal levels or in a mutated state, contributes to the carcinogenic process through dysregulation of cell growth and differentiation.

premalignancy An epithelial region that is histologically abnormal but not fully malignant in appearance or behavior and that is at risk for neoplastic progression in the future.

retinoid receptor A cytoplasmic or nuclear protein that binds retinoids and functions in retinoid signal transduction.

retinoids A chemically diverse group of natural and synthetic compounds that are related to vitamin A and bind a specific receptor or set of receptors.

second primary tumor A tumor that occurs in a patient who has been cured of a prior cancer and that is of a different histology and/or occurs in a separate location from the original cancer.

tumor suppressor gene A gene that normally functions as a physiologic inhibitor of abnormal clonal expansion, preventing the outgrowth of cells that have undergone oncogenic mutations.

C ancer prevention efforts have been a long and arduous process. As the biological basis for carcinogenesis continues to be elucidated, different strategies for prevention have emerged. The success of recent clinical trials designed to prevent cancer in patients who are at increased risk of cancer (cancer "chemoprevention" trials) suggests that chemoprevention is a rational and appealing treatment strategy. Success in the prevention of epithelial cancers suggests that chemopreventive agents can interrupt the carcinogenic process. This article focuses on current chemoprevention research both laboratory and clinical. Chemopreventive agents, how they might interrupt the biological effects of genetic changes to inhibit abnormal epithelial cell growth and differentiation, and the genetic events associated with epithelial carcinogenesis are discussed and the usefulness of intermediate biomarkers as markers of premalignancy is reviewed. Finally, chemoprevention trials are analyzed with emphasis on strategies of trial design and clinical outcome and future directions in chemoprevention are proposed that are based on recently acquired mechanistic insight into carcinogenesis and chemoprevention.

I. INTRODUCTION

Epithelial cancers have historically been a cause for frustration by both patients and practitioners. Since the mid-1970s, the mortality rate from epithelial malignancies has improved only slightly despite advancements in cancer therapeutics. Although some patients will present with early stage epithelial malignancies, the majority of these patients will present with locally advanced or metastatic disease. Surgical intervention with adjuvant treatment, including radiotherapy and/or chemotherapy, has offered some improvements in long-term survival rates. However, local recurrence and especially the development of

second primary tumors have impacted both morbidity and mortality in this patient population. Thus, a novel approach to these epithelial cancers is needed. Epithelial carcinogenesis is a multistep process in which an accumulation of genetic events leads to a progressively dysplastic cellular appearance, deregulated cell growth, and finally carcinoma.

II. CHEMOPREVENTION

Chemoprevention can be defined as the use of specific natural or synthetic chemical agents to reverse, suppress, or prevent carcinogenic progression to invasive cancer. Sporn first defined the term chemoprevention in 1976. Cancer chemoprevention is a rapidly developing field that approaches carcinogenesis from a different perspective. Previously, early detection techniques were employed to reduce morbidity and mortality with respect to cancer treatment. In lung cancer, this included early chest X-ray and sputum cytology analysis in individuals at high risk. Despite these early detection techniques, overall mortality did not improve. Chemoprevention bridges basic biologic research with clinical chemical intervention and attempts to halt the process of carcinogenesis. Its principles are based on the concepts of field cancerization and multistep carcinogenesis. In field cancerization, diffuse epithelial injury results from carcinogen exposure in the aerodigestive tract, genetic changes, and premalignant and malignant lesions in one region of the field translate into an increased risk of cancer developing in the entire field. Multistep carcinogenesis describes a stepwise accumulation of alterations, both genotypic and phenotypic. Arresting one or several of the steps may impede or delay the development of cancer. This has been described particularly well in studies involving precancerous and cancerous lesions of the head and neck, which focus on oral premalignant lesions (leukoplakia and erythroplakia) and their associated increased risk of progression to cancer. As the new millennium begins, exciting new techniques to fight cancer are being devised, including biologic interventions and genetic manipulations. Intermediate markers of response are needed to assess the validity of these approaches in a timely and cost-efficient manner.

III. BIOLOGICAL BASIS OF EPITHELIAL CARCINOGENESIS

A. Field Cancerization

Field cancerization was originally described by Auerbach in 1953. In the upper aerodigestive tract (UADT), the surface epithelium, or field, is exposed in large amounts to environmental carcinogens, predominantly tobacco smoke. Pathologic evaluation of the epithelial mucosa of the UADT located adjacent to carcinomas frequently reveals hyperplastic and dysplastic changes. These premalignant changes found in areas of carcinogen-exposed epithelium adjacent to tumors are termed "field cancerization" and suggest that these multiple foci of premalignancy could progress concurrently to form multiple primary cancers. Second primary tumors (SPTs) have become the leading cause of mortality in head and neck cancer and this best illustrates the concept of field cancerization. Multiple genetic abnormalities have been detected in normal and premalignant epithelium of the lung and UADT in high-risk patients. In limited studies, when primary tumors and SPTs are analyzed for p53 mutations, evidence supports the independent origin of these tumors. Mutations of p53 can occur in only one of the tumors or distinct mutations occur between the primary and SPT. Continued work in analyzing molecular characteristics of primary and second primary cancers is needed.

B. Multistep Carcinogenesis

Pathological observations in field cancerization gave rise to the hypothesis of multistep carcinogenesis, which proposes that neoplastic changes evolve over a period of time progressing from normal, to hyperplastic, to dysplastic, and finally to fully malignant phenotypes. Elucidating the mechanism of multistep carcinogenesis has awaited the integration of molecular biological techniques into pathologic evaluation of epithelial lesions. This has led to the discovery of genetic abnormalities in premalignant and malignant epithelial cells. Studies have identified different carcinogenic stages, including initiation, promotion, and progression. Initiation involves direct DNA binding and damage by carcinogens and is rapid and irreversible. Promotion leads to premalignancy and is generally irreversible involving epigenetic mechanisms. Progression is the period between premalignancy and the cancer and is generally irreversible involving genetic mechanisms. The stages of promotion and progression are prolonged. Genetic damage appears to accumulate during neoplastic transformation, and specific genes have been discovered that, when altered, may play a role in epithelial carcinogenesis. These include both tumor suppressor genes and protooncogenes, which encode proteins that are involved in cell cycle control, signal transduction, and transcriptional regulation. Tumor suppressor genes inhibit clonal expansion by suppressing cell growth and genomic mutability. Some tumor suppressors that have been linked to epithelial carcinogenesis include p53, retinoblastoma (Rb), DCC (deleted in colorectal carcinoma), MCC (mutated in colorectal carcinoma), and APC (adenomatous polyposis coli) genes. Over 500 genes that play vital roles in cell signaling and growth control are altered in cancer cells and, as protooncogenes, may be involved in the process of neoplasia. These include ras, the myc (C-, N-, and L-myc), erbB [erbB1 (epidermal growth factor receptor), erbB2 (her2/neu), erbB3 (her3), and erbB4/her4]. Chromosomes, also extensively damaged during epithelial carcinogenesis, are detected in the form of nuclear DNA adducts, cytoplasmic DNA fragments, or micronuclei and chromosomal abnormalities, which include aneuploidy as well as intrachromosomal deletions and amplifications. Future studies designed to discover genes disrupted by these chromosomal lesions may reveal both known and novel tumor suppressor genes and oncogenes, which play a role in epithelial carcinogenesis.

IV. BIOLOGICAL BASIS OF CHEMOPREVENTION

Chemoprevention trials are based on the hypothesis that interruption of the biological processes involved in carcinogenesis will inhibit this process and, in turn, reduce cancer incidence. This hypothesis provides a framework for the design and evaluation of chemoprevention trials, including the rationale for the selection of agents that are likely to inhibit biological processes and the development of intermediate markers associated with carcinogenesis. DNA damage associated with epithelial malignancies is thought to occur partly through oxidative processes induced by free radicals. Aberrant epithelial proliferation and differentiation are hallmarks of premalignant lesions. Treatment approaches include interrupting any of these processes. Development of intermediate markers for chemoprevention trials is crucial. Because treatment-induced improvements in cancer incidence require years to evaluate, monitoring intermediate markers that are both modulated by chemoprevention treatment and correlate with a reduction in cancer incidence would allow a more expeditious evaluation of potentially active chemopreventive agents. Premalignant lesions are a potential source of intermediate markers, and if disappearance of these lesions correlates with a reduction in cancer incidence, then markers of premalignancy will serve as intermediate end points for chemoprevention trials. Future studies in chemoprevention will continue to test this hypothesis.

V. CHEMOPREVENTION TRIALS

Cancer chemoprevention is still investigational, although its role in oncologic practice continues to expand. Prevention in cancer has become more prominent as frustration over the failures of current therapeutic modalities has grown. A variety of chemopreventive agents have been studied in over 40 randomized trials since 1990. Some clinical activity has been demonstrated proving the potential utility of this method of cancer prevention. Still, large randomized trials are needed before chemoprevention agents can be fully integrated into standard oncologic practice. Major trials are listed in Table I.

A. Trial Design

Chemoprevention trials are conducted in three phases similar to other clinical trials. Phase I trials determine the toxicity of an agent alone or in combination with other agents. However, in latter phases, the ideal end point of chemoprevention trials is a reduction in cancer incidence as patients who are enrolled in study are free of cancer as opposed to traditional phase II studies. Because cancer incidence is extremely low among the general population with no known cancer risk factors, demonstrating a treatment-induced reduction in cancer incidence among the general population requires large randomized studies, which are expensive and time-consuming.

The time and resources required for chemoprevention trials can be significantly reduced by targeting high-risk populations and utilizing potential intermediate biomarkers. This point is best illustrated by ongoing trials of chemoprevention of upper aerodigestive tract cancer. In these studies, patients are definitively treated for a stage I or II cancer of the UADT. Although recurrence is a concern, development of second primary tumors is the leading cause of cancer-related death following treatment in early stage disease as reported by Vikram. Therefore, the end points in these trials are the occurrence of SPTs and survival. SPTs occur at a rate of 3–7% per year in these patients. To test whether a given chemopreventive agent has an effect, if a cancer incidence rate of 6% is used, it is necessary to follow 1000 patients for a period of 5 years. As of September 1, 1999, the Retinoid Head and Neck Second Primary Trial had completed accrual with 1384 registered patients and 1191 patients randomized and eligible. Interim analysis performed in May 2000 indicated significantly higher recurrence rates in active smokers vs former smokers and significantly higher smoking related SPT rates in active smokers vs never smokers, with intermediate rates for former smokers. This trial will be unblinded and definitively analyzed in September 2002, when all randomized patients have completed active therapy.

The risk of SPTs is much lower in most other epithelial cancers. For patients who have undergone resection of a breast cancer, the risk of a SPT is 0.8% per year. When compared to UADT cancer chemoprevention trials, breast cancer chemoprevention trials require up to 5 to 10 times more patients with longer clinical follow-up. As 5000–10,000 patients are required for these trials, this is still less than the 20,000 or more required to conduct a study in the general population.

Intermediate end points can reduce the duration of studies as far as cost and resources. By utilizing bio-

TABLE I
Completed Randomized Chemoprevention Trials

Author	Study setting	Design	Number	Intervention	Outcome
Head and neck					
Hong (1986)	Oral leukoplakia	Phase IIb	44	Isotretinoin (1–2 mg/kg/day)	Positive
Stich (1988)	Oral leukoplakia	Phase IIb	65	Vitamin A (200,000 IU/week)	Positive
Han (1990)	Oral leukoplakia	Phase IIb	61	Retinamide (40 mg/day)	Positive
Lippman (1993)	Oral leukoplakia	Phase IIb (maintenance)	70	Isotretinoin (0.5 mg/kg/day)	Positive
Chiesa (1993)	Oral leukoplakia	Phase IIb (maintenance)	80	Fenretinide	Positive
Hong (1990)	Prior SCC	Phase III	103	Isotretinoin (50–100 mg/m^2/day)	Positive
Lung					
Heimberger (1988)	Metaplasia (sputum)	Phase IIb	73	Vitamin B$_{12}$ (500 μg/day); folic acid (10 mg/day)	Positive
Arnold (1992)	Metaplasia (sputum)	Phase IIb	150	Etretinate (25 mg/day)	Negative
Van Poppel (1992)	Micronuclei (sputum)	Phase IIb	114	β-Carotene (20 mg/day)	Positive
Lee (1993)	Metaplasia (biopsy)	Phase IIb	87	Isotretinoin (1 mg/kg/day)	Negative
Pastorino (1993)	Prior NSCLC	Phase III	307	Retinyl palmitate (300,000 IU/day)	Positive (SPT)
Kurie (2000)	Metaplasia/dysplasia	Phase IIb	82	4-HPR	Negative
Lippman (2000)	Prior NSCLC	Phase III	1166	Isotretinoin (30 mg/day)	Negative
Colorectal					
Bussey (1982)	FAP	Phase IIb	36	Vitamin C (3 g/day)	Positive (polyp)
McKeown-Eyssen (1988)	Resected adenoma	Phase IIb	137	Vitamins C (400 mg/day) and E (400 mg/day)	Negative
Decosse (1989)	FAP	Phase IIb	58	Vitamins C (4 g/day) and E (400 mg/day); fiber (22.5 g/day)	Positive (polyp)
Gregoire (1989)	Prior colon cancer	Phase IIb	30	Calcium (1200 mg/day)	Negative (LI)
Stern (1990)	Prior FAP	Phase IIb	31	Calcium (1200 mg/day)	Negative (LI)
Labayle (1991)	FAP	Phase IIb	10	Sulindac (100 mg three times/day)	Positive (polyp)
Wargovich (1992)	Resected adenoma	Phase IIb	20	Calcium (2000 mg/day)	Positive (LI)
Paganelli (1992)	Resected adenoma	Phase IIb	41	Vitamins A (30,000 IU/day), E (70 mg/d), and C (1 g/day)	Negative (LI)
Alberts (1992)	Resected adenoma	Phase IIb	100	WBF (2.0 or 13.5 g/day); calcium (250 or 1500 mg/day)	Negative (LI)
Nugent (1993)	FAP	Phase IIb	14	Sulindac (200 mg twice a day)	Positive (polyp)
Giardiello (1993)	FAP	Phase IIb	22	Sulindac (150 mg twice a day)	Positive (polyp)
MacLennan (1993)	Resected adenoma	Phase IIb	378	Fat (<25% of calories); WBF (11 g/day); β-carotene (20 mg/day)	Negative (polyps)
Bostick (1993)	Resected adenoma	Phase IIb	21	Calcium (1200 mg/day)	Negative (LI)
Roncucci (1993)	Resected adenoma	Phase IIb	209	Vitamins A (30,000 IU/day), C (1 g/day), and E (70 mg/day); lactulose (20 g/day)	Positive (vitamins> lactulose)
Gann (1993)	U.S. male physicians	Phase III	22,071	Aspirin (325 mg qod)	Negative
Steinbach (2000)	FAP	Phase IIb	77	Celecoxib 100 mg twice a day Celecoxib 400 mg twice a day	Negative Positive
Schatzkin (2000)	Resected adenoma	Phase IIb	2079	High fiber, low fat, counseling	Negative
Alberts (2000)	Resected adenoma	Phase IIb	1429	Wheat bran, 2.0 or 13.5 g daily	Negative
Skin					
Moriarty (1982)	Actinic keratoses	Phase IIb	50	Etretinate (75 mg/day)	Positive
Watson (1986)	Actinic keratoses	Phase IIb	15	Etretinate (75 mg/day)	Positive
Kligman (1991)	Actinic keratoses	Phase IIb	527	Topical tretinoin (0.05%)	Negative
Kligman (1991)	Actinic keratoses	Phase IIb	455	Topical tretinoin (0.10%)	Positive
Moon (1993)	Prior BCC/SCC	Phase III	524	Isotretinoin (5–10 mg/day), retinol (25,000 IU/day)	Negative
Greenberg (1990)	Prior BCC/SCC	Phase III	1805	β-Carotene (50 mg/day)	Negative
Tangrea (1992)	Prior BCC	Phase III	981	Isotretinoin (10 mg/day)	Negative

continues

TABLE I—*Continued*

Author	Study setting	Design	Number	Intervention	Outcome
Moon (1993)	Prior actinic keratoses	Phase III	2298	Retinol (25,000 IU/day)	Positive
Clark (1996)	Prior BCC/SCC	Phase III	1312	Selenium (200 mcg)	Negative
Esophagus/stomach					
Munoz (1985)	Geographic high risk (Huixan)	Phase IIb	610	Retinol (50,000 IU/week); riboflavin (200 mg/week); zinc (50 mg/week)	Negative (dysplasia) Positive (micronuclei)
Zaridze (1993)	Geographic high risk (Uzbekistan) (oral leukoplakia and/or chronic esophagitis)	Phase IIb	532	Riboflavin (80 mg/week); vitamins A (100,000 IU/week) and E (80 mg/week); β-carotene (40 mg/day)	Negative
Blot (1993)	Geographic high risk (Linxian)	Phase III	29,584	Multiple vitamins/minerals	Positive (stomach)
Li (1993)	Geographic high risk (Linxian, dysplasia)	Phase III	3318	Multiple vitamins/minerals	Negative
Bladder					
Alfthan (1983)	Superficial tumors (resected)	Phase IIb	32	Etretinate (25–50 mg/day)	Positive
Pederson (1984)	Superficial tumors (resected)	Phase IIb	73	Etretinate (50 mg/day)	Negative
Studer (1984)	Superficial tumors (resected)	Phase IIb	86	Etretinate (25–50 mg/day)	Positive
Cervix					
Byrne (1986)	Dysplasia (CIN 2,3)	Phase IIb	26	HLI (0.8 × 10^6 IU/week)	Negative
Yliskoski (1990)	Dysplasia (CIN 1,2)	Phase IIb	20	HLI (9 × 10^6 IU/day)	Negative
Frost (1990)	Dysplasia (CIN 2)	Phase IIb	10	IFN-α2b (4 × 10^6 IU/day)	Negative
de Vet (1991)	Dysplasia (CIN 1-3)	Phase IIb	278	β-Carotene (10 mg/day)	Negative
Butterworth (1992)	Dysplasia (CIN 1,2)	Phase IIb	235	Folic acid (10 mg/day)	Negative
Chu (1993)	Dysplasia (CIN 1,2)	Phase IIb	298	Folic acid (5 mg/day)	Negative
Meyskens (1993)	Dysplasia (CIN 2,3)	Phase IIb	301	Topical tretinoin (0.372%)	Positive (CIN 2)
Breast					
BCPT	LCIS, high-risk factors	Phase III	13,388	Tamoxifen 20 mg daily	Positive–early stop
Powles (1998)	Family history	Phase III	2494	Tamoxifen 20 mg for 8 years	Negative
Veronesi (1999)	Previous hysterectomy	Phase III	5408	Tamoxifen 20 mg for 5 years	Negative

markers that highly predict the development of cancer rather than assessing the actual development of cancer, chemoprevention trials can be designed to test the effects of potential agents in a smaller population in a shorter period of time.

B. Chemopreventive Agents

Approximately 2000 natural and synthetic agents have been shown in experimental systems to have chemopreventive activity. Agents that have been studied in clinical trials include retinoids, *N*-acetylcysteine, β-carotene, calcium, α-tocopherol, selenium, tamoxifen, finasteride, and nonsteroidal anti-inflammatory drugs (NSAIDs.) Of the group, the retinoids have been studied most extensively as

chemopreventive agents. Vitamin A was first noted to be an essential nutrient in 1913, and its deficiency was associated with changes in epithelial histology in 1925. Since that time, it has been shown that vitamin A deficiency is associated with bronchial metaplasia and an increased incidence of cancer. Vitamin A exists as preformed vitamin A (retinol esters, retinol, and retinal) and provitamin A carotenoids (β-carotene and metabolic precursors of retinol). Retinoids occur in natural (all-*trans* retinoic acid or ATRA, 13-*cis* retinoic acid or 13-cRA, 9-*cis* retinoic acid or 9-cRA, retinyl palmitate) and synthetic [fenretinide or *N*- (4-hydroxyphenyl)retinamide (4-HPR)] forms. They are important for normal cell growth and differentiation, as well as for the regulation of apoptosis. In preclinical models, they have been shown to suppress or reverse epithelial carcinogenesis in lung, oral cavity, esophagus, bladder, skin, mammary gland, prostate, and liver tissues. Clinical trials have studied naturally occurring retinoids, including tretinoin or ATRA, its stereoisomer isotretinoin or 13-cRA, and the retinoid-related molecule β-carotene. Synthetic retinoids that have demonstrated clinical activity in chemoprevention trials include retinyl palmitate, fenretinide or 4-HPR, and etretinate. A retinoid that will be studied in future clinical trials is the naturally occurring ATRA stereoisomer 9-cRA. Of all chemopreventive agents, retinoids have the best-defined mechanism of action. Retinoids function as ligands for intracellular receptors. Cytosolic receptors for retinol (CRBP) and retinoic acid (CRABP) bind retinoids and appear to regulate the transfer of retinoids into the nucleus. Nuclear retinoid receptors were discovered in 1987 and are believed to mediate the effects of retinoids and are members of a larger steroid superfamily of nuclear receptors that includes glucocorticoid, thyroid, vitamin D, progesterone, and estrogen receptors, among others. There are two families of retinoid nuclear receptors, RAR and RXR, and each family consists of three members: α, β, and γ forms. These receptors can exist as heterodimers or homodimers. RARs bind ATRA and 9-cRA, and RXRs bind 9-cRA and bexarotene (Targretin). Liganded nuclear receptors function as transcription factors that bind DNA and regulate the expression of genes that mediate retinoid cell functions, including growth, differentiation, and apoptosis. Retinoid nuclear receptors associate with inhibitory corepressors or stimulatory coactivators that after their transcriptional activities. Some retinoids, including 4-HPR, which has potent apoptosis-inducing activity, do not bind retinoid receptors. Other retinoids have not demonstrated any ability to bind either family of nuclear receptors (carotenoids), whereas their metabolites do (13-cRA, and retinol). Whether these retinoids are metabolized to another form that can bind to known nuclear receptors or bind to as yet undiscovered receptors is unknown. Studies have shown intracellular interconversion of 13-cRA to ATRA, demonstrating the importance of retinoid metabolism in determining the biological effects of retinoid treatment.

The nuclear retinoid receptor RAR-β seems to have a major role in UADT carcinogenesis. Important observations of RAR-β made in various studies include its absence in many head and neck carcinomas and lung cancer cell lines and its ability to suppress tumorigenesis. When upregulated with isotretinoin treatment, increased RAR-β expression and clinical response correlate in 40 to 90% of cases. Thus, RAR-β is the best indicator to date of retinoid chemoprevention efficacy in human head and neck carcinogenesis and a good biomarker for continued research. Surprisingly though, strong intratumoral RAR-β expression has been associated with a poorer outcome in early stage lung cancer. Thus, the biological mechanism and clinical outcome still need further investigation.

C. Trial Results

1. UADT Trials

The upper aerodigestive tract has served as a good model for chemoprevention and its utility. Premalignant oral lesions include erythroplakia and dysplastic leukoplakia. Retinoids, β-carotene, vitamin E, and selenium have shown activity in the reversal of oral premalignancy, but only retinoids have demonstrated positive results in randomized trials.

Isotretinoin, retinal (a synthetic retinamide), and fenretinide were used in these randomized trials. Of these agents, the best characterized is isotretinoin, which has been studied in two related randomized trials. In 1986, Hong reported a placebo-controlled, double-blind study of 44 patients randomized to receive 13-cRA (1–2 mg/kg/day) or placebo for 3 months and followed for 6 months. The clinical and histologic major response rates to 3 months' treatment with high-dose isotretinoin were 67 and 54%, respectively ($P = 0.0002$ and 0.01), after 6 months of follow-up; clinical and histologic rates of response to placebo were 10%. Toxicity was severe with the high-dose regimen, and more than 50% of treated patients relapsed within 2 to 3 months after discontinuing therapy.

A second trial was instituted to examine the effects of low-dose maintenance isotretinoin or β-carotene for 9 months following 3 months of high-dose induction therapy with isotretinoin. Sixty-six patients completed the first phase of the study, and the premalignant disease progression rates were 8% in patients who received low-dose isotretinoin and 55% in patients who received β-carotene ($P < 0.001$). The percentage of patients whose lesions decreased in size was 33% in patients treated with isotretinoin and 10% in patients treated with β-carotene. Carcinoma developed in seven patients who received β-carotene and only one who received isotretinoin. This study not only confirmed the activity of isotretinoin demonstrated in the first study, but also showed that isotretinoin is superior to β-carotene in this setting and revealed that low-dose maintenance therapy with isotretinoin may yield better long-term effects than a short course of high-dose therapy. However, a 10-year update of the study revealed no differences in cancer rates between the two groups. These studies established the rationale for the treatment of premalignant disease with chemopreventive agents.

These findings were further elaborated by studies that examined the effects of retinoid treatment in head and neck cancer patients who had been cured of their primary disease. A placebo-controlled, randomized trial of 103 patients who received high-dose isotretinoin (50–100 mg/m^2 for 12 months) following surgery and/or radiotherapy for early stage disease revealed that isotretinoin reduced the rate of SPT development after 32 months ($P = 0.005$), but this effect decreased after a median follow-up of approximately 5 years ($P = 0.04$). The treatment had no effect on local, regional, or distant recurrence or overall survival rates. In addition to reversing oral premalignancy, treatment with retinoids reduced the incidence of SPTs, the major cause of mortality in head and neck cancer patients. This effect diminished with time after concluding treatment. Many patients had side effects to the retinoid, which points to the need for developing better tolerated, more efficacious therapies. To further evaluate the retinoid effect on SPTs, a randomized, double-blind, multiinstitutional trial was launched examining the effect of low-dose 13-cRA in previously definitively treated patients with early stage head and neck cancer. Patients received 30 mg of 13-cRA per day for 3 years and are followed for 4 years documenting any end points, recurrences, or SPTs. This trial is planned to be unblinded in 2002. These results, positive or negative, will help establish a new standard in head and neck cancer chemoprevention.

Another study examined the effect of a second-generation retinoid, etretinate, in patients with early stage head and neck squamous cell carcinoma treated with surgery or radiation. This randomized study followed 316 patients who were randomized to receive etretinate, 50 mg/day for the first month, followed by 25 mg/day in the following months, or placebo for 24 months. There were no significant differences regarding local, regional, and distant metastases at 5 years. Treatment was discontinued in 33% of patients taking etretinate and 23% taking placebo ($P < 0.05$) because of toxicity. This study failed to show any effect in prevention of SPTs with etretinate.

Adjuvant therapy in advanced head and neck cancer has also been examined. Trials used a combination of 13cRA (50 mg/m^2/day), interferon-α (3 MU/m^2/t.i.w.), and α-tocopherol (1200 IU/day) given for 12 months. In a phase II study of 45 evaluable patients with definitively treated stage III/IV head and neck cancer, 39 have no evidence of disease with only 6 recurrences at 21 months median follow-up. The 2-year disease-free survival of the study is 84%. This suggests that perhaps in patients with a higher risk of developing recurrence or SPTs, more aggressive therapies for prevention are warranted.

EUROSCAN, a large phase III study encompassing 2592 patients, reported no benefit of chemopreventive agents in patients with head and neck or lung cancer in terms of survival, event-free survival, or SPT. In the EUROSCAN study, patients were randomized to receive supplementation with retinyl palmitate, N-acetylcysteine, both drugs in combination, or placebo for 2 years. Sixty percent of patients had a history of head and neck cancer and 40% had a history of lung cancer. Patients were grouped as current/former (93.5%) smokers and never (6.5%) smokers. However, data regarding smoking status, verification thereof (cotinine levels), and its impact relative to SPTs and recurrence were not presented. Further research and studies are needed to formulate a risk model in head and neck cancer, which can help identify that section of the general population highest at risk for development of cancer.

2. Lung Trials

The rationale for prevention of lung cancer is similar to that in head and neck cancer. In both diseases, chronic exposure to tobacco is the major risk factor and dysplastic epithelial lesions are thought to represent a premalignant stage. Preclinical data indicate that retinoids reverse dysplastic bronchial epithelial lesions. Despite these data, placebo-controlled, randomized trials in smokers have revealed that retinoid treatment adds no significant benefit to the effects of smoking cessation and reversal of bronchial metaplasia. In light of results demonstrating that retinoids reduce SPTs in patients who have had a lung cancer resected (see later), bronchial metaplasia may not accurately reflect the chemopreventive effects of retinoids on bronchial epithelium. Research is underway to identify intermediate markers that predict retinoid chemopreventive effects on bronchial epithelial cells.

In resected NSCLC patients, SPTs occur at the rate of 2–4% per year. Similar to its effects in head and neck cancer patients, retinoid treatment reduces the incidence of SPTs in lung cancer patients who have undergone resection. In the only completed trial addressing this question, 307 patients whose stage I NSCLC were completely resected were randomized to receive 12 months of treatment with retinol palmitate (300,000 IU a day) or no treatment. At a median of 46 months follow-up, patients who received retinol palmitate had a 35% lower incidence of SPTs than the control group (3.1% vs 4.8%). As in studies of head and neck cancer patients, retinoid treatment had no observed effect on survival duration or the rate of primary disease recurrence. EUROSCAN, as mentioned earlier, also showed no chemopreventive benefit in lung cancer patients. These trials in NSCLC patients point out the need to further investigate the effects of different retinoids in this setting and to extend these trials to include patients whose small cell lung cancer (SCLC) has been cured, who have SPTs rates twofold higher than in patients who have been treated for early stage head and neck cancer.

Trials in lung cancer chemoprevention have demonstrated the importance of smoking status and use of these agents. The Alpha-Tocopherol, Beta Carotene (ATBC) Cancer Prevention study was a randomized, double-blind, placebo-controlled primary-prevention trial in which 29,133 Finnish male smokers received α-tocopherol 50 mg a day alone, β-carotene 20 mg a day alone, both α-tocopherol and β-carotene, or placebo. These men were between 50 and 69 years of age and all smoked five or more cigarettes a day. Patients were followed for 5–8 years. Lung cancer incidence, the primary end point, did not change with the addition of β-tocopherol alone, nor did overall mortality. However, both groups who received β-carotene supplementation (alone or with α-tocopherol) had an 18% increase in the incidence of lung cancer. There appeared to be a stronger adverse effect from β-carotene in those men who smoked more than 20 cigarettes a day. This trial raised the serious issue that pharmacologic doses of β-carotene could potentially be harmful in active smokers.

The β-Carotene and Retinol Efficacy Trial (CARET) confirmed results of the Finnish trial. This randomized, double-blinded, placebo-controlled trial tested the combination of 30 mg β-carotene and 25,000 IU retinyl palmitate against placebo in 18,314 men and women age 50–69 years at high risk for lung cancer; 14,254 had at least a 20 pack-year smoking history and were either current or recent former smokers. Four thousand and sixty men had extensive occupational exposure to asbestos. This trial was stopped after 21 months because no benefit and even possibly harm were found. Lung cancer incidence, the primary end point, increased 28% in the active intervention group. Overall mortality also increased 17% in this group. Given these results, as well as those of the ATBC trial, high-dose β-carotene is not recommended for high-risk patients who continue to smoke.

The Physicians Health Study, a randomized, double-blind, placebo-controlled trial studied 22,071 healthy male physicians: 11,036 received 50 mg of β-carotene on alternate days and 11,035 received placebo. The use of supplemental β-carotene showed virtually no adverse or beneficial effects on cancer incidence or overall mortality during a 12-year follow-up.

In China, a study evaluating β-carotene, α-tocopherol, and selenium in the prevention of gastric and esophageal cancer showed a nonsignificant decrease in the risk of lung cancer in a small cohort of patients.

Subgroup analysis of the aforementioned studies, especially ATBC and CARET, have provided few explanations for the increase in lung cancer incidence. It seems β-carotene has a harmful effect only in high-risk heavy smokers or those with previous exposure to asbestos. Current recommendations are for these people to avoid supplemental β-carotene in large doses. Including the results of EUROSCAN mentioned previously, much work is needed before chemoprevention agents can be instituted in lung cancer. Currently, an ECOG trial is studying patients with stage I lung cancer and the effect of daily selenium supplementation.

3. Colorectal Trials

Colorectal cancer is associated with premalignant lesions, including polyps and dysplastic epithelium. Large polyps with villous elements and dysplastic epithelia are more likely to progress to carcinoma than small, tubular polyps. The premalignant stages of colon carcinogenesis present an evaluable process for chemoprevention trials.

The agents most widely used in colorectal cancer chemoprevention trials are NSAIDs and calcium salts. In phase II trials, the NSAID sulindac achieved a statistically significant decrease in both mean polyp number and diameter compared to placebo. Aspirin also shows promise in colon cancer prevention. Epidemiologic studies suggest that aspirin inhibits colon carcinogenesis. The effects of low-dose aspirin on colon cancer incidence were examined in the large-scale U.S. Physicians Health Study. This study revealed that aspirin had no effect on polyp or cancer incidence, but the trial's premature closing because of the finding of a statistically significant effect on myocardial infarction incidence most likely limited the power of this study to detect a modest effect of aspirin in preventing colon cancer. Despite evidence of colorectal cancer prevention, NSAIDs still require more investigation. Agent specificity, mechanism of action, and dose and duration of treatment, in addition to adverse side effects, have made recommendations for prevention difficult. Better understanding of the role of aspirin and other NSAIDs in colon cancer chemoprevention awaits further randomized, placebo-controlled trials.

Cyclooxygenase-2 (COX-2) inhibitors have shown promise. Forms of the COX enzyme demonstrated include COX-1, which is constitutively expressed, and COX-2, which is overexpressed in inflammatory cells and sites of inflammation. Most NSAIDs inhibit both enzymes. Inhibition of COX-2 specifically reduces untoward side affects such as ulcers and gastritis. In familial adenomatous polyposis (FAP), patients develop hundreds of polyps in their colon due to mutation of the adenomatous polyposis coli (APC) gene. Strong evidence for the activity of COX-2 inhibitors in the treatment and prevention of FAP has been demonstrated in mouse models and, more recently, human patients. In a recent double-blind, placebo-controlled study, 77 patients with FAP received Celebrex, a COX-2 inhibitor, 100 mg or 400 mg twice daily or placebo for 6 months. Patients who received 400 mg twice daily had a 28% reduction in the mean number of colorectal polyps and a 31% reduction in polyp burden, or the sum of polyp diameters. Based on these studies, trials to assess the prevention of adenoma development in adolescents with preclinical FAP will be needed.

Fiber in the prevention of colon cancer has been examined in several studies. The Polyp Prevention Trial studied 2079 patients with a history of colorectal adenomas randomized to receive counseling, a low-fat, high-fiber diet rich in fruits and vegetables, or to continue their current diet without counseling. Colonoscopy after 1 and 4 years found no difference in the incidence of recurrent adenomas. Another study by the Phoenix Colon Cancer Prevention Physician's Network studied 1429 patients with a history of colorectal adenoma. These patients were randomized to receive supplemental wheat bran, 2.0 or 13.5 g a day. Again, no difference in the incidence of recurrent adenomas was found between the two groups. Currently, there is no prospective evidence that fiber supplementation is effective for colorectal cancer prevention.

Calcium salts are available in several forms (gluconate, citrate, and carbonate). Randomized trials testing the effects of calcium as a chemopreventive agent have used cellular proliferation rates within colonic mucosal crypts as an index of response in resected colon cancer patients. Three of the four randomized trials performed to date have shown an increase in cellular proliferation rates within colonic mucosal crypts as an index of response in resected colon cancer patients. Three of the four randomized trials performed to date have shown an increase in cellular proliferation with calcium treatment. A randomized, double-blind trial tested the effect of dietary supplementation with calcium carbonate in 930 patients with a recent history of colorectal adenomas. The calcium carbonate-treated group was found to have a lower risk of recurrent adenoma. The results of this study, which were modestly significant, continue to support the investigation of calcium carbonate as a possible chemopreventive agent. If calcium is found to be an effective treatment in colorectal cancer chemoprevention, then intermediate end points other than cellular proliferation will be needed for future trials.

4. Skin Trials

Chemoprevention of skin cancer has been reported in two large trials using selenium and retinols. The objective of the selenium study was to determine whether supplemental selenium would decrease the incidence of cancer, specifically basal cell and squamous cell carcinomas of the skin. This multicenter, double-blind, randomized trial evaluated 1312 patients ages 18–80 years having a history of skin cancer who were given 200 μg of selenium (0.5 g high selenium brewer's yeast tablet) or placebo daily. Selenium had no effect on skin cancer incidence. However, secondary end point analyses revealed that selenium supplementation was associated with significantly lower incidences of total nonskin cancer and total nonskin and overall cancer mortality rates. In addition, lung cancer, prostate cancer, and colon cancer incidences were significantly reduced. Future trials will test the efficacy of selenium in lung and with α-tocopherol in prostate cancer.

Retinoids have demonstrated activity in the reversal of actinic keratoses, a premalignant skin disorder. Trials have tested either topical tretinoin or various retinoids given systemically. Small-scale trials in patients at high risk for skin cancers such as xeroderma pigmentosa or in renal transplant patients have shown that prolonged treatment with high-dose isotretinoin or etretinate reduced the incidence of invasive skin cancers. In a phase III trial, 2297 patients who were at a lower risk for skin cancer, including patients with actinic keratoses, received oral retinol (25,000 IU) or placebo daily for 5 years. Retinol treatment was effective in reducing the incidence of squamous cell skin cancer, but not basal cell carcinoma. However, in patients with a prior skin cancer, three phase III trials that tested the effects of retinol, β-carotene, and low-dose isotretinoin demonstrated that these retinoids had no effect on the incidence of SPTs. Further studies are needed to validate the effects of these agents in skin and other cancers.

5. Breast Trials

Like UADT and lung cancers, breast cancer provides a model to study the effects of chemopreventive agents. Chemoprevention strategies in breast cancer target the development of SPTs, which occur at a rate of 0.8% per year, as well as preventing breast cancer in high-risk patients. Pooled data from over 40 randomized adjuvant trials revealed that tamoxifen, given over prolonged periods, reduces the incidence of SPTs by 39% in postmenopausal women who have undergone resection. Observing that tamoxifen reduced the incidence of contralateral breast cancer when used as adjuvant therapy, investigators hypothesized that a possible benefit could exist in the prevention of breast cancer in high-risk patients. This initiated several large studies, including the U.S. Breast Cancer Prevention Trial (BCPT) or NSABP P-1 (National Surgical Adjuvant Breast and Bowel Project) trial that was launched in 1992. They studied 13,388 patients who were at increased risk for breast cancer: greater than age 60 years, elevated Gail assessment in those aged 35–59 years, and patients with a history of lobular carcinoma *in situ*. Patients were randomized to take tamoxifen or placebo for 5 years. This trial was stopped early and unblinded after interim analysis results demonstrated a 50% reduction in new tumors. Two other studies, the Royal Marsden Hospital (RMH) Tamoxifen Chemoprevention Trial with 2494 patients and the Italian Tamoxifen Prevention Trial with 5408 patients, are still blinded because preliminary results did not indicate a reduction in breast cancer incidence. The Italian study, a multicenter, double-blind, placebo-controlled trial, evaluated the effect of taking tamoxifen for 5 years in healthy women. The RMH study included women age 30 to 70 years with a family history of breast cancer.

Another trial, MORE, is studying 3 years of treatment with raloxifene to prevent osteoporosis. It too has reported a reduction in breast cancer incidence in women taking raloxifene. Currently, the NSABP-P2 or STAR (Study of Tamoxifen and Raloxifene) is ongoing in the United States. It will enroll tens of thousands of patients to help determine whether a difference exists in treatment between the two drugs. Raloxifene is another type of SERM, which binds with high affinity to estrogen receptors and preliminarily has shown a marked effect on estrogen receptor-positive tumors. The final results of these trials are still pending.

Fenretinide, a synthetic vitamin A derivative, has been studied in breast cancer since 1979. A phase III trial initiated in 1987 randomized 2972 women with a history of stage I breast cancer to receive 200 mg of fenretinide daily or no intervention for 5 years in an attempt to reduce contralateral breast cancer. Although no significant difference was found between the two groups after a median of 8 years, there was a trend for benefit in premenopausal women. This has led to a current trial studying the effect of tamoxifen and fenretinide in premenopausal women at increased risk for breast cancer.

Other strategies for chemoprevention trials in breast cancer include studying the effects of lutenizing hormone-releasing hormone (LHRH) agonists in high-risk premenopausal women as well as aromatase inhibitors in postmenopausal women.

6. Esophageal/Gastric Trials

Esophageal carcinoma has been associated with tobacco and alcohol exposure in the United States and with nutrient deficiencies and exposure to N-nitrous compounds in China. Randomized chemoprevention studies in China, which tested the effects of combinations of agents such as retinol, riboflavin, zinc, and vitamin E, have revealed a reduction in micronuclei frequency but not in the incidence of premalignant lesions in the esophagus. A cooperative study with the United States in Linxian, China, studied the effects of one of four combinations of vitamins/minerals for 5 years (retinol and zinc, riboflavin and niacin, vitamin C, molybdenum and β-carotene, vitamin E and selenium). No statistically significant relationships were correlated with the intervention. However, in secondary analysis, selenium, β-carotene, and vitamin E use was associated with a statistically significant lower mortality rate in all cancers, predominantly gastric cancer. No effect was seen with esophageal cancer. The interpretation of these studies is made difficult by the use of readily available vitamin supplements in the control arm, blurring potential differences from the treatment arm. This represents an inherent flaw in trials utilizing vitamin supplements and dietary intervention.

Other trials include examining the effects of vitamin/mineral supplementation in patients with esophageal dysplasia; 3,318 patients with defined histologic evidence received treatment for 6 years and demonstrated lowered mortality as well as a reduced risk of esophageal or gastric dysplasia. Other trials currently ongoing are comparing gastric dysplasia and treatment of Helicobacter pylori and chronic atrophic gastritis with oltipraz treatment.

7. Bladder Trials

Previous studies using retinoids to prevent recurrence and SPTs in bladder cancer patients have been small and limited by high toxicity. Two trials with prolonged low-dose etretinate appeared to have some effect. One double-blind, placebo-controlled trial studied 30 patients with superficial bladder tumors and the preventive effect of etretinate. A reduction in recurrence was seen in the treated group. Another trial, which was multicenter and randomized, evaluated 79 patients with superficial papillary bladder tumors with 25 mg of etretinate or placebo daily. Time to first recurrence was similar in the two groups; however, the interval to subsequent tumor recurrence was significantly longer in the treated group. Some mild toxicity was experienced in these trials and, although small, indicate beneficial effects of retinoids in prevention. Better tolerated retinoids such as fenretinide are being used in ongoing bladder cancer trials, and combinations of these with other treatment modalities, such as intravesical chemotherapy, NSAIDs, and oltipraz, are under investigation.

8. Cervical Trials

Cervical cancer has well-recognized premalignant dysplastic stages that are accessible for study. Interferon, folic acid, β-carotene, and retinoids have been used in the treatment of cervical dysplasia, and only retinoids have yielded positive results. Nutritional studies have helped define micronutrients of interest (folate, carotenoids, vitamin C, vitamin E). Other interesting medications under evaluation include retinoids [4-hydroxyphenylretinamide (4-HPR), retinyl acetate gel, topical all-trans retinoic acid], polyamine synthesis inhibitors [α-difluoromethylornithine (DFMO)], and nonsteroidal anti-inflammatory drugs (ibuprofen). Phase I chemoprevention studies of the cervix have tested retinyl acetate gel and all-trans retinoic acid. Topical all-trans retinoic acid has been shown to increase the histological regression rate in women with moderate cervical intraepithelial hyperplasia (CIN 2). Phase II trials of all-*trans* retinoic acid, β-carotene, and folic acid have been and are being carried out, whereas phase III trials of all-*trans* retinoic acid have been completed and have shown significant regression of CIN 2 but not CIN 3. Clearly, further studies are warranted to formulate chemoprevention strategies in cervical cancer.

9. Prostate Trials

Chemoprevention in prostate cancer is a relatively new area of research. The Prostate Cancer Prevention Trial (PCPT) was launched in 1993 with its principle end point being a reduction of biopsy-proven prostate cancer incidence. Patients included 18,882 males age 55 years and older who are received finasteride, 5-α-reductase inhibitor, 5 mg or placebo daily for 7 years. The trial is still blinded and will achieve its primary end point in 2004. Selenium and vitamin E have been observed to decrease prostate cancer incidence in several trials. Therefore, the National Cancer Institute will launch a trial entitled "SELECT." This phase III trial will enroll more than 32,000 men and assess prostate cancer prevention with selenium, vitamin E, selenium and vitamin E, and placebo. Results of this trial, which will last over 10 years, will help elucidate new strategies in prostate cancer chemoprevention.

10. Other Cancers

Studies of retinoids in other cancers such as hepatocellular carcinoma have been described as well. A prospective randomized study reported in 1996 studied 89 patients who were definitively treated for primary hepatoma. Patients received polyprenoic acid (600 mg daily) or placebo for 12 months. There was a significant decrease in recurrence as well as second primary hepatomas in the retinoid-treated group. At 38 months, 27% of treated patients had recurrence or SPT versus 49% in the placebo group ($P = 0.04$). Further studies are needed to verify these encouraging results.

VI. FUTURE DIRECTIONS

A. Risk Models

Treatment of epithelial malignancies is moving toward prevention. Since the early 1980s, many patients at high risk for epithelial cancers, mostly those with premalignant lesions or a history of epithelial malignancy, have been enrolled in chemoprevention trials. While this accounts for a substantial number of patients, the vast majority of epithelial malignancies arise in patients with no history of either of these risk factors. This population is, at present, unrecognizable and is therefore not entering chemoprevention trials. While this accounts for a substantial number of patients, the vast majority of epithelial malignancies arise in patients with no history of either of these risk factors. This population is, at present, unrecognizable and is therefore not entering chemoprevention trials. This points out the need to develop a risk model to use in identifying high-risk people from the general population.

Developing a risk model will require the identification of markers that will predict the likelihood of cancer development. Ongoing research will determine the cancer risks associated with the presence of premalignant epithelial lesions and the genetic abnormalities they contain. These studies will be advanced by improved techniques in the diagnosis of premalignant epithelial foci. Spectroscopic analysis of epithelial tissues performed at endoscopy can differentiate normal, dysplastic, and malignant areas. This technique is based on fluorescent emission spectra of epithelial cells following laser excitation and this reflects differences between normal and malignant cells in their endogenous flavins, riboflavins, and other fluorophors. These endoscopic techniques will aid in the identification and acquisition of premalignant tissue for histologic and genotypic analyses. By using this technique, genetic events that are associated with malignant progression can be analyzed, including changes in chromosomal ploidy, micronuclei, proliferation antigens, point mutations in ras and p53, amplification of the myc or erbB-2 genes, and deletions incorporating these markers into ongoing chemoprevention trials in patients with prior malignancies, clinical correlation will reveal the power of these markers to predict the likelihood of an SPT. To determine whether these variables can be used in a model to predict cancer risk among the general population with no history of cancer, prospective studies must be performed. Because cancer risk among the general population is low, population sample size for these studies will be extremely large and will require years of clinical follow-up. Analysis of biopsy material and patient examinations will be extremely expensive to carry out. However, these studies are necessary to the construction of a framework on which chemoprevention trials can be built. Not until high-risk patients are identified can potential chemopreventive agents be tested.

B. Intermediate End Points

Work is underway to identify cellular and molecular markers that change during chemopreventive treatment and correlate with a treatment-induced reduction in cancer incidence. Intracellular pathways activated or inhibited by chemopreventive agents offer potential intermediate markers of response. Of the pathways known to be important in mediating the effects of chemopreventive agents, the retinoid pathway is the best characterized. Cytoplasmic and nuclear retinoid receptors are key elements of retinoid signal transduction. *In vitro* studies have shown that the expression of RARs is activated within hours of retinoid treatment. A growing body of evidence reveals that the activated expression of specific RARs is crucial to the process of retinoid-induced tumor differentiation. For example, in P19 murine teratocarcinoma cells, retinoid refractoriness correlates with aberrant RAR-α expression. The mechanism by which retinoids induce tumor differentiation may be different from that of their chemopreventive effects. Growth inhibition, apoptosis, reversal of dysplasia, and stabilization of the DNA damage process are potential mechanisms of retinoid actions. In acute promyelocytic leukemia patients, tretinoin induces differentiation of promyelocytic cells within weeks. The minimum duration of retinoid treatment necessary to prevent epithelial cancers is not known. If months of treatment are required, then events other than receptor activation may be necessary for retinoid-induced chemoprevention. In addition to retinoid receptors, specific growth factors, their receptors, and carbohydrate antigens have been shown to be modulated by retinoid treatment *in vitro* and may be important in mediating retinoid effects in epithelial cells. Previous studies have shown that retinoid treatment downregulates the expression of transforming growth factor α, epidermal growth factor receptor, and fibroblast growth factor-4. To examine the roles

of these and other biological events as potential intermediate markers for chemoprevention trials, prospective clinical studies that correlate treatment-induced changes in these cellular components with clinical outcome are needed.

Premalignant lesions are another source of intermediate end points. Phenotypic analysis of hyperplastic and dysplastic changes can be performed by light microscopy and immunostaining for proliferation antigens such as proliferating cell nuclear antigen and nuclear protein that binds the Ki-67 antibody. Analysis of genetic changes associated with premalignancy offers a potentially more objective means of diagnosis. For example, mutations in p53 have been found in preneoplastic lesions associated with most epithelial cancers. Because mutations can occur over a large region of the p53 gene, a mutation at a specific site, involving an alteration to a specific nucleotide, may be considered a clonal marker. Thus, disappearance of a clonal marker during treatment with a chemopreventive agent could represent regression of a premalignant lesion and may have prognostic value. Work is underway to develop the ability to detect the presence of such clonal markers in sputum, urine, and stool. This will pave the way to testing their usefulness as intermediate markers in chemoprevention trials.

C. Chemopreventive Agents

There is a long list of potentially effective chemopreventive agents that await clinical trials. As shown in Table I, the list includes a broad range of compounds, including vitamins, minerals, antioxidants, anti-inflammatory agents, and steroid hormone antagonists. As single agents alone, these compounds will provide material for important clinical trials over at least the next decade.

Retinoids have undergone extensive development as chemopreventive agents. In addition to 13-cRA, another retinoic acid stereoisomer, 9-cRA, has been developed for clinical trials. 9-cRA is able to bind and activate both RAR and RXR receptor families. Because of its novel nuclear receptor affinities, *9-cis* RA may have biochemical effects that other retinoic acid stereoisomers do not have. In addition, synthetic retinoids have been developed that have receptor-specific activity. These agents may have greater efficacy than natural retinoids if particular receptors are implicated in epithelial carcinogenesis. One site in which this may prove true is UADT. RAR-β expression is lower in cancers in this region than in adjacent histologically normal mucosa. In UADT cancer patients, treatment with retinoic acid leads to a chemopreventive response that occurs in UADT cancer patients who have undergone resection. The mechanisms by which retinoids induce a chemopreventive effect in the UADT and lung are unknown, but insight was provided by *in vitro* experiments that showed that RAR-β appears to suppress cell growth. In a lung cancer cell line, overexpression of RAR-β through stable transfection led to a suppression of growth and tumorigenicity in nude mice. Thus, novel retinoids that target RAR-β may be more efficacious than other retinoids in UADT and lung cancer chemoprevention trials. Recently though, several studies have suggested an adverse effect of retinoids in current smokers producing a higher incidence of lung cancer. If RAR-β regulates growth in epithelial cells of the lung and UADT, then the RAR-β gene might be considered as a therapeutic agent in gene therapy trials in the future. The settings in which RAR-β might be most efficacious are unknown, but trials in lung cancer prevention should be considered. The rationale for its use in prevention trials rests on the observation that benign bronchial epithelial cells are more responsive to the growth suppressive effects of retinoids than lung cancer cells, suggesting that retinoid receptors may have greater biological activity in benign bronchial epithelium than in lung cancer cells. Trials such as these await the development of vectors that can safely and effectively deliver genes of interest to the target tissues.

Specific gene mutations found in premalignant lesions, such as ras and p53 point mutations, may offer additional opportunities for intervention at the molecular level. For example, posttranslational farnesylation of mutant ras is necessary for activation of its transforming properties. FTIs block the enzyme farnesyltransferase or its substrate, farnesyl. Although the technology to deliver efficiently peptides or proteins in clinical trials has not yet been developed, this is the goal of several ongoing studies. Similarly, *in vitro* studies suggest that changes in mutant p53 phosphorylation can induce wild-type p53 properties. Such an approach might be considered to restore p53 tumor suppressor activities within tumor cells.

Another direction in chemoprevention trials that may prove fruitful is combination therapy. Combining agents that mediate their effects through different pathways might enhance the ultimate chemopreventive effect. For example, agents that decrease the accumulation of intracellular-free radicals, such as oltipraz, might be combined with retinoids that activate a separate pathway, i.e., the modulation of cell growth and differentiation. Other agents have enhanced the effects of retinoids. In tumor differentiation models, for example, the effects of retinoids are augmented by agents such as phorbol esters or cyclic AMP, which activate protein kinase C (PKC) and protein kinase A, respectively. In a human teratocarcinoma cell line, activation of these kinases enhanced the effects of retinoic acid on RAR-β activation, demonstrating coupling of these kinase pathways with retinoid receptors. In addition to retinoid receptors, another mechanism through which retinoids and kinases might couple is transforming growth factor-β (TGF-β). Intracellular TGF-β production is increased by either retinoic acid treatment or PKC activation. Thus, retinoid and protein kinase pathways converge on TGF-β. Transforming growth factor-β has been shown to induce profound growth suppression in many cell types. Studies that illuminate the convergence of different intracellular pathways by molecules that mediate growth suppression, such as retinoid receptors and TGF-β, provide a basis for combination therapy. Combination therapy might be used in the design of future chemoprevention trials. These trials might await the development of agents that interact with specific kinase pathways. One drug that should be considered in future chemoprevention trials is bryostatin, a PKC activator that is now entering phase I trials. Other agents that could potentially be effective preventive agents in high-risk patients because of their favorable side effect profiles include farnesyltransferase inhibitors, which inhibit ras, monoclonal antibodies and small molecules such as tyrosine kinase inhibitors to epidermal growth factor or vascular endothelial growth factor. Cyclooxygenase of lipoxygenase inhibitors and other NSAIDs need to be further studied as chemopreventive agents. Immunotherapy with interferon-α combinations is also under investigation. These agents all have promise in high-risk patients as primary prevention agents or in the adjuvant setting.

VII. SUMMARY

Since the mid-1980s, the goal of treatment for epithelial cancers has begun to shift from the eradication of metastatic disease to the prevention of cancer. Along these lines, advancements have been made in the prevention of UADT cancer by treatment with retinoids as well as the use of tamoxifen in breast cancer and targeting COX-2 in FAP colon cancer. Further advances in epithelial cancer prevention await the development of cancer risk models and intermediate markers that can be incorporated into the design of chemoprevention trials. These needs may be met through advancements in our understanding of genetic events that occur during epithelial carcinogenesis, such as point mutations of ras and p53. Pathways activated or inhibited by chemopreventive agents may offer additional intermediate markers of response, including retinoid receptor expression, which increases following retinoid treatment, epidermal growth factor, and cyclooxygenase. Prospective phase III clinical trials are necessary to examine these possibilities and to establish eventually chemoprevention strategies as standard of care in health policy.

See Also the Following Articles

CHEMOPREVENTION, PRINCIPLES OF • COLORECTAL CANCER: MOLECULAR AND CELLULAR ABNORMALITIES • HEAD AND NECK CANCER • LUNG CANCER: MOLECULAR AND CELLULAR ABNORMALITIES • MOLECULAR EPIDEMIOLOGY AND CANCER RISK • MULTISTAGE CARCINOGENESIS

Bibliography

Bollag, G., and McCormick, F. (1992). GTPase activating proteins. *Semin. Cancer Biol.* **3**, 199–208.

Brison, O. (1993). Gene amplification and tumor progression. *Biochim. Biophys. Acta* **1155**, 25–41.

Cho, K. R., and Vogelstein, B. (1992). Suppressor gene alterations in the colorectal adenoma-carcinoma sequence. *J. Cell. Biochem.* **16G,** 137–141.

Decensi, A., and Costa, A. (2000). Recent advances in cancer chemoprevention, with emphasis on breast and colorectal cancer. *Eur. J. Cancer* **36,** 694–709.

Fisher, B., Costantino, J. P., Wickerham, D. L., *et al.* (1998). Tamoxifen for prevention of breast cancer: Report of the National Surgical Adjuvant Breast and Bowel Project P-1 Study. *J. Natl. Cancer Inst.* **90,** 1371–1388.

Harris, C. C., and Hollstein, M. (1993). Clinical implications of the p53 tumor-suppressor gene. *N. Engl. J. Med.* **329,** 1318–1326.

Hong, W. K. (2000). Chemoprevention in the 21st century: Genetics, risk modeling, and molecular targets. David A. Karnofsky Memorial Award Lecture, *J. Clin. Oncol.* **18**(21 suppl.), 95–185.

Hong, W. K., and Sporn, M. B. (1997). Recent advances in chemoprevention of cancer. *Science* **278**(5340), 1073–1077.

Hong, W. K., Lippman, S. M., Itri, L. M., *et al.* (1990). Prevention of second primary tumors with isotretinoin in squamous-cell carcinoma of the head and neck. *N. Engl. J. Med.* **323**(12), 795–801.

Kim, E. S., Hong, W. K., and Khuri, F. R. (2000). Prevention of lung cancer: The new millennium. *Chest Surg. Clin. North Am.* **10**(4), 663–690.

Lippman, S. M., Brenner, S. E., and Hong, W. K. (1994). Cancer chemoprevention. *J. Clin. Oncol.* **12,** 851–873.

Lippman, S. M., Lee, J. J., Karp, D. D., *et al.* (2001). Phase-III intergroup trial of isotretinoin to prevent second primary tumors in stage-I non-small-cell lung cancer. *J. Natl. Cancer Inst.* **93**(8), 605–618.

Lippman, S. M., Lee, J. J., and Sabichi A. L. (1998). Cancer chemoprevention: Progress and promise. *J. Natl. Cancer Inst.* **90**(20), 1514–1528.

Sabichi, A. L., Lerner, S. P., Grossman H. B., and Lippman, S. M. (1998). Retinoids in chemoprevention of bladder cancer. *Curr. Opin. Oncol.* **10,** 479–484.

van Zandwijk. N., Dalesio, O., Pastorino, U., *et al.* (2000). EUROSCAN, a randomized trial of vitamin A and N-acetylcysteine in patients with head and neck cancer or lung cancer. For the European Organization for Research and Treatment of Cancer Head and Neck and Lung Cancer Cooperative Groups. *J. Natl. Cancer Inst.* **92**(12); 977–986.

Weinberg, R. (1991). Tumor suppressor genes. *Science* **254,** 1138–1146.

Chemotherapy: Synergism and Antagonism

Ting-Chao Chou

Memorial Sloan-Kettering Cancer Center

I. Combination Chemotherapy of Cancer
II. General Equation for Dose–Effect Analyses
III. Quantitation of Synergism and Antagonism
IV. Data Analysis for Synergism and Antagonism
V. Mechanism of Synergism and Antagonism

GLOSSARY

additive effect (CI = 1) the combined effect predicted by the mass-action law principle.

antagonism (CI > 1) the production of smaller than expected additive effect.

augmentation another term for potentiation.

combination index (CI) A quantitative measure of the degree of drug interaction for a given endpoint of the effect measurement.

dose-reduction index (DRI) A measure of how much the dose of each drug in a synergist combination may be reduced at a given effect level compared with the doses of each drug alone.

enhancement Another term for potentiation.

isobologram (ED$_{50}$-isobol, ED$_{75}$-isobol, ED$_{90}$-isobol, etc.) a graph indicating the equipotent combinations of various doses; it can be used to illustrate additism, synergism, or antagonism.

median-effect dose (D_m) the dose that produces 50% effect such as ED$_{50}$, IC$_{50}$, LD$_{50}$, IC$_{50}$, or LD$_{50}$. It is a potency parameter and is obtained from the x-intercept of the median-effect plot.

median-effect equation $f_a/f_u = (D/D_m)^m$, a general equation for dose–effect relationship derived from the mass-action law principle that takes into account both the potency (D_m) and the shape (m) of dose–effect curve, where f_a and f_u are the fractions affected and unaffected, respectively.

potentiation A condition in which one of two drugs is not effective by itself, but increases the effect of the other drug.

synergism (CI < 1) the production of a greater than expected additive effect.

therapeutic index (TI) A measure of selectivity of effect representing the ratio of the median-effect doses for toxicity in relation to that of the therapeutic effect.

Combination therapy with multiple drugs or with multiple modalities is common practice in the treatment of cancer. When anticancer agents with similar or different modes of actions are combined, the outcome can be synergistic, additive, or antagonistic. Depending on the shapes of the dose–effect curves for each drug, mixed outcomes may ensue at different doses or different effect levels. Selective synergism against tumor may increase therapeutic efficacy, decrease toxicity toward the host due to dose reduction, and minimize or delay the development of drug resistance due to less selective pressure at a lower dose required for a given effect.

I. COMBINATION CHEMOTHERAPY OF CANCER

A. Goals of Drug Combinations

The improved end results of combination chemotherapy in cancer frequently cannot be predicted from mechanisms of actions or modes of actions alone and the conclusions obtained *in vitro* not always can be extrapolated to *in vivo* or in human. However, *in vitro* analyses have the advantage of flexibility, accuracy, rapidity, and economic features that allow quantitative assessment of synergism, additive effect, or antagonism under various conditions.

Presently used clinical protocols for cancer combination therapy are still mainly obtained empirically and from comparison of statistics. Accumulation of experience in clinical settings is invaluable but is a slow and expensive process, and rational design of protocols through *in vitro* prospective studies is an important development.

B. Pitfalls in Synergy Interpretation

There are several pitfalls in evaluating synergism or antagonism in drug combination. Contrary to what is often presumed, an additive effect (i.e., in the absence of synergism or antagonism) is not the simple arithmetic sum of the effect of two drugs. For example, if a given cancer treatment of drug 1 and drug 2 each inhibits a biological system 50 and 60%, respectively, the combined effect (if additive) cannot be 110% inhibition since it exceeds 100%. Furthermore, calculation of the additive effect by the fractional product method of Webb may also lead to erroneous conclusions. By using Webb's method, for example, the above case is calculated by $[1 - (f_a)_{1,2}] = [1 - (f_a)_1] [1 - (f_a)_2]$, thus $[1 - (f_a)_{1,2}] = (1 - 0.5) (1 - 0.6) = 0.2$ and, therefore, $(f_a)_{1,2} = 1 - 0.2 = 0.8$ which indicates the combined inhibition of 80%. The pitfall is that this calculation does not take into account the shape(s) of the dose–effect curves of each drug. As is well known, hyperbolic- and sigmoidal-shaped curved can make a great difference in the outcome of drug combination but in the above calculation, it is ignored.

In clinical studies, the term "therapeutic synergy" is used when two drugs in combination produce a therapeutic effect (e.g., complete remission of cancer) greater than the result of each drug alone. In this case, both the therapeutic end result and the toxicity to the host are simultaneously considered. Although potency is taken into account, the shapes of dose–effect curves are ignored. This type of clinical evaluation is frequently nonquantitative due to limitations in the patient settings where endpoints of measurement are subjective or when the dose–effect relationship parameters are not available. Therefore, therapeutic synergy is often an issue of selectivity of effects (i.e., efficacy vs toxicity) rather than the issue of synergism. Therapeutic synergy may be a result of real synergy, an additive effect, or even a moderate antagonistic effect when there are nonoverlapping toxicities of two drugs.

Combination treatment protocols vary greatly for different cancers. Hodgkin's disease, for example, utilizes the well-known regimen MOPP [mechlorethamine, vincristine (Oncovin), procarbazine, and prednisone]. Therapy for non-Hodgkin's lymphomas, for example, employs CVP (cyclophosphamide, vincristine, and prednisone) and many alternative regimens which may include doxorubicin (adriamycin), etoposide, methotrexate, or cytarabine. Sequential combination therapy with methotrexate and 5-fluorouracil has been widely used in the treatment of adenocarcinoma of the gastrointestinal tract, breast, and head and neck carcinoma. Biochemical modulation of 5-fluorouracil with leucovorin, trimetrexate, triazinate, dipyridamole, phosphonacetyl-L-aspartic acid (PALA), and hydroxyurea is also under study.

II. GENERAL EQUATION FOR DOSE–EFFECT ANALYSES

A. The Median-Effect Equation of the Mass-Action Law

In order to have an equation that is generally applicable in dose–effect analysis, it is essential that the equation has a sound theoretical basis, e.g., not empirically obtained but explicitly derived from physical-chemical models. In addition, for flexibility, the equation should be mechanism nonspecific since the detailed mechanisms of most drugs are unknown. The general equation for dose–effect analysis was derived during 1974–1976 by Chou using enzyme kinetic models. By taking the ratios of reaction velocities in the presence and absence of the inhibitors of various types of inhibition (competitive, noncompetitive, and uncompetitive) and on various reaction mechanisms (e.g., sequential, ordered, ping-pong, random) with one to n substrates and/or products. After canceling out kinetic constants, the median-effect equation was obtained which was given by

$$f_a/f_u = (D/D_m)^m, \qquad (1)$$

where D is the dose (or concentration) of a drug, f_a is the fraction affected by D (percentage inhibition/ 100), and f_u is the fraction unaffected (i.e., $f_u = 1 - f_a$). D_m is the median-effect dose (ED_{50} or IC_{50}) that inhibits the system under study by 50% and m is the coefficient signifying the shape of the dose–effect relationship, where $m = 1$, >1, and <1 indicate hyperbolic, sigmoidal, and negative sigmoidal dose–effect curves, respectively, for an inhibitory drug. These and other glossaries are given in Table I. Equation (1) is the simplest possible form for relating the dose (right side) and the effect (left side) deduced from several hundred equations derived from the mass-action law models. Rearranging Eq. (1) gives

$$D = D_m \left[f_a/(1 - f_a) \right]^{1/m} \qquad (2)$$

and

$$f_a = 1/[1 + (D_m/D)^m]. \qquad (3)$$

Therefore, the dose and the effect are interchangeable since the dose (D) for any given degree of effect (f_a) in Eq. (2), can be determined if D_m and m values are known. Likewise, in Eq. (3), the effect (f_a) for any given dose (D) can be determined if D_m and m values are known.

B. The Median-Effect Plot

For x percentage inhibition, the dose D is designated as D_x. The D_m and m values are readily determined by the median-effect plot, $x = \log (D)$ vs $y = \log (f_a/f_u)$, which is based on the logarithmic form of Eq. (1) as defined by Chou:

$$\log (f_a/f_u) = m \log D - m \log D_m, \qquad (4)$$

where m is the slope and $\log (D_m)$ is the x-intercept of the median-effect plot. Equation (4) has the form of classical straight line equation $y = m_x + b$. The conformity of the data to the median-effect plot can be readily manifested by the linear correlation coefficient (r) of the median-effect plot in which $r = 1$ indicates perfect conformity.

III. QUANTITATION OF SYNERGISM AND ANTAGONISM

The observed experimental effect if greater or smaller than the expected additive effect is then termed synergism or antagonism, respectively. If the definition of an additive effect is not clear, then the attempt to determine synergism or antagonism will be in vain or can be erroneous. The derived equations for multidrug combination defines the expected additive effect.

The isobologram concept for graphical representation of the concentrations of two drugs that produce the same effect (iso effect) was extensively discussed by Loewe and others in the 1950s. However, the theoretical basis was not clearly defined until its equation was explicitly derived from the mass-action law principle in the early 1980s. The usefulness and limitations of the isobologram can now be defined and its construction can be readily carried out with or without the use of a microcomputer, as will be shown later in this article.

The fractional product method for predicting an additive effect was introduced by Webb in 1963. This method is simple, but without knowing its limitations it can be easily misused. This method indicates

$$[1 - (f_a)_{1,2}] = [1 - (f_a)_1] [1 - (f_a)_2]. \qquad (5)$$

Thus, based on Eq. (5), if drug 1 inhibits 50% and drug 2 inhibits 60%, then the combined additive effect should be 80% inhibition since $[1 - 0.5] [1 - 0.6] = 0.20$ and $1 - 0.2 = 0.8$. The limitations of this method are twofold. First, it does not take into account the shape of dose–effect curves (e.g., sigmoidal and hyperbolic). Second, it is valid only for two drugs that have hyperbolic dose–effect curves (i.e., Michaelis–Menten type but not Hill type) and the effects of two drugs should be totally independent (i.e., mutually nonexclusive) as described later. Therefore, the applicability of Webb's method is severely limited.

A. Combination Index-Isobologram Equation

Based on systematic analysis of various combinations involving two drugs in enzyme kinetic systems, Chou and Talalay derived the classical isobologram equations as

$$\frac{(D)_1}{(D_x)_1} + \frac{(D)_2}{(D_x)_2} = 1 \qquad (6)$$

for two drugs and

$$\sum_{j=1}^{n} \frac{(D)_j}{(D_x)_j} = 1 \qquad (7)$$

for multiple drugs (n drugs).

Using the median-effect principle as shown by Eq. (2), $(D_x)_1$, $(D_x)_2$, or $(D_x)_n$ in the denominators can be readily calculated, and $(D)_1$, $(D)_2$, $(D)_2 \ldots (D)_n$ in the numerator are the experimental doses of each drug alone that in combination also produce $x\%$ inhibition.

For determination of degrees of synergism or antagonism, the combination index (CI) was introduced where

$$CI = \frac{(D)_1}{(D_x)_1} + \frac{(D)_2}{(D_x)_2} \qquad (8a)$$

for two drugs, and

$$CI = \sum_{j=1}^{n} \frac{(D)_j}{(D_x)_j} \qquad (8b)$$

for n drugs. For both Eq. (8a) and Eq. (8b), CI <1, = 1, and >1 indicate synergism, an additive effect, and antagonism, respectively.

It should be noted that Eqs. (5–7) are derived based on the assumption that each drug in the combination has the same or similar mode of action (i.e., mutually exclusive). For two drugs that act totally independently (i.e., mutually nonexclusive), the isobol or CI equation becomes

$$CI = \frac{(D)_1}{(D_x)_1} + \frac{(D)_2}{(D_x)_2} + \frac{(D)_1(D)_2}{(D_x)_1(D_x)_2}. \qquad (9)$$

It has been shown earlier that when both drugs have hyperbolic dose–effect curves (i.e., $m = 1$) and when CI = 1, Eq. (9) and Eq. (5) become identical. Equation (9) depicts a conservative isobologram when it is set to be 1 (unity). Since the equation is the sum of three terms instead of two terms for two drugs [e.g., Eq. (8a)], the equation is termed a conservative isobologram equation.

B. Computerized Determination of Combination Index and Simulation of F_a–CI Plot

Synergism or antagonism can be most efficiently presented in the form of a CI table since it is quantitative and a condensed form of information. It can also be presented in two versions of graphics. The isobologram is dose oriented and the combination index plot (F_a–CI plot) is effect oriented. Both yield identical conclusions. A f_a–CI plot shows a combination index (synergism or antagonism) at all effect levels whereas an isobol plot shows synergism or antagonism at several effect levels (e.g., ED_{50}, ED_{70}, ED_{90}, etc.). Isobols may be visually too complex if more than three effect levels are used.

A specific example of data analysis will be given later. The algorithm for computerized simulation of synergism and antagonism of two drugs D_1 and D_2 with f_a equals to $x\%$ inhibition singly, and also in combination, is shown below where $(D_x)_{1,2} = (D)_1 + (D)_2$ and $(D)_1/(D)_2 = P/Q$:

$$CI = \frac{(D)_1}{(D_x)_1} + \frac{(D)_2}{(D_x)_2} + \frac{\alpha(D)_1(D)_2}{(D_x)_1(D_x)_2}.$$

Therefore,

$$CI = \frac{(D_x)_{1,2}[P/(P + Q)]}{(D_m)_1\{(f_{a_x})_1/[1 - (f_{a_x})_1]\}^{1/m_1}}$$

$$+ \frac{(D_x)_{1,2}[Q/(P + Q)]}{(D_m)_2\{(f_{a_x})_2/[1 - (f_{a_x})_2]\}^{1/m_2}} \quad (10)$$

$$+ \frac{\alpha[(D_x)_{1,2}]^2[P/(P + Q)][Q/(P + Q)]}{(D_m)_1\{(f_{a_x})_1/[1 - (f_{a_x})_1]\}^{1/m_1}(D_m)_2\{(f_{a_x})_2/[1 - (f_{a_x})_2]\}^{1/m_2}},$$

where $(D_x)_{1,2} = \{(f_{a_x})_{1,2}/[1 - (f_{a_x})_{1,2}]\}^{1/m_{1,2}}[(D_m)_{1,2}]$ and $(f_{a_x})_1 = (f_{a_x})_2 = (f_{a_x})_{1,2}$ (i.e., isoeffective).

For mutually exclusive drugs, $\alpha = 0$
For mutually nonexclusive drugs, $\alpha = 1$
Diagnosis: CI = 1, additive; CI < 1, synergistic; and
    CI > 1, antagonistic.

C. Computerized Construction of Isobols

For the construction of isobologram, the denominator for Eq. (6) can be readily obtained from Eq. (2). For more than three drug combinations, n drug can be partitioned into:

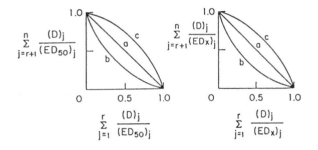

D. Dose-Reduction Index

A synergistic drug combination allows the possibility of achieving a given effect with lower doses of each drug. Consequently, toxicity toward the host may be avoided or reduced when the dose is reduced. This is of particular significance since nearly all cancer chemotherapeutic agents have strong side effects and their usefulness is limited by toxicities. The dose-reduction index is related to the combination index by

$$CI = \frac{(D)_1}{(D_x)_1} + \frac{(D)_2}{(D_x)_2} = \frac{1}{(DRI)_1} + \frac{1}{(DRI)_2}, \quad (11)$$

where $(DRI)_1 = (D_x)_1/(D)_1$ and $(DRI)_2 = (D_x)_2/(D)_2$.

DRI is a more restricted conditional constant than CI since DRI is not only influenced by the effect level selected but also by the combination ratio of drugs that have been selected.

E. Combination of More Than Two Drugs

For combinations of more than two drugs, inclusion of the assumption of the mutually nonexclusive mode of action makes the equation very complex. Since the exclusivity among drugs is frequently unknown, for simplicity and for consistence with the classical isobol concept it is suggested that CI be calculated based on the mutually exclusive assumption. This assumption should be clearly indicated in the analysis or when drawing synergism or antagonism conclusions.

IV. DATA ANALYSIS FOR SYNERGISM AND ANTAGONISM

A. Experimental Design

There are several basic requirements in experimental design for the determination of synergism or antagonism: (i) Each drug alone should have dose–effect relationships. Both potency (D_m) and shape (m) are essential for determining synergism or antagonism. If one of the two drugs has no effect by itself, then synergism/antagonism cannot be determined. Instead, potentiation (augmentation, enhancement) or inhibition (suppression) can be determined. (ii) In order to determine the potency and shape, at least three (or preferably more) data points are required for each drug alone. For combinations, in contrast, any number of data points can be used for CI calculations. (iii) The basic rule of mass-action law should be obeyed. The linear correlation coefficient of the median-effect plot should be reasonably good, e.g., $r > 0.90$ for *in vitro* experiments and $r > 80$ for *in vivo* experiments. Some drugs have biphasic mode of actions and others may have multimodality of effects. In some special cases an increase in dose may lead to a decrease in effect. These abnormalities yield a negative slope and contradict the mass-action law principle.

Conservation in experimental data points is particularly important for *in vivo* studies for economic reasons.

A constant ratio combination design at the IC_{50} ratio is recommended for the most efficient drug combination studies, which are usually arranged into a diagonal scheme as shown in Table I. However, serial dilutions of a combination mixture can be varied in any way, not necessarily corresponding to the single drug dilutions.

For three drug combinations, its is suggested that $D_1{:}D_2{:}D_3 = a{:}b{:}c$ *to be first selected so that a:b:c is approximated* to $(IC_{50})_1{:}(IC_{50})_2{:}(IC_{50})_3$. It is also suggested that two drug combinations for components drugs be carried out simultaneously so that single drug data can be shared and reused. Two drug combination ratios should correspond to three drug ratios so that

TABLE I
A Two Drug Combination with Cisplatin + Topotecan (10:1) on 833K Testicular Teratocarcinoma Cells in a 96-hr Incubation XTT Assay (from Chou *et al.*, 1994)

Data (μM) for Drug A:
  Cisplatin ($\bigcirc$)
    Number of data points: 6

Dose	Fraction affected
0.05	0.0554
0.10	0.2327
0.20	0.3005
0.50	0.5592
1.00	0.8214
2.00	0.9528

Calculations with standard error
X-intercept:	-0.49477 ± 0.00044
Y-intercept:	0.72152 ± 0.06135
Slope, m:	1.45830 ± 0.12271
D_m:	0.32006
r:	0.98613

Data (μM) for Drug B:
  Topotecan ($\square$)
    Number of data points: 6

Dose	Fraction affected
0.01	0.0686
0.02	0.2127
0.05	0.3726
0.10	0.7854
0.20	0.9396
0.50	0.9906

Calculations with standard error
X-intercept:	-1.33363 ± 0.01107
Y-intercept:	2.46366 ± 0.14291
Slope, m:	1.84733 ± 0.12249
D_m:	0.04638
r:	0.99132

Data for Mixture ($\triangle$)
  Ratio: 10:1
    Number of data points: 5

Dose	Fraction affected
0.055	0.3040
0.110	0.4130
0.220	0.6754
0.550	0.9240
1.100	0.9770

Calculations with standard error
X-intercept:	-0.93609 ± 0.02674
Y-intercept:	1.48631 ± 0.08280
Slope, m:	1.58779 ± 0.13380
D_m:	0.11585
r:	0.98952 $\longrightarrow$

The median-effect equation (Chou, 1976)

$$f_a/f_u = (D/D_m)^m$$
$$\downarrow$$
$$f_a = 1/[1 + (D_m/D)^m]$$

$m = 1$ Hyperbolic

$m > 1$ Sigmoidal

$m < 1$ Negative sigmoidal

[Shape]$\rightarrow$Sigmoidicity

[Potency]$\rightarrow$$IC_{50}$ (in the unit as specified above)

[Conformity]$\rightarrow$Linear correlation coefficient

(continues)

TABLE I—*Continued*

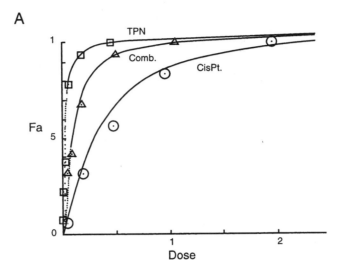

A

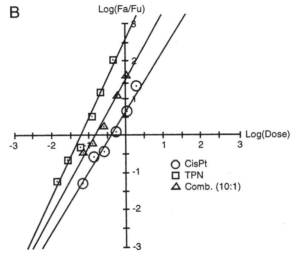

B

CI Values for a mixture of A and B in a 10:1 Ratio

F_a	Dose A	Dose B	CI exclusive	CI Nonexclusive
0.05	0.0164	0.0016	0.5629	0.6308
0.10	0.0264	0.0026	0.5590	0.6286
0.15	0.0353	0.0035	0.5573	0.6279
0.20	0.0439	0.0044	0.5564	0.6278
0.25	0.0527	0.0052	0.5559	0.6280
0.30	0.0617	0.0061	0.5557	0.6283
0.35	0.0713	0.0071	0.5556	0.6288
0.40	0.0815	0.0081	0.5556	0.6294
0.45	0.0928	0.0092	0.5558	0.6300
0.50	0.1053	0.0105	0.5561	0.6308
0.55	0.1195	0.0119	0.5565	0.6317

(continues)

TABLE I—*Continued*

F_a	Dose A	Dose B	CI exclusive	CI Nonexclusive
0.60	0.1359	0.0136	0.5570	0.6327
0.65	0.1555	0.0155	0.5577	0.6339
0.70	0.1795	0.0179	0.5585	0.6354
0.75	0.2103	0.0210	0.5597	0.6371
0.80	0.2521	0.0252	0.5612	0.6393
0.85	0.3140	0.0314	0.5633	0.6424
0.90	0.4202	0.0420	0.5668	0.6470
0.95	0.6728	0.0672	0.5737	0.6560
0.97	0.9403	0.0940	0.5797	0.6634
0.99	1.9027	0.1902	0.5954	0.6822

CI Values for Actual Experimental Points of a Mixture of Drug A
(Cisplatin) and Drug B (Topotecan) in a 10:1 Ratio

F_a	Dose A	Dose B	CI exclusive	CI Nonexclusive
0.304	0.05	0.005	0.4444	0.4910
0.413	0.10	0.010	0.6584	0.7621
0.6754	0.20	0.020	0.6680	0.7777
0.924	0.50	0.050	0.5605	0.6391
0.977	1.00	0.100	0.5222	0.5899

Dose Reduction Index Table

F_a	Dose A alone	Dose B alone	Dose reduction index	
			Drug A	Drug B
0.05	0.0425	0.0094	2.577	5.714
0.10	0.0709	0.0141	2.687	5.349
0.15	0.0974	0.0181	2.757	5.134
0.20	0.1237	0.0219	2.812	4.978
0.25	0.1506	0.0255	2.857	4.853
0.30	0.1790	0.0293	2.898	4.746
0.35	0.2093	0.0331	2.935	4.651
0.40	0.2423	0.0372	2.970	4.564
0.45	0.2789	0.0416	3.004	4.482
0.50	0.3200	0.0463	3.038	4.403
0.55	0.3672	0.0517	3.073	4.326
0.60	0.4226	0.0577	3.108	4.248
0.65	0.4893	0.0648	3.145	4.169
0.70	0.5722	0.0733	3.186	4.085
0.75	0.6798	0.0840	3.231	3.996
0.80	0.8281	0.0982	3.283	3.895
0.85	1.0515	0.1186	3.348	3.777
0.90	1.4440	0.1523	3.436	3.625
0.95	2.4105	0.2283	3.582	3.393
0.97	3.4709	0.3044	3.690	3.237
0.99	7.4766	0.5580	3.929	2.932

(continues)

TABLE I—*Continued*

Dose Reduction Indices for Actual Experimental Points of a Mixture of
Drug A (Cisplatin) and Drug B (Topotecan) in
a 10:1 Ratio

| | | | Dose reduction index | |
F_a	Dose A alone	Dose B alone	Drug A	Drug B
0.304	0.1813	0.0296	3.627	5.924
0.413	0.2515	0.0383	2.514	3.834
0.6754	0.5289	0.0689	2.644	3.448
0.924	1.7748	0.1793	3.549	3.586
0.977	4.1852	0.3529	4.185	3.529

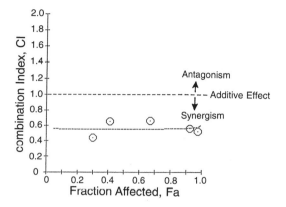

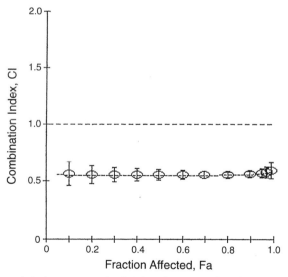

This graph is the computer-simulated combination index plot at
$f_a = 0.1, 0.2 \ldots 0.9, 0.95, 0.97,$ and 0.99 along with their mean ± 95%
confidence intervals. Confidence intervals (95%) are calculated by serial
deletion of data points (including no deletion) of the combinations ($n = 6$
steps of iterations). The linear correlation coefficient (r) of the median-
effect plot is the primary statistic. The 95% confidence interval of the
combination index is the secondary statistic.

(*continues*)

TABLE I—*Continued*

Effect level		Cisplatin (μM)	Topotecan (μM)	Mixture (10:1)
ED30.4	○	0.1813	0.0296	0.055
ED41.3	□	0.2515	0.0383	0.110
ED67.54	△	0.5289	0.0689	0.220
ED92.4	X	1.7748	0.1793	0.550
ED97.7	+	4.1852	0.3529	1.100

Normalized Isobolograms for the Following Effect Levels Will Be Generated

Normalized classical isobologram (A) and nonnormalized classical isobologram (B): Two versions of isobolograms using the same set of data and both based on mutually exclusive isobologram equation.

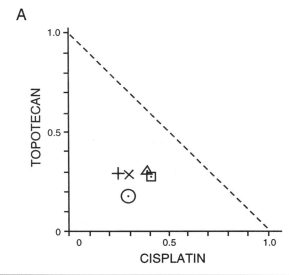

	ED50 ○	ED70 □	ED90 △
Drug A	.32006	.57223	1.44407
Drug B	.04638	.07338	.15238
Mixture Pt1	.11585	.19755	.46228

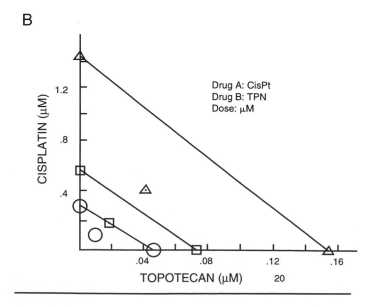

Drug A: CisPt
Drug B: TPN
Dose: μM

20

$D_1:D_2 = a:b$, $D_2:D_3 = b:c$, and $D_1:D_3 = a:c$. In this design the effect of D_1 on ($D_2 + D_3$), D_2 on ($D_1 + D_3$), and D_3 on ($D_1 + D_2$) can also be analyzed.

B. Example of Computerized Data Analysis

Experimental data for two drug combination using cisplatin (an alkylating agent) and topotecan (an inhibitor DNA topoisomerase I) are used for computerized synergism/antagonism analysis as shown in Table I. Dose–effect relationships of each drug alone or their combination (10:1 molar ratio) are obtained from studies of inhibition of 833K teratocarcinoma cell growth using a protein staining XTT assay carried out in 96-well microculture plates. Percentage inhibition is determined at the end of a 96-hr exposure to the drug(s).

V. MECHANISM OF SYNERGISM AND ANTAGONISM

A. Complexity in Synergism and Antagonism

It is no longer sufficient just to mention that two drugs are synergistic or antagonistic since they can be antagonistic at one effect level (e.g., at 50% inhibition) and synergistic at another effect level (e.g., at 90% inhibition). At one combination ratio they may be additive and at another combination ratio they may be antagonistic. Other factors such as treatment regimens, conditions factors (such as modulators, pH, oxygen tension, cell cycle transverse, and endpoint of measurement) may also affect synergistic or antagonistic outcomes. Each conclusion may be specific for particular experimental conditions. Furthermore, extrapolation of *in vitro* experimental results to *in vivo* therapy and extrapolation of animal data to human clinical situations require appropriate conservative predictions.

Quantitative drug combination studies are practical only *in vitro* and to a limited extent in animals. Human clinical data, due to heterogeneous patient populations, disease stage, previous treatments, end point of measurement, limited dose range, etc., usually cannot be used for quantitative synergy determinations. Therefore, in experimental design, it is im-

portant to control the route of administration, the desired plasma concentration range, and area under the concentration curve (AUC) in clinical situations.

B. Schedule Dependency

Because of differences in uptake, metabolism, onset or duration of action, pharmacokinetic behavior, and the mechanism of action of different drugs, simultaneous exposure with multiple drugs may yield a more desirable therapeutic result than a sequential order of drug exposure, e.g., D_1 preceding D_2 or vice versa, separated by a selected time interval. The degrees of synergism or antagonism (in CI values) can be determined under specified conditions as described earlier.

C. Combination Ratios

For initial *in vitro* studies it is suggested that equipotent concentrates of each drug at their IC_{50} values be used for drug combinations so that the contribution of effect of each drug would be about equal. In the case where a drug may produce severe toxicity (e.g., cardiotoxicity of adriamycin, renal toxicity of cisplatin, etc.), one may design a combination ratio that emphasizes one drug (e.g., high doses of arabinosylcytosine or methotrexate) and deemphasizes the other. Using different combination ratios in one experiment may yield different outcomes of synergism or antagonism (in CI values), although these differences are frequently not significant.

Instead of a diagonal scheme of design for a constant ratio of combinations, one may also use a checkerboard (Latin square) design which consists of several constant ratios. The optimal combination ratio of maximal synergy may be projected in large-scale experiments.

D. Selectivity of Synergism and Antagonism

Synergism against tumor target and antagonism toward host vulnerable host tissues (e.g., bone marrow and gut epithelium) would be ideal but such a desirable selectivity is difficult to obtain. If a drug combination is equally synergistic against the tumor and the host, the desirability of the drug combination may be

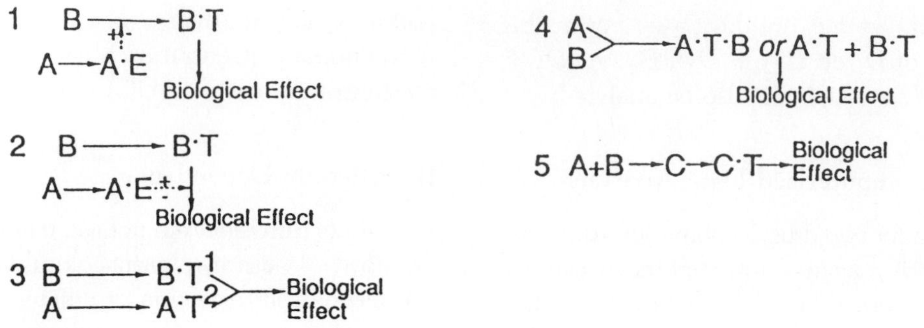

FIGURE 1 Examples of different classes of drug interactions. A, B, and C represent drugs in their final active form (e.g., vinblastine, ara-CTP, methotrexate polyglutamates); E is an effect macromolecule (e.g., nucleoside kinase, p-glycoprotein); T, T1, and T2 are target macromolecules or membranes (e.g., DNA, DNA topoisomerase, tubulin); and A · E and B · T, etc., are complexes (covalently or noncovalently bound). The dotted arrow and the ± symbol represent inhibition or enhancement of action.

canceled out. Various approaches may be use to exploit the safety window including the use of modulators (Fig. 1).

See Also the Following Articles

ESTROGENS AND ANTIESTROGENS • MALIGNANT MESOTHELIOMA • PURINE ANTIMETABOLITES • PYRIMIDINE ANTIMETABOLITES • RESISTANCE TO INHIBITOR COMPOUNDS OF THYMIDINE SYNTHASE

Bibliography

Bertino, J. R., Savicki, W. L., Lindquist, C. A., and Gupta, V. S. (1977). Schedule-dependent antitumor effects of methotrexate and 5-fluorouracil. *Cancer Res.* **37,** 327.

Bertino, J. R. (1982). Keynote address: Chemotherapy and cancer care. *Int. J. Oncol. Biol. Phys.* **8,** 109.

Chou, T.-C., and Chou, J. (1987). "Dose Effect Analysis with Microcomputers." Software for IBM-PC. Biosoft, Cambridge, U.K.

Chou, T.-C., and Rideout, D. C. (eds.) (1991). "Synergism and Antagonism in Chemotherapy." Academic Press, San Diego.

Chou, T.-C., and Talalay, T. (1984). Quantitative analysis of dose–effect relationships: The combined effects of multiple drugs or enzyme inhibitors. *Adv. Enzyme Regul.* **22,** 27.

Chou, T.-C., Rideout, D. C., Chou, J., and Bertino, J. R. (1991). Chemotherapeutic synergism, potentiation, and antagonism. *In* "Encyclopedia of Human Biology" (R. Dulbecco, ed.), Vol. 2, p. 371. Academic Press, San Diego.

Chou, T.-C., Motzer, R. J., Tong, Y., and Bosl, G. J. (1994). Computerized quantitation of synergism and antagonism of taxol, topotecan and cisplatin against teratocarcinoma cell growth: A rational approach to clinical protocol design. *J. Natl. Cancer Inst.* **86,** 1517.

Loewe, S. (1953). Antagonism and antagonist. *Pharmacol. Rev.* **9,** 237.

Webb, J. L. (1961). Effect of more than one inhibitor. *In* "Enzyme and Metabolic Inhibitors." Vol. 1, p. 66 and p. 488. Academic Press, New York.

Chromosome Aberrations

Krzysztof Mrózek
Clara D. Bloomfield
Roswell Park Cancer Institute, Buffalo, New York

GLOSSARY

banding pattern An arrangement of alternating, more and less intense (darker and lighter) transverse bands in chromosomes. The banding pattern can be obtained by various chromosome staining techniques, of which the G-banding method is most widely used. Each pair of autosomes (see definition of karyotype) and chromosomes X and Y are characterized by unique banding patterns allowing for their unambiguous identification. The banding patterns of chromosomes are the same in all individuals of a given species and, within the same organism, are identical in all cells from different tissues.

chromosomes Structures of the nucleus composed of chromatin containing DNA and proteins. Chromosomes accommodate genes. The number and the morphology of chromosomes are best studied during cell division, in metaphase or late prophase, when chromosomes contract and become easily discernible. Each chromosome contains a centromere (primary constriction) and two arms, the shorter of which is designated p and the longer q.

clonal chromosome aberration An identical structural abnormality or gain of the same chromosome present in at least two metaphase cells, or a missing chromosome detected in a minimum of three cells.

deletion (del) The loss of genetic material, usually as a result of two breaks within the same chromosome arm (interstitial deletion). One break may lead to a terminal deletion–loss of chromatin distal to the breakpoint. In theory, true terminal deletions are rare because they are unstable and lead to gradual shortening of the deleted chromosome due to the absence of a telomere, a specialized structure located at the end of each chromosome arm that maintains structural integrity of a chromosome during DNA replication.

inversion (inv) The rotation 180° of a chromosome segment resulting from two breaks within one chromosome. If the breaks take place in the same chromosome arm (i.e., the centromere is not present within the inverted fragment), the inversion is named paracentric; if the breaks occur on the opposite sides of the centromere (i.e., in p and q arms), the inversion is called pericentric.

karyotype The chromosome complement representative for a given cell population, arranged according to size, location of the centromere, and banding patterns of individual chromosomes. A normal human karyotype contains 46 chromosomes, including 22 pairs of homologous chromosomes called autosomes, numbered from 1 to 22, and a pair of sex chromosomes designated X and Y (XX in females and XY in males). The description of the karyotype always contains the following items separated by commas: the total number of chromosomes, the constitution of sex chromosomes, and, in case of an abnormal karyotype, abnormalities of sex chromosomes followed by aberrations of autosomes listed in increasing numerical order.

translocation (t) The relocation of genetic material between two or more chromosomes. A reciprocal translocation involves the exchange of segments between chromosomes without a microscopically detectable loss of chromatin. Unbalanced translocations result in net gain or loss of genetic material.

Chromosome aberrations are any deviations from the normal diploid number of 46 chromosomes in the human karyotype (numerical chromosome aberrations) or are any changes in chromosome structure (structural chromosome aberrations) that can be detected by microscopic analysis. Depending on the type of aberration, chromosome abnormalities may result in the transposition of genes, loss or gain of genetic material, or both. In cancer, chromosome aberrations are acquired during the process of tumorigenesis and are confined to tumorous tissue, not being present in the remaining cells of the patient's body. In most types of cancer that have been adequately studied, chromosome aberrations are present in the majority of cases and their distribution is highly nonrandom. Chromosome aberrations have been divided with regard to their specificity and postulated significance in the neoplastic process into two main categories: primary and secondary abnormalities. Primary aberrations, strongly correlated with a particular tumor type and sometimes detected as the only karyotypic change, are assumed to play an important role in the earliest stages of tumor development (tumor initiation). Secondary abnormalities, although also

nonrandom, are less specific and are believed to be later events contributing to the process of tumor progression. The molecular dissection of many primary aberrations has led to the identification of genes involved in the malignant process. Even though the molecular consequences and pathogenetic significance of other recurrent aberrations have not been elucidated to date, the detection of chromosome aberrations often has clinical usefulness since many of them constitute unique tumor markers of diagnostic and prognostic value.

I. INTRODUCTION

The concept that acquired alterations of genetic material may lead to malignant transformation dates back to the end of the nineteenth century when the first observations of asymmetrical cell divisions and unequal distribution of chromatin in cancer cells were made. The causative role of chromosome aberrations in the genesis of cancer was postulated by Boveri in 1914, long before the correct number of chromosomes in the human karyotype was established. For many years Boveri's somatic mutation theory of cancer could not be verified experimentally due to methodological difficulties. Various improvements in the study of mammalian chromosomes, including the application of colchicine as a mitotic inhibitor to arrest cell division in metaphase and the use of hypotonic solutions to help spreading of chromosomes, led to the discovery of the first consistent chromosome aberration in human malignancy. This was a diminutive chromosome, typical of chronic myeloid leukemia (CML), called the Philadelphia chromosome after the city in which it was described by Nowell and Hungerford in 1960. It was not until the 1970s, however, when the era of modern cancer cytogenetics began with the introduction of chromosome banding techniques. These techniques enabled not only the identification of individual chromosomes but also precise characterization of numerical and even subtle structural chromosome aberrations. Further improvements in the accuracy of description of chromosome aberrations as well as detection of certain chromosome aberrations in nondividing, interphase cells can be achieved by the use of recently developed methods combining cytogenetic and molecular genetic technologies, namely fluorescence *in situ* hybridization and comparative genomic hybridization.

II. THE MAJORITY OF HUMAN CANCERS ARE KARYOTYPICALLY ABNORMAL

Ongoing, extensive cytogenetic studies have revealed that the majority of malignant, as well as benign, tumors display chromosome aberrations. However, the frequencies with which abnormal karyotypes are detected at the time of diagnosis vary among different neoplastic diseases. In such diseases as chronic myeloid leukemia (CML) or non-Hodgkin's lymphoma (NHL), 80 to 95% of cases have abnormal karyotypes, whereas in acute myeloid (AML) and lymphoblastic (ALL) leukemias, about two-thirds of all cases display recognizable chromosome changes. In contrast, in some other entities, especially those characterized by low mitotic activity of the neoplastic cells like Hodgkin's disease or those difficult to culture *in vitro* like prostatic adenocarcinoma, most tumors do not exhibit clonal abnormalities. Instead, in these cancers, single cells with unique, nonclonal chromosome aberrations can sometimes be detected cytogenetically. It has been demonstrated by *in situ* hybridization techniques that these nonclonal aberrations may in fact represent clonal populations of chromosomally aberrant cells that have failed to enter mitosis *in vitro*.

The existence of tumors in which no aberration can be detected cytogenetically does not disprove the somatic mutation theory of cancer. Sometimes chromosome aberrations in cancer cells cannot be detected due to the overgrowth of reactive, nonneoplastic cells that preferentially divide *in vitro*, thus leading to false-negative results of cytogenetic study. In other instances, the degree of resolution of standard cytogenetic analysis may be too low to visualize subtle rearrangements, such as reciprocal translocations or insertions of tiny segments between similarly banded regions or deletions or duplications of segments smaller than the length of a single band. Nonetheless, such submicroscopic rearrangements may involve several genes since, on average, a single

chromosomal band contains 10^6–10^7 bp. Finally, a proportion of karyotypically normal tumors may solely contain gene mutations and these, of course, cannot be detected using cytogenetic methods.

III. MECHANISMS OF GENERATION OF CHROMOSOME ABERRATIONS

Table I contains examples of the major types of numerical and structural chromosome aberrations that can occur in human cancer. Numerical chromosome changes result from disturbances in the mitotic spindle apparatus during cell division. In the process called *nondisjunction*, chromosomes of a given pair fail to separate in the normal way during anaphase, and two daughter cells with an abnormal number of chromosomes (aneuploid cells) are created. One cell contains an addition copy of the chromosome (trisomy); the second has only one of the two homologous chromosomes (monosomy). The latter aberration also may be the outcome of a phenomenon designated anaphase lag, when one chromosome does not move fast enough to one of the opposite poles of the cell, and consequently is not included within the new nuclear membrane. The causes of numerical aberrations remain largely enigmatic.

All different kinds of structural chromosome aberrations are initiated by DNA breakage and result from erroneous DNA repair processes leading to abnormal reconfiguration of broken chromosome ends. Chromosome breaks may be caused by exogenous factors including ionizing radiation, viruses, and chemical mutagenic agents interacting with DNA, as well as by endogenous enzyme systems participating in normal physiologic and developmental processes of DNA replication, transcription, and recombination.

The exact mechanisms creating specific cancer-associated chromosome aberrations are not yet well understood. There is, however, experimental evidence supporting the view that the generation of genomic rearrangements is not a completely random process. It appears that the structure of the DNA in the vicinity of breakpoint regions may determine in some instances the type of carcinogenic aberration. For example, it has been shown that in many cases of B- or T-cell lymphoma- or leukemia-specific translocations

TABLE I

Selected Examples of Cytogenetic Nomenclature Describing Numerical and Structural
Cancer-Associated Chromosome Aberrations[a]

Chromosome aberration	Description
−7	Monosomy of chromosome 7; only one copy of chromosome 7 present. Aberration frequent in MDS, AML, and idiopathic myelofibrosis in children.
+11	Trisomy of chromosome 11; three copies of chromosome 11 present. Recurrent aberration in AML, MDS, and infantile fibrosarcoma.
+8,+8	Tetrasomy of chromosome 8; four copies of chromosome 8 present. A rare recurrent change in AML.
add(19)(p13)	Additional genetic material (add) of unknown origin adjoined to band 19p13 of the short arm (p) of chromosome 19. Recurrently observed in malignant fibrous histiocytoma, ovarian carcinoma, and Hodgkin's disease.
del(20)(q11q13)	Interstitial deletion (del) of the long arm (q) of chromosome 20. The segment between bands 20q11 and 20q13 has been lost. Recurrent aberration in MDS, AML, and myeloproliferative disorders.
del(17)(p11)	Terminal deletion (del) of the short arm of 17 resulting in loss of the segment distal to the breakpoint at band 17p11. Recurrent aberration in colorectal adenocarcinoma, lung carcinoma, and NHL.
der(16)t(1;16)(q12;12)	Derivative chromosome (der) 16 created by an unbalanced translocation (t) between chromosomes 1 and 16. When the der(16)t(1;16) replaces one normal chromosome 16 (Fig. 2E), it results in partial trisomy of the segment of the chromosome 1 long arm distal to band 1q12 and in loss of genetic material from the long arm of chromosome 16 distal to band 16q12. This and similar rearrangements (with breakpoints assigned differently but always leading to trisomy 1q and loss of a portion of 16q) are recurrent, presumably secondary, aberrations in Ewing's sarcoma, peripheral neuroepithelioma, rhabdomyosarcoma, myxoid liposarcoma, Wilms' tumor, retinoblastoma, breast cancer, endometrial adenocarcinoma. ALL, AML, MDS, and multiple myeloma.
der(1;7)(q10;p10)	Derivative chromosome (der) resulting from an unbalanced whole arm translocation between chromosomes 1 and 7. This chromosome consists of the whole short arm of chromosome 7 and the whole long arm of chromosome 1. When it replaces a normal chromosome 7, der(1;7) leads to monosomy of 7q and trisomy of 1q. Recurrently observed in secondary MDS and AML.
dic(9;12)(p11;p12)	Dicentric chromosome (dic) created by a translocation between chromosomes 9 and 12. This chromosome contains whole long arms, centromeres, and portions of short arms proximal to the breakpoints in both chromosomes involved. Segments distal to 9p11 and 12p12 have been lost. Recurrently seen in pre-B ALL.
dmin	Double-minute chromosome (dmin). This is a small chromosome, without a centromere or banding pattern, usually resulting from gene amplification. Particularly often seen in neurogenic neoplasms.
dup(12)(q13q24)	Duplication (dup) of the segment between bands 12q13 and 12q24. The clone with such an aberration is trisomic for the duplicated segment of chromosome 12. Recurrently observed in NHL.
hsr(11)(q13)	Homogeneously staining region (hsr), i.e., region without any banding pattern, in band q13 of chromosome 11. Hsrs are usually caused by gene amplification.
i(12)(p10)	Isochromosome (i) of the short arm of chromosome 12. This symmetrical chromosome results from transverse misdivision of the centromere (instead of the normal longitudinal division) and is composed of two copies of the short arm of chromosome 12. The long arm (12q) has been lost. The break occurred within the centromere in a band designated as 12p10. An extra i(12)(p10) is the most common chromosome aberration in male germ cell tumors (GCT); it is occasionally seen in AML or MDS developing in patients with concurrent or preceding GCT.
ins(3;3)(q26;q21q26)	Insertion (ins) of a segment between bands 3q21 and 3q26 of one chromosome 3 into the homologous chromosome 3 at 3q26. Of note, the band to which the segment is inserted is specified first followed by a semicolon and bands bordering the inserted fragment. Recurrent aberration in MDS and AML.
inv(14)(q11q32)	Paracentric, i.e., within the same arm, inversion (inv) of chromosome 14. The segment of the long arm between bands 14q11 and 14q32 has been rotated 180°. Recurrently seen in T-cell chronic lymphoproliferative disorders and T-cell NHL.
inv(16)(p13q22)	Pericentric inversion (inv) of chromosome 16 (Fig. 2C). The segment between bands 16p13 (in the short arm) and 16q22 (in the long arm), containing the centromere, has been inverted. Recurrent aberration characteristic for AML FAB M4Eo.
mar	Marker chromosome (mar). This is a structurally rearranged chromosome in which no part can be identified.
t(4;11)(q21;q23)	Reciprocal translocation (t) between chromosomes 4 and 11 with breakpoints at 4q21 and 11q23. This translocation is balanced; no apparent loss of genetic material has taken place. Note that the chromosome with the lower number (or the sex chromosome) is always specified first. Consistent aberration in ALL.
r(1)(p12q42)	Ring chromosome (r) created by breakage and reunion of bands 1p12 and 1q42. The segments of the chromosome 1 short and long arms distal to band 1p12 and band 1q42, respectively, have been lost.

[a]Abbreviations: MDS, myelodysplastic syndrome; AML, acute myeloid leukemia; NHL, non-Hodgkin's lymphoma; ALL, acute lymphoblastic leukemia; FAB, French–American–British cooperative study group classification of acute leukemias.

involving immunoglobulin *(IG)* or T-cell receptor *(TCR)* genes, the breakpoint regions contain recombinase signal sequences. This suggests that these translocations were created as a result of mistakes in the physiologic reactions of *IG* or *TCR* V-D-J joining or *IG* heavy chain class switch recombination, catalyzed by recombinase complexes. In the generation of other translocations that do not involve *IG* or *TCR* genes, such as t(9;22)(q34;q11) or translocations involving band 11q23, repetitive DNA sequences have been implicated. Additionally, such factors as spatial proximity of specific chromosome segments in the interphase nucleus or high transcriptional activity of certain genes, thought to be associated with a relatively open chromatin conformation and increased susceptibility to rearrangements, may also play a role in the induction of chromosome abnormalities. Moreover, the formation of structural, as well as numerical, chromosome aberrations can be increased dramatically by chemical agents inhibiting DNA topoisomerases, the family of enzymes critical for the preservation of the integrity and stability of chromosome structure.

IV. PRIMARY AND SECONDARY CHROMOSOME ABERRATIONS

Although cases with a single chromosome aberration are not unusual, especially in the leukemias and certain types of malignant and benign solid tumors of mesenchymal origin, very often the tumor karyotype is complex, i.e., contains several structural or numerical aberrations or both concurrently. An example of such a complex karyotype found in a malignant soft tissue is depicted in Fig. 1. With the accumulation of cytogenetic data it has become obvious that not all chromosome changes have equal importance in oncogenesis. Consequently, chromosome aberrations have been divided with regard to their specificity and postulated significance in the neoplastic process into two main categories: primary and secondary abnormalities.

Primary aberrations are strongly correlated with a particular tumor type, are sometimes detected as the only karyotypic change, and are assumed to play an essential role in the earliest stages of tumor development (tumor initiation). Selected examples of pri-

mary chromosome changes, detected predominantly in leukemias, NHL, and mesenchymal solid tumors, are provided in Table II. Postulated primary chromosome aberrations in malignant epithelial solid tumors, in which delineation of primary aberrations is in general more difficult due to the fact that these cancers are usually studied in advanced clinical stages and often have very complex karyotypes, include deletions of the short arm of chromosome 3 in lung carcinomas, nonpapillary renal cell carcinomas and breast cancer; t(X;1)(p11;q21) in papillary renal cell carcinomas; deletions of the long arm of chromosome 6 in salivary gland carcinomas; monosomy of chromosome 9 or deletion of its long arm in transitional cell carcinomas of the bladder; and del(10)(q24) in adenocarcinoma of the prostate.

Secondary abnormalities, although also nonrandom, are less specific. They are believed to be later events, occurring in cells already carrying a primary chromosome change and contributing to the process of tumor progression, defined as the stepwise acquisition of new phenotypic features by cancer cells leading to more aggressive biologic and clinical behavior of the neoplasm over time. Probably the most extensively studied entity with the nonrandom acquisition of secondary chromosome changes associated with acceleration of the disease course is CML. Three-fourths of CML patients with the t(9;22)(q34;q11) as a primary abnormality develop additional aberrations correlated with the progression to a more malignant disease stage (blast crisis). The secondary aberrations seen most frequently in CML are (in decreasing order): an extra copy of der(22)t(9;22)(q34;q11) (Philadelphia chromosome), trisomy 8 (+8), isochromosome for the long arm of chromosome 17 [i(17)(q10)], +19, +21, −Y, +17, −7, −17, and t(3;21)(q26;q22). Each of these aberrations has been detected either as the only change in addition to the (9;22) or in various combinations of two or more additional abnormalities. By definition, the occurrence of all aforementioned secondary aberrations is not restricted to CML. Trisomy 8 as a secondary abnormality seems to be the most widespread among tumor types being recurrently observed in AML, ALL, myelodysplastic syndromes (MDS), colorectal adenoma, clear cell sarcoma of tendons and aponeuroses (Fig. 1). Ewing sarcoma, myxoid liposarcoma, and

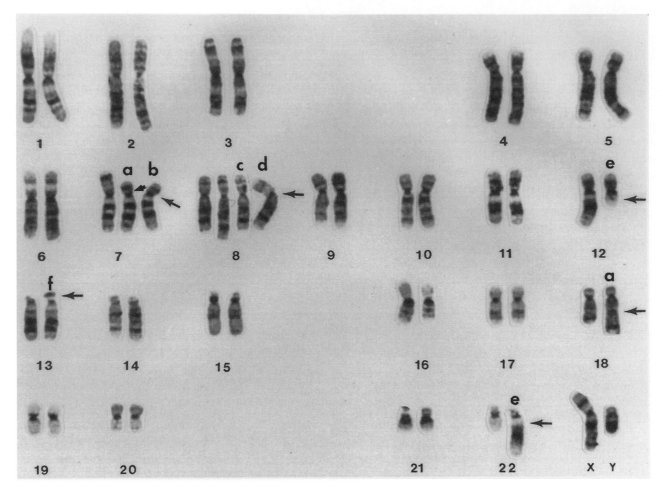

FIGURE 1 The G-banded abnormal karyotype of a clear cell sarcoma of tendons and aponeuroses: 49,XY,t(7;18)(p11.2;q21.3), +der(7)t(7;18) (p11.2;q21.3), +8, +der(8;17)(q10;q10),t(12;22)(q13;q12.2), add(13)(p13). This is an example of a complex karyotype with both numerical (an extra copy of an intact chromosome 8, indicated by the letter c) and structural chromosome changes. The latter include a reciprocal translocation between chromosomes 12 and 22[t(12;22)(q13;q12.2), indicated by the letters e] that constitutes a highly specific, primary aberration in this type of malignant soft tissue tumor. The remaining structural aberrations are presumably secondary cytogenetic rearrangements. They include another reciprocal (balanced) translocation [t(7;18)(p11.2;q21.3), indicated by the letters a]; an extra copy of one of the derivative 7 and 18; an unbalanced whole arm translocation between the long arms of chromosomes 8 and 17 [der(8;17)(q10;q10), indicated by the letter d] leading to tetrasomy of 8q and trisomy of 17q; and additional material of unknown origin adjoined to band 13p13 [add(13)(p13), indicated by the letter f]. Arrows indicate breakpoints in structural abnormalities. [Modified from Mrózek, K., Karakousis, C. P., Perez-Mesa, C., and Bloomfield, C. D. (1993). Translocation t(12;22)(q13;q12.2-12.3) in a clear cell sarcoma of tendons and aponeuroses. *Genes Chromosomes Cancer* **6**, 249. Copyright 1993 Wiley-Liss, Inc.]

synovial sarcoma. Among many other secondary cytogenetic rearrangements, various structural aberrations of chromosome 1, often leading to trisomy of its long arm [e.g., i(1) (q10), dup(1)(q11-21q31-44), der (16)t(1;16) (q11-21; q11-13) or der(1;16)(q10;q10)], are the most common.

V. PATHOGENETIC CONSEQUENCES OF CHROMOSOME ABERRATIONS

Despite a relatively large variety of different kinds of chromosome aberrations, examples of which are presented in Table I, each aberration usually results in

TABLE II

Selected Examples of Primary Chromosome Aberrations, and Genes Involved, That Display High Specificity in Human Malignant Diseases and Are of Diagnostic Value

Malignancy type[a]	Type of chromosome aberration	Gene involved (chromosome location)	
Acute myeloblastic leukemia with maturation, FAB M2	t(8;21)(q22;q22)	ETO (8q22)	AML1 (21q22)
Acute promyelocytic leukemia, FAB M3	t(15;17)(q22;q11-12)	PML (15q22)	RARA (17q12)
Acute myelomonocytic leukemia with eosinophilia, FAB M4Eo	inv(16)(p13q22)	MYH11 (16p13)	CBFB (16q22)
Acute monocytic leukemia, FAB M5a	t(9;11)(p22;q23)	AF9 (9p22)	ALL1 (11q23)
Chronic myeloid leukemia; acute lymphoblastic leukemia FAB L1, L2, never L3; acute myeloblastic leukemia without (FAB M1) and with (FAB M2) maturation	t(9;22)(q34;q11)[b]	ABL (9q34)	BCR (22q11)
Pre-B acute lymphoblastic leukemia, FAB L1	t(1;19)(q23;p13)	PBX1 (1q23)	E2A (19p13)
Burkitt's lymphoma; acute lymphoblastic leukemia, FAB L3	t(8;14)(q24;q32)	MYC (8q24)	IGH (14q32)
	t(8;22)(q24;q11)	MYC (8q24)	IGL (22q11)
	t(2;8)(p12;q24)	IGK (2p12)	MYC (8q24)
Non-Hodgkin's lymphoma, Ki-1-positive anaplastic large cell	t(2;5)(p23;q35)	ALK (2p23)	NPM (5q35)
Non-Hodgkin's lymphoma, follicular	t(14;18)(p32;q21)	IGH (14q32)	BCL2 (18q21)
Meningioma, acoustic neuroma	−22	NF2 (22q12)	
Papillary carcinoma of the thyroid gland	inv(10)(q11q21)	RET (10q11)	PTC (10q21)
Ewing's sarcoma; peripheral neuroepithelioma	t(11;22)(q24;q12)	FLI1 (11q24)	EWS (22q12)
	t(21;22)(q22;q12)[c]	ERG (21q22)	EWS (22q12)
	t(7;22)(p22;q12)	ETV1 (7p22)	EWS (22q12)
Clear cell sarcoma of tendons and aponeuroses (malignant melanoma of soft parts)	t(12;22)(q13;q12)	ATF1 (12q13)	EWS (22q12)
Desmoplastic small round-cell intraabdominal tumor	t(11;22)(p13;q12)	WT1 (11p13)	EWS (22q12)
Myxoid extraskeletal chondrosarcoma	t(9;22)(q22;q12)	TEC (9q22)	EWS (22q12)
Myxoid liposarcoma	t(12;16)(q13;p11)	CHOP (12q13)	FUS (16p11)
Alveolar rhabdomyosarcoma	t(2;13)(q35;q14)	PAX3 (2q35)	FKHR (13q14)
	t(1;13)(p36;q14)	PAX7 (1p36)	FKHR (13q14)
Synovial sarcoma	t(X;18)(p11;q11)	SSX1, SSX2 (Xp11)	SYT (18q11)
Lipoma	t(3;12)(q28;q15)[d]	LPP (3q28)	HMGIC (12q15)

[a]FAB, French–American–British cooperative study group classification of acute leukemias.
[b]The translocation in chronic myeloid leukemia differs from that in acute leukemias at the molecular level.
[c]Translocation not detected cytogenetically.
[d]Translocations between 12q15 and several chromosomes other than chromosome 3 have been reported.

one of three possible outcomes: (a) reduction of chromosomal segments within a chromosome or between chromosomes that leads to a recombination of genes, (b) loss of genetic material from the entire chromosome or part of it, or (c) gain of a whole chromosome(s) or a chromosomal segment.

A. Gene Relocation

The first type of outcome, gene relocation, can be brought about by reciprocal translocations, by inversions, by insertions, and sometimes by interstitial deletions. There are two major consequences of these chromosome aberrations.

1. Activation of a Cellular Protooncogene through Juxtaposition to the Vicinity of a Highly Transcriptionally Active Gene

This mechanism involves predominantly, but not exclusively, translocations and inversions that affect *IG* or *TCR* genes. Aberrations affecting *IG* or *TCR* genes occur in neoplasms originating in the lymphatic system, namely B- and T-cell acute and chronic lymphocytic leukemias and NHL. In most cases, the protein products of genes activated in this manner remain unchanged and are identical to their nontranslocated counterparts. Many of these proteins are putative transcription factors, including the product of the first oncogene shown to be implicated in lymphomagenesis, MYC. The MYC gene is activated by the t(8;14) (q24;q32) or by less frequent variant translocations, namely t(2;8)(p12;q24) and t(8;22) (q24;q11). These translocations are typical of Burkitt's lymphoma and its leukemic counterpart, ALL L3. The consequent constitutive expression of MYC disrupts a delicate balance in a transcriptional network of at least four proteins (myc, max, mad, and mxil) that is implicated in the regulation of a number of other critical genes and presumably leads to the unrestricted proliferation of cells carrying the translocation and to oncogenesis.

The consequences of another translocation, the t(14;18)(q32;q21), characteristic of follicular lymphoma, are different. This translocation results in overexpression of BCL2, a putative oncogene whose protein product represses programmed cell death (apoptosis). Thus increased levels of the bcl2 protein result in the prolonged survival of cells with the t(14;18) that presumably allows the acquisition of additional genomic mutations required for the multistep process of lymphomagenesis.

Although juxtaposition to IG or TCR appears to be the most prevalent way of activating oncogenes involved in neoplasms that originate in the immune system, alternative mechanisms also exist. The TAL1 gene (also known as TCL5 or SCL), demonstrated to be overexpressed in leukemia cells of a significant proportion of cases of childhood T-cell ALL, constitutes an interesting example. This gene can be activated by two mechanisms. Occasionally, the reciprocal translocation t(1;14)(p32;q11) juxtaposes TAL1 (mapped to band 1p32) to the α or δ locus of TCR at 14q11 and its expression is increased. In the majority of patients, however, it is a submicroscopic, interstitial deletion in the short arm of chromosome 1 that juxtaposes the coding exons of the TAL1 gene to the regulatory region of another upstream located gene called SIL.

2. Creation of Fusion Genes Encoding Chimeric Proteins

Gene fusion appears to be the main outcome of recurring translocations, inversions, and insertions occurring in neoplastic diseases originating outside the immune system, e.g., acute and chronic myeloid leukemias, MDS, and soft tissue sarcomas. With lower frequency, gene fusions have also been observed in ALL, NHL, and malignant solid tumors of epithelial origin. Since the breakage and the reunion occur within introns of the genes involved, the fusion leads to production of a functional chimeric protein with presumed oncogenic properties. Some hybrid proteins display excessive tyrosine kinase activity. Examples include fusion of the tyrosine kinase gene (ALK) with a nuclear phosphoprotein gene (NPM) caused by the t(2;5)(p23;q35), typical of Ki-1-positive anaplastic lymphoma, and fusion of the oncogene ABL with the BCR locus by t(9;22)(q34;q11). The latter translocation, or its variants, occurs in almost all cases of CML, in a subset of ALL, and in rare cases of AML. Although cytogenetically indistinguishable, t(9;22) is different in CML and ALL at the molecular level. The breakpoint in the BCR gene is more proximal in ALL than in CML and the bcr-abl protein is of a smaller size in ALL.

The majority of gene fusions thus far characterized create chimeric transcription factors indicating that disturbances in transcription control play a principal role in the etiology of cancer. An interesting model has been suggested by the molecular dissection of several translocations highly specific for rare soft tissue sarcomas (see Table II). In five distinct tumor types, the translocation fuses one of two closely related genes containing an RNA-binding domain (EWS or FUS) with a transcription factor gene (FLI1, ERG, ETV1, ATF1, WT1 or CHOP) or an orphan nuclear receptor gene (TEC). In all translocations, the DNA-binding domain of the transcriptional activator gene is retained and fused with the N-terminal domain and promoter region of the EWS or FUS gene. The latter genes are known to be ubiquitously expressed. Thus it appears that in sarcomas, the target specificity of the transcriptional activation of fusion proteins depends on the gene providing the DNA-binding domain, whereas the increased, untimely, or tissue inappropriate expression of the fusion gene is driven by the partner gene supplying the N-terminal domain and promoter region. Interestingly, two of the genes involved in sarcoma translocations, namely *FUS* and *ERG*, have been shown to be fused with each other by t(16;21)(p11;q22), a recurrent translocation detected in some patients with AML.

B. Loss of Genetic Material

Loss of genetic material may occur as a result of whole chromosome loss (monosomy) or such structural aberrations as interstitial and terminal deletions, unbalanced translocations, and isochromosomes. Consistently lost chromosomal regions may contain tumor suppressor genes (TSGs), the inactivation of which promotes the neoplastic process by causing disturbances in the cell's growth control. The normal functions of the TSGs and how their loss or mutation contributes to malignant transformation are largely unknown, but it appears that some TSGs act as negative regulators of gene transcription. In contrast to carcinogenesis mediated by activation or alteration of oncogenes, which usually requires involvement of only one of the two copies (alleles) of an oncogene (dominant mode of action), tumorigenesis brought about by loss of function of TSGs is recessive at the cellular level, i.e., tumor development can occur only when both alleles of a TSG in the same somatic cell are inactivated.

Most TSGs identified thus far play important pathogenetic roles in rare hereditary forms of cancer (e.g., retinoblastoma, Wilms' tumor) or inherited conditions predisposing to cancer development (e.g., Li-Fraumeni syndrome, neurofibromatosis) in which affected persons inherit one copy of a mutated gene from one of the parents and carry it in every somatic cell. As a consequence, such persons develop tumors with significantly highly frequencies because only one additional somatic mutation is necessary to inactivate the remaining allele of the TSG. Cytogenetic and molecular genetic studies of patients with germline mutations in TSGs led to cloning or mapping to particular chromosome bands of the vast majority of currently known TSGs. For example, discoveries of constitutional deletions of bands 13q14 and 11p13 in occasional patients with hereditary forms of retinoblastoma and Wilms' tumor, respectively, pinpointed the location of the *RB1* gene to band 13q14 and the *WT1* gene to band 11p13, and facilitated cloning of these TSGs. Further studies revealed that loss and/or mutation of *RB1* and other TSGs are not restricted to rare familial forms of a cancer but also are involved in sporadic (nonhereditary) tumors of the same type as well as in some sporadic cancers that are not typical for persons heterozygous for germline mutations in TSGs. Perhaps the most frequently affected gene in human oncogenesis is *TP53*, a TSG mapped to 17p13. In common sporadic epithelial carcinomas, loss of function of a single TSG is usually not sufficient for malignant transformation, and several TSGs are lost and/or mutated simultaneously in addition to other genomic rearrangements.

C. Gain of Chromosome Material

The third type of outcome may be achieved by the addition of an extra whole chromosome (trisomy) or chromosomes (two extra homologous chromosomes, tetrasomy; three, pentasomy; and so on). Structural abnormalities leading to a gain of chromosome segments include a duplication or triplication or a segment within a chromosome, isochromosomes, or unbalanced translocations. Presumably these rearrangements exert their oncogenic effect by adding another active copy of an oncogene or oncogenes (dose effect), but such a mechanism has not yet been demonstrated experimentally. The genes that are rearranged in association with almost all the recurrent trisomies in human cancer are unknown. The only exception is the *ALL1* gene (also called *MLL, HRX, HTRX1*) which has been shown recently to undergo partial tandem duplication in the majority of AML patients with trisomy 11 as a sole abnormality. Preliminary results indicate that in this case only one of three chromosomes 11 carries the partially duplicated *ALL1* gene.

Amplification of a large number of copies of an oncogene or oncogenes may be accomplished by formation of double minutes (dmin) or homogeneously staining regions (hsr). Both dmin and hsr are especially common, although not restricted to, tumors of the nervous system: 15% of cytogenetically abnormal astrocytomas contain dmin and one-half of neuroblastomas have dmin or hsr. It has been shown that the oncogene MYCN, mapped to band 2p24.1, is consistently amplified in neuroblastoma. The number of MYCN copies ranges from five to several hundred.

VI. CHROMOSOME PATTERNS OF NEOPLASTIC DISEASES

The rapidly growing cancer cytogenetics literature contains descriptions of chromosome aberrations detected in over 22,000 cases of various neoplastic diseases. The main conclusion emerging from overview of this immense amount of data is that chromosome aberrations do not occur at random. Distinct types of leukemia, lymphoma, and solid tumors are characterized by different patterns of cytogenetic abnormalities. Although, for technical reasons, the available cytogenetic data are heavily biased toward hematologic disorders (approximately two-thirds of abnormal karyotypes published to date have been obtained from patients with leukemias, MDS, and myelo- or lympho-proliferative syndromes), some generalizations as to the predominant type of genetic lesions characteristic of tumors of diverse embryonal origin can be made. The majority of leukemias, lymphomas, and some sarcomas exhibit reciprocal translocations as the principal type of genetic lesion (examples are provided in Tables I and II and Figs. 1 and 2). These lead to activation or fusion of genes controlling cell growth, differentiation, and programmed death (apoptosis). On the other hand, epithelial cancers and neurogenic tumors appear to be characterized predominantly by deletions, unbalanced translocations, and loss of whole chromosomes, suggesting that loss and inactivation of TSGs is crucial in these cancers' pathogenesis. In male germ cell tumors, gain of material from the short arm of chromosome 12, most frequently in the form of i(12)(p10), appears to be the most consistent cytogenetic change. The aforementioned generalizations do not mean, of course, that loss of function of TSGs is not operative in some leukemias, lymphomas, and sarcomas or that balanced translocations or inversions resulting in gene fusion cannot be found in selected tumors of epithelial origin.

Many cytogenetic–clinicopathologic associations have been established. Table II presents examples of chromosome aberrations, and the genes involved, that are highly specific for a given neoplastic disease. All of these aberrations represent primary changes due to their specificity for the respective disease and the fact that they have been occasionally seen as the sole abnormalities. For a more complex list of specific cytogenetic rearrangements in cancer and in-depth discussion of their significance and clinical value, the reader is referred to the review articles and books cited at the end of this article.

VII. CLINICAL VALUE OF CANCER CYTOGENETICS

In addition to providing insights into genetic mechanisms of tumorigenesis and pinpointing the chromosomal location of cancer-relevant genes, cytogenetic analysis has become a valuable tool in clinical practice. It is especially important in diagnosis, predicting the clinical course (prognosis) and guiding the management of patients with hematologic malignancies. In solid tumors, the significance of chromosome analysis is at present mainly diagnostic. The discovery of acquired clonal aberrations in the specimens obtained from bone marrow, lymph nodes, ascitic or pleural fluids, or tumor masses very often confirms the neoplastic nature of the disease. This is particularly true in cases where several structural or numerical chromosome changes are found concurrently, in the same clone. The interpretation of some simple clonal aberrations occurring as a sole abnormality, such as trisomy 7, sex chromosome loss, or t(14;18)(q32;q21), may be sometimes more difficult since they are occasionally observed in nonneoplastic tissues.

The presence of characteristic chromosome aberrations may aid in the differential diagnosis between tumor types sharing common features. For instance, histopathologic and clinical features of the childhood small round-cell tumors, including neuroblastoma, rhabdomyosarcoma, Ewing sarcoma and neuroepithelioma, and occasionally NHL, are often very similar, thus making the correct diagnosis difficult to establish. Since each of the aforementioned disorders displays a distinctive pattern of chromosome aberrations,

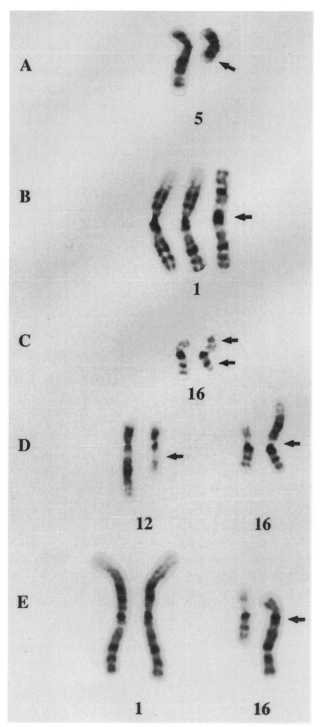

cytogenetic analysis may yield crucial information for diagnosis.

In acute leukemias, the distinction between myeloid and lymphoid lineages is of utmost importance in choosing remission induction therapeutic regimens. Results of cytogenetic investigations may corroborate or refute lineage assignment established on the basis of morphlogic, cytochemical, and immunophenotyping studies because many recurrent primary chromosome aberrations are seen exclusively in AML or ALL (examples are provided in Tables I and II). Moreover, several chromosome aberrations are highly specific for a particular clinicopathologic syndrome. Probably the strongest association exists between the t(15;17)(q22;q11-12) and acute promyelocytic leukemia (APL); essentially every patient with APL has this translocation, its rare variant t(11;17)(q23;q11-12), or the molecular rearrangement of genes involved in the t(15;17), namely retinoic acid receptor gene α (RARα), mapped to 17q11-12, and promyelocytic leukemia gene (PML), mapped to 15q22. The accuracy of diagnosis in the case of APL has profound consequences for the management of such patients. First, the majority of APL patients suffer from bleeding complications due to disseminated intravascular coagulopathy that may lead to fatal bleeding into the central nervous system or lungs. The finding of the t(15;17), especially in cases without classic morphologic features of APL (variant APL), alerts the physician and enables early introduction of treatment preventing death from such complications. Second, it has been shown that the anomalous protein produced by the chimeric gene PML–RARα, formed as

FIGURE 2 G-banded partial karyotypes demonstrating selected types of structural aberrations. (A) Interstitial deletion of the long arm of chromosome 5 - del(5)(q14-15q33). This and other deletions of 5q (with different breakpoints but always leading to loss of band 5q31) are frequently found in MDS and in AML developing mainly in patients previously exposed to genotoxic agents, including chemotherapeutic drugs and radiation. (B) Extra isochromosome of the long arm

of chromosome 1 - i(1)(q10). This rearrangement results in tetrasomy for 1q. The isochromosome of 1q is a recurrent, presumably secondary, abnormality in ALL, AML, NHL, Hodgkin's disease, chronic lymphoproliferative disorders, and in various solid tumors including carcinomas, sarcomas, germ cell neoplasms, and malignant neurogenic tumors. (C) Pericentric inversion of chromosome 16 - inv(16)(p13q22). This is a primary chromosome aberration highly specific for acute myelomonocytic leukemia with eosinophilia. (D) Reciprocal translocation between chromosomes 12 and 16 - t(12;16)(q13.3;p11.2). This is a primary abnormality pathognomonic (i.e., seen exclusively in and thus diagnostic for) myxoid and round cell liposarcoma. (E) Unbalanced translocation between chromosomes 1 and 16 - der(16)-t(1;16)(q12;q12). Two normal copies of chromosome 1 are present. A recurrent, presumably secondary, aberration in many tumor types (see Table I). Arrows indicate breakpoints.

the consequence of the t(15;17), has the ability to block the differentiation of promyelocytes and prolong their survival leading to the outgrowth of APL cells. These effects can be reversed by all-*trans*-retinoic acid. This drug has proved to be very effective in inducing complete remission (CR) in APL patients with the t(15;17), but not in patients with other morphologic subtypes of acute leukemia or different cytogenetic aberrations.

Cytogenetic findings have been shown repeatedly to constitute independent prognostic factors in AML, in ALL, and, to a somewhat lesser extent, in chronic lymphocytic leukemia and NHL. In general, in all aforementioned groups of diseases, an exclusively normal karyotype of a tumor specimen at diagnosis signifies a relatively favorable prognosis, whereas the presence of multiple structural and numerical abnormalities predicts an aggressive disease course and poor outcome. Numerous correlations between specific chromosome aberrations and different parameters such as CR rate, CR duration, and overall survival have been and are being reported. Obviously, a detailed review of these associations is beyond the scope of this article; relevant information may be found in the publications listed in the bibliography. It is worthy of note that because prognostic factors are highly dependent on the therapy used and because treatment strategies are being improved constantly, a clear need for a continuous study of relationships between cytogenetic subgroups and clinical outcome exists. An abnormality conferring an unfavorable prognosis with one therapeutic scheme may lose its adverse prognostic significance or even become a favorable prognostic determinant when another treatment is used. Furthermore, accumulation of more data on the less frequent recurrent aberrations, whose clinical import is at present unknown, will enable evaluation of their prognostic significance in the future.

Acknowledgments

The authors gratefully acknowledge Professor Albert de la Chapelle for critical reading of the manuscript. This work was supported in part by the Coleman Leukemia Research Fund.

See Also the Following Articles

CHRONIC MYELOGENOUS LEUKEMIA • C-MYC PROTOONCOGENE • RECOMBINATION: MECHANISMS AND ROLES IN TUMORIGENESIS

Bibliography

Heim, S., and Mitelman, F. (1995). "Cancer Cytogenetics," 2nd Ed. Wiley-Liss, New York.

Kirsch, I. R. (ed.) (1993). "The Causes and Consequences of Chromosomal Aberrations." CRC Press, Boca Raton, FL.

Knudson, A. G. (1993). Antioncogenes and human cancer. *Proc. Natl. Acad. Sci. USA* **90,** 10914.

Ladanyi, M. (1995). The emerging molecular genetics of sarcoma translocations. *Diagn. Mol. Pathol.* **4,** 162.

Mitelman, F. (1994). "Catalog of Chromosome Aberrations in Cancer," 5th Ed. Wiley-Liss, New York.

Mitelman, F., Kaneko, Y., and Berger, R. (1994). Report of the committee on chromosome changes in neoplasia. *In* "Human Gene Mapping 1993: A Compendium" (A. J. Cuticchia, and P. L. Pearson, eds.), p. 773. Johns Hopkins University Press, Baltimore.

Mrózek, K., and Bloomfield, C. D. (1996). Cytogenetics of non Hodgkin's lymphoma and Hodgkin's disease. *In* "Neoplastic Diseases of the Blood" (P. H. Wiernik, G. P. Canellos, J. P. Dutcher, and R. A. Kyle, eds.), 3rd Ed., p. 835. Churchill-Livingstone, New York.

Rabbits, T. H. (1994). Chromosomal translocations in human cancer. *Nature* **372,** 143.

Rodriguez, E., Sreekantaiah, C., and Chaganti, R. S. K. (1994). Genetic changes in epithelial solid neoplasia. *Cancer Res.* **54,** 3398.

Sandberg, A. A. (1990). "The Chromosomes in Human Cancer and Leukemia," 2nd Ed. Elsevier, New York.

Sandberg, A. A., and Bridge, J. A. (1994). "The Cytogenetics of Bone and Soft Tissue Tumors." RG Landes Company, Austin.

Chronic Lymphocytic Leukemia

Michael J. Keating

University of Texas M. D. Anderson Cancer Center

GLOSSARY

B cell or B lymphocytes A cell that is the backbone of the humoral immune system and the only cell that can produce antibodies.

staging The clinicopathologic assessment of a tumor based on the size of the primary lesion, the extent of spread to regional structures, and the presence or absence of distant metastases.

C hronic lymphocytic leukemia (CLL) is an accumulative disease usually of B lymphocytes that occurs predominantly in older patients. It is the most common form of leukemia in Caucasians but is less common in Hispanics and is rare in Japan and other Asian countries. There is a 26-fold difference between the highest incidence, which is in Canada, and the lowest, which is in Japan. The male/female ratio is usually of the order of 2:1. In the United States, black populations have the same incidence as Caucasians. There is no increase in the incidence of CLL at the time, but patients are more recently being diagnosed at a younger age and at an earlier stage because of the increasing use of screening blood tests as health checks and for preoperative evaluation.

Encyclopedia of Cancer, Second Edition
Volume 1

I. CAUSATION

As opposed to other leukemias, there is no evidence relating exposure to radiation with the risk of CLL or to support a relationship between electromagnetic field (EMF) and causation of CLL. Benzene, although established as a carcinogen for acute myelogenous leukemia, is not associated with CLL. There is no increase of the likelihood of developing CLL among gasoline service station workers or other petroleum workers.

A number of studies have noted an association of all types of leukemia in farming. Some studies have suggested an increased risk of CLL and farm-related activities. No specific causative agent, however, has ever been established.

II. GENETICS OF CHRONIC LYMPHOCYTIC LEUKEMIA (CLL)

Familial clustering of CLL is more common than for other leukemias. First-degree relatives of patients with leukemia are more commonly found to have CLL subsequently than other leukemias. This is often associated with "anticipation," which is the worsening severity or earlier age of onset of CLL in successive generations. No particular CLL gene has been identified within the families. Studies of the ATM gene (mutated in ataxia telangiectasia) suggest that heterozygotes for ATM abnormalities have an increased likelihood of developing CLL. Patients with ataxia telangiectasia have a 100-fold risk of developing cancer. CLL patients with ATM mutations have a more aggressive disease and a shorter survival than others.

III. CLL CYTOGENETICS

The Philadelphia chromosome translocation is found in 95% of cases of chronic myelogenous leukemia. No equivalent chromosome change is found in CLL. However, approximately two-thirds of patients have deletions of chromosome 13 at the site 13q14, in proximity to the Rb1 gene. However, Rb1 is not the gene deletion that is associated with CLL and, in all probability, leukemia-associated tumor suppressor genes exist at this site.

IV. SECOND MALIGNANCIES IN CLL

As CLL advances, it is associated with increasing impairment of the immune system. Hypogammaglobulinemia becomes common, and T-cell abnormalities are widespread, such as a slow and impaired response to mitogens. In addition, there is diminished recognition of CLL cells in autologous mixed lymphocyte populations. A number of studies have suggested that different cancers are more common in CLL (5–15% of cases) than in other control populations, perhaps related to impaired immune surveillance. The increased risk of second malignancies such as non-Hodgkin's lymphoma (NHL), Hodgkin's disease (HD), multiple myeloma, lung cancer, soft tissue sarcomas, and skin cancers, including melanoma, ranges from 1.1 to 3.18. The largest review of patients with CLL treated with fludarabine (a purine analog with marked immunosuppressive activity) noted an increased risk of second cancers of 1.65.

V. ORIGIN OF CLL

More than 95% of cases with chronic lymphocytic leukemia involve B lymphocytes. Small, resting, long-lived B cells accumulate. These have a characteristic pattern of coexpression of the CD5 molecule with mature B-cell surface antigens. The phenotype can be easily identified, as these cells express CD19, CD23, CD21, CD24, and CD40 as well as CD5 with a dim expression of CD20 and variable expression of CD22. CD5-positive B cells are normally present in high numbers in fetal life and at the time of birth and infancy. Subsequently, the numbers decrease to less than 10% of B lymphocytes. CD5-positive B cells are increased in rheumatoid arthritis, following allogeneic bone marrow transplantation and possibly in cases of disseminated lupus erythematosus. The role of CD5-positive B cells is assumed to be related to the regulation of natural autoantibodies. Immunoglobulin expression on the surface (sIgM and/or D) is dim and sometimes undetectable. The cells are monoclonal with expression of either κ or λ light chains. B-CLL cells appear to be anergic with a poor response to stimulants. CD79b, which is part of the bcr complex, has a missing extracellular domain in most CLL patients. The use of IgH chain variable reagent (Vh) genes in CLL is not random. A few genes are overexpressed, especially the Vh1-69 gene. This gene is present in 20% of all patients.

Patients with CLL have high levels of somatic mutations, suggesting that they have been triggered into terminal differentiation and function as memory cells. The development of memory cells occurs in the germinal center. It is now hypothesized that there are two major subgroups of CLL. A number of patients do not have hypermutation of the immunoglobulin genes and are considered to be naive CD5-positive B cells. The other major subset has hypermutated gene memory B cells. The memory cells have a very low expression of CD38, whereas naive B-CLL cells have a higher expression of CD38. Clinical studies have demonstrated that the memory cell subsets of B-cell CLL have an excellent prognosis, whereas naive B-cell CLL patients are more likely to develop progressive disease. CD38 is not as strong a predictor for survival as immunoglobulin gene hypermutation.

VI. DEFECTIVE APOPTOSIS

Characteristic of CLL cells is defective apoptosis *in vivo*. Survival of CLL B cells is approximately 10 times that of normal B cells. B-CLL cells do not exhibit increased apoptosis after CD95 (Fas receptor) ligation. Overexpression of the Bcl 2 protein is noted in almost all cases of CLL, despite absence of the t(14;18) translocation. CLL cells commonly also express Bax and Bak proteins without appreciable levels of Bcl-XL and Bad. Two-thirds of patients with CLL express the antiapoptotic protein, MCL 1. Apoptosis is more prominent when CLL cells are studied *in vitro* than *in vivo*. CLL cells express the CD40 molecule. CD40 ligation inhibits apoptosis due to agents such as fludarabine. A number of associations of cytokines with differentiation, activation, proliferation, and apoptosis have been described. However, no clear association

exists between any combination of cytokines and clinical behavior. A number of cytokines such as interleukin (IL)-6, IL-10, and IL-8 have been associated with a poor prognosis when elevated in plasma. Also, elevated levels of tumor necrosis factor are associated with shorter survival.

VII. PROGNOSTIC CHARACTERISTICS

An important contribution to understanding of CLL was developed with the staging systems of Rai and Binet (Table I). These two staging systems have allowed the separation of patients into low-, intermediate-, and high-risk groups of patients. The staging systems are based on number of involved lymphoid sites, such as lymph nodes, liver, and spleen, and impairment of marrow function. The Rai staging system is more widely accepted in the United States, whereas the Binet system is used in Europe. Staging systems have allowed comparison of different patient populations and clinical trial results. An important contribution has been the separation of a subset of patients with "smoldering CLL." Patients who have a low lymphocyte count at the time of diagnosis with an adequate hemoglobin, platelet count, and Binet stage A who are then observed to have a lymphocyte doubling time of greater than 12 months with a nondiffuse bone marrow pattern have a survival the same as age- and sex-matched segments of the population. Younger patients with CLL have the same prognostic characteristics but have a longer survival compared to older patient populations. A variety of other characteristics have been associated with a poor prognosis, including atypical appearance of the lymphocytes, hypogammaglobulinemia, and elevated serum levels of soluble CD23 and β-2-microglobulin. The β-2-microglobulin level has been confirmed widely to be important in prognosis. In addition, thymidine kinase has additional prognostic information when combined with β-2-microglobulin. The β-2-microglobulin level also predicts probability of response to chemotherapy. An important morphologic subset of CLL is mantle cell CLL. This group of

TABLE I
The Rai and Binet Staging System

Staging system	Stage	Modified three-stage system	Clinicohematological features	Median survival (years)
Rai	0	Low risk	Lymphocytes in PB and BMM	>10
	I		Lymphocytosis + lymphoadenopathy	7
		Intermediate risk		
	II		Lymphocytosis + splenomegaly and/or hepatomegaly ± lymphoadenopathy	7
	III		Lymphocytosis + anemia (hemoglobin <110 g/liter ± lymphoadenopathy ± splenomegaly ± hepatomegaly	1.5
		High risk		
	IV		Lymphocytosis + thrombocytopenia (platelets <100 × 10^9/liter) ± anemia ± lymphoadenopathy ± splenomegaly ± hepatomegaly	
Binet	A		Lymphoid areas involved <3	>10
	B		Lymphoid areas involved ≥3	5
	C		Anemia (hemoglobin <100 g/liter) and/or thrombocytopenia (platelets <100 × 10^9/liter)	2

patients has a leukemic phase of mantle cell lymphoma. They have low to absent CD23 expression and characteristically a translocation 11:14 with a high expression of bcl1 protein (cyclin D1). The prognosis in this subset of patients is very poor.

VIII. TREATMENT OF CLL

CLL is unique in that the first decision regarding treatment is whether the patient requires therapy. Many patients with early stage, low tumor burden CLL will not have any evidence of progressive disease for many years. Patients with early stage disease, particularly those with smoldering CLL, have a very low likelihood of having significant morbidity or mortality from their disease. The National Cancer Institute Working Group (NCIWG) on CLL has developed a series of recommendations for initiation of treatment and evaluating response to treatment for patients (Table II). Basically, patients with advanced stage disease or bulky tumors or symptomatic disease are recommended for treatment. Because CLL is a disseminated disease, systemic therapy is indicated. The traditional approach to treatment has been with alkylating agents such as chlorambucil or cyclophosphamide with or without corticosteroids. Evaluation of response has been heterogeneous with a variety of criteria for response used over many years. Now that the NCIWG criteria are

being applied, it is possible to evaluate the outcome of a variety of treatment strategies.

In the 1980s, purine analogs fludarabine (Fludara) and 2-chlorodeoxyadenosine (2-CDA) and pentostatin were all demonstrated to have significant activity in CLL. In the United States, Fludara has been primarily investigated and approved for the management of CLL. 2-CDA has been more widely used in Europe. The primary role of pentostatin at the present time is in the management of hairy cell leukemia.

Comparative clinical trials have demonstrated that fludarabine is more potent than chlorambucil with or without prednisone in the management of CLL. In a North American intergroup study, the complete response rate was 20% for Fludara vs 4% for CLB vs an overall response rate of 63% vs 37%. The remission duration was also significantly longer for Fludara-treated patients. A variety of other treatment combinations, including anthracyclines, have been utilized in the management of CLL, but purine analogs are emerging as major building blocks for the treatment of CLL. More recently, combinations of Fludara and alkylators such as FC (Fludara + cyclophosphamide) have been developed. The response rates, particularly in patients who have had previous therapy, are higher than have been reported with single agents. Other agents that have demonstrated activity include Nelarabine. Major complications of the management of CLL are the incidence of infections which become

TABLE II
Comparison of NCI-WG and IWCLL Guidelines for CLL

	NCI	IWCLL
Diagnosis		
Lymphocytes ($10^3/\mu l$)	>5	a. ≥10 and B phenotype or bone marrow involved
Atypical cells	<55%	b. <10 and both of above
Duration of lymphocytosis	≥2 months	Not stated
Bone marrow lymphocytes	≥30%	Not stated
Staging	Rai, correlate with Binet	>30
Eligibility for trials	active or bulky disease, progression	IWCLL
		A. >50 × $10^3/\mu l$ lymphocytes
		Doubling time <12 months, diffuse marrow pattern
		B, C. all patients
Response criteria		
Complete response		
Physical examination	Normal	Normal
Symptoms	None	None
Lymphocytes	≤4 × $10^3/\mu l$	<4 × $10^3/\mu l$
Neutrophils	≥1.5 × $10^3/\mu l$	<1.5 × 10^3l
Platelets	>100 × $10^3/\mu l$	>100 × 10^3l
Hemoglobin	>11%/dl	Not stated
Bone marrow lymphs	<30%	Normal
Bone marrow biopsy	No nodules or infiltrates	Nodules or infiltrates permitted
Nodular partial response	CR with BM nodules or infiltrates	
Partial response		
Physical examination (nodes, liver, spleen)	≥50% decrease	Downshift in stage
Plus ≥1 of		
Neutrophils	≥1.5 × $10^3/\mu l$	
Platelets	>100 × $10^3/\mu l$ or 50% improvement	
Hemoglobin	>11 g/dl	Not stated
Duration of CR or PR	≥2 months	Upshift in stage
Progressive disease		
Physical examination (nodes, liver, spleen)	≥50% increase or new site	
Circulating lymphocytes	≥50% increase	No change in stage
Other	Richter's syndrome	
Stable disease	All others	

more common as the stage of the disease and increased amount of prior therapy is administered. Major infections initially are sinobronchial infections, which are more common in patients with low gammaglobulin levels. As the disease progresses, gram-negative organisms, cytomegalovirus, *Pneumocystis carinii*, and fungi become more prominent.

IX. MONOCLONAL ANTIBODIES IN CLL

Two monoclonal antibodies, Rituximab and alemtuzimab, have been developed for the management of B-

cell malignancies. While initially Rituximab had a low level of activity at conventional doses in CLL, regimens using a higher dose intensity have achieved response rates up to 75%. Rituximab is active against CD20, which is expressed dimly on the surface of CLL cells. Campath-1H (alemtuzimab) has been extensively investigated for a number of years in Europe. However, a pivotal clinical trial has demonstrated that the drug has significant activity in patients refractory to fludarabine, leading to its approval in the United States and Europe. Alemtuzimab is a monoclonal antibody developed against CD52, which is present in high intensity in the majority of cases of CLL.

Both Rituximab and alemtuzimab are chimeric

antibodies with more than 95% of the murine antibody being replaced by a humanized antibody. Chimeric antibodies have a low incidence of antimouse (HAMA) or antirat (HARA) antibody production. Postulated mechanisms of action are complement lysis, antibody dependency cellular cytotoxicity (ADCC), and activation of intercellular signal transduction pathways leading to apoptosis.

Monoclonal antibodies have now been combined with chemotherapy regimens to provide very high complete remission rates in previously untreated patients with CLL when used either as simultaneous or sequential therapy. In addition, Campath-1H has been utilized for the management of minimal residual disease and is able to achieve clearing of the marrow as demonstrated by flow cytometry and preliminary chain reaction for immunoglobulin heavy chain rearrangement.

X. BONE MARROW TRANSPLANTATION

Both autologous (auto) and allogeneic (allo) stem cell transplantations (SCT) have been explored in CLL. Initially, these were not considered viable because, before purine analogs, treatment was unable to provide sufficient clearance of blood or bone marrow

to harvest autologous stem cells. Auto SCT is becoming increasingly applied as an intensification or remission induction strategy. The results are better the earlier the patients receive the auto SCT. Whether there is any survival advantage for auto SCT is uncertain. Long-term follow-up needs to be obtained before conclusions can be drawn.

Until recently, allo SCT was not used extensively in CLL because of the age of the patients. A number of studies have now evaluated ablative allo SCT in CLL. These have obtained high complete remission rates with a long-term survival fraction of approximately 50%. Following the discovery that prior treatment with fludarabine decreased the likelihood of allo SCT patients developing significant graft vs host disease (GVHD), nonablative regimens have been developed for the treatment of CLL. This has allowed allo SCT to be applied to patients into their 70s. It appears that the long-term survival of nonablative SCT is equivalent to ablative SCT.

XI. GENE THERAPY

Adenoviral vectors enable CD154 (the mouse gene for CD40 ligand) to be inserted into CLL cells. This heightens the expression of costimulatory molecules on the surface of CLL cells and makes them more effec-

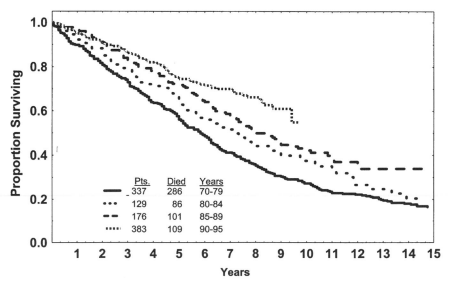

FIGURE 1 Improved survival of previously untreated CLL patients over time.

tive antigen-presenting cells. A pilot study of a small number of patients has demonstrated that this form of gene therapy can obtain substantial reductions in white blood cell count and lymph node size and expand the T-cell population, which is active against CLL. This strategy shows promise for developing specific immunotherapy against CLL. DNA vaccination is also emerging as a possibility following initial experiments in patients with follicular lymphoma.

XII. CONCLUSIONS

In the 1990s there was an explosion of new information regarding the biology and immunology of CLL. In addition, application of new treatments has led to higher response rates with longer remission durations. Evidence from MDACC suggests that a survival advantage is now emerging for CLL patients (Fig. 1). How much of this is due to earlier diagnosis and how much is due to the effect of therapy are uncertain at the present time. The extended range of options provides optimism that the natural history of CLL will be altered for the first time.

See Also the Following Articles

ACUTE LYMPHOBLASTIC LEUKEMIA IN ADULTS • ACUTE LYMPHOBLASTIC LEUKEMIA IN CHILDREN • ACUTE MYELOCYTIC LEUKEMIA • BCL-2 FAMILY PROTEINS AND THE DYSREGULATION OF PROGRAMMED CELL DEATH • CHRONIC MYELOGENOUS LEUKEMIA • GRAFT VERSUS LEUKEMIAS AND GRAFT VERSUS TUMOR • MONOCLONAL ANTIBODIES: LEUKEMIA AND LYMPHOMA • STEM CELL TRANSPLANTATION

Bibliography

Blair, A., and Zahm, S. H. (1995). Agricultural exposures and cancer. *Environ. Health Perspect.* **103** (Suppl 8):205–208.

Caligaris-Cappio, F. (2000). Biology of chronic lymphocytic leukemia. *In* "Reviews in Clinical Experimental Hematology" (R. Foa and A. V. Hoffbrand, eds.), p. 5. Accademia Nazionale di Medicina, Genova.

Cheson, B. D., Bennett, J. M., Kay, N., *et al.* (1996). National Cancer Institute-Sponsored Working Group guidelines for chronic lymphocytic leukemia: Revised guidelines for diagnosis and treatment. *Blood* **12**, 4990–4997.

Copur, M. S., Ledakis, P., Muhvic, J., *et al.* (2001). Fludarabine for chronic lymphocytic leukemia. *N. Engl. J. Med.* **344**, 1166–1168.

Damle, R. N., Wasill, T., Fais F., *et al.* (1999). Immunoglobulin V gene mutation status and CD38 expression as novel prognostic indicators in chronic lymphocytic leukemia. *Blood* **94**, 1840–1847.

Esteve, J., and Montserrat, E. (2000). Hematopoietic stem-cell transplantation for B-cell chronic lymphocytic leukemia: Current status. *In* "Reviews in Clinical Experimental Hematology" (R. Foa and A. V. Hoffbrand, eds.), p. 167. Accademia Nazionale di Medicina, Genova.

Hamblin, T. J., Davis Z., Gardiner, A., *et al.* (1999). Unmutated immunoglobulin VH genes are associated with a more aggressive form of chronic lymphocytic leukemia. *Blood* **94**, 1848–1854.

Hisada, M., Biggar, R. J., Greene, M. H., Fraumeni, J. F., Jr., and Travis, L. B. (2001). Solid tumors after chronic lymphocytic leukemia. *Blood* **98**, 1979–1981.

Keating, M. J., and O'Brien, S. (2000). Conventional management of chronic lymphocytic leukemia. *In* "Reviews in Clinical Experimental Hematology" (R. Foa and A. V. Hoffbrand, eds.), p. 118. Accademia Nazionale di Medicina, Genova.

Molica, S. (2001). Prognostic factors in chronic lymphocytic leukemia. *In* "Chronic Lymphoid Leukemias" (B. D. Cheson, ed.), p. 231. Dekker, New York.

Montserrat, E., Vinolas N., Reverter, J. C., and Rozman, C. (1988). Natural history of chronic lymphocytic leukemia: On the progression and prognosis of early stages. *Nouv Rev Fr Hematol* **30**, 359–361.

Rai, K. R., and Gupta, N. (2000). Monoclonal antibodies in chronic lymphocytic leukemia. *In* "Reviews in Clinical Experimental Hematology" (R. Foa and A. V. Hoffbrand, eds.), p. 134. Accademia Nazionale di Medicina, Genova.

Sgambati, M. T., Linet, M. S., and Devesa, S. S. (2001). Chronic lymphocytic leukemia: Epidemiological, familial, and genetic aspects. *In* "Chronic Lymphoid Leukemias" (B. D. Cheson, ed.), p. 231. Dekker, New York.

Stilgenbauer, S., Lichter, P., and Dohner, H. (2000). Genetic features of B-cell chronic lymphocytic leukemia. *In* "Reviews in Clinical and Experimental Hematology" (R. Foa and A. V. Hoffbrand, eds.), p. 48. Accademia Nazionale di Medicina, Genova.

Wierda, W. G., Cantwell M. J., Woods, S. J., Rassenti, L. Z., Prussak, C. E., and Kipps, T. J. (2000). CD40-ligand (CD154) gene therapy for chronic lymphocytic leukemia. *Blood* **96**, 2917–2924.

Yuille, M. R., Houlston, R. S., and Catovsky, D. (1998). Anticipation in familial chronic lymphocytic leukaemia. *Leukemia* **12**, 1696–1698.

Chronic Myelogenous Leukemia: Etiology, Incidence, and Clinical Features

Bayard Clarkson

Memorial Sloan-Kettering Cancer Center

GLOSSARY

BCR/ABL Chimeric gene created by the Philadelphia chromosome translocation of the second exon of protooncogene c-abl from chromosome 9 to the breakpoint clust region on chromosome 22.

p210$^{BCR/ABL}$ The 201-kDa product of the chimeric BCR/ABL gene; a tyrosine kinase that is thought to cause chronic myelogenous leukemia in humans.

phosphorylation A process by which a phosphate group is transferred from ATP to tyrosine, serine, or threonine amino acid residues on a protein; a mechanism by which many proteins acquire altered activity.

signal transduction A series of ordered biochemical reactions by which a signal initiated at the cell surface is transmitted inside the cell to elicit specific cellular responses.

tyrosine kinase An enzyme that catalyzes the transfer of a high-energy phosphate group from ATP to a tyrosine residue on a protein, very often then modulating the activity of the target proteins.

Chronic myelogenous leukemia (CML) is a chronic form of leukemia originating in a primitive myeloid stem cell in which the leukemic cells retain the capacity for differentiation and are able to perform the essential functions of normal hematopoietic cells that they replace in the marrow. Leukemic cells have a pronounced tendency to undergo further malignant transformation with loss of ability to differentiate in later stages of the disease. Although commonly

Encyclopedia of Cancer, Second Edition
Volume 1

included among other myeloproliferative disorders, CML is a distinct entity that is easily recognized because the leukemic cells have a distinctive cytogenetic abnormality, the Philadelphia (Ph) chromosome.

I. HISTORY

Chronic myelogenous leukemia was recognized as a clinical entity around the middle of the last century and was the first type of leukemia to be described. The original case reports from Edinburgh in 1845 were entitled: "Case of hypertrophy of the spleen and liver in which death took place from suppuration of the blood" and "Case of disease of the spleen in which death took place in consequence of the presence of purulent matter in the blood." About the same time in Berlin, Virchow, then an intern, published his classic papers entitled, "Weisses Blut" and "Weisses Blut and Milztumoren" in which he recognized that the "white blood" and splenic enlargement did not represent a suppurative process, but rather were manifestations of a distinct disease entity, thereafter called leukemia. Based on his clinical and pathological studies, he later distinguished between a predominantly splenic form of leukemia (CML) and one in which lymphadenopathy was more prominent [chronic lymphocytic leukemia [CLL]]. A decade later, Friedreich first described acute leukemia, but it was not until near the turn of the century that further conceptual advances and improvements in staining techniques permitted a definitive distinction between acute and chronic forms of leukemia and between myelogenous leukemias and lymphocytic leukemias and lymphomas.

In the ensuing years, CML was gradually distinguished from myelofibrosis and other myeloproliferative diseases on the basis of differing clinical and pathological features, but the first real clue as to its pathogenesis was the landmark discovery in 1960 of an abnormally small chromosome in leukemic cells, thereafter designated the Philadelphia chromosome. It soon became apparent that about 90% of patients who presented with clinical features of CML had the Ph chromosome in most of their bone marrow cells during metaphase, but about 10% with similar clinical manifestations did not; the subsequent literature has customarily referred to Ph-positive and Ph-negative CML. A decade after the Ph chromosome was first described, and shortly after the introduction

of chromosome banding techniques, the Ph chromosome was identified as a modified 22 chromosome. A few years later, Rowley showed that the Ph anomaly was not due to a simple deletion, but rather resulted from translocation of the distal segment of the long arm of chromosome 22 to the distal portion of the long arm of chromosome 9 [t(9;22) (q34; q11)]. Although it was generally assumed that the translocation was reciprocal, this was not confirmed at the molecular level until another decade had passed when it was demonstrated that the c-abl oncogene was transposed from its normal position (q34) on chromosome 9 to a specific breakpoint cluster region (bcr) on chromosome 22 (q11). The transposed c-abl and rearranged bcr gene on 22q11 form a new fusion bcr-abl gene that transcribes a novel chimeric 8.5-kb mRNA, which in turn encodes a hybrid 210-kDa phosphoprotein p210$^{bcr-abl}$.

Some patients lacking a morphologically detectable Ph chromosome on cytogenetic analysis can be shown by molecular analysis to have a so-called "masked" Ph chromosome; the clinical features and molecular changes of such patients are indistinguishable from those of Ph-positive CML patients. Other Ph-negative patients are simply misdiagnosed and have other myeloproliferative disorders, but a few patients still remain who are truly Ph negative, lacking the characteristic gene rearrangement. The latter patients comprise only a few percent of the total patients initially suspected of having CML and they generally respond less well to treatment and have a shorter survival than Ph-positive patients. About 5% of Ph-positive patients have variant translocations involving other chromosomes, but almost all the variants, both simple and complex, also result in juxtaposition of abl from chromosome 9 and the rearranged bcr gene on chromosome 22 to form a fused bcr-abl gene. Moreover, the clinical course of patients with variant translocations appears to be the same as those with the standard 9;22 translocation; thus the bcr-abl juxtaposition is closely correlated with the clinical disease.

The Philadelphia chromosome was the first example of a specific cytogenetic abnormality consistently associated with a human neoplasm, and for more than a decade after it was discovered it remained the only example. However, rather than being unique as many investigators proposed at the time, CML pointed the way to general verification of the somatic mutation theory of cancer, which was originally proposed in

1914. The evidence of course is now compelling that all human cancers result from one or more specific genetic defects, although some can only be detected by molecular methods of analysis.

II. ETIOLOGY, INCIDENCE, AND CLINICAL FEATURES

The t(9,22) translocation characteristic of CML is acquired, as the Ph chromosome is not found in the majority of lymphocytes nor in the fibroblasts of skin or marrow of CML patients. Moreover, monozygous twins of patients with CML rarely develop CML, and only rare instances of familial occurrence have been reported. The etiology of CML is unknown. The majority of patients with CML have no history of excessive exposure to ionizing radiation or chemical leukemogens, but the incidence does increase progressively with exposure to increasing doses of radiation. This has been noted following chronic exposure in radiologists who practiced without adequate shielding, in patients who received radiation treatments for ankylosing spondylitis or uterine or cervical cancer, and in subjects exposed to a single massive dose of radiation, as in the atomic bomb explosions in Japan in 1945. After acute or subacute exposure to large radiation doses there is a variable latent period of about 4 to 11 years, after which the incidence of both acute myeloid leukemia and CML increases in an approximately linear relationship to the radiation dose. In the atomic explosion survivors, the peak incidence of CML occurred about 10 years after the explosion and was about 50 times that of nonexposed subjects; younger individuals (<15 years of age) developed leukemia earlier than older ones (>30 years). The rate then declined, but still exceeded the national average 15 years later.

The incidence of CML in the United States and most Western countries is about 1.5 per 100,000 population per year and accounts for about 15% of all cases of leukemia; about 4500 new cases are diagnosed in the United States each year. CML is slightly more frequent in men than women, but the course of the disease is the same. The median age is about 50; it is rare in children and the incidence increases progressively with age to over 8 per 100,000 in octogenarians. In children with CML in whom the Ph chromosome is present (i.e., about 5% of total CML patients), the disease characteristics and course of the disease are similar to that in adults, although children may respond better to intensive treatment and bone marrow transplantation.

A rare juvenile form of CML (JCML) occurs in young children that has a more rapidly progressive course and in which the leukemic cells lack the Ph chromosome. Subsets of patients also have neurofibromatosis, monosomy 7, or other chromosomal abnormalities. JCML was previously thought to be due to the excessive secretion of hemopoietic cytokines, such as GM-CSF or interleukin 1 by monocytes, but more recent studies have shown that there is no increased production of hemopoietic cytokines in some patients with JCML, but that the progenitor cells are selectively hypersensitive to stimulation by GM-CSF (but not by G-CSF or IL-3). Polymorphisms of GM-CSFR α and β chains are common in both JCML patients and normal controls, but pathogenic point mutations of GM-CSFR are infrequent in JCML and do not appear to be responsible for the hypersensitivity of the JCML progenitors to GM-CSF. In JCML there is excessive clonal proliferation of the leukemic progenitors in the absence of addition of exogenous growth factors, and the cells respond aberrantly to numerous growth and inhibitory factors. JCML thus appears to have quite a different pathogenesis and course than Ph+ CML.

Based on the occurrence of CML in patients with chromosome mosaicism and in those heterozygous for G6PD, there is good evidence that the leukemic population arises from a single cell because the Ph anomaly has been found to be restricted to just one of their dual cell lines. The clonal origin of CML and most other myeloproliferative disorders has been confirmed using X chromosome gene probes and various other molecular methods. The presence of the Ph chromosome in erythrocyte, granulocyte, monocyte, B lymphocyte, and megakaryocyte precursors indicates that the original transformation occurred in an ancestral stem cell common to these cell types. The Ph chromosome is absent in the majority of mature lymphocytes, although in about 20–25% of patients in chronic phase some of the B cells contain the Ph marker, and early B-cell progenitors predominate in about 25% of patients in blastic transformation. T lymphocytes have only rarely been reported to be Ph+ during either the chronic or blastic phases of the disease, but bilineal (T lymphoid/myeloid) Ph+ progenitors may be involved in some cases of blastic transformation, and quadralineal involvement [B cells (CD19$^+$), T cells (CD3$^+$), myeloid (CD13$^+$), and erythroid (glycophorin A$^+$)] was reported in one patient with Ph+ acute lymphoblastic leukemia (ALL).

It is still not known why leukemic cells in CML have a proliferative advantage over normal cells. At diagnosis the leukemic population has usually reached several trillion cells and almost completely replaced the normal hematopoietic cells in the bone marrow. Normal stem cells survive, at least during the chronic phase of the disease, but are largely suppressed by the leukemic cells and thus produce very few normal mature cells. In the chronic stage of the disease, leukemic cells retain the capacity to differentiate almost normally, and the biochemical and functional defects exhibited by leukemic cells are not of sufficient severity to prevent them from carrying out their essential normal functions.

III. CLINICAL AND PATHOLOGICAL FEATURES

During the chronic phase of the disease, leukemic cells function fairly normally and are able to support life largely in the absence of normal hematopoietic cells that they have replaced. Many patients at diagnosis are asymptomatic. Symptoms occur when the spleen becomes grossly enlarged, white blood cells (WBC) become sufficiently elevated to cause leukostasis, significant anemia develops, or abnormalities of the platelets result in thrombotic or hemorrhagic complications. In the absence of extreme blood cell counts or other unusual manifestations such as hyperbasophilia, patients have few symptoms because the leukemic cells are able to carry out all their normal functions fairly effectively, such as transporting oxygen, killing invading microorganisms, and maintaining hemostasis.

The most obvious and consistent clinical laboratory feature of CML is an otherwise unexplained leukocytosis. If the disease is detected early, WBC may be only minimally elevated, but as the disease progresses, it may rise to 10^5/mm^3 or even higher than 10^6/mm^3. The marrow is characteristically hypercellular, and in the chronic phase the differential counts of both marrow and blood show a spectrum of mature and immature granulocytes similar to those found in normal marrow. In most cases, neutrophilic granulocytes predominate, but increased numbers of eosinophils and/or basophils are common and occasionally monocytosis also occurs. About half of patients have some degree of thrombocytosis at diagnosis, accompanied by increased numbers of megakaryocytes in the marrow and often with fragments of megakaryocytic nuclei in the blood. There may be no anemia at diagnosis in early stage disease, but progressively severe anemia is common as the disease advances, usually accompanied by extreme degrees of leukocytosis if uncontrolled by therapy. Unless there are complicating features such as bleeding and development of iron deficiency, the anemia is normochromic and normocytic. Shortened red cell survival may occur in patients with massive splenomegaly and/or hepatomegaly, but autoimmune hemolysis is not seen in uncomplicated CML. Some patients, especially those with enlarged spleens, may have circulating nucleated erythrocyte precursors in the blood, but this finding is usually not prominent. The ratio of myeloid/erythroid cells is usually greatly increased from the normal ratio of ~3:1 in newly diagnosed patients with CML, but may return toward normal after treatment. The percentages of lymphocytes in both marrow and blood are also decreased in comparison to normal subjects, but the absolute lymphocyte count is usually normal with normal proportions of B and T cells.

To appreciate the magnitude of the increased cell production in CML, it is worthwhile to consider some basic parameters of hematopoiesis. The bone marrow of a normal 70-kg adult contains approximately 10^{12} hematopoietic cells, of which about one-half are granulocyte precursors, one-third to two-fifths are erythroblasts, and the remainder are other cells, including megakaryocytes and lymphocytes. The total volume of marrow in a 70-kg adult is about 3700 ml, but only about one-fourth of this marrow space consists of "red" marrow occupied by hematopoietic tissue (mainly located in the central skeleton), whereas the other three-fourths is composed of yellow, fatty marrow. Because even the "red" marrow is composed of one-half to two-thirds adipose tissue, the actual volume of marrow occupied by hematopoietic tissue is only about 500 to 600 ml.

With greatly increased demand as in severe, uncompensated hemolytic anemia, the red marrow may expand enormously, displacing the fatty marrow and filling the entire skeletal marrow space; in extreme cases, red cell production may be increased to its maximum limit of about 10–12 times normal. In advanced, uncontrolled chronic-phase CML, a comparable or even greater expansion of granulopoiesis can occur because extramedullary hematopoiesis is a regular feature of the disease. In untreated patients, depending on how advanced the disease is at diagnosis, the cellularity of the marrow is usually increased 3- to 5-fold compared to normal, with the cells in the most crowded marrows almost completely replacing the normal fatty component and cramming the available marrow space. Not only is the cell density increased severalfold, but hematopoiesis expands into the long bones and other parts of the skeleton normally occupied by fatty marrow, as in hemolytic anemias. In addition, extramedullary hematopoiesis in uncontrolled disease may become extreme with massive enlargement of the spleen and sometimes the liver and other organs. If one considers the total expansion of granulopoiesis involving the skeletal marrow, blood, and extramedullary sites, it should hardly be surprising that a 5- to 10-fold expansion of the normal myeloid mass in untreated CML commonly occurs and that an even greater expansion can occur in patients with very advanced disease who have massive splenomegaly and sometimes involvement of the liver, lymph nodes, and other organs. The main reason for the expanded myeloid mass is that leukemic progenitor cells, especially granulocyte progenitors, continue to proliferate after exceeding the cell density limit in the marrow at which normal progenitor cells curtail cell production, but the biochemical pathways involved and the specific abnormalities caused by Bcr-Abl that are responsible for this overproduction are not yet well defined. There are several reports that Bcr-Abl downregulates an important cyclin-dependent kinase inhibitor, p27^{Kip1}. Because p27^{Kip1} appears to have a critical role in regulating stem and progenitor cells, its dysregulation may be at least partially responsible for the expanded progenitor cell compartment in CML. Regulation of leukemic and normal hematopoietic cell growth is extremely complex, and while knowledge is increasing as to how cytokines, chemokines, cyclins, and cellular interactions function in controlling the growth and differentiation of stem cells and progenitor cells at different stages of

development, understanding of how the controls operate and interact is still incomplete.

Leukemic cells in chronic-phase CML have a striking propensity for further transformation. After a variable duration of the chronic phase, averaging about 3 to 4 years, the disease enters an accelerated or blastic phase. Such malignant progression occurs in about 80% of patients and probably would eventually occur in all of them if they did not die of other complications of the disease or of unrelated causes. No single mutation has been identified that is responsible for disease progression but rather a number of additional genetic events have been implicated, most commonly an additional Ph chromosome, trisomy of chromosome 8 or 19, and isochromosome 17. The Ph chromosome is almost always preserved in the blastic phase, and only rare cases of blastic transformation have been reported with loss of the Ph chromosome and/or the deletion of bcr-abl sequences. In the accelerated phase, some of the cells are still able to undergo partial or even complete differentiation, whereas in the blastic phase the majority of cells are arrested at the blastic level of differentiation. The direction of differentiation is variable in the accelerated and blastic phases, and transitional forms may occur among the three phases.

IV. CYTOKINETIC ABNORMALITIES

Although there is considerable variability among patients, cytokinetic studies performed during the chronic phase of CML have shown that while the DNA synthesis time of both blood and marrow myelocytes in CML is about the same as that of normal myelocytes, the earlier leukemic precursors (i.e., blasts and promyelocytes) have lower mitotic indices, a lower fraction of cells in DNA synthesis, longer generation times, and the mature leukocytes have longer transit times in the blood than comparable normal cells. Stryckmans found a relationship between the WBC count and the fraction of cells in S phase as measured by the [^{3}H]thymidine-labeling index (LI) in chronic-phase CML. When the WBC was >40,000 cells/mm^{3}, the mean myeloblast LI was about 20%, whereas after treatment, when the WBC was <20,000/mm^{3}, the average myeloblast LI was 46% or in the same range as that of myeloblasts in normal subjects. When treatment was discontinued and the disease relapsed, the LI of the CML myeloblasts again decreased and similar findings were found for CML CFU-c. Stryckmans also observed that unlike the myeloblasts and CFU-c, the LI of CML myelocytes was not influenced by the leukocyte count, and he suggested that both CML and normal myelocytes may no longer be under regulatory control.

The slower proliferative parameters of the CML precursors are thus closely related to the high cell density in the marrow. All cells, both normal and neoplastic, are of course inhibited in their growth at high cell densities, although the density at which growth arrest occurs varies greatly among different cell populations, and the mode of growth inhibition may also differ depending on the conditions. The general tendency of Ph+ populations is to undergo progressive expansion, but CML patients often show stabilization of their WBC counts and the size of their spleens for many months without treatment, although the levels at which these parameters stabilize may vary considerably among patients. CML cells are thus still subject to feedback regulation, although the curtailment of cell production occurs at higher than normal cell densities.

Although many immature cells are usually present in the blood in CML and their fraction in S phase is similar or only slightly lower than that in the marrow because their mitotic index is almost invariably lower in the blood, the immature cells must usually return to the marrow or spleen in order to divide. The rate of cell production is similar in the marrow and spleen, and in patients with extensive splenic involvement, the majority of circulating immature granulocytes may originate in the spleen. The size of the total blood granulocyte pool (TBGP) in CML patients may be 10 to 100 times greater than normal; both the circulating granulocyte pool (CGP) and the marginated granulocyte pool (MGP) are grossly expanded.

Blood granulocyte levels have sometimes been observed to undergo cyclical fluctuations in normal individuals, although most normal people do not have obvious oscillations, probably because of the damping action of granulocyte reserves in the marrow. Pronounced cyclic oscillations have been observed following injury to the marrow by cytotoxic drugs and in cyclic neutropenia. Cyclic oscillations of the blood granulocytes have also been observed in CML, and although there is considerable variability among patients, both the amplitudes and the lengths of the cycles in CML are usually much greater than in normal subjects or patients with neutropenia, suggesting that a greater than normal number of divisions occurs between division of the CML stem cells and the appearance of nondividing mature cells. In addition, the occurrence of cyclic oscillations in CML provides strong evidence that leukemic cells retain at least partial responsiveness to normal regulatory controls, although the response threshold is of course set at a much higher level than normal. The periodic oscillations of the neutrophils in CML, as well as in cyclic neutropenia in both humans and gray collies, are usually accompanied by similar oscillations in the cells of other lineages (i.e., platelets, reticulocytes, and monocytes). Moreover, the cell density waves have also been noted to extend back to involve precursor cells in multiple lineages, thus providing additional evidence that periodic oscillations both in (nonleukemic) cyclic neutropenia and in CML originate in stem cells. However, it is still uncertain whether the fluctuations are mainly due to variable rates of stem cell proliferative activity or self-renewal or to a variable incidence of apoptosis in stem cells and perhaps also in their committed progeny.

V. LIFE SPAN AND PROGRAMMED CELL DEATH

Using a variety of isotopic labeling procedures, it has been consistently observed that mature granulocytes in chronic-phase CML have a markedly slower rate of disappearance from the blood than normal mature granulocytes. It has often been presumed that this indicates that they have a longer life span, but interpretation of the slow granulocyte disappearance rate in CML is confounded by the presence of many circulating immature granulocytes and by abnormal granulocyte traffic and distribution patterns in CML. By irradiating the immature cells to minimize their contribution, the blood transit time of CML polymorphonuclear cells was still 2 to 4 times longer than normal, and the granulocyte turnover rate was also usually found to be substantially increased in CML (1 to 14 times normal). Cross-transfusion experiments also showed that normal mature granulocytes transfused into CML patients disappear normally and that

CML mature granulocytes transfused into cancer patients disappear more slowly than normal; the explanation for these observations may be at least partly due to the fact that the CML circulating granulocytes are not fully mature.

Once committed to differentiation, all hematopoietic cells have finite life spans and normally undergo programmed cell death at prescribed times depending on the lineage and environmental factors. Numerous reports demonstrate that apoptosis is inhibited under a variety of conditions in cell lines expressing $p210^{bcr-abl}$ and in v-abl transfected cells with activated tyrosine kinase activity, as well as in progenitors and granulocytes obtained directly from CML patients. While some investigators have suggested that the decreased rate of programmed cell death may be the primary mechanism responsible for expansion of the leukemic clone in CML, this claim has not been generally accepted, and the effects of bcr-abl in inhibiting apoptosis appear to be quite complicated. Contradictory or inconclusive results have been reported concerning the roles of p53, c-myc, bcl-2, bcl-X_L, and CD95/Fas-R in inhibiting apoptosis in bcr-abl-containing cells, but because a variety of cell lines were used and the experimental conditions differed considerably, this is hardly surprising. Cell lines hyperexpressing bcr-abl or having many additional genetic abnormalities are often imperfect models for fresh human CML cells. Most, but not all, studies have shown that CML CD34+ cells and granulocytes are more resistant to apoptosis than comparable normal cells, and this conclusion is in keeping with the older cytokinetic labeling studies conducted in patients that showed that CML mature neutrophils had a significantly slower disappearance rate than normal. However, the cell kinetic measurements included incompletely mature neutrophils prematurely released into the blood, so one would expect them to have a longer life span than more fully mature normal bands and polymorphonuclear cells. Even if one assumes that CML cells do survive longer than normal, without exception all of the detailed cytokinetic-labeling studies performed *in vivo* have concluded that prolonged life span alone cannot possibly account for the enormous progressive expansion of the CML population and that the expansion is primarily due to greatly increased cell production.

VI. MORPHOLOGIC, BIOCHEMICAL, AND FUNCTIONAL ABNORMALITIES OF CML CELLS

Numerous subtle morphological, biochemical, and functional abnormalities of the leukemic cells have been described. The most common morphological abnormalities observed by light microscopy include hypersegmentation, hyposegmentation, abnormal lobulation and ring-shaped nuclei of polymorphonuclear leukocytes, Pelger-like leukocytes, binucleate myelocytes, multinuclearity and karyorrhexis of erythroblasts, and large mononuclear forms, multiple small separated nuclei, and micro forms of the megakaryocytes. Dysplastic changes occur in the chronic phase of CML more frequently than in normal subjects and become more prominent as the disease approaches an accelerated or blastic phase; in particular the appearance of hyposegmented neutrophils and micromegakaryocytes appears to herald blastic transformation. Another frequent abnormality occurring in CML is the presence of both eosinophilic and basophilic granules in the same cell. According to Mlynek and colleagues, these bigranulated cells are not found in normal subjects and are thought to demonstrate lineage infidelity in CML. Electron microscopic studies have also revealed that maturation is faulty in developing CML cells. Especially significant is the observation that there is asynchrony in maturation of the cytoplasm and the nucleus, with the cytoplasm generally maturing more rapidly than the nucleus. CML promyelocytes, myelocytes, and Pelger–Hüet-like granulocytes may show well-developed cytoplasmic organelles and granules, whereas the nucleus remains immature compared to a normal cell at the same stage of development, and similar nuclear/cytoplasmic asynchrony with lagging nuclear maturation is also commonly observed in developing CML megakaryocytes.

A large number of biochemical and functional abnormalities have been reported in CML granulocytes, most of which appear to be mutually linked. In general, the abnormalities are quantitative rather than qualitative and represent mean values of the total mature granulocyte population. Biochemical abnormalities include low neutrophil alkaline phosphatase (NAP) activities, subnormal contents of lactoferrin and lysozyme, hypersialylation of the membrane protein due to increased activity of a specific sialyltransferase, reduced total gangliosides and neutral glycosphingolipid content of the cell membrane compared to normal neutrophils, and quantitative changes in many of the cellular proteins, including granule proteins and some of the plasma membrane protein constituents.

Functional defects of CML polymorphonuclear neutrophils include delayed emigration to extravascular sites, impaired phagocytic and bacteriocidal activities, reduced motility, defective chemotaxis and abnormal electrophoretic mobility, impaired internalization of certain proteins such as concanavalin A, and subnormal adhesiveness to glass and nylon surfaces. CML progenitors also adhere less well to bone marrow stroma and are less responsive to stromal-derived regulatory signals than normal progenitors; the decreased adhesion to stromal elements undoubtedly is a significant factor in the premature release of immature cells into the bloodstream. The marrow stroma provides a microenvironment that is clearly essential for maintaining hematopoiesis, but its structure and the factors controlling the production and release of cells and the homing and circulation of stem cells are very complex. It was first reported in 1969 that the marrow and fibroblasts do not have the Ph chromosome and are therefore not part of the transformed clone, and this observation has been repeatedly confirmed. It has been reported that variable proportions of endothelial cells in CML patients contain the bcr-abl fusion gene, suggesting they may be derived from a common hemangioblastic progenitor cell. However, detection of the bcr-abl fusion gene relied entirely on fluorescence *in situ* hybridization (FISH), and only two patients displayed colocalization signals that were well above the background level of false-positive results. Other studies have also supported the concept that multipotent stem cells may exist that exhibit "plasticity" (e.g., neural stem cells forming blood cells and bone marrow-derived cells forming muscle cells), but further work is needed to better define the true nature of these multipotent stem cells and their relation to stem cells that appear to be restricted to hematopoiesis, at least in normal physiologic conditions.

Several investigators have emphasized that many if not all of the biochemical and functional abnormalities of CML leukocytes, including impaired adhesiveness, extravascular emigration, phagocytic and bacteriocidal activities, neutrophil alkaline phosphatase (NAP) activities, hypersialylation, and reduced lacto-

ferrin and lysozyme contents, are mutually linked characteristics related to the degree of neutrophil maturation. For example, band forms have lower NAP activities and are less capable of adhering, emigrating, and phagocytizing than segmented forms, marrow segmented cells phagocytize less actively than circulating segmented cells, and the density of sialoproteins decrease and adhesiveness increases as the neutrophil matures. Therefore, even among morphologically indistinguishable normal polymorphonuclear cells there is heterogeneity in the degree of maturation (i.e., marrow vs circulating polymorphonuclear cells). The asynchronous nuclear/cytoplasmic maturation of CML cells coupled with their premature release from the marrow can result in a proportion of circulating polymorphonuclear cells that appear morphologically mature and to closely resemble normal mature neutrophils but that are not strictly comparable. This can lead to false conclusions from investigations seeking to find differences in survival, apoptosis, or various biochemical or functional parameters between CML and normal cells that are assumed to be comparable but that actually differ significantly in their state of maturation. Various abnormalities of stromal elements have been described in the marrow of CML patients, but it is not yet clear how important these abnormalities are in the overall evolution of the disease. Many of the abnormalities of CML granulocytes return to normal when the disease is brought into hematologic remission by treatment; moreover, some abnormalities can also modulate *in vitro*. For example, NAP activity is uniformly low in patients with CML at diagnosis, but increases during infections or when the leukocyte count is reduced with chemotherapy. CML granulocytes have also been shown to recover NAP activity *in vitro* by treatment with exogenous granulocyte growth factors (e.g., rhG-CSF). Thus many of the leukocyte abnormalities that have been described in CML appear to be mutually linked, are quantitative rather than qualitative, and tend to return to normal when the disease is brought into hematologic remission by treatment; many abnormalities may simply reflect the premature release of incompletely mature marrow bands and polymorphs into the blood in CML.

In attempting to correlate the molecular, biochemical, and biological changes induced by the multifunctional bcr-abl protein, it is important to recognize that the biological changes are pleiotropic, usually quite subtle, often interconnected, and that in the aggregate, they cannot all be explained by simply focusing on one mechanism such as dysregulation of the cell cycle, reduced programmed cell death, increased self-renewal of stem cells, or impairment of any single property such as cell adhesion or anchorage dependence. The signaling pathways controlling apoptosis, differentiation, maturation, proliferation, and other cell processes are intimately interrelated, and considered in this context, it is quite reasonable to expect that the biological abnormalities would be both pleiotropic and mutually linked.

VII. MOLECULAR AND SIGNALING ABNORMALITIES

In the t(9,22) translocation, the c-abl oncogene is transposed from its normal position on chromosome 9 (q34) to a 5.8-kb major breakpoint cluster region (M-bcr) on chromosome 22q11, forming a fusion bcr-abl gene. Although the precise point of breakage within bcr in CML patients may vary and atypical bcr-abl transcripts have been noted, the majority of breakpoints in the M-bcr region occur between exons b2 and b3 or between b3 and b4 so that the chimeric bcr-abl gene may include bcr exon b3. About 10% of patients have dual expression of b2a2 and b3a2 transcripts, and rare patients have been reported with b2/a3 or b3/a3 transcripts. There have been numerous attempts to correlate the exact site of the M-bcr breakpoint with the duration of the chronic phase of CML, but the results have been conflicting and overall no clear-cut or consistent difference in survival has been observed.

The bcr-abl gene transcribes a novel 8.5-kb mRNA, which in turn encodes a p210-kDa protein that, unlike the normal c-abl protein, is phosphorylated on tyrosine and has increased intrinsic protein tyrosine kinase activity compared to that of the normal c-abl protein. Because the tyrosine kinase activity of the Abelson murine leukemia virus product p160v-abl was known to be necessary for cellular transformation, it was suggested that the p210bcr-abl tyrosine kinase may have an important role in the pathogenesis of CML, and now a large amount of experimental evidence supports this suggestion.

Breakpoints for the related bcr-abl gene encoding the p190bcr-abl protein (often referred to as p185bcr-

abl in the literature) found in Ph-positive acute leukemias are located in a 20-kb region (known as minor bcr or m-bcr) at the 3 prime end of the first bcr intron so that the first exon of the bcr gene (e1) is joined directly to the second abl exon, resulting in an e1a2 fusion in p190bcr-abl. The p210bcr-abl protein contains either 902 or 927 bcr amino acids depending on the breakpoint in M-bcr (including sequences from the first 11 or 12 exons of bcr), whereas the p190bcr-abl protein contains only 426 or 436 bcr amino acids. The p190bcr-abl protein has about fivefold higher tyrosine kinase activity than p210bcr-abl, which correlates with the former's much more frequent association with an acute rather than a chronic form of leukemia, and with its greater transforming potency both in *in vitro* and in animal experimental systems.

Chronic neutrophilic leukemia, also known as neutrophilic–chronic leukemia (CML-N), is a rare myeloproliferative disorder first described in the mid-1920s, which is characterized by a moderate nonprogressive neutrophilic leukocytosis with infrequent circulating immature myeloid cells, an excess of mature myeloid cells in the marrow, a normal or elevated NAP score, absent or minimal splenomegaly, and absence of any underlying infection or other condition capable of provoking a leukemoid reaction. CML-N has a more indolent course than classical CML, and blastic transformation usually occurs much later or not at all. Six patients with presumed CML-N have been reported who had a t(9,22) chromosome translocation and a rare bcr-abl rearrangement with a 3 prime bcr breakpoint between exons e19 and e20 (originally designated bcr exons c3 and c4). This breakpoint, named μ-bcr, is located distally to the M breakpoint of classical CML and encodes a 230-kDa fusion protein that has an additional 180 amino acids compared to p210bcr-abl.

At least three major forms of bcr-abl fusion proteins have been recognized and it appears that the inclusion or exclusion of bcr exons is largely responsible for determining the disease phenotype caused by these proteins. The smallest fusion protein, p190bcr-abl (m-bcr breakpoint), predominantly causes acute lymphoblastic leukemia and is only rarely associated with CML, AML or other diseases, such as multiple myeloma or B-cell lymphomas. It has been suggested that the lack of bcr domains encoded by sequences downstream of bcr exon e1 may be irrelevant to the mechanism by which signal transduction is deregulated by p190bcr-abl in lymphoid precursors, but may be more restrictive or inefficient in CML progenitors. p210bcr-abl (M-bcr) is the commonest fusion protein; it most frequently causes classical CML, but can also be associated with ALL, AML (usually FAB M4 or M5), or rarely other diseases such as essential thrombocythemia. The largest bcr-abl fusion protein, p230bcr-abl (μ-bcr), includes over 90% of bcr amino acids, lacking only the C-terminal two-thirds of the GAPrac domain. In one study comparing the leukemogenic activity of p190, p210, and p230 *in vitro* and *in vivo* in mice, p230 exhibited the lowest intrinsic tyrosine kinase activity, p210 was intermediate, and p190 had the highest activity (i.e., 7-, 5.4-, and 3.7-fold increase, respectively, relative to c-abl). The three forms of bcr-abl were equally potent in inducing a similar type of a polyclonal CML-like myeloproliferative syndrome in mice when 5FU-treated donors were used, leading to the authors' contention that the more benign clinical course observed in patients with CML-N might be due to other variables than p230. However, because less than a dozen CML-N patients have been reported and most had a very indolent disease, it may well be that murine transduction/transplantation models in which p230 is overexpressed in stem cells or early progenitor cells surviving 5FU do not accurately reflect the (presumably) lower expression of p230 in the clinical setting, and one must be cautious in extrapolating interpretation of the results of the murine models to CML-N. In other studies using primary bone marrow cells as targets for bcr-abl oncogenes, p185/p190bcr.abl was the most potent in inducing lymphoid tumors in SCID mice, whereas p230-expressing cells differentiated into the myeloid lineage and did not form tumors.

Unexpectedly, using highly sensitive reverse transcriptase–polymerase chain reaction assays, bcr-abl transcripts were found in the blood cells of 22/73 normal healthy adults and 1/22 children, but not in 22 samples of cord blood. This surprising finding was subsequently confirmed in the circulating leukocytes of 12 of 16 healthy adults with 11 showing e1/a2 transcripts (p190) and 4 b2/a2 or b3/a2 transcripts (p210). The same aberrant transcripts were also found in many non-CML cell lines, both hematopoietic and non-hematopoietic. The significance of these observations is unclear, but among the possible explanations offered are that additional (unspecified) changes are required for progression to overt leukemia, that normal, healthy individuals have some as yet unidentified surveillance mechanism to prevent expansion of these "benign" bcr-abl-containing cells, or, as appears most likely, that the fusion gene occurred in a later precursor incapable of extensive expansion.

c-abl was first identified as a protooncogene in the genome of the Abelson murine leukemia virus, which specifically targets early B cells. The v-abl gene is derived by recombination of c-abl with the viral Gag gene, which replaces the SH3 domain, a negative regulatory domain, creating a fusion protein with unregulated high kinase activity. The viral Gag sequence also provides a myristoylation signal causing v-abl to localize predominantly at the plasma membrane. The protein tyrosine kinase activity of c-abl is normally tightly regulated, and both the deregulation of kinase activity and the abnormal cellular localization of v-abl and Bcr-abl are important elements governing the transforming potency of these fusion proteins.

The normal p140c-abl protein is localized both to the cytoplasm and to the nucleus, and c-abl binds specifically to DNA, suggesting that this may be critical to its normal biological function. In contrast, the chimeric p210bcr-abl and other abl transforming proteins are only present in the cytoplasm and lack the ability to bind DNA. bcr sequences not only deregulate abl tyrosine kinase, but also activate an actin filament-binding function associated with c-abl. Based on observations in fibroblasts, it was proposed that the normal function of bcr is related to maintenance of the cytoskeleton and that the chimerization of bcr and abl permits abl to bind to actin microfilaments. Because actin fibers are vital elements involved in maintaining cell shape and in regulating many cellular functions and interactions, dysregulation of actin could have a critical role in altering cell growth and maturation. Domain 1 of bcr, consisting of 63 amino acids, is a coiled-coil oligomerization domain that forms a homotetramer, and tetramerization of bcr-abl through this first bcr domain was found to be correlated both with the activation of tyrosine kinase and with the F-actin-binding function of abl. The reciprocal abl/bcr fusion gene is expressed in about two-thirds of CML patients, but although all the junctions in the bcr-abl transcripts are in-frame and should allow for functional abl/bcr fusion proteins to be translated, the presence of abl/bcr proteins could not be detected in cells from CML patients. Other studies have also indicated that c-abl may have an important role in maintaining the cytoskeleton and normal cytoskeletal processes. One study showed that a membrane pool of c-abl in fibroblasts is activated both by PDGF and EGF, that cells expressing oncogenic src proteins increased c-abl kinase activity 10- to 20-fold, and that src and fyn kinases directly phosphorylated c-abl *in vitro*. In another report, both bcr-abl and v-src oncoproteins were found to support normal erythroid development in fetal liver erythroid progenitors from EpoR$-/-$ mice; these embryos die around 13–15 days of embryogenesis as a result of severe anemia attributable to the absence of red cell maturation. It thus appears from recent studies that c-abl may serve as a downstream target for both activated receptor tyrosine kinases and src kinases, and moreover that terminal differentiation in at least the erythroid lineage may not require a signal unique to a specific cytokine receptor, but may respond to a generic signal by other activated protein tyrosine kinases, such as bcr-abl.

c-abl is expressed throughout murine gestation and ubiquitously in adult mouse tissues, with the highest levels in thymus, spleen and testes. Mice homozygous for mutated c-abl become runted and die within a few weeks after birth, and many have thymic and splenic atrophy and lymphopenia. c-abl is thought to be involved in the regulation of several important cell functions, including cell interactions, proliferation, differentiation, DNA repair, and apoptosis. Both p53 and the p53-related p73 protein can participate in the apoptotic response to DNA damage, but they appear to operate by different mechanisms. Whereas the p53 apoptotic pathway is apparently independent of c-abl, the p73 pathway requires c-abl kinase to stabilize and activate p73. In experiments using single or double knockout Abl ($-/-$) and p53 ($-/-$) mice and mouse embryo fibroblasts (MEF), doubly deficient mice died during embryogenesis, but in MEF cells, c-abl was observed to have a positive effect on cell growth in the absence of p53, but a negative effect in p53 ($+/+$) cells.

The abl sequences of bcr-abl genes are unchanged except for loss of the first exon, and this loss alone does not endow c-abl with the ability to transform cells. However, bcr first-exon sequences potentiate tyrosine kinase activation and transforming ability when they are fused to the second exon of c-abl, presum-

ably by specifically interfering with the negative regulation of abl-encoded tyrosine kinase. bcr has been reported to have a novel type of kinase activity, which is confined to a segment encoded by the first exon. The abl-binding domain is localized in the first exon of bcr, and bcr sequences bind specifically to the SH2 (src homology region 2) regulatory domain of abl in a nonphosphotyrosine-dependent manner. The protein fragments appear to fold back on each other to form a second link at the SH2 regions, and this binding appears to be essential for bcr-abl-mediated transformation. Bap-1, a member of the 14-3-3 family of proteins, interacts with c-bcr and bcr-abl and may function in the regulation of c-bcr and contribute to the transforming activity of bcr-abl.

VIII. PROTEIN PHOSPHORYLATION AND REGULATION OF HEMATOPOIESIS

Proteins with SH2 domains are well known to be important in growth factor-mediated intracellular signaling and oncogenesis. The SH3 domain of c-abl suppresses its intrinsic transforming activity while the SH2 domain is required for transformation; point mutations in the abl SH2 domain have been shown to coordinately impair phosphotyrosine binding and transforming activity. This suggests that SH2–phosphotyrosine interactions may be involved in transformation by nonreceptor tyrosine kinases, probably by localizing activated kinases to the cell membrane where they phosphorylate a complex of membrane-associated substrates; assembly of this multiprotein complex could then facilitate the transmission of positive growth signals. The tertiary structure of the SH2 domain of c-abl has been determined. It is a compact domain with an obvious putative phosphotyrosine-binding site, and while comparison with other SH2 sequences shows a common mode of phosphotyrosine binding, subtle differences in structure appear to allow sufficient latitude to control the specificity of binding of different peptides. A phosphopeptide library has been used to determine the sequence specificity of the peptide-binding sites of SH2 domains. SH2 and SH3 domains serve as recognition modules that target proteins to specific sites containing phosphotyrosine residues or Pro-x-x-Pro motifs, respectively. Phosphorylation of different tyrosines within tyrosine kinases controls kinase activity in opposing ways. For example, phosphorylation of Tyr-527 in the C-terminal tail region of src kinases suppresses kinase activity, whereas phosphorylation of Tyr-416, which is in a centrally located "activation segment," releases blockage of the peptide substrate-binding site and enhances catalytic activity. The SH2 and SH3 domains of src kinases regulate kinase activity at least in part by influencing the rate at which the autophosphorylation of Tyr-416 occurs; the control mechanisms are complicated and involve multiple conformational changes in different sites of the proteins.

The v-abl oncogene has substantially greater transforming ability than bcr-abl because the negative regulatory SH3 (src homology region 3) domain is deleted in the v-abl product, p160v-abl, and because the upstream fusion of viral gag sequences provides for N-terminal myristoylation, thereby directing localization of the protein to the inner cell membrane. Both p210 and p185/p190 bcr-abl oncoproteins have an intact SH3 domain and are not myristoylated at the N terminus. Based on the comparative transforming abilities of various bcr-abl constructs, it appears that fusion of bcr first exon sequences upstream of the second exon of c-abl may functionally mimic deletion of the SH3 domain and the effects of the myristoylation localization signal by inhibiting the negative regulation of the tyrosine kinase domain of abl. However, deletion of SH3 coupled with a gag-encoded myristoylation consensus sequence is about 10-fold more effective in activating the transforming potential of c-abl in Rat 1 fibroblasts than bcr-abl fusion. Whereas p160v-abl readily transforms NIH/3T3 fibroblasts, p210bcr-abl has limited transforming ability for fibroblasts, despite the fact that the transfected cells adequately express p210bcr-abl. However, if myristoylated viral gag sequences are fused to bcr-abl, the gag-bcr-abl protein then has significant transforming ability. It appears that if a myristoylation site or hydrophobic domain is lacking, the protein is not anchored to the cell membrane but remains in the cytoplasm where it is less effective in inducing transformation.

Thus the transforming potential of abl oncoproteins appears to be related not only to increased tyrosine kinase activity, but also to localization to the cell membrane where the protein may more readily interact with critical membrane-associated substrates, such as growth factor receptors and phosphoinositides. The normal c-Abl can shuttle between the cytoplasmic and nuclear compartments, whereas Bcr-Abl is generally restricted to the cytoplasm. Most studies have suggested that c-Abl contributes to the activation of apoptosis whereas Bcr-Abl inhibits apoptosis, but it has been reported that when Bcr-Abl is entrapped in the nucleus by mutation or treatment with STI571 and leptomycin B, the nuclear Bcr-Abl may activate rather than suppress apoptosis.

In NIH/3T3 cells, bcr-abl was found to abrogate only the anchorage requirement but not the serum requirement for growth. Abi-2 is a novel protein that contains a SH3 domain and proline-rich sequences critical for binding to c-abl. Abi-2 interacts with both the SH3 domain and carboxy-terminal sequences of abl tyrosine kinase and modulates the transforming capacity of oncogenic abl. The destruction of Abi proteins requires tyrosine kinase activity and is dependent on the ubiquitin proteasome pathway. Oncogenic forms of abl and src tyrosine kinases trigger destruction of the Abi proteins that antagonize abl, thereby enhancing the oncogenic potential of abl; significantly, expression of Abi is lost in cell lines and bone marrow cells from patients with aggressive bcr-abl leukemias.

Phosphorylation and dephosphorylation of key regulatory proteins have pivotal roles in signal transduction in eukaryotic organisms. Protein tyrosine kinases (PTKs) are less numerous than protein serine or threonine kinases, but many of the former function as receptors and signal transducers for growth factors of hematopoietic as well as other types of cells. The state of phosphorylation of specific regulatory proteins involving tyrosine residues is thought to be critically important in controlling many essential cell functions, such as gene expression, metabolism, cytoskeletal architecture, cell division, and differentiation in many types of cells, including hematopoietic cells. Activation of growth factor receptors promotes a cascade of intracellular phosphorylations that ultimately result in a wide range of cellular responses. Protein tyrosine phosphatases (PTPs) interact with the tyrosine kinases in a complex fashion, probably acting in concert to regulate enzymatic activity; several phosphatases have important roles in regulating hematopoiesis.

Saccharomyces cerevisiae has 114 conventional protein kinase genes out of 6217 genes (1.8%) but no bona fide PTKs, whereas the C. *elegans* genome encodes 400 protein kinase catalytic domains out of 19,099 genes (2.1%), of which 92 are PTKs (23%). Based on public human EST (expressed sequence tag) databases, Hunter predicted that the human genome probably encodes >1100 protein kinases with ~150 PTKs if it is assumed the human genome has about 80,000 genes. (More recent estimates suggest there may be only ~35,000 human genes.) Hunter points out that the lack of bona fide PTKs in the yeasts and their presence in one of the simplest multicellular eukaryotes strongly suggest that protein-tyrosine phosphorylation evolved hand in hand with multicellularity in response to a need for intercellular communication, and that in keeping with this idea, the majority of PTKs have a role in transmembrane signaling in response to ligands that bind to surface receptors. The state of phosphorylation of specific regulatory proteins involving tyrosine residues is thought to be critically important in controlling many essential cell functions, such as gene expression, metabolism, cytoskeletal architecture, cell division, and differentiation in many types of cells, including hematopoietic cells. Activation of growth factor receptors promotes a cascade of intracellular phosphorylations that ultimately result in a wide range of cellular responses. Protein tyrosine phosphatases (PTPs) interact with the tyrosine kinases in a complex fashion, probably acting in concert to regulate enzymatic activity. Several phosphatases have already been shown to have important roles in regulating hematopoiesis. For example, SHP-1 (PTP1C) is a negative regulator of growth factor-mediated signaling in hematopoietic cells, and it has been reported that defective expression of SHP-1 is common in polycythemia vera and may contribute to the pathogenesis of this disease. SHP-1 also has key roles in modulating several other types of hematopoietic cells; to give another example, SHP-1 deficient (motheaten) me/me mice have a severe myeloproliferative disorder with a massive pulmonary infiltration of granulocytes and macrophages. It has been reported that p62^{dok-1} is a major substrate of SHP-1; SHP-1-deficient macrophages from me/me mice manifest constitutive tyrosine phosphorylation of p62^{dok-1}, which is correlated with growth factor independent survival of the macrophages.

IX. ABNORMALITIES OF PROTEIN PHOSPHORYLATION

Until a few years ago, little was known about the specific abnormalities in the signaling pathways that might be caused by p210bcr-abl and other bcr-abl oncoproteins. As indicated earlier, the signal transduction pathways are highly complex, and it has been difficult not only to identify the most important immediate target proteins that are constitutively phosphorylated by p210bcr-abl, but also to unravel the ensuing protein interactions and cascade of pleiotropic signals that are activated. Early studies using antiphosphotyrosine antibodies detected several putative substrates of p210$^{bcr-abl}$, but these were not well characterized. More recently, a large number of proteins have been reported to be tyrosine phosphorylated in cells expressing p210$^{bcr-abl}$, including p190, p160bcr, p125FAK, p120Cbl, p95Vav, p93Fes, p68paxillin and other focal adhesion proteins, p67Syp, p52Shc and p46Shc, p38Crkl, p30Bap-1, SHIP1 and SHIP2, and SHP2. Most of these studies were conducted in rodent, simian, or human cell lines transfected with bcr-abl or in established cell lines derived from CML patients that have multiple other chromosomal abnormalities in addition to t(9,22) (e.g., K562 and RWLeu4); their physiological significance with regard to the pathogenesis of chronic-phase CML is uncertain. Only a few studies used primary CML or Ph+ ALL blasts or CML peripheral blood granulocytes. The most prominent P-tyr proteins that are constitutively phosphorylated in primary CML progenitor cells and/or precursors by p210$^{bcr-abl}$ are: p190Rho-Gap, p155SHIP2, p145SHIP1, p110c-cbl, p62dok1, p56c-lyn, p56SHC, p42/44ERK1/2, and p39c-CRKL.

Alteration in gene expression has also been studied in various animal and human cell lines expressing bcr-abl proteins. A large number of genes, both known (i.e., MYC, BCL-2, GRAME, integrin α_6, Cyclin D2, CSCP, OSMRβ, DD9, MYC, BCL-2, GRAME, KIR, MPPI, BCL-6, R-PTPμ, DDM, DD1, DD221, and DDW) and unknown, have been reported to be overexpressed or underexpressed, but the results differ greatly in different cell lines, and again the physiological significance of these observations with regard to the evolution of the clinical disease is uncertain.

It is known that the sustained activation of discrete

signaling pathways in some types of cells results in differentiation, whereas transient activation is not associated with differentiation but rather leads to a proliferative response; in other cell types, the converse is observed. Thus different cell types may respond differently depending on prior developmental events such as their content of specific responsive transcription factors.

The control of hematopoiesis and the signaling pathways involved are highly complex, and the information is still far too incomplete to be able to design an accurate model of all the protein–protein, protein–lipid, and other interactions in normal hematopoiesis or CML. However, there is increasing evidence that the increased tyrosine kinase activity of p210$^{bcr-abl}$ has an essential role in causing untimely and inappropriate constitutive tyrosine phosphorylation of a number of proteins involved in critical signaling pathways, especially including the c-kit pathway.

Thus in CML it may be postulated that the stem cells or primitive committed progenitors are at a particularly susceptible stage of development that renders them especially responsive to constitutive, sustained bcr-abl-induced downstream hyperactivation of components of critical regulatory pathways that are ordinarily activated by low-level, transient extracellular stimulation by kit ligand and other cytokines. The affected short-circuited pathways presumably control and coordinate multiple diverse cell processes, including proliferation, differentiation, maturation, and programmed cell death, processes that are normally tightly regulated and highly integrated. Perturbation of these key pathways in stem cells or primitive progenitor cells would be expected to seriously disrupt orderly hematopoiesis and could also explain all of the subsequent subtle, pleiotropic biological abnormalities characteristically observed in later maturing cell compartments that have collectively been designated "discordant maturation." While it is reasonable to assume that such a general unifying hypothesis can explain all of the manifestations of the chronic phase of CML, innumerable unanswered questions remain concerning the details of the normal signaling pathways and the specific aberrations induced by bcr-abl. Many laboratories are now engaged in trying to understand the highly complex normal circuitry, the interactions between different signaling pathways, and the specific changes caused by bcr-abl, and within the next few years a clearer picture should emerge.

See Also the Following Articles

ACUTE LYMPHOBLASTIC LEUKEMIA IN ADULTS • ACUTE LYMPHOBLASTIC LEUKEMIA IN CHILDREN • ACUTE MYELOCYTIC LEUKEMIA • BCR-ABL • CHRONIC LYMPHOCYTIC LEUKEMIA • CYTOKINES • GRAFT VERSUS LEUKEMIAS AND GRAFT VERSUS TUMOR • MONOCLONAL ANTIBODIES: LEUKEMIA AND LYMPHOMA • SIGNAL TRANSDUCTION MECHANISMS INITIATED BY RECEPTOR TYROSINE KINASES

Bibliography

Clarkson, B., and Strife, A. (1993). Linkage of proliferative and maturational abnormalities in chronic myelogenous leukemia and relevance to treatment. *Leukemia* **7,** 1683–1721.

Clarkson, B. D., Strife, A., Wisniewski, D., Lambek, C., and Carpino, N. (1997). New understanding of the pathogenesis of CML: A prototype of early neoplasia. *Leukemia* **11,** 1404–1428.

Era, T., and Witte, O. N. (2000). Regulated expression of P210 Bcr-Abl during embryonic stem cell differentiation stimulates multipotential progenitor expansion and myeloid cell fate. *Proc. Natl. Acad. Sci. U.S.A.* **97,** 1737–1742.

Faderl, S., Talpaz, M., Estrov, Z., O'Brien, S., Kurzrock, R., and Kantarjian H. M. (1999). The biology of chronic myeloid leukemia. *New Engl. J. Med.* **341,** 164–172.

Hunter, T. (2000). Signaling—2000 and beyond. *Cell* **100,** 113–127.

Melo, J. V. (1996). The molecular biology of chronic myeloid leukaemia. *Leukemia* **10,** 751–756.

Minot, J. B., Buckman, T. E., and Isaacs, R. (1924). Chronic myelogenous leukemia: Age, incidence, duration and benefit derived from irradiations. *J. Am. Med. Assoc.* **82,** 1489.

Pear, W. S., Miller, J. P., Xu, L., Pui, J. C., Soffer, B., Quackenbush, R. C., Pendergast, A. M., Bronson, R., Aster, J. C., Scott, M. L., and Baltimore, D. (1998). Efficient and rapid induction of a chronic myelogenous leukemia-like myeloproliferative disease in mice receiving P210 bcr/abl-transduced bone marrow. *Blood* **92,** 3780–3792.

Sawyers, C. L. (1999). Medical progress: Chronic myeloid leukemia. *New Engl. J. Med.* **340,** 1330–1340.

Schindler, T., Bornmann, W., Pellicena, P., Miller, W. T., Clarkson, B., and Kuriyan, J. (2000). Structural mechanism for STI-571 inhibition of Abelson tyrosine kinase. *Science* **289,** 1938–1942.

Chronic Myelogenous Leukemia: Prognosis and Current Status of Treatment

Bayard Clarkson

Memorial Sloan-Kettering Cancer Center

GLOSSARY

BCR/ABL Chimeric gene created by the Philadelphia chromosome translocation of the second exon of protooncogene c-abl from chromosome 9 to the breakpoint cluster region on chromosome 22.

p210$^{BCR/ABL}$ The 201-kDa product of the chimeric BCR/ABL gene; a tyrosine kinase that is thought to cause chronic myelogenous leukemia in humans.

phosphorylation A process by which a phosphate group is transferred from ATP to tyrosine, serine, or threonine amino acid residues on a protein; a mechanism by which many proteins acquire altered activity.

signal transduction A series of ordered biochemical reactions by which a signal initiated at the cell surface is transmitted inside the cell to elicit specific cellular responses.

tyrosine kinase An enzyme that catalyzes the transfer of a high-energy phosphate group from ATP to a tyrosine residue on a protein, very often then modulating the activity of the target proteins.

The overall median survival of patients with Ph-positive chronic myelogenous leukemia (CML) in chronic phase from diagnosis treated with conventional chemotherapy has varied from around 3–5 years in different series, with a range of less than a year to over 20 years. Survival after development of an accelerated phase is usually less than a year and after blastic transformation only a few months, although patients with lymphoblastic transformation may live longer with appropriate chemotherapy.

I. PROGNOSTIC FACTORS

In a multi-institutional study of disease features at diagnosis in nonblastic CML, the most important characteristics associated with shortened survival were older age, male sex, large spleen, high platelet count, high percentages of blasts in blood and marrow, high percentages of eosinophils and basophils, presence of nucleated red cells in the blood, a high serum lactic dehydrogenase (LDH) level, and a low hematocrit. Based on a Cox model using five variables—sex, spleen size, platelet count, hematocrit, and percentage of circulating blasts—patients could be segregated into a high-risk group who had an actuarial mortality of 30% during the first 2 years after diagnosis and an annual risk of 30% thereafter, while the most favorable group had a 2-year actuarial mortality of 9%, an average annual risk thereafter of 17%, and a median survival of 52 years. Additional factors reported to be associated with an unfavorable prognosis in other series are black race, cytogenetic abnormalities in addition to the Ph chromosome, rapid white blood cell (WBC) doubling time, poor response to chemotherapy, liver enlargement, and myelofibrosis.

II. CONVENTIONAL AND INTENSIVE CHEMOTHERAPY

In the classic paper by Minot in 1924, the median survival of untreated CML patients was reported to be 31 months from the onset of symptoms, but this early series probably included some patients in transition from the chronic phase to an accelerated or blastic phase. Since the mid-1920s, the results of most of the therapies attempting to improve survival have been disappointing. Although the clinical manifestations of the chronic phase can usually be readily controlled by many different types of cytotoxic drugs and most patients are able to lead normal lives during the early part of the disease, conventional chemotherapy with commonly used drugs, such as busulfan or hydroxy-urea, given in relatively low doses rarely cause cytogenetic remissions and at best have only a modest effect in improving overall survival. In a large randomized clinical trial in Germany comparing busulfan and hydroxyurea in CML, the median survival of busulfan-treated patients was 45.4 months, whereas that of the hydroxyurea group was 58.2 months ($p = 0.008$).

It was first reported in the mid-1970s that it was possible to induce cytogenetic remissions in chronic-phase CML with intensive chemotherapy and splenectomy in a significant fraction of patients (i.e., with temporary disappearance of Ph-positive cells from the bone marrow). However, these remissions were almost invariably short and further follow-up showed that there was only a relatively small survival advantage for patients having remissions. Since these initial reports, many intensive treatment protocols, with or without splenectomy, have been tried during the chronic phase of CML, but these trials also resulted in only marginal or no prolongation of survival. A number of drugs capable of inducing myeloid cell differentiation (e.g., retinoic acid, HMBA, bryostatin, Vitamin D derivatives) have been shown to cause differentiation and/or growth inhibition of human CML or other types of leukemia cells *in vitro*, and several studies have reported selective effects on CML cells *in vitro*. Several trials combining chemotherapy and differentiation agents in myelodysplastic syndromes or leukemia have been reported, but none of these trials in CML (or in other types of leukemia) have shown the same degree of therapeutic benefit that has been demonstrated for retinoic acid in acute promyelocytic leukemia (APL). Interestingly, one patient with CML in promyelocytic blast crisis had a transient response to all-*trans* retinoic acid similar to that observed in APL.

III. INTERFERON

Treatment with interferon (INF)-α alone appears to prolong survival by about a year compared to busulfan or hydroxyurea, and some patients (~5–35% of patients in different series), especially those with favorable prognostic indices (ie., low score using Sokal or newer prognostic scoring systems), have complete cytogenetic remissions (CCR). A smaller percentage (~5–7%) of patients have quite durable complete remissions that persist even after stopping treatment. However, using polymerase chain reaction (PCR) detection assays, small numbers of leukemic cells can still be detected in the majority of patients having long-term cytogenetic remissions, and longer follow-up will be required to ascertain whether the disease will eventually recur. It has been reported that it is possible to quantitate residual disease in CML patients receiving interferon by competitive PCR with good correlation with the clinical response, but again, all 398 "remission" samples were positive in variable degree for bcr-abl transcripts. Interferon is not devoid of toxicity, and many patients are unable to tolerate the unpleasant side effects for the long periods of treatment required to obtain durable responses. Whereas some of the early clinical trials of INF-α in CML showed little or no survival advantage over conventional chemotherapy, several large trials comparing interferon with hydroxyurea and/or busulfan showed improved survival with interferon treatment. However, other large clinical trials have not shown as great an advantage of interferon over hydroxyurea or as high a percentage of complete cytogenetic remissions with interferon as in the trials referenced earlier, which may have excluded disproportionate numbers of patients with unfavorable prognostic features.

The mechanism by which IFN inhibits growth of normal and CML progenitor cells is still uncertain and is probably very complex; several possible mechanisms have been proposed, and it appears it may affect multiple gene transcription and protein phosphorylation events. Other studies suggest that the therapeutic activity of IFN may be mediated through the activation of dendritic cells, by Fas-R-mediated induction of apoptosis, or by inducing degradation of bcr-abl mRNA and thus reducing the effective tyrosine kinase dosage.

Combined treatment with interferon-α and low-dose cytarabine (arabinosylcytosine) appears to be better than interferon alone. In the largest multi-institutional study in 237 patients so far reported conducted in France beginning in 1988 and ending in 1991, the combined treatment resulted in 66% complete hematologic remissions and 28% complete CCR (compared to 20% CCR with interferon alone). In the latest French trial begun in 1991 involving 721 patients of whom 360 were randomly assigned to IFN–cytarabine and 361 to IFN alone, the former group had a significantly higher incidence of CCR ($p < 0.01$) and their 3-year estimated survival rate was 85.7% compared to 79.1% for the IFN alone group. Because the early results of three current clinical trials comparing IFN alone with IFN–cytarabine appear to be similar to those of the earlier French trials, it appears reasonable to conclude that combining cytarabine with IFN leads to improved results. Other cytotoxic drugs, including homoharringtonine, idarubicin, and etoposide, are also now being tried in combination with IFN, but it is too early to draw any conclusions.

IV. BONE MARROW TRANSPLANTATION

Presently the only consistently curative treatment for CML is supralethal doses of chemotherapy and/or total body irradiation followed by syngeneic or allogeneic bone marrow transplantation, but this option is only available to approximately one-quarter of patients who have an HLA-matched sibling or an unrelated HLA-matched donor. Of patients in chronic phase who were treated with allogeneic-related donor bone marrow transplants, approximately 50–60% overall have had actual or projected long-term survival (usually > 5–7 years) with better results in younger patients and those transplanted within a year of diagnosis. In the largest single-institution experience with the longest follow-up, a survival rate of 70% at 10 years has been reported. The early results of correlative studies using cytogenetic methods and RT-PCR to detect small numbers of residual Ph+ cells in patients in complete hematologic remissions following transplant were inconsistent and sometimes contradictory. However, with more experience and the development of more accurate fluorescence in situ hybridization (FISH) and competitive PCR assays, these methods have become more reliable in monitoring minimal residual disease following transplantation and in predicting the likelihood and rapidity of hematologic relapse. As might be expected, patients who remain RT-PCR and/or FISH negative for several years or longer after transplants have an increasing likelihood of being cured, but even some patients in whom persistent low-level bcr-abl transcripts are detected (without progressively increasing) may remain in clinical remission for extended periods.

It became apparent in early trials that patients who developed graft-versus-host disease (GVHD) following allogeneic transplantation had a lower incidence of relapse than those who did not, and much effort has been given to try to separate and augment a graft-versus-leukemia (GVL) response from GVHD. Several reports suggest that such adaptive immunotherapy may succeed at least in part in that durable remissions have sometimes been obtained by the infusion of donor lymphocytes in chronic-phase CML patients who have relapsed after allogeneic transplantation. However, donor lymphocyte infusions may also cause an appreciable incidence of GVHD, which may be severe or even fatal, and marrow aplasia has also been reported.

The survival of recipients (who lack HLA-matched siblings) of transplants from unrelated HLA-matched donors identified by bone marrow registries is generally substantially lower than recipients of related donor transplants, although certain immunologically distinct HLA subtypes and good-risk recipients fare better than others. Granulocyte-colony stimulating factor (G-CSF)-stimulated peripheral blood stem cells (PBSC) have largely replaced bone marrow stem cells in most transplant centers, as there is now good evidence that PBSC engraft and function more rapidly in producing neutrophils and platelets and also appear less likely to cause GVHD.

V. AUTOLOGOUS TRANSPLANTS

There have been numerous attempts to treat patients without histocompatible donors in both blastic and chronic phases of the disease with marrow ablative intensive chemotherapy and/or irradiation regimens followed by autologous stem cell transplantation. Various methods have been tried to preferentially eliminate residual Ph+ progenitor cells in the graft while sparing normal stem cells. These have included various cytotoxic drugs, antisense molecules against bcr-abl junction peptide sequences, peptide-based vaccines using b3a2 junctional peptides or generation of dendritic cells to stimulate a selective antileukemic cytotoxic T lymphocyte (CTL) response, and cold or radiolabeled antibodies directed against surface antigens such as CD33 or AC133. Investigators in Vancouver have employed a cell culture system in attempts to selectively expand normal primitive progenitors [i.e., amplification of long-term culture initiating cells (LTC-IC) in cultures initiated with CML-derived $CD34^+ CD38^-$ cells] and have reported that while Ph+ colony-forming cells are also amplified, Ph+ LTC-IC disappeared regardless of the cytokines present. However, because other investigators have reported that Ph+ progenitor cells may survive in long-term culture under certain conditions, there is still some question as to the reliability of cell culture methods for selectively eliminating early Ph+ progenitors that are capable of reproducing the disease. It is still uncertain which of the proposed purging methods is optimal or whether any of those so far tried are sufficiently selective and reliable to consistently eliminate all Ph+ progenitors in the autograft.

It appeared from the initial clinical trials that few patients were cured by autologous stem cell transplantation, as the majority of patients who survived the procedure still had Ph+ cells in the marrow detectable by cytogenetic or PCR analysis. Retroviral marking of donor cells showed that residual Ph+ progenitors remaining in the autologous transplant (despite in vivo or in vitro purging attempts) may contribute to relapse as well as residual leukemic cells surviving in the patient. An early meta-analysis showed that the 3-year posttransplant leukemia-free survival was less than 5%. However, more recent reports suggest that survival may be prolonged and that a significant number of patients in the chronic phase undergoing autologous transplantation may have more durable remissions. Thus while improved methodology has resulted in some improvement with perhaps 15 to 25% of patients remaining in CCR after autografting, the follow-up is still too short in the majority of patients to be certain how many are actually cured or whether the survivors will develop late complications as a consequence of high-dose chemotherapy and/or irradiation. Interestingly in this regard, in contrast to the increased incidence of acute myelogenous leukemia (AML) and myelodysplasia syndromes (MDS) occurring in patients with other malignancies (e.g., Hodgkin's disease and ovarian cancer) who have been treated with high doses of irradiation or cytotoxic drugs, no increased incidence of acute leukemia or myelodysplasia has yet been noted in CML survivors of allografts in the largest series with the longest follow-up at the Fred Hutchison Cancer Center in Seattle. A possible explanation for this difference is that the very high doses of TBI (i.e., 1200–1500 Gy) and/or cytotoxic drugs such as busulfan, cyclophosphamide, or etoposide used to eradicate the Ph+ clone also effectively eliminate any stem cells (normal or Ph+) that are susceptible to irradiation or drug-induced transformation, unlike the situation in Hodgkin's disease or solid tumors treated with more localized irradiation and nonlethal drug doses where many damaged stem cells survive and can later cause leukemia.

VI. RESULTS AND FUTURE DIRECTIONS

Because there is still an appreciable early mortality and a relatively high incidence of complications including chronic GVHD associated with allogeneic bone marrow transplantation (BMT), the advisability of this form of treatment is still controversial in older patients who are less able to tolerate the intensive treatment. In an analysis of a large German study comparing hydroxyurea (HU), interferon, and BMT, there was a significant survival advantage for HU or interferon during the first 4 years after diagnosis and for BMT starting 5.5 years after diagnosis. The survival advantage for BMT was greater in patients with intermediate or high-risk prognostic features than in those with low-risk features. In efforts to further increase curability with reduced toxicity, investigators at Seattle and elsewhere are currently exploring a number of new approaches in clinical BMT protocols. These include nonablative (i.e., low-dose TBI ∼2 Gy) plus immuno-therapy; leukemia-specific targeted isotopic or toxin-conjugated antibodies directed against minor tissue-specific antigens to enhance selective purging of residual leukemic cells in autologous transplants; pretargeting methods employing streptavidin and biotin to increase antibody binding to the leukemia cells; and various adoptive immunotherapy protocols posttransplant to reduce the incidence of relapse and/or GVHD. Some of the early results appear promising, and doubtless there will be further advances in stem cell transplantation methodology, immunotherapy, and leukemia-specific therapies in the future.

Nevertheless, despite enormous efforts during the past several decades to improve treatment, only a minority of patients with chronic phase CML are presently being cured with BMT protocols, and it is doubtful if older patients will ever be able to tolerate the aggressive treatment required to eradicate the Ph+ clone. The results are even worse for patients in the accelerated or blastic phases of the disease or for those presenting with Ph+ acute leukemia, and such patients are rarely amenable to cure with any type of treatment. It is not known why Ph+ acute and chronic leukemias are so refractory to therapies that have proven successful in some other types of leukemia and disseminated lymphomas with other genetic abnormalities, but it is quite evident that there is still a very pressing need for more selective, less toxic, and more effective treatment.

VII. NOVEL THERAPIES FOR CML

A number of potential "molecularly rationale" therapies have been suggested for Ph+ and other leukemias that are not generally curable with conventional chemotherapy, including some mentioned earlier as possible approaches for selectively eliminating leukemic progenitors from the marrow *ex vivo* for use in autologous bone marrow transplantation protocols. Among the approaches that have been suggested are the use of ribozymes; antisense oligonucleotides complementary to the junction sequence of bcr-abl; tyrosine kinase inhibitors with specificity for bcr-abl kinase activity; inhibition of other functional domains of abl or bcr-abl proteins (besides the kinase domain) that might serve as targets for specific therapies, such as the abl SH2 domain or the first exon of bcr; inhibiting Grb2 interactions with bcr-abl or Ras; or some form of specific immunologic therapy. The presence of unique amino acid sequences across the bcr-abl fusion breakpoint suggested that it might be possible to develop a specific immunological approach to CML. Although the p210$^{bcr-abl}$ protein is not expressed on the cell surface, peptide sequences may be presented in the context of HLA molecules for recognition by T cells that might augment an immune response to leukemia cells or perhaps kill them. One study sought to determine if CML-specific amino acid sequences could be presented by HLA molecules and, if so, if these HLA bearing cells could serve as targets of specific T cells from normal or leukemia patients. Based on these studies, a vaccine was prepared and a clinical trial was initiated to try to prevent recurrence after bone marrow transplantation, but it is too soon to know if this immunological approach will be successful in preventing relapses.

VIII. TYROSINE KINASE INHIBITORS

As noted earlier, because the increased protein tyrosine kinase (PTK) activity of the oncogenic bcr-abl fusion proteins has been shown to be essential for transformation, many investigators have examined various PTK inhibitors, hoping to find one that will selectively inhibit bcr-abl kinase. One of the most potent and selective inhibitors of bcr-abl kinase activity discovered so far is Novartis compound ST1571 (formerly Ciba-Geigy compound CGP57148), which has been undergoing clinical trials in patients with CML under the leadership of Dr. Brian Druker at the University of Oregon. ST1571 acts as a competitive inhibitor of

ATP at the ATP-binding site of the tyrosine kinase domains of both normal abl and bcr-abl. It is much less inhibitory to most other PTKs that have been tested with the notable exceptions of two normal receptor PTKs; c-kit and PDGF-R. In the phase I trial that was carried out in patients in whom treatment with interferon had failed or who could not tolerate interferon, the dose was gradually escalated attempting to reach therapeutically effective levels, without encountering serious toxicity. While it is too soon to draw any final conclusions, the early results are very promising. Ninety-eight percent (53/54) of patients who were treated for at least 4 weeks with (single daily oral) doses of 300 mg or greater had complete hematologic remissions, 31% had major cytogenetic responses, and 7 had complete cytogenetic remissions. In 2 of the 7 CCRs, the cells tested negative for Bcr-Abl by FISH analysis and one patient tested negative for Bcr-Abl by the RT-PCR. ST1571 was well tolerated and no serious toxicities that could be ascribed to the drug were reported; the commonest adverse effects included nausea, myalgias, edema, diarrhea, and fatigue. Patients with a shorter duration of disease prior to therapy appeared to respond best.

ST1571 has also produced responses in CML patients in blast crisis. Responses occurred in 55% (21/38) of patients in myeloid blast crisis, 4 of whom had complete hematologic remissions, and in 70% (14/20) of patients with lymphoblastic blast crisis, again with 4 complete responses. STI571 is currently being tested in conjunction with other agents in bcr-abl-positive cell lines on the likely assumption that CML cells will probably develop resistance to a single agent such as ST1571. According to Druker, few patients in chronic phase have yet shown clear evidence of developing resistance to ST1571 while on continuing therapy, but patients in blastic phase frequently develop resistance, often quite rapidly. A novel mechanism of resistance to ST1571 has been reported for the bcr-abl-positive human leukemic line KU812 in nude mice. α_1 acidic glycoprotein (AGP), which is produced by the liver, was found to bind ST1571 and to significantly inhibit its biological activity; moreover, erythromycin was found to compete with ST1571 for binding AGP and to increase the biological activity of ST1571 both *in vivo* and *in vitro*. Several other mechanisms of resistance to ST1571 have been reported, but the encouraging results of the clinical trials so far nevertheless represent a very significant advance in the attempt to develop highly selective therapies directed at specific oncogenic proteins. In future studies, we can anticipate that there will be further improvements in developing even more potent specific inhibitors of abl kinase and that additional vulnerable targets will be identified for developments of other specific inhibitors of $p210^{bcr-abl}$, other oncogenic proteins, and oncogenes. Once several inhibitors of different oncogenic mutational sites become available, it should be possible to combine them to induce long-term remissions or possibly even cures of CML, as has already proved possible in the majority of patients with acute promyelocytic leukemia and in children with acute lymphoblastic leukemia.

See Also the Following Articles

ACUTE LYMPHOBLASTIC LEUKEMIA IN ADULTS • ACUTE LYMPHOBLASTIC LEUKEMIA IN CHILDREN • ACUTE MYELOCYTIC LEUKEMIA • BCR-ABL • CHRONIC LYMPHOCYTIC LEUKEMIA • GRAFT VERSUS LEUKEMIAS AND GRAFT VERSUS TUMOR • MONOCLONAL ANTIBODIES: LEUKEMIA AND LYMPHOMA • SIGNAL TRANSDUCTION MECHANISMS INITIATED BY RECEPTOR TYROSINE KINASES • STEM CELL TRANSPLANTATION

Bibliography

Chronic Myeloid Leukemia Trialists' Collaborative Group. (1997). Interferon alpha versus chemotherapy for chronic myeloid leukemia: A meta-analysis of seven randomized trials. *J. Natl. Cancer Inst.* **89,** 1616–1620.

Drobyski, W.R., Hessner, M.J., and Klein, J.P. (1999). T-cell depletion plus salvage immunotherapy with donor leukocyte infusions as a strategy to treat chronic-phase chronic myelogenous leukemia patients undergoing HLA-identical sibling marrow transplantation. *Blood.* **94,** 434–441.

Druker, B.J., *et al.* (2001). Efficacy and safety of a specific inhibitor of the Bcr-Abl tyrosine kinase in chronic myeloid leukemia. *N. Engl. J. Med.* **344,** 1031–1037.

Hansen, J.A., Gooley, T.A., and Martin, P.J. (1998). Bone marrow transplants from unrelated donors for patients with chronic myeloid leukemia. *N. Engl. J. Med.* **338,** 962–968.

Hasford, J., *et al.* (1998). A new prognostic score for survival of patients with chronic myeloid leukemia treated with interferon alfa. Writing Committee for the Collaborative CML Prognostic Factors Project Group. *J. Natl. Cancer Inst.* **90,** 850–858.

Kano, Y., Akutsu, M., Tsunoda, S., Mano, H., Sato, Y., Honma, Y., and Furukawa, Y. (2001). In vitro cytotoxic effects of a tyrosine kinase inhibitor STI571 in combination with commonly used antileukemic agents. *Blood.* **97,** 1999–2007.

Cisplatin and Related Drugs

Pieter Pil
Stephen J. Lippard
Massachusetts Institute of Technology

GLOSSARY

apoptosis A suicidal process resulting in cell death that requires active gene transcription and translation. It is believed to occur by a well-defined pathway that can be activated by events such as severe, irreparable DNA damage.

cisplatin The common name for *cis*-diamminedichloroplatinum(II), a widely used anticancer drug. It is sold under the trade name Platinol.

cytotoxicity The ability of a compound to kill cells.

drug resistance The ability of cells to withstand challenges by compounds which in previous generations were lethal.

genotoxicity The ability of a compound to damage DNA.

HMG domain A DNA-binding motif present in a number of proteins. Its approximately 75-amino-acid sequence is associated with DNA binding, which is often accompanied by bending of the double helix.

interstrand cross-link A covalent linking of DNA bases from opposite strands of the helix.

intrastrand cross-link A covalent linking of DNA bases from the same strand of the helix.

C isplatin, as the platinum compound cis-diamminedichloroplatinum(II) is generally known, is an important chemotherapeutic agent for testicular cancer, including advanced forms of the disease.

Long-term survival is experienced in more than 90% of cisplatin-treated patients with solid tumors of the testes. Cisplatin is also effective in the treatment of ovarian, head and neck, and bladder cancers, although for these cancers it is curative at lower rates than observed for testicular tumors. The compound is believed to exert its cytotoxic effects by coordinating to DNA where it inhibits both replication and transcription and induces programmed cell death. The biological activity of cisplatin cannot be explained solely on the basis of its ability to damage DNA, however, because the geometric isomer trans-diamminedichloroplatinum(II) also binds DNA, but is ineffective as a chemotherapeutic agent. Stereochemical differences in the adducts formed by the two isomers imply that the antitumor activity of cisplatin arises from the formation of a specific structural motif on DNA which, in turn, triggers a cellular response leading to cell death. To investigate this possibility, attention has turned to identifying cellular proteins that recognize cisplatin–DNA lesions with the ultimate aim of understanding how such interactions might lead to the selective toxicity of the drug to tumor cells.

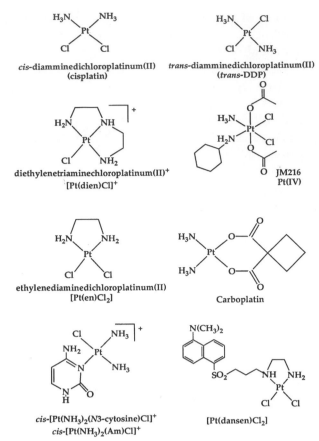

FIGURE 1 Structures of platinum compounds discussed in this article.

I. INTRODUCTION

The general theory behind classical chemotherapy is to treat the patient with compounds that affect rapidly dividing cells, while leaving other cells unharmed. This strategy eliminates many fast-growing cells: cancer cells, hair cells, bone marrow cells, epithelial cells lining the digestive tract, and so forth. Certain anticancer drugs do not affect all rapidly growing cells, but instead are particularly effective against a specific subset of tumors. Among such compounds is the platinum coordination compound cis-diamminedichloroplatinum(II) (see Fig. 1), also known as cisplatin, which in combination chemotherapy provides a cure for most patients with testicular cancer, including those with advanced disease. The use of cisplatin to treat testicular cancer is unique among the management of solid tumors in that 90% of those afflicted with the disease are expected to survive. Cisplatin is also effective against cancers of the ovaries, cervix, head and neck, lungs, and bladder, among others, and

recently has shown activity when used as first-line chemotherapy against breast cancer. Despite the curative effect of cisplatin on testicular cancer, which annually accounts for fewer than 0.6% of all new cancer cases, treatment with this drug is usually only palliative for other tumors.

The discovery of the antitumor activity of cisplatin is one of the classic stories of serendipity in scientific research. The compound, originally known as Peyrone's chloride, was first synthesized in 1845 and had its structure deduced one century ago. Its effects on biological systems were not discovered until 1965, however. The seminal discovery was made by the biophysicist Barnett Rosenberg, who was studying the effects of electric fields on *Escherichia coli* bacterial cultures. The bacteria stopped dividing and grew into long filaments because of contamination of the cultures by platinum from the electrodes. The compounds responsible for this inhibition of cell division were identified, one of which was cisplatin. Since it was known that agents able to inhibit cell division sometimes could be used as anticancer agents, cisplatin was tested and found to exhibit antitumor activity in mice (see Fig. 2). Human trials of cisplatin commenced shortly thereafter, culminating with the approval of the drug at the end of 1978 by the Food and Drug Administration (FDA) for the treatment of genitourinary tumors. Today it is one of the most widely used and successful chemotherapeutic drugs.

Extensive research has been carried out to understand the mechanism of action of the drug. Such knowledge might lead not only to the development of anticancer compounds effective against a wider range of tumors, but also to agents with fewer toxic side effects than cisplatin. Toxicity resulting from cisplatin administration includes kidney damage, hearing loss, peripheral nerve damage, severe nausea and vomiting, and bone marrow suppression. These side effects have been successfully mitigated in clinical practice. Prehydrating the patient with physiological saline prior to cisplatin infusion has reduced kidney damage, whereas careful dosage control, currently no more than 120 mg/m^2 per administration, has limited the incidence of hearing loss and nerve damage. Bone marrow suppression has been reduced with the use of bone marrow growth factors and novel anti-nausea drugs have been used to alleviate the nausea and vomiting that accompany cisplatin treatment. Even though the clinical consequences of cisplatin treatment are currently well defined, the mechanisms by which the drug exerts its cytotoxic effects are not fully understood.

CONTROL SARCOMA 180

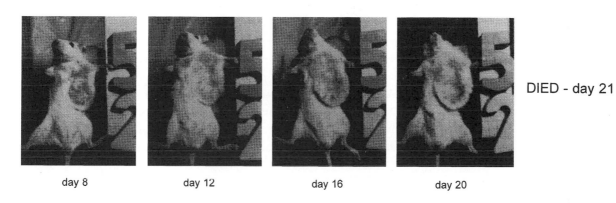

day 8　　　day 12　　　day 16　　　day 20　　　DIED - day 21

TREATED - SINGLE INJECTION CIS - $Pt(II)\ (NH_3)_2Cl_2$ - 8 mg/kg - DAY 8

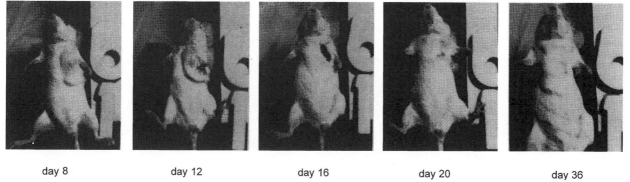

day 8　　　day 12　　　day 16　　　day 20　　　day 36

FIGURE 2 Early experiments with mice illustrating the remarkable ability of cisplatin as a cure for solid tumors. (Top) The fate of a mouse given a solid sarcoma 180 tumor. (Bottom) Another mouse treated similarly except for a single dose of cisplatin on day 8 [reproduced with permission from B. Rosenberg (1980). *In* "Metal Ions in Biology" (T. G. Spiro, ed.), Vol. 1, pp. 1–29. Wiley, New York].

Cisplatin is administered intravenously as a solution in physiological saline. In the blood, the high (~100 mM) concentration of chloride ion retards the rate of hydrolysis of the drug. The neutral compound then enters the cell by what is generally assumed to be passive diffusion, although some evidence indicates that cells may be able to regulate their uptake of the drug. Inside the cell, a much lower concentration of chloride ion (~3–20 mM) facilitates hydrolysis of the chloride ligands, resulting in a positively charged, aquated, electrophilic species capable of bifunctional coordination. These activated molecules can react, by ligand substitution, with macromolecules in the cell, including DNA, RNA, and proteins (see Fig. 3). In this manner, the drug accumulates at similar levels in the tumor and tissues such as kidney, liver, brain, and bone marrow.

The coordination of cisplatin to RNA and proteins is not thought to be fundamental to its mechanism of action for two main reasons. The first is that any single damaged protein or RNA molecule is expendable; it can be replaced by newly synthesized material, as evidenced by studies revealing that 5 mM cisplatin inhibited DNA synthesis, but not RNA or protein synthesis. The second reason is that only a small fraction of protein (1 out of 3×10^3–10^4) and RNA molecules (1 out of 10 to 1 out of 1000) is damaged in human HeLa cells treated with cisplatin at its mean lethal concentration. Cisplatin is capable of inhibiting DNA transcription, however, suggesting the possibility that, even though total RNA and protein synthesis may appear unchanged, the levels of specific RNA or protein species could be altered.

The best evidence that DNA is the key target responsible for cisplatin cytotoxicity is the enhanced sensitivity of DNA repair-deficient cells, both prokaryotic and eukaryotic, to the drug. In yeast, the cytotoxicity of cisplatin correlates rather well with its genotoxicity. Furthermore, cell lines derived from testicular tumors are hypersensitive to a whole array of chemotherapeutic agents, including cisplatin, which have in common the property that they interact directly with DNA. This sensitivity was not observed for agents that do not interact directly with DNA.

II. INTERACTION OF CISPLATIN WITH DNA

The coordination of cisplatin to DNA occurs mainly through the N7 atoms of purines (see Fig. 4), which are exposed in the major groove of the double helix and are not involved in base-pair hydrogen bonding. The resulting adducts can be grouped into six major categories: 1,2-intrastrand d(GpG) adducts between adjacent guanines, 1,2-intrastrand d(ApG) adducts between an adjacent adenine and guanine, intrastrand adducts between purines separated by one or more in-

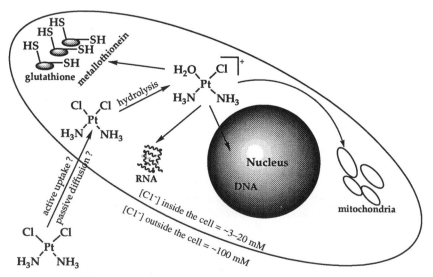

FIGURE 3 The cellular uptake of cisplatin and its targets.

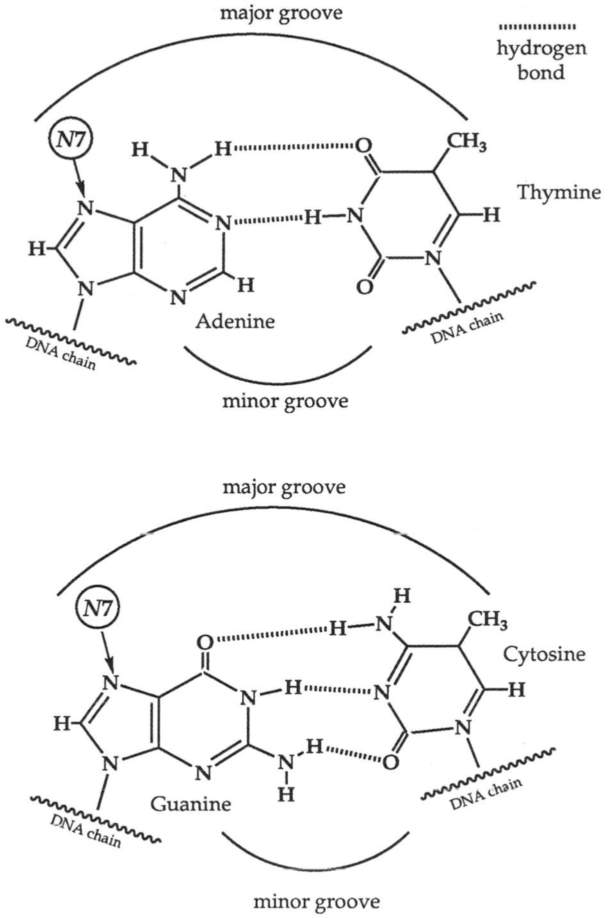

major groove

hydrogen
bond

Thymine

Adenine

minor groove

major groove

Cytosine

Guanine

minor groove

FIGURE 4 The DNA base pairs. Cisplatin coordinates to the N7 atoms of the purine (guanine and adenine) bases, which are located in the major groove.

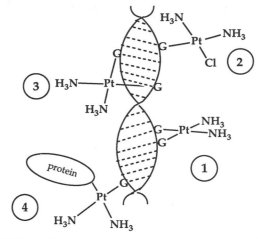

FIGURE 5 DNA double helix showing the adducts formed by cisplatin: (1) intrastrand cross-link [this adduct, observed for adjacent guanosine residues as depicted, also occurs for the dinucleotide d(ApG)]; (2) monofunctional adduct; (3) interstrand cross-link; and (4) protein–DNA cross-link.

tervening bases, interstrand adducts linking the two strands of the DNA double helix, monofunctional adducts coordinated to a single purine, and protein–DNA cross-links, where cisplatin coordinates a protein molecule and a nucleobase (see Fig. 5). Some of these cross-links may involve coordination to cytosines, although purines are preferred. It is interesting to note that d(GpA) 1,2-intrastrand adducts are very rare.

Immunochemical studies on DNA isolated from leukocytes taken from patients treated with cisplatin by using antisera raised to specific platinum lesions revealed that intrastrand d(GpG) adducts constituted 65% of the total adduct pool, d(ApG) adducts made up 22%, and interstrand or intrastrand cross-links between guanines separated by one or more intervening

bases accounted for 12%, whereas cisplatin adducts coordinated monofunctionally were found at a frequency of less than 1%. These numbers are similar to those obtained for salmon sperm DNA platinated *in vitro* and analyzed by HPLC, which gave 50% d(GpG) adducts, 28% d(ApG) adducts, 10% interstrand or long range intrastrand cross-links, and 2% monofunctional adducts. The majority of adducts are clearly intrastrand adducts, with DNA interstrand cross-links and DNA–protein cross-links accounting for only a small fraction of the platinum on the DNA. Until the antitumor mechanism of cisplatin is elucidated fully, however, all adducts remain potential candidates for the lesion(s) mediating the activity of the drug.

Understanding how cisplatin coordination to DNA might effect cell death has been facilitated by the existence of a clinically inactive geometric isomer, *trans*-diamminedichloroplatinum(II) (see Fig. 1), also known as *trans*-DDP. Like cisplatin, *trans*-DDP coordinates to DNA, but because of steric constraints, this compound is unable to cross-link adjacent purines. This inability of *trans*-DDP to form the 1,2-intrastrand d(GpG) and d(ApG) adducts observed for cisplatin suggests that the structures of these adducts may be fundamental to the cytotoxic mechanism of cisplatin. Analysis of DNA modified globally with *trans*-DDP by HPLC following enzyme digestion revealed that 40% of the adducts span two guanines and 50% link a guanine to a cytosine. These adducts include both intra- and interstrand cross-links, with the intrastrand cross-links containing at least one intervening nucleotide. *trans*-DDP appears to form interstrand cross-links more slowly than cisplatin, but over time more interstrand cross-links accumulate with the *trans* isomer. The interstrand adducts formed by *trans*-DDP were observed to form preferentially between guanines and their complementary cytosine residues. Thus, the DNA adducts formed by *cis*- and *trans*-DDP are quite distinct.

The structures of adducts formed by cisplatin and *trans*-DDP with DNA have been studied by various methods, including single-crystal X-ray diffraction (X-ray crystallography), nuclear magnetic resonance (NMR), several forms of gel electrophoresis, and various other methods. X-ray crystallography revealed the structure of cisplatin coordinates to the dinucleotide d(pGpG), where platinum coordination to the N7 atoms of the guanines forced these bases to destack (see Fig. 6). Less destacking takes place in a cisplatin-modified DNA double helix, as deduced from

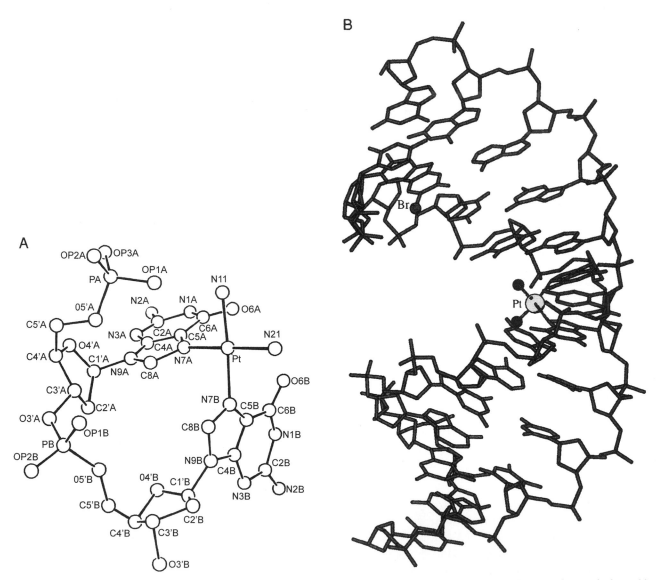

FIGURE 6 (A) The structure of cisplatin coordinated to the dinucleotide d(pGpG). Notice the destacking of guanine bases, which would normally be parallel to one other. Adapted from Sherman *et al.* (1988). *J. Am. Chem. Soc.* **110,** 7368–7381. (B) The structure of cisplatin coordinated to d(GpG) in the duplex d(CCTCTG*G*TCTCC) · d(GGAGACCAGAGG) where the G*G* denotes the platinum-binding site. Adapted from Takahara *et al.* (1995). *Nature* **377,** 649–657.

the gel electrophoretic mobilities of site-specifically platinated DNA molecules. Such an analysis revealed that cisplatin d(GpG) and d(ApG) 1,2-intrastrand cross-links, and the d(GpTpG) 1,3-intrastrand cross-link, bend the DNA helix in the direction of the major groove by approximately 34°. The degree of helix unwinding for the d(GpG) and d(ApG) adducts was 13°, whereas the unwinding induced by the d(GpTpG) adduct was greater at 23°. A similar analysis of what might be one of the major adducts of *trans*-DDP, the d(GpTpG) 1,3-intrastrand cross-link, revealed that platination induces a nondirectional point of flexibility into the DNA helix. The unwinding of DNA globally modified by *trans*-DDP, examined by agarose gel electrophoresis, is 9°. A cisplatin interstrand cross-link spanning two diagonally opposed guanine residues in a 22-bp double-stranded DNA fragment was estimated to bend the helix by 55° toward the major groove, with no unwinding. Monofunctional platinum adducts do not bend DNA, but the model compound [Pt(dien)Cl]Cl (see Fig. 1), which has only one labile chloride and can only coordinate to one nucleophile, unwinds the DNA helix by about 6°. A recent study on a selfcomplementary dodecanucleotide modified with cisplatin at one of two d(GpG) sites revealed the formation of a stable DNA hairpin. This result suggests the possibility that, *in vivo*, cisplatin might stabilize the formation of cruciform structures in palindromic regions, which is interesting since the DNA cruciform-binding protein HMG1 recognizes platinated DNA (see below). A structure of the cisplatin d(GpG) 1,2-intrastrand cross-link in duplex DNA has recently been determined by X-ray crystallography (see Fig. 6).

The kinetics of cisplatin binding to DNA have been studied by ^{195}Pt NMR spectroscopy. The rate-limiting step of the reaction is hydrolysis of the first chloride ion, followed quickly by coordination to DNA to form monofunctional adducts (cisplatin half-life, 2 hr). These transient monofunctional adducts, which also had half-lives on the order of 2 to 3 hr, then reacted with an additional DNA base to form bifunctional cross-links. The rate of formation of bifunctional adducts from monofunctional ones, the so-called "rates of closure," is affected by the superhelical density of the DNA helix, being faster for supercoiled as compared to relaxed DNA. As determined from an investigation of *trans*-DDP by ^{195}Pt

NMR spectroscopy, the rate at which this inactive compound coordinates to DNA differs little from that observed for cisplatin, suggesting that the different biological effects of the two are not the result of dissimilar DNA-binding kinetics.

III. EFFECTS OF CISPLATIN ON DNA REPLICATION

One of the central tenets of cancer chemotherapy is that compounds which reduce the rate at which a cell can divide, either by inhibiting replication or by blocking biological pathways involved in DNA synthesis and the cell cycle, can be used as antitumor agents. Such compounds can have profound effects on rapidly dividing cells, especially tumor cells. Given this dogma, it is not surprising that extensive efforts have been devoted to studying the effects of cisplatin on DNA replication.

In vitro studies on a number of DNA polymerases, including enzymes of viral, prokaryotic, and eukaryotic origins, revealed that cisplatin and *trans*-DDP adducts block their progression. The activities of bacteriophage T7 polymerase, T4 polymerase, *E. coli* DNA polymerase I, and *E. coli* DNA polymerase III holoenzyme on site-specifically platinated templates have been examined. These polymerases were all stopped by cisplatin d(GpG) and d(ApG) 1,2-intrastrand adducts and by d(GpCpG), 1,3-intrastrand adducts. Varying degrees of bypass replication, which resulted when the polymerase was able to translocate past the lesion on the template strand, were observed. On average, bypass replication occurred about 10% of the time, with d(GpG) adducts allowing the least amount of translesion synthesis, and the d(GpCpG) adducts permitting 25% bypass. DNA globally modified with *trans*-DDP blocked replication synthesis by *E. coli* DNA polymerase I. DNA damaged with the monofunctional binding platinum model compound chlorodiethylenetriamineplatinum(II) chloride (see Fig. 1) did not inhibit the progression of *E. coli* DNA polymerase I, whereas DNA adducts formed by a new class of monofunctional platinum antitumor drugs (see Section XIV) inhibited the progression of both T7 DNA polymerase and *E. coli* DNA polymerase I.

The effects of platinum-damaged DNA templates on replication have also been examined by using polymerases purified from eukaryotic sources. DNA polymerase α derived from both calf thymus and *Drosophila melanogaster* was blocked at d(GpG) and d(ApG) adducts, but not at monofunctional adducts. As observed for viral and prokaryotic polymerases, d(GpG) adducts blocked polymerase progression to a greater extent than d(ApG) adducts. The increased bypass replication occurring with d(ApG) adducts correlates well with the increased mutagenicity of this adduct when compared to the d(GpG) adduct, suggesting that such replication occurs with reduced fidelity. In addition, these observations indicate that even though d(ApG) and d(GpG) cisplatin adducts distort the DNA helix in a similar manner, these distortions must be somewhat different in detail.

More recently, the effects of cisplatin on replication by the eukaryotic DNA polymerase ε, purified from calf thymus, have been examined. This polymerase, like DNA polymerase α, is required for chromosomal DNA replication and is believed to play a role in DNA repair. The progression of polymerase ε was blocked by d(GpG) intrastrand adducts, as well as by monofunctional cisplatin adducts on guanines. Furthermore, it was observed that this polymerase was actually sequestered on the DNA at the sites of cisplatin damage and was thus prevented from beginning replication on other templates. These results suggest that replication may be inhibited not only by the blockage of polymerase progression, but that the rate of replication may be reduced further by the sequestering of the polymerase.

By using SV40 as a model minichromosome, cisplatin and *trans*-DDP were found to be equally effective at inhibiting replication *in vivo* when equal amounts of platinum were coordinated to the viral genome. The *trans*-DDP adducts appeared to be repaired much more efficiently so that, over time, the inhibition by this inactive isomer was less than that of cisplatin. A similar inhibition for *trans*-DDP and cisplatin was observed in mouse L1210 leukemia cells. The effective inhibition of DNA replication by *trans*-DDP suggests that the clinical activity of cisplatin is not derived solely from its ability to inhibit DNA replication. Furthermore, it is unclear how blocking replication leads to cell death, or if indeed it has this effect.

IV. EFFECTS OF CISPLATIN ON TRANSCRIPTION

Transcription is the synthesis of RNA from a DNA template. The ability of cisplatin DNA adducts to block transcription has been studied both *in vitro* and *in vivo*. The latter studies employed plasmids containing reporter genes that were transfected into a variety of cells.

An *in vitro* experiment revealed that cisplatin adducts block the progression of *E. coli* RNA polymerase only if present on the template strand, but not when located on the nontranscribed strand. Another study found that both d(ApG) and d(GpG) adducts blocked transcription by *E. coli* RNA polymerase and wheat germ RNA polymerase II. As before, these adducts terminated RNA synthesis only if they were present on the transcribed strand.

In one study using reporter genes transfected into monkey cells, it was found that low levels of cisplatin reduced the rate of transcription. Interestingly, when stronger promoters were used cisplatin damage led to a more complete inhibition of transcription, whereas the expression of genes under the control of weaker promoters was relatively insensitive to the drug. In this same assay, *trans*-DDP was ineffective at inhibiting the transcription of genes from strong promoters, whereas on the weaker promoters it reduced gene expression in a manner similar to that of cisplatin. Additional analysis showed that the effects of cisplatin on the stronger promoters were not due to an increased formation of d(GpG) intrastrand cross-links.

A similar study carried out in human HeLa cells yielded a more startling result. Cisplatin treatment of cells containing plasmids with reporter genes actually enhanced the level of gene expression for some promoters, while reducing the level of expression for others. A similar result was observed for a chloramphenicol acetyltransferase (CAT) gene under the control of the HIV-1 long terminal repeat (LTR) promoter. In order to obtain cisplatin-enhanced transcription with this LTR construct in resistant ovarian carcinoma cells, an increased drug concentration was required. The reasons for this enhancement of transcription remain unknown. One possibility is that cisplatin adducts present on the constructs actually enhance the rate of transcription by bending the DNA, signaling the initiation of transcription. In *E. coli*, synthetic curved DNA sequences function as transcriptional activators. Such bending may attract proteins required for transcription and may aid in the binding of RNA polymerase and the formation of a transcription complex. In addition to being dependent on promoter strength, the sensitivity of gene transcription to cisplatin parallels the size of the gene being transcribed, which could be the result of an increased presence of potential platinum binding sites.

The observed inhibition of transcription by cisplatin suggests that this process may play a role in the antitumor mechanism. For example, cisplatin could block the transcription of genes vital to tumor growth, tumor cell homeostasis, or of genes encoding inhibitors of self-destructive apoptosis. In addition, given the differential effects of cisplatin on genes transcribed from various promoters, it is possible that platinum adducts upset the delicate balance of gene transcription in such a manner as to lead to the death of the cancer cell.

V. EFFECTS OF CISPLATIN ON MITOCHONDRIA

Mitochondria are small subcellular organelles intimately involved with aerobic energy metabolism and pH homeostasis. Each mammalian cell contains hundreds of self-replicating mitochondria, which in turn contain several copies of mitochondrial DNA, a 16-kb double-stranded circular molecule. The mitochondrial genome encodes proteins vital to the oxidative phosphorylation pathway. Since DNA can be covalently modified by cisplatin, it is not surprising that mitochondrial DNA is a target for platinum adduct formation. Indeed, when the platinum content of a mouse liver mitochondrial fraction was compared to that of the nuclear fraction, the concentration of cisplatin was found to be much higher in the former. In human melanoma cells grown as xenografts in nude mice, cisplatin levels on mitochondrial DNA were 50 times greater than on chromosomal DNA.

The presence of platinum on a mitochondrial genome probably inhibits its replication and transcription, an effect that would be potentiated by the apparent lack of any mitochondrial DNA repair systems. Mitochondrial damage could lead to deficiencies in energy conversion, as well as in pH homeostasis, which could be of considerable toxicity to the cell. Cisplatin treatment of melanoma cells resulted in a 60% decrease in the mitochondrially encoded NADH-ubiquinone reductase, along with decreases in cellular ATP levels and intracellular pH.

Despite the evidence that cisplatin has profound effects on mitochondria, it is not known whether these organelles are a primary target responsible for the cytotoxic effects of the drug. At present, we can only speculate that mitochondrial DNA damage probably contributes to cell death following cisplatin treatment.

VI. CISPLATIN AND DNA REPAIR

Since DNA damage is believed to the fundamental to the mechanism of cisplatin, possibly by inhibiting replication, transcription, or a combination of the two, the effects of DNA repair systems on platinum adducts have been examined in some detail. Repairing DNA damage resulting from cisplatin treatment may be one way that a cell can increase the probability of its survival. In *E. coli*, mutants lacking in either the *uvr* genes that mediate excision repair or the *rec* genes that mediate recombination are extremely sensitive to the toxic effects of cisplatin. Characterized best is the *E. coli* UvrABC excision repair system. Here, the proteins UvrA and UvrB bind at the site of damage and recruit the protein UvrC. The resultant complex incises the DNA on the damaged strand at the eighth phosphodiester bond 5′ and at the fourth phosphodiester bond 3′ to the site of platinum damage. UvrD in conjunction with DNA polymerase I then removes the damaged oligonucleotide, and the polymerase fills in the gap, which is then sealed covalently by DNA ligase. This process is known as excision repair because it involves the excision of the damaged DNA as an oligonucleotide.

The UvrABC excinuclease system can repair many forms of DNA damage, including cisplatin cross-links, apurinic sites, psoralen cross-links, and thymine dimers. The rates at which UvrABC excision repair takes place on some of the DNA adducts formed by cisplatin were examined by using DNA fragments containing site-specific platinum adducts. This study revealed that the d(GpCpG) 1,3-intrastrand adduct is incised 3.5 times more efficiently than the d(GpG) 1,2-intrastrand adduct. Interestingly, the adduct incised with the lowest efficiency, namely the d(GpG) 1,2-intrastrand adduct, is the one that is the most prevalent both *in vivo* and *in vitro*. Whereas *trans*-DDP adducts appear to be repaired more efficiently *in vivo* in *E. coli*, they are not as readily incised *in vitro* by UvrABC excinuclease as cisplatin adducts, suggesting that the *in vivo* repair of these adducts may occur via a different pathway. This conclusion is supported by previous work, which revealed that *E. coli* mutants blocked in excision repair have enhanced sensitivity to cisplatin, but not to *trans*-DDP.

Studies on the repair of cisplatin adducts in mammalian cells have been more difficult to carry out and interpret because of a limited understanding of the processes involved at the protein level. Cisplatin treatment of cells leads to increased poly(ADP-ribosyl)ation of proteins in the nucleus. This covalent modification is catalyzed by poly(ADP-ribose) polymerase, which is activated by DNA strand breaks. It plays a role in the activation of DNA repair systems, suggesting that the presence of cisplatin adducts induces repair systems.

It has been proposed, based on experimental observations, that cisplatin adducts, in contrast to DNA adducts produced by *trans*-DDP or monofunctional platinum adducts, are poorly repaired in eukaryotic cells. Making matters unclear, others observed that cisplatin and *trans*-DDP adducts appeared to be repaired at similar rates. To resolve this discrepancy, investigators have analyzed repair by using *in vitro* systems. In a study examining the effects of cisplatin and *trans*-DDP on replication *in vitro*, it was noted that preincubation of the platinated templates in cytosolic extracts restored by 30% the replication of templates damaged with *trans*-DDP, but not with cisplatin. Furthermore, by using an *in vitro* excision repair assay, it was shown that the extracts employed contained a repair activity for *trans*-DDP adducts. By using the same *in vitro* excision repair assay, it was found that both cisplatin and *trans*-DDP adducts are repaired, with the *trans*-DDP adducts being repaired twice as fast at the same levels of DNA damage. The repair activity observed for both kinds of adducts was much reduced in XP complementation group A cells, suggesting that repair occurs via the same pathways.

By using these *in vitro* excision repair synthesis assays

with mammalian cell extracts, it was noted that the repair activity for cisplatin adducts resulted in the removal of minor adducts instead of the major 1,2-intrastrand adducts. The major DNA adduct of cisplatin, the d(GpG) 1,2-intrastrand adduct, was refractory to repair in these assays. Pretreatment of the template with UvrABC enzyme prior to its introduction into the extract allowed repair to take place, suggesting that mammalian cells do not recognize and efficiently incise the d(GpG) 1,2-intrastrand adducts. In subsequent studies employing a more sensitive *in vitro* human excision repair system and site-specifically cisplatin-modified DNA templates, it was demonstrated that both d(GpG) 1,2-intrastrand adducts and d(GpTpG) 1,3-intrastrand adducts are excised in fragments of 27–29 nucleotides. The rate of incision of this human excinuclease was estimated to be up to twice as fast for the 1,3 adduct as compared to the more common 1,2 adduct. In general, these studies provide evidence that the clinical efficacy of cisplatin may stem in part from the formation of adducts that are poor substrates for repair. One caveat must be kept in mind when analyzing the results of *in vitro* repair assays, however. The levels of repair activity thus calculated do not necessarily correspond to the levels of adduct removal occurring *in vivo* because some repair mechanisms may not be functional in cell extracts.

The rates at which cisplatin adducts are removed from genomic DNA have been determined for specific genes. Cisplatin intrastrand adducts appear to be removed faster from the coding regions of a gene than from its noncoding regions, and adducts present on the transcribed strand are removed preferentially. These studies have all used UvrABC excinuclease to assay the presence of adducts following cisplatin treatment, however, so it is possible that adducts, such as 1,2-intrastrand cross-links, which are poorly recognized by the enzyme, escaped detection. These adducts may be poorly repaired *in vivo*, regardless of their location in the genome.

VII. INTERACTIONS OF CELLULAR PROTEINS WITH CISPLATIN-DAMAGED DNA

Cisplatin may be active as an antitumor drug and its geometric isomer *trans*-DDP inactive because the structures of adducts formed by the two compounds are recognized and processed differentially by cellular proteins. Such proteins might be involved in repairing DNA damage, in a manner similar to the *E. coli* UvrABC system, or they might be involved in the activation of apoptotic pathways, among many possibilities. A first step in excision repair is presumed to be the detection of an adduct by a damage recognition protein. By using gel mobility shift and Southwestern blot assays, the existence of proteins in mammalian and yeast cellular extracts capable of binding to cisplatin adducts with high affinity and specificity was established, providing some of the most exciting new results in the cisplatin field in recent years. No proteins recognizing DNA damaged with *trans*-DDP have been identified to date, even though evidence suggests that adducts of this compound may be repaired more rapidly than those of cisplatin.

In gel mobility shift assays, electrophoresis separates proteins bound to a DNA probe from the free DNA probe based on the increased size of the protein–DNA complex. Comparison of results obtained from gel mobility shifts by various investigators is complicated by the use of different cell extracts, but it appears that the observed changes in mobility are due to the binding of several proteins. In one case, the protein responsible for one of the bands in the mobility shift was found to bind to DNA damaged with either ultraviolet (UV) light or cisplatin and was absent from the human xeroderma pigmentosum complementation group E (XPE) cell line. Because XPE cells are deficient in DNA repair, which leads to high levels of UV-induced skin cancer in afflicted individuals, it appears that this protein may play a role in DNA repair. It may be a damage recognition protein, recruiting the necessary repair enzymes to the site of damage. Although this protein was absent from the repair-deficient XPE cells, its level was actually increased in cisplatin-resistant HeLa cells. This observation is consistent with a potential role in repair, for these resistant HeLa cells showed more efficient DNA repair. The purified protein responsible for the observed mobility shift had a molecular weight of 125 kDa and its binding depended on the presence of unmodified cysteine residues.

Another platinum damage binding activity was identified in extracts prepared from HeLa and hamster V79 cells. This protein had an estimated molec-

ular mass of 91 kDa and bound only DNA modified with cisplatin, and not DNA damaged with *trans*-DDP or UV light. The protein was calculated to bind with a dissociation constant on the order of 10^{-10} M and was shown to recognize cisplatin d(GpG) and d(ApG) 1,2-intrastrand adducts, but not d(GpTpG) 1,3-intrastrand adducts. The binding of the protein to platinated DNA could be abolished by the presence of 1 mM $HgCl_2$, suggesting the potential involvement of cysteine residues in binding. Unlike the 125-kDa protein, however, this protein was present at equal levels in cisplatin-resistant V79 and HeLa cells. This result is similar to that obtained with clinically more relevant sensitive and cisplatin-resistant ovarian cancer cell lines, where no differences in platinated DNA-binding activities were observed.

Preincubating cell extracts with antibodies against human single-stranded DNA binding protein (HSSB) before using the extracts in gel shift experiments allowed one group to identify HSSB as being able to bind to platinated DNA. HSSB, which consists of three polypeptide subunits (molecular masses 70, 34, and 11 kDa), may bind to the underwound DNA resulting from platinum damage. No differences in the levels of HSSB were found among pairs of sensitive and resistant cervical carcinoma, ovarian carcinoma, and testicular carcinoma cell lines.

Cisplatin damage-specific DNA-binding proteins have also been identified using Southwestern blots. In this method, proteins present in extracts are separated according to molecular weight by SDS-PAGE, followed by the electrophoretic transfer of the resolved proteins to a nitrocellulose membrane. This membrane is then treated with a binding solution containing radioactively labeled DNA damaged with cisplatin, together with unlabeled nonspecific competitor DNA. Proteins that bind specifically to platinum-damaged DNA can then be identified by autoradiography and their molecular weights estimated. By using this method, cellular extracts from human cell lines were found to contain several proteins recognizing platinated DNA. Cisplatin-damaged DNA-binding proteins were observed with molecular masses in the 90- to 100-kDa range and also in the 30-kDa range. Because Southwestern blots involve an electrophoresis step under denaturing conditions (SDS-PAGE), proteins which require multiple subunits for binding, such as HSSB, or whose binding relies on complex three-dimensional structure may not be detected.

Following the identification of cisplatin-damaged DNA-binding proteins by Southwestern blotting, an *E. coli* phage human B-cell cDNA expression library was screened under similar conditions. Two clones encoding large portions of the same protein were isolated. The encoded protein was named structure-specific recognition protein 1 (SSRP1). In a Southwestern blot assay, it bound specifically to DNA damaged with cisplatin. A full-length clone of SSRP1 was isolated by the hybridization screening of other cDNA libraries. Its deduced amino acid sequence revealed an 81-kDa protein with a preponderance of charged residues and a region of homology to the high mobility group 1 (HMG1) protein in a DNA-binding motif referred to as the HMG domain. SSRP1 is the human homolog of a mouse protein which has been shown to bind to the V(D)J sequences involved in generating antibody diversity. It is also the homolog of a transcription factor that binds to the first intron enhancer region of the rat and chicken collagen II gene.

On the assumption that the HMG domain was responsible for the specific binding to cisplatin-modified DNA, the ability of recombinant rat HMG1, which consists essentially of two such domains, to interact with platinated DNA was examined. HMG1 was found to bind with a 100-fold greater affinity to cisplatin-damaged DNA than to unmodified DNA. The protein did not bind to DNA modified with *trans*-DDP or the monofunctional platinum compound [Pt(dien)Cl]Cl and recognized cisplatin d(ApG) and d(GpG) 1,2-intrastrand lesions, but not d(GpTpG) 1,3-intrastrand adducts. This adduct recognition profile is the same as that previously observed in gel shifts with crude mammalian cellular extracts.

By using antibodies cross-reactive to HMG1 and HMG2, it was shown that both of these proteins bind platinated DNA, and that together these proteins account for the binding activity observed previously in the 30-kDa region on Southwestern blots. HMG1 and HMG2 were also identified as cisplatin damage-binding proteins by using DNA modified with the drug attached to cellulose and incubating this material with cellular extracts. The proteins were analyzed by SDS-PAGE and found to be 26.5, 28, 90, and 97 kDa in size. The identity of the 26.5- and 28-kDa proteins as HMG2 and HMG1, respectively, was confirmed by N-terminal sequencing. When the effects of cisplatin on isolated chicken erythrocyte nuclei were examined, the drug was found to cross-link selectively HMG1 and HMG2 to the internucleosomal linker DNA. HMG1 is an abundant, highly conserved protein, the actual cellular role of which remains unknown, with strong affinity for cruciform DNA. It is possible that the bending and unwinding induced by cisplatin adducts resemble, in some way, the bending and unwinding present in a cruciform DNA molecule.

The DNA-binding unit of HMG1 can be reduced to a single 75-amino-acid HMG-domain motif and still maintain its specificity for DNA damaged with cisplatin. This result identifies the HMG domain as being able to discriminate between DNA damaged with cisplatin and unmodified DNA or DNA damaged with clinically inactive platinum compounds. Furthermore, because a single HMG domain can mediate binding to platinated DNA, one expects that any protein containing one or more of these motifs will have some affinity for platinated DNA (see Table I). Indeed, such appears to be the case with the proteins examined to date. In addition to the HMG-domain-containing SSRP, HMG1, and HMG2 proteins, the human rRNA transcription factor hUBF (which contains six HMG domains), the testis-specific transcription factor SRY (which contains a single HMG domain), and the mitochondrial transcription factor mtTF1 (which contains two domains) bind to DNA damaged with cisplatin.

Recently, the methodology used to isolate SSRP1 was employed to screen a yeast (*Saccharomyces cerevisiae*) genomic DNA expression library in an attempt to identify functional homologs to human cisplatin-adduct-binding proteins. An 80-kDa protein, Ixr1, with two tandem HMG domains was thus isolated. Despite having little homology with any human proteins apart from its HMG domains, it shared 56 identical residues with yeast ARS-binding factor 2 (ABF2), the yeast homolog of HMG1. When a yeast strain lacking a functional IXR1 gene was examined for sensitivity to cisplatin, it was twofold less sensitive compared to the parental strain expressing Ixr1. This decrease in sensitivity was accompanied by a three-fold diminution in the number of platinum–DNA le-

TABLE I
Listing of Selected HMG Domain Proteins

Name	Pt/DNA Binding	HMG domains	M_r (kDa)	Species	Function
hSSRP1	Yes	1	81	Human	Unknown, binds to DNA modified with cisplatin
T160	Likely	1	81	Mouse	Binds V(D)J recombination sequences, hSSRP1 homolog
CIIDBP-r	Likely	1	81	Rat	Binds collagen promoter, hSSRP1 homolog
CIIDBP-c	Likely	1	81	Chicken	Binds collagen promoter, hSSRP1 homolog
dSSRP1	Likely	1	81	Drosophila	hSSRP1 homolog, function unknown
hUBF	Yes	6	97	Human	Transcription factor for rRNA transcription
Ixrl	Yes	2	80	Yeast	Transcription repressor, binds DNA modified with cisplatin
LEF-1	Yes	1	44	Human	Transcription factor binds T-cell receptor enhancer
TCF-1α	Unknown	1	55	Human	Transcription factor for T-cell receptor enhancer
HMG1	Yes	2	28	Human, rat	Unknown, binds DNA cruciforms, bends DNA
HMG2	Yes	2	26.5	Human	Unknown
SRY	Yes	1	24	Human	Testes-determining transcription factor
mtTF1	Yes	1	24	Human	Transcription factor in mitochondria
ABF2	Likely	2	20	Yeast	Required for mitochondrial DNA maintenance
NHP6A,B	Unknown	1	11	Yeast	Appears to be the yeast homolog of HMG1

sions by comparison to the strain expressing Ixr1. The absence of Ixr1 did not alter the response of this strain to DNA damage with *trans*-DDP or UV irradiation, indicating that the observed increase in resistance was specific for cisplatin.

The diminished cisplatin sensitivity of cells lacking Ixr1 is the first result directly correlating a protein containing an HMG domain and an effect on the activity of cisplatin *in vivo*. It suggests that, in mammalian cells, HMG-domain-containing proteins might have similar effects. One possibility by which the presence of a protein such as Ixr1 might contribute to the toxicity was suggested early on (see Fig. 7). In this model, the protein binds to the platinum adducts and camouflages them from removal by cellular repair mechanisms, allowing the adducts to persist, and enhancing cisplatin cytotoxicity. In the absence of adduct-specific-binding proteins, the platinum damage is located by repair systems, and the adducts are removed, improving the rate of cell survival. Support for this model in human cells comes from a study employing an *in vitro* human repair assay, in which it was shown that the addition of HMG1 to the assay inhibited specifically the excision of d(GpG) and d(ApG) 1,2-intrastrand adducts.

Whereas in yeast there is a direct link between an HMG-domain protein and cellular sensitivity to cis-

platin, evidence for a similar link in mammalian cells is equivocal. The 125-kDa factor lacking in XPE cells appears to be present at higher levels in cisplatin-resistant HeLa cells, suggesting that it may be a damage

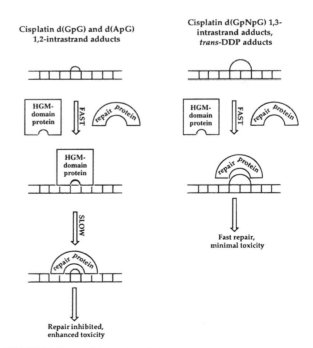

FIGURE 7 Model for the inhibition of cisplatin adduct repair in the presence of HMG-domain proteins. Adapted from G. Chu (1994), *J. Biol. Chem.* **269**, 787–790.

recognition protein involved in repair. It is unknown, however, whether this so-called XPE factor contains an HMG domain. To date, researchers have found no correlation between the levels of HMG1, SSRP1, or HSSB and the levels of resistance present in various cell lines. These proteins are present in all tissues and cell lines examined, which does not correlate well with the observed tissue-specific effects of cisplatin. Even though these results suggest, prima facie, that binding of HMG-domain proteins to cisplatin is fortuitous, it is possible that such binding is responsible for the observed anticancer effects of cisplatin. Binding of these proteins in sensitive and resistant cells may be regulated differentially, either by covalent posttranslational modifications or by interactions with other cellular partner proteins.

In the simplest analysis, the specific binding of proteins to platinated DNA is a sign that some cisplatin adducts, in particular the abundant d(ApG) and d(GpG) 1,2-intrastrand adducts, mimic naturally occurring DNA structures and conformations. Since they resemble naturally occurring DNA structures, the adducts may escape repair and effect their cytotoxic activity by inhibiting replication, transcription, or both. This simple theory explains why the d(GpG) adduct, the major cisplatin adduct, which is recognized by HMG1, is not repaired by cell extracts that repair the d(GpTpG) 1,3-intrastrand cross-link, which is not recognized. It is consistent with the observation that yeast cell extracts are unable to remove adducts from cisplatin-damaged DNA efficiently, and with the observation that *trans*-DDP adducts, which are not recognized by HMG-domain proteins, are repaired both *in vitro* and *in vivo*.

VIII. RESISTANCE TO CISPLATIN

One of the major obstacles to cancer chemotherapy is that the cytotoxicity of the agents employed selects those cells able to withstand assault; eventually, only resistant cells remain. Drug resistance is a serious problem in chemotherapy, accounting for its failure to cure the majority of cancer patients. For example, almost all advanced ovarian cancers respond initially to cisplatin-containing chemotherapy regimens, but only 50% have a complete response and only 25% of pa-

tients with advanced ovarian cancer are cured. Similarly, when bladder cancer patients are treated with cisplatin, 36% will achieve a complete remission, but of these, 68% will eventually relapse because of the development of resistance. These patients will ultimately succumb to their disease. The levels of resistance responsible for these relapses are usually only on the order of two- to fourfold. These levels of resistance may not appear to be very high, but for cisplatin, which is routinely used in dosages at the limit of its systemic toxicity, they completely eliminate clinical effectiveness.

In addition to the development of acquired resistance, some tumors are intrinsically resistant in that they do not respond to chemotherapy from the very beginning of treatment. Given this current state of affairs, there is an enormous need to discover and develop novel drugs that will allow for the curative treatment of resistant tumors. The achievement of this goal would be greatly facilitated by a complete molecular understanding of the resistance phenomenon. Such an understanding is made difficult by the varied nature of resistance, which is multifactorial (see below). Perhaps it will be easier to learn why some cells are very sensitive to cisplatin.

IX. MECHANISMS OF RESISTANCE

To understand resistance of cisplatin, researchers have focused on molecular events governing the phenomenon. Two caveats must be kept in mind when attempting to study the basis for resistance. The first is that part of the resistance phenomenon may be due to mechanisms operating at the organismic rather than cellular level. For example, a murine mammary tumor that was cisplatin resistant *in vivo* was no longer resistant when cultured *in vitro*. In addition, resistance of human small cell lung cancer lines did not correlate with the effects of cisplatin on the tumors in patients. The second caveat is that cells made resistant *in vitro* by growing them in the presence of cisplatin often show levels of resistance much higher than the two- to threefold observed for tumors *in vivo*, implying that mechanisms not normally operative are at work.

Many factors appear to govern the development of

TABLE II
Summary of Cisplatin Resistance Mechanisms

Increased levels of sulfur-containing macromolecules react with
    cisplatin and sequester the drug

The rate of cisplatin transport into the cell is reduced by unknown
    mechanisms, resulting in lower intracellular levels of cisplatin and
    reduced levels of DNA damage.

Enhanced DNA repair systems allows for more efficient removal of
    platinum adducts from DNA, eliminating blockages to replication
    and transcription

Alterations in the levels of HMG-domain proteins result in the
    decreased accumulation of cisplatin adducts on the DNA

The cell increasingly tolerates cisplatin adducts on its DNA

DNA sequence modifications, in particular a decrease in guanine
    content, take place in critical control regions, reducing the level
    of cisplatin targets and the number of platinum adducts that form

resistance, not all of which contribute equally, if at all, in every resistant tumor and cell line. In general, resistance involves several potential mechanisms, including reduction in cellular cisplatin accumulation, elevated levels of molecules such as glutathione, metallothionein, and possibly rRNA, which can sequester cisplatin, increased levels of repair activity to remove cisplatin–DNA adducts, the tolerance of platinum adducts on the DNA, and possibly DNA sequence modifications in critical regulatory regions. Furthermore, the resistance phenotype may involve alterations in the levels of proteins which specifically recognize cisplatin DNA adducts (see earlier). Table II summarizes these resistance mechanisms, any combination of which may be operative in different cells. Some, or possibly all, of these mechanisms may involve the expression of oncogenes such as *c-fos*, *c-myc*, and Ha-*ras*. The importance of oncogene expression in resistance has been demonstrated for *ras* and *fos*. In the presence of an inactivating suppresser *ras* mutant, cisplatin sensitivity was restored to a resistant line. In the case of *fos*, an anti-*fos* ribozyme was used to reduce the expression of the oncogene, resulting in the restoration of cisplatin sensitivity.

X. DECREASED CISPLATIN UPTAKE

Several experiments have revealed that cell signaling pathways can affect cisplatin uptake, suggesting that the drug does not necessarily migrate across the membrane by passive diffusion alone. Keeping cisplatin out of the cell in the first place reduces the amount of subsequent cytotoxic damage to DNA and other cellular components, and allows the cell to survive challenges with higher drug concentrations. It is thus not surprising that, when selected with cisplatin, those cells with impaired platinum uptake will be more likely to survive. Reducing cisplatin accumulation appears to be a major mechanism of acquired resistance. In one study, variants of an ovarian carcinoma line with increasing resistance showed decreasing levels of cisplatin accumulation, which could be measured only 5 min following treatment. The decreased uptake observed was not due to the increased efflux of cisplatin nor was there an alteration in cellular glutathione levels. Similar decreases in platinum uptake have been noted for a variety of other cisplatin-resistant cell lines. Cisplatin uptake can also be controlled at the organismic level. For example, the levels of platinum adducts present in leukocytes correlate well with disease response. The higher the levels of adducts on the DNA of leukocytes, the higher the likelihood of a disease response. Attempts to increase the uptake of cisplatin have been made by using platinum(II) compounds with different ligands, as well as platinum(IV) compounds, with some success. Cisplatin-resistant cells have also been treated with the drug under hyperthermic conditions, which are believed to alter the structure of the cell membrane, allowing more cisplatin to enter the cell.

XI. METALLOTHIONEINS AND GLUTATHIONE

Once cisplatin has crossed the cell membrane and entered the cytoplasm, it encounters a variety of molecules with which it can react before reaching DNA. By increasing the levels of sulfur-rich molecules such as the protein metallothionein and the cysteine-containing tripeptide glutathione, the cell can reduce the likelihood that cisplatin will form DNA adducts. Elevating intracellular thiol levels might thus be a mechanism by which cells can become resistant to cisplatin. Researchers have examined the levels of metallothioneins and glutathione in resistant and sensitive cells. It appears that some resistant cells have increased their levels of these molecules, whereas others had the same levels found in sensitive cells.

Metallothioneins, which normally function in zinc homeostasis and heavy metal (e.g., mercury or cadmium) detoxification, were overexpressed in some, but not all, bladder tumor samples in a study on tissue from patients who had not responded to cisplatin therapy. In human small cell lung cancer lines, the levels of both the metallothionein proteins and its mRNA appeared to correlate with the level of resistance, and a resistant testicular tumor cell line was 1.9-fold resistant to the cytotoxic effects of cadmium chloride, suggesting that it had an increased level of metallothionein. A clinical application of this knowledge was suggested when it was shown that pretreatment with bismuth, which increases cellular metallothionein levels, reduced the nephrotoxicity of cisplatin in mice. Resistance can obviously result from other factors as well because other cell lines examined had levels of metallothionein that did not correlate with their levels of cisplatin resistance.

As with metallothionein, the levels of glutathione may be higher in resistant compared to sensitive cells. For example, in ovarian tumor cell lines that showed 30- to 1000-fold increases in resistance to cisplatin, levels that can only be obtained *in vitro* by lengthy selection in the presence of high levels of cisplatin, glutathione levels were increased by 13- to 50-fold over the sensitive parental lines. In a human small cell lung cancer cell line that was 8.6-fold resistant to cisplatin, levels of glutathione were 2.5-fold higher than for the parental line. Not unexpectedly, given the multifactorial nature of resistance, other resistant cell lines had levels of glutathione similar to their sensitive counterparts, and in one case even had lower levels. In an attempt to reduce the resistance of cells expressing increased levels of glutathione, researchers treated such cells with the glutathione synthesis inhibitor buthionine sulfoximine. Such treatment reduced the levels of cisplatin resistance in some cell lines, but not in others.

XII. RESISTANCE AND REPAIR

Treating a cell with cisplatin concentrations that overwhelm both the mechanisms that reduce cellular uptake and those that use nonessential molecules to sequester the drug before it reaches the DNA should result in DNA damage. Resistant cells are able to overcome this DNA damage in several ways. They may have more efficient repair systems operating, they may better be able to tolerate platinum on their DNA without needing to repair it, and they may have undergone mutations that reduce the binding of cisplatin to critical control elements. The importance of DNA repair in cisplatin resistance is underscored by the extreme sensitivity of repair-deficient xeroderma pigmentosum fibroblasts to the drug. Furthermore, the SUSA cell line, derived from a testicular teratoma that is exquisitely sensitive to cisplatin, is deficient in the repair of cisplatin adducts, as determined by the immunochemical quantitation of adducts on SUSA genomic DNA.

In a study that examined the gene-specific repair of cisplatin adducts, it was found that the rates of intrastrand adduct removal were the same for resistant and sensitive ovarian cancer cell lines, but that the resistant cell lines were better able to remove interstrand cross-links. Enhanced DNA repair has been observed for resistant ovarian carcinoma cells, both by noting a faster rate of decrease in the number of adducts present on genomic DNA and by seeing enhanced repair of transfected plasmid DNA containing the CAT reporter gene. In a cisplatin-resistant murine leukemia cell line, higher levels of proliferating cell nuclear antigen (PCNA), a protein associated with DNA repair synthesis, were noted. Interestingly, levels of the mRNA for the human repair gene ERCC1 were severalfold higher in tumor tissue from ovarian cancer patients who were clinically resistant to platinum-based therapy. As with the other mechanisms that can contribute to cisplatin resistance, enhanced DNA repair is by no means a hallmark of resistance in every cell line examined, and the presence of repair activity can depend on whether the resistance of a cell line stems from *in vivo* or *in vitro* adaptation.

Cellular resistance to cisplatin in ovarian carcinoma cells can even be accompanied by an apparent decreased rate of adduct removal when compared to the drug-sensitive parental line. Such an observation suggests that some resistant cells may be able to tolerate higher levels of platinum adducts on their DNA or that, in these cells, the cytotoxicity of cisplatin is potentiated by repair-related events.

XIII. RESISTANCE AND DNA SEQUENCE MODIFICATIONS

Other than by repair, it is possible that resistant cell lines could reduce the levels of cisplatin bound to critical control regions by altering the base content of such regions to favor sequences with reduced affinity for cisplatin. In the case of the SV40 virus, cisplatin preferentially attacks regulatory DNA elements, the so-called GC box, that control both viral transcription and replication. By selecting the SV40 virus in the presence of cisplatin and sequencing the GC-box elements of surviving SV40 viruses, it was found that the resistant viral strains had lost some of the GC content of these elements, reducing the binding sites available for the drug in this region. Whether such alterations take place in cellular genomes is not known, but given both the mutagenicity of cisplatin and its affinity for runs of guanines, it would not be surprising that selection in the presence of the drug may favor mutations in critical control regions that reduce the likelihood of platinum binding. Such GC-rich regions have been observed 5′ to cellular genes, particularly oncogenes. The combined introduction of mutations and selection by cisplatin could account for the appearance of stable cellular resistance at the genetic level which remains for long periods of time, even when the cells are grown in the absence of cisplatin.

XIV. NOVEL PLATINUM COMPOUNDS

Since the identification of the potent antitumor activity of cisplatin in the late 1960s, hundreds of platinum compounds have been synthesized and examined for antitumor activity in a variety of cell and animal screens. Most of the platinum compounds demonstrating antitumor activity obeyed the structure–function relationship first defined by Cleare and Hoeschele. Molecules exhibiting anticancer drug activity were observed to be neutral platinum(II)

complexes of the form cis-$[PtA_2X_2]$ in which A is an amine/ammine ligand and X is a labile anionic leaving group.

The intensive quest for platinum drugs with a broader activity spectrum and fewer side effects than cisplatin has produced several promising new compounds, one of which, carboplatin (see Fig. 1), has been approved by the FDA. Carboplatin, which is hydrolyzed more slowly than cisplatin, yields the same active aquated intracellular metabolite as cisplatin, resulting in a similar DNA adduct spectrum and cytotoxic mechanism. This similarity in mechanism is supported by the effectiveness of both compounds against the same tumors, and essentially complete tumor cross-resistance. The reduction in the rate at which carboplatin is hydrolyzed decreases its systemic toxicity when compared to cisplatin, and the drug can be administered at fourfold higher levels, with only myelosuppression being dose limiting.

More recently, attention has focused on platinum(IV) dicarboxylate compounds, in particular mixed ammine/amine Pt(IV) complexes such as bis(acetato)(ammine)dichloro(cyclohexylamine)platinum(IV) (JM216, see Fig. 1). These molecules are reduced *in vivo* to their Pt(II) counterparts following the hydrolysis of the carboxylates and eventually form adducts on DNA similar to those of cisplatin. The benefit of using these Pt(IV) dicarboxylates over cisplatin or carboplatin is that they allow for oral administration with good bioavailability and a reduced emetic potential, eliminating the need for costly and uncomfortable intravenous administrations in an inpatient setting. Even though ingest JM216 appears to have antitumor activity comparable to intravenously administered cisplatin or carboplatin, there is some evidence that it may circumvent transport determined acquired resistance to cisplatin, possibly from its different pharmacokinetic properties. Compound JM216 is currently undergoing clinical trials in the United Kingdom and the United States.

Both carboplatin and JM216 form bifunctional adducts on DNA in a manner similar or identical to cisplatin, suggesting that, despite improvements in toxicity and bioavailability, these compounds will be no more successful than the parent drug in the treatment of refractory cancers. In an attempt to overcome the clinical limitations which result from the formation of similar DNA adduct pools, platinum(II) compounds of the form cis-$[Pt(NH_3)_2(Am)Cl]^+$ (see Fig. 1) have been synthesized. Here Am is a derivative of pyridine, pyrimidine, purine, or aniline. The compounds clearly do not follow the expected structure–function relationship for platinum anticancer drugs. They are cationic and can bind only monofunctionally, but demonstrate antitumor activity $in\ vivo$. When studied $in\ vitro$, one of these compounds, cis-$[Pt(NH_3)_2(4\text{-}Br\text{-}py)Cl]^+$, was very different from cisplatin, forming monofunctional adducts on DNA that did not bend the helix but unwound it by 10°. Nevertheless, these compounds were able to inhibit both DNA replication and the progression of DNA polymerases $in\ vitro$. Since the DNA adducts formed by this new class of compounds are clearly very different from those of cisplatin and cisplatin-like drugs such as carboplatin and JM216, it is possible that they will allow a wider range of previously resistant tumors to be treated with platinum.

Other approaches to designing new platinum drugs have included attempts to target the delivery of cisplatin-like compounds to cancerous cells. This task could be performed by conjugation to molecules such as sugars, antibodies, or hormones, which localize preferentially to the tumor. Platinum(II) with lipophilic ligands encapsulated in liposomes has been studied as a way to increase platinum dosage and to reduce toxicity to nontarget cells.

XV. FUTURE OUTLOOK

Extending the success obtained with cisplatin in the treatment of testicular cancer, even in a limited sense, to other cancers would have a major impact on overall survival rates. To develop new drugs toward this end will require a better understanding of the molecular basis for the activity of cisplatin and its particular effectiveness against testicular cancers. In the years that have passed since the biological effects of cisplatin were first discovered, much progress has been made in this area. We now know that the likely cellular target for cisplatin is DNA, and the chemistry of the interactions between these two molecules is well understood. The mechanisms contributing to the acquired resistance of tumor cells are beginning to emerge, and already this information is being translated into clinical practice.

After decades of synthesis, chemists have found only a very few molecules capable of reproducing the antitumor activity of cisplatin. Even though these compounds reduce some of the side effects observed for cisplatin, they do not widen appreciably the scope of tumors amenable to curative treatment. One possible exception may be the cis-$[Pt(NH_3)_2(Am)Cl]^+$ compounds, which appear to behave very differently from cisplatin in their interactions with DNA.

Perhaps the best new opportunity for improving our understanding of how cisplatin cytotoxicity is mediated, both at a structural and mechanistic level, is the study of the cellular proteins which recognize cisplatin adducts on DNA. Knowledge of whether and how such proteins play a role in mediating the antitumor activity of cisplatin may lead to efforts in raising or lowering their levels in attempts to sensitize resistant cells. The use of easily manipulated yeast and bacterial systems and protein homologs will enhance the rate at which such an understanding evolves. Even in the absence of knowledge about the roles of these proteins, their ability to recognize selectively the majority of adducts of antitumor–active platinum complexes suggests a rational approach to drug design. These proteins could be used in screens of DNA-damaging agents in order to identify molecules forming structures similar to those of cisplatin. Such a screen might identify potential compounds, not necessarily platinum based, worthy of further analysis for antitumor activity.

Finally, the majority of studies on the mechanism of cisplatin have employed cell lines derived from tumors not normally treated with cisplatin, such as cervical carcinomas and leukemias. Recently, more effort has gone into establishing testicular tumor cell lines, derived from tissue that is exquisitely sensitive to cisplatin. Analyzing the effects of cisplatin on these sensitive cells in great detail may also aid in the elucidation of the mechanism of action of cisplatin.

Acknowledgment

This work was supported by a grant from the National Cancer Institute.

See Also the Following Articles

CHEMOTHERAPY: SYNERGISM AND ANTAGONISM • ENDOME-
TRIAL CANCER • ESOPHAGEAL CANCER: TREATMENT • FO-
LATE ANTAGONISTS • GERM CELL TUMORS

Bibliography

Andrews, P. A., and Howell, S. B. (1990). *Cancer Cells* **2,** 35–43.

Bruhn, S. L., Toney, J. H., and Lippard, S. J. (1990). *Prog. Inorg. Chem.* **38,** 477–516.

Chu, G. (1994). *J. Biol. Chem.* **269,** 787–790.

Cleare, M. J., and Hoeschele, J. D. (1973). *Bioinorg. Chem.* **2,** 187–210.

Comess, K. M., and Lippard, S. J. (1993). Molecular aspects of platinum–DNA interactions. *In* "Molecular Aspects of Anticancer Drug–DNA Interactions," Vol. 1, pp. 134–168. Macmillan, London.

Dabholkar, M., and Reed, E. (1993). *Cancer Chemother. Biol. Resp. Mod.* **14,** 86–97.

Eastman, A. (1991). *Cancer Treat. Res.* **57,** 233–249.

Lepre, C. A., and Lippard, S. J. (1990). Interaction of platinum antitumor compounds with DNA. *In* "Nucleic Acids and Molecular Biology." Springer-Verlag, Heidelberg.

Loehrer, P. J., and Einhorn, L. H. (1984). *Ann. Int. Med.* **100,** 704–713.

c-mos Protooncogene

Nicholas T. Schulz

University of Pittsburgh School of Medicine

GLOSSARY

cell division control 2 (cdc2) A gene coding for a 34-kDa protein ($p34^{cdc2}$) that regulates the entry of a cell into mitosis. Initially isolated in the fission yeast *Schizosaccharomyes Pombe*.

cyclin An ~50-kDa protein whose level fluctuates during the cell cycle. First characterized in sea urchin embryos.

cytostatic factor (CSF) An activity isolated from mature oocytes able to arrest cells at metaphase of meiosis II.

maturation (or mitosis) promoting factor (MPF) A cytosolic factor that can induce G_2/M-arrested oocytes to enter meiosis in the absence of protein synthesis. Demonstrated to be a complex of $p34^{cdc2}$ and cyclin.

Moloney murine sarcoma virus (Mo-MSV) A retrovirus that causes fibrosarcomas in mice, rats, and hamsters.

transgenic mouse A mouse whose genome has been altered prior to embryonic development in order to study the effects of aberrant gene expression.

The discovery of oncogenes represents the most significant advance in our understanding of the molecular basis of cancer. These genes are altered forms of normal cellular genes or "protooncogenes." The c-*mos* gene is the first protooncogene to be molecularly cloned and have its transforming activity demonstrated. The protein product, $p39^{mos}$, is a serine/threonine kinase. To understand how this oncogene contributes to neoplastic transformation, this article (1) discusses the normal function of the protooncogene, (2) discusses the place of the c-*mos* gene in meiosis/mitosis, (3) examines how aberrant expression brings about transformation, and (4) examines the effect of overexpression and nonexpression ("knockout") of this gene in transgenic mice.

I. INTRODUCTION

This article describes the properties of the *mos* oncogene as well as how this gene might affect neoplastic transformation. The transformed phenotype constitutes a subset of normal cellular functions. Examining the molecular biology of the transformed cell, comparing it to that of a normal cell, can elucidate the molecular basis of malignancy. Understanding the control of cell proliferation hinges on an appreciation of cell cycle control. The role of *mos* in cell cycle control as well as that of other oncogenes will be discussed. It is hoped that the insight gained from studying *mos* will serve as a paradigm in elucidating the role other oncogenes play in the molecular biology of cancer.

II. FUNCTION OF THE *c-mos* PROTOONCOGENE

The *mos* oncogene was discovered as part of the genome of the acute transforming, replication-defective retrovirus, Moloney murine sarcoma virus (Mo-MSV). Infection by Mo-MSV causes fibrosarcomas in mice, rats, and hamsters. The *mos* protooncogene, isolated from the mouse genome, was the first cellular protooncogene shown to have transforming activity. The gene contains no introns, and the only posttranscriptional modification detected is polyadenylation. Sensitive and specific RNA detection assays (S1 nuclease and RNAse protection) are necessary to identify *mos* transcripts in a variety of tissues. *mos* expression is high in gonadal tissue and in early embryogenesis. In adult tissue, the only site that *mos* is expressed is in maturing germ cells. By *in situ* hybridization, expression is detected in growing and maturing oocytes and this persists through ovulation, although expression is not evident in fertilized eggs.

The amino acid sequence of *Xenopus mos* compared to human, mouse, and chicken *mos* reveals that it is less well conserved between species than other protooncogenes. For example, between chicken and human the *src* protooncogene shares 90% homology, whereas the *mos* protooncogene shares approximately 60%. Most of the conserved regions are in the sequences shared among the *src* kinase family members.

The expression of *mos* during oocyte maturation provides an opportunity to test how and when *mos* functions in this developmental process. By microinjecting DNA sequences complementary to the sense sequences present (antisense), one can block the expression of a cell's native RNA. Such antisense experiments may demonstrate not only if a particular gene is necessary for a biological process, but may demonstrate where in the process it is required. When one injects sense and antisense *mos* oligodeoxyribonucleotides into maturing mouse oocytes, only the antisense molecules inhibit polar body emission. This indicates that depletion of *mos* blocks meiotic maturation.

The morphology of the antisense-treated oocytes interrupted in maturation is quite remarkable. Sense-injected oocytes undergo normal maturation and polar body extrusion. Antisense-injected oocytes undergo germinal vesicle breakdown (GVBD) and metaphase chromosome condensation, but are arrested at a stage when cytoplasmic particulates and mitochondria have migrated over the nucleus during GVBD. Normally, these particulates redistribute to the cytoplasm after GVBD. Thus, depletion of *mos* during maturation interrupts this developmental process at a specific stage of cytoskeletal morphogenesis.

In order to pinpoint precisely where in oocyte maturation *mos* functions, it is important to recapitulate some of the experiments done with the South African frog: *Xenopus laevis*. This frog provides large numbers of large, easily studied oocytes at morphologically distinct stages of oocyte maturation. This availability of large numbers of oocytes at each developmental stage provides the opportunity to determine the dynamics of *mos* expression. When *mos* mRNA is assayed, it is present throughout oogenesis and early embryonic development. Surprisingly, the *mos* protein, p39^{mos}, is only present in maturing oocytes. This demonstrates that *mos* RNA translation is very tightly regulated. The developmental process that occurs during this interval is reentry into meiosis, meiosis I, and arrest at metaphase II of meiosis. This suggests that p39^{mos} is involved in meiosis.

In vertebrates, fully grown oocytes are naturally arrested at the first meiotic prophase. In *Xenopus*, this arrest is released by progesterone and is followed by the appearance of the cytoplasmic activity called maturation (or mitosis) promoting factor (MPF). This activity is responsible for germinal vesicle (or nuclear membrane) breakdown (GVBD) and chromosome condensation. MPF was originally described as a cytosolic factor that, upon microinjection into G_2/M-arrested oocytes, could induce them to enter meiosis in the absence of protein synthesis. As with mouse oocytes, p39^{mos} is required for *Xenopus* oocyte maturation. The injection of fully grown oocytes with *mos* antisense DNA blocks GVBD induced by progesterone. An important difference between mouse and *Xenopus* is that mouse oocyte maturation proceeds past GVBD. This difference suggests that *mos* is required not only at the beginning of maturation, but also at later stages of meiosis.

The work of Wasserman and Masui demonstrates that early stages of progesterone-induced maturation are sensitive to protein synthesis inhibitors. In later stages, maturation becomes protein synthesis independent. This corresponds to the activation of MPF from its inactive precursor, pre-MPF. Thus, the addition of MPF directly to oocytes abrogates the protein synthesis requirement. This led Wasserman and Masui to conclude that *de novo* synthesis of an *initiator* was required to start maturation. The expression of p39^{mos} only during maturation suggested that *mos* may be that initiator. Indeed, there is a rapid increase in p39^{mos} synthesis after progesterone treatment, preceding the time when oocyte maturation becomes protein synthesis independent or when MPF is activated. By injecting *mos* RNA directly into fully grown oocytes, it is possible to demonstrate that its overexpression induces maturation. Studies by Watanabe and colleagues indicate that even though the *mos* product is stable in unfertilized, mature oocytes, within 30 min after fertilization all p39^{mos} disappears. This explains the absence of the product in fertilized eggs.

The properties of calcium sensitivity and absence after fertilization in dividing embryos correlate with those of the activity cytostatic factor (CSF). CSF was first characterized by Masui and Markert and is also associated with mature oocytes. This activity is believed to be responsible for arresting vertebrate oocytes at metaphse II of meiosis. Masui and Clarke showed that CSF injected into one cell of a two-cell, cleaving embryo arrests it at metaphase of mitosis. The similarity of p39^{mos} with CSF led Sagata and col-

leagues to address whether p39^{mos} is responsible for CSF activity. In these experiments, one cell of a two-cell embryo injected with *mos* RNA was arrested in cleavage at metaphase of mitosis and displayed CSF activity. Moreover, it is possible to show that antibodies directed against *mos* can neutralize CSF activity extracted from mature oocytes. Thus, p39^{mos} is responsible for arresting oocytes at metaphase II of meiosis. This activity is also required for the stabilization of MPF.

Further success in the characterization of p39^{mos} stems from two observations. First, CSF-arrested mitotic cells have larger than normal spindles. Second, taxol, a drug that binds to and stabilizes microtubules and spindles, arrests dividing embryos at metaphase and thus resembles CSF in activity. This raises the question of whether p39^{mos} may be associated with the polymerization and stabilization of microtubules and spindle. Microtubule assembly is a dynamic process, and it is possible that the presence of p39^{mos} in oocytes is catalytic in promoting spindle assembly. Its programmed proteolysis after fertilization would then cause spindle depolymerization. Work by Zhou and colleagues indicates that p39^{mos} not only polymerizes with tubulin into microtubules *in vitro*, but that α- and β-tubulin are major substrates of *mos* kinase phosphorylation *in vitro*. Thus, p39^{mos} is a microtubule-associated kinase and may interact or influence the formation and stability of microtubules as spindles. The dramatic interruption of the movement of cytoplasmic particulates observed in maturing mouse oocytes depleted of *mos* would be consistent with the *mos* product functioning directly or indirectly in microtubule assembly.

III. CELL CYCLE, MITOSIS, AND MEIOSIS

There are two major control points within the cell cycle. These points are defined by arrested stages in the cell cycle due to nutrient limitations or hormonal blocks. One occurs late in G_1, just before S phase (G_1/S). The second major control point occurs at the end of G_2 and regulates entry into mitosis (G_2/M). Genetic analysis of the fission yeast *Schizosaccharomyces pombe* has uncovered the presence of cell division cycle (*cdc*) genes which has shed light on how these control points serve to coordinate DNA synthesis and mitosis. Study of conditional *cdc* mutations has allowed ordering the time and interdependence of the gene functions and shows that each step is dependent on the successful completion of earlier steps.

The fission yeast *cdc2* gene encodes a 34-kDa protein termed p34^{cdc2}, which is a serine kinase. The structure of this protein is well conserved among eukaryotes, pointing to the central role this gene plays in cell cycle control. In a striking example of conservation of function, Lee and Nurse identified the human homolog of *cdc2* by selecting for a gene from a human cDNA library that could complement mutations in the *cdc2* gene of fission yeast.

Another gene, *cdc13*, is also required for the induction of mitosis in *S. pombe*. Importantly, its product has been shown to complex with p34^{cdc2}. The significance of this association requires background in a different class of proteins active in mitosis. A 50-kDa protein is present during the embryonic cell cycle of sea urchins which accumulates before the first mitotic division and then disappears at the end of mitosis. This protein is designated cyclin because of the cycling nature of its appearance. Two types of cyclins, referred to as A and B, have been identified. These cyclin proteins are homologous to the *cdc13* product of fission yeast. The complex of *cdc13* and p34^{cdc2} is analogous to MPF.

MPF, therefore, is a universal regulator of M phase and G$_2$/M transition in both meiosis and mitosis in eukaryotes. MPF purified from amphibian and starfish eggs has been shown to be a protein kinase that phosphorylates H1 histone and appears to be identical to the growth-associated H1 kinase that was known to appear during mitosis in a number of organisms. It has been postulated that high and low levels of MPF activity define the two major control points in the cell cycle: high levels are found during mitosis and low levels are found during interphase. The cell cycle is organized so that transitions are initiated by changes in the activity of the p34^{cdc2} and cyclin protein complexes.

The first half of this article described mechanisms of cell cycle control revealed by the study of genes in yeast and the characterization of activities that occur in maturing oocytes of vertebrates and invertebrates. There is a direct connection with protooncogenes in that CSF is the *mos* protooncogene product and, therefore, a direct regulator of MPF and the metaphase stage of meiosis. It is not yet known whether the *mos* protooncogene product functions during mitosis, but there is probably a mitotic gene product with an equivalent activity. The *mos* product is therefore the first protooncogene shown to be functioning at a major control point of the cell cycle.

IV. *c-mos* AND TRANSFORMATION

Transformed cells display a spectrum of characteristics ranging from, but not including, senescence (cells that are morphologically normal and nontumorigenic, displaying contact inhibition, but growing continuously in culture) to a high degree of transformation (cells that display anchorage-independent growth and are very tumorigenic in animals). One hypothesis of the dynamics of tumor progression proposes that the transition to a more transformed phenotype is caused by an accumulation of genetic errors. These errors result in more oncogenes being activated or suppressor genes being inactivated. Compared to nontransformed cells, transformed cells display a high degree of genetic instability. This in and of itself can account for tumor progression and it is likely that some properties of the transformed phenotype increase as genetic instability increases.

The *mos* oncogene provides a unique insight into the molecular basis of transformation. Like many other oncogenes, *mos* was discovered as part of an acute transforming retrovirus, Mo-MSV. As previously mentioned, this replication-defective virus causes fibrosarcomas in mice, rats, and hamsters. Acute infection of tissue culture fibroblasts with Mo-MSV, however, does not result in the transformation of all cells. A large percentage of fibroblasts infected with Mo-MSV round up and show evidence for premature chromatin condensation, ring chromosome formation, and chromosome pulverization. These rounded, floating cells are growth arrested, whereas the cells that remain attached develop as transformed cells. The transformed cells are anchorage independent, grow in semisolid agar to high saturation density, and show a disruption of the cytoskeleton, changes typical of the transformed phenotype. These acutely infected cells express a 10-fold higher level of *mos* product than stably transformed cell populations. The *mos* oncogene product expressed in transformed cells represents only 0.0005% of the total cellular protein, indicating extraordinary efficiency as an oncoprotein.

Given the normal function of p39^{mos}, the major question to be addressed is how *mos* expression in somatic cells can result in transformation. The *mos* product may only function during meiosis. It may be that unscheduled, constitutive expression of p39^{mos} in somatic cells causes the expression of the meiotic phenotype during interphase. Because microtubule polymerization/depolymerization is a dynamic process, even a low level of p39^{mos} would be expected to influence microtubule formation. The identification of spindle polymerization as a potential *mos* function suggests that an aberrant formation of the mitotic spindle may be responsible for transformation. Another explanation may be that since *mos* stabilizes MPF, the aberrant spindle forms may also stabilize MPF.

Let us examine how the inappropriate expression of *mos* and the corresponding mitotic or meiotic phenotype may explain certain hallmarks of the transformed phenotype. Altered nuclear morphology present in transformed cells might represent an incompletely "penetrant" phenotype of mitotic cell rounding and GVBD as high levels of MPF induce GVBD and chromosome condensation. Loss of contact inhibition could correspond to a phenotype that normally occurs during cytokinesis as daughter cells cannot growth arrest when they are in contact. A very important property of transformed cells is genetic instability. The constitutive presence of MPF activity during late S phase may result in premature chromosome condensation which generates free DNA ends. Such structures, in lower eukaryotes, are highly recombinogenic. This could explain the genetic instability as manifest by chromosomal translocations observed in tumor cells.

Another specific substrate or pathway that *mos*-mediated transformation has been associated with is mitogen-activated protein kinase (MAPK). It has been demonstrated that Mos activates MAPK. This protein is a kinase known to be constitutively activated in a number of transformed cell lines. Thus, MAPK acts as a common pathway for transformation by some oncogenes. To further investigate the role of MAPK, Okazaki and Sagata overexpressed a mutant of a protein (MEK1) that phosporylates MAPK in NIH/3T3 cells already transformed by *mos*. The presence of this dominant-negative mutant caused the cells to revert to a nontransformed phenotype. This demonstrates that transformation by *mos* can be suppressed by blocking its action on wild-type MAPK. When, however, the wild-type isoform of MEK1 is co-expressed, transformation is markedly enhanced. This shows that *mos*-induced transformation is mediated via the MAPK pathway in NIH/3T3 cells.

mos may also serve as a paradigm when examining other oncogenes that may function at control points in the cell cycle. Oncogenes such as p21^{ras} also activate maturation, and p60^{c-src} is specifically phosphorylated by p34^{cdc2} during mitosis. Under these conditions, p60^{src} is activated as a tyrosine kinase. Daar and colleagues have shown that activated p21^{ras} displays CSF activity and, therefore, also functions at a major cell cycle control point, suggesting that it might transform by a mechanism similar to *mos*. This may help explain how certain oncogenes may "cooperate" to produce a more transformed phenotype. Because microtubule formation is dynamic, increasing the amount of one oncoprotein or activating additional oncogenes with catalytic microtubule polymerization activity could cause a progressive increase in the degree of transformation.

V. TRANSGENIC *mos* AND *mos*-LESS MICE

The role of oncogenes in carcinogenesis has been explored through the use of transgenic animals. In such animals a genetic sequence is inserted into the host genome. In the case of most transgenic animals the gene is inserted and expressed in a nonphysiological manner. The effects of the inappropriate expression on embryogenesis and eventual phenotype are then studied. In the case of "knockout" mice, a gene is targeted and replaced by a nonfunctioning counterpart. In these animals, the phenotype is studied for the significance of a gene's absence.

Most transgenic animals created to study the function of an oncogene involve the insertion of an oncogene coupled to a site-specific promoter. In this way the site of tumor formation is directed by the promoter sequence used to express the oncogene. For example, when a mouse mammary tumor virus promoter is linked to the c-myc oncogene, an increased incidence of mammary tumors is observed in stochastic fashion. In contrast, when an IgG enhancer is used with c-myc, lymphoid neoplasms develop. An insulin promoter linked to the SV40 large T antigen produces pancreatic β cell tumors. These model systems have not yielded transgenic animals displaying patterns of tumors resembling those seen in familial neoplasia syndromes. Yet it is such a pattern that is observed in transgenic mice bearing the c-mos oncogene. These mice contain the murine *mos* oncogene coupled to a ubiquitous promoter, the Moloney virus long terminal repeat (LTR). These mice present tumors in a pattern such as is found in the human autosomal dominant neoplastic syndrome multiple endocrine neoplasia (Table I).

Pheochromocytomas and medullary thyroid carcinomas (MTC) are principal manifestations of the autosomal dominant neoplastic syndrome, multiple endocrine neoplasia type 2 (MEN 2). Pheochromocytomas are adrenal tumors that originate as small nodules of hyperplastic cells in the adrenal medulla. The precursor lesion of MTC is C-cell hyperplasia. The C cell is the cell type in the thyroid responsible for the elaboration of calcitonin. Both of these tumors are neural crest derivatives. The pathology of both of these MEN 2 neoplasms is multifocal. It is interesting to note that both of these tumor types and precursor lesions are found in *mos* transgenic mice.

More interesting, however, is that not all *mos* transgenic mice show similar patterns of tumor presentation. As demonstrated in Table II, the first line of mice studied primarily manifests pheochromocytomas. In contrast, the second display MTC. The third line displays an incidence of tumors no higher than that of normal controls. Thus, the same transgene, when integrated into three different sites, produced three distinct tumor presentation patterns.

These first three transgenic lines all use the same background of mouse (FVB/N). When a different background, B6C3 (and a different integration site for the transgene), is used, a mouse is obtained displaying both tumor types (line 4). The variation of tumor presentation pattern between the transgenic lines is similar to that observed in humans with MEN 2. In the human syndrome, the tumor presentation pattern is consistent within a kindred (analogous to mouse background). The most commonly observed pattern of tumor formation in humans with MEN 2 is the presence of both medullary thyroid carcinomas and pheochromocytomas, as in the line 4 animals.

This line-dependent variation of neural crest tumor presentation is quite curious and suggests that the transgene integration site or background of the animal plays a role in the type of tumor induced. To evaluate this variance of penetrance, the first three *mos* transgenic FVB/N lines were crossed with a different background of mouse, BALB/c (Table III).

The progeny of the first two crosses shows essentially the same tumor phenotype as on the FVB/N background. Quite remarkably, however, the mice of the line 3 × BALB/c cross display a high frequency of both pheochromocytomas and medullary thyroid C-cell carcinomas. Neither of these neoplasms is displayed in the parental line 3 animals, suggesting that the integration site and/or background is responsible for this variation. Of interest are preliminary results involving line 3 crosses to yet another background, C3H. When C3H mice are crossed to line 3 transgenic, the phenotype observed is reminiscent of the human familial tumor syndrome MEN 1, with a high incidence of pituitary adenomas and pancreatic islet cell hyperplasia being seen.

The variation of tumor presentation patterns seen is similar to that observed in humans with MEN 2. The most commonly observed patterns of tumor for-

TABLE I
Characteristics of Human Multiple
Endocrine Neoplasia

MEN	MEN 2 (a + b)
Autosomal dominant	Autosomal dominant
Pancreatic islet cell tumors	Medullary thyroid carcinoma
Pituitary adenomas	Pheochromocytomas
Hyperparathyroidism	Mucosal ganglioneuromas
Mapped to chromosome 11	Hyperparathyroidism
	Mapped to chromosome 10

TABLE II

Percentage of Transgenic c-mos Mice with Tumors

Transgenic mouse line	Pheos only (%)	MTC only (%)	Both (%)	Total (%)
1	58	0	4	62
2	0	63	4	67
3	2	0	0	2
4	23	13	32	68

mation in humans with MEN 2 is the presence of both medullary thyroid carcinomas and pheochromocytomas, as observed in the line 4 animals. A far less common form of MEN 2 is exhibited by patients who present solitary medullary thyroid carcinomas. These patients never develop pheochromocytomas, which is very similar to the presentation observed in the line 2 mos transgenic animals.

The differences in tumor presentation patterns in the various lines may be attributable to variations in the level of transgene expression or may reflect earlier activation of expression in the target organs of the tumor-bearing lines. This could be due to the transgene integration site or the genetic background used. As illustrated in Table III, the interaction of transgene with genetic background can influence the penetrance of the phenotype. The tumor phenotypes of the progeny of the FVB/N mos transgenic lines crossed with BALB/c may change because of alterations in transgene expression. Alternatively, it may be that a second genetic event may be suppressed in line 3 or predisposed to in the progeny.

These transgenic lines provide an opportunity to study the genetic and molecular bases of tumor induction and may help in elucidating the mechanism

of tissue targeting in the human syndromes. This model for MEN is one where tumor phenotype and penetrance are background dependent. Although the promoter used (MoLTR) results in ubiquitous expression, tumors of only neural crest origin (pheochromocytomas, C-cell carcinomas of the thyroid, pituitary adenomas, and islet cell tumors) are found. This indicates that mos, in order to affect transformation, may require a substrate specific to neuroectodermal tissue.

MEN 2 has been assigned to chromosome 10 by linkage studies whereas mos is located on human chromosome 8. Mulligan and colleagues have shown the presence of missense mutations in the RET protooncogene in 20 of 23 patients with MEN 2A. The genetic mutations or genes responsible for MEN 2B and MEN 1 remain unknown. However, the marked similarity between the pathologies of MEN 2 and the mos transgenic mice suggests that the Mos-LTR transgene may function in the same pathway that gives rise to MEN 2.

Thus far, this article has discussed the effect of overexpression of mos and the effects it has on tumor formation in tissues and in transgenic animals. Equally important is studying the effects that the absence of

TABLE III

Tumor Incidence in Offspring of c-mos Transgenic Mice Crossed to BALB/c Mice

Cross	Pheos only (%)	MTC only (%)	Both (%)	Total (%)
1 × BALB/c	51	2	12	65
2 × BALB/c	0	52	16	68
3 × BALB/c	7	33	20	60

the gene has on an organism. The advent of technologies such as stem cell culture and homologous recombination has made it feasible to examine the function of a gene by targeting the host gene and inactivating it. This is first accomplished in stem cell culture and, once an allele has been inactivated, the cells are injected into embryos to produce chimeric animals. If the cells that end up giving rise to gonadal tissues are derived from the injected pluripotent cells, germline transmission of gene "knockout" is achieved. Crossing two animals heterozygous for the knockout allows one to obtain animals with both alleles inactivated. It is this experiment that two groups, Colledge and colleagues and Hashimoto and colleagues, have accomplished.

In these *mos* knockout mice, the fertility of the female mice is markedly reduced. This is consistent with the ability of p39^{mos} to stabilize oocytes at meiosis II. Lacking this stabilization, the oocytes undergo spontaneous parthenogenetic activation, yielding teratomas. In contrast, male mice lacking *c-mos* are as fertile as their control littermates. Hence, although one detects the expression of *c-mos* in maturing normal spermatozoa, its function is either not required or is redundant. Neither males nor females show growth malformations, indicating that *c-mos* is not necessary for normal fetal development. The only obvious pathology that any adult mice displays is the presence of ovarian cysts and teratomas, as mentioned, presumably the result of parthenogenetic activation of mature oocytes.

VI. CONCLUSIONS

The discovery of oncogenes has revolutionized the way we think about cancer. These genes represent a class of normal, physiological functions whose inappropriate expression produces malignant transformation. The *c-mos* gene is the first protooncogene to have been molecularly cloned and to have its transforming activity demonstrated. It is also one of the first oncogenes whose function as a protooncogene has been elucidated. By understanding the function of *mos*, we have shown how it can affect cell cycle control. Comparing malignant transformation with normal function allows us to realize that properties

recognized as hallmarks of malignancy are actually a subset of normal cellular physiology. The explosion of the number of known oncogenes points to how much remains to be learned about the function of these protooncogenes and, by extension, how they effect transformation.

Although much has been learned about *mos*, much remains to be explained. As the experiments in mice show, although *mos* is expressed during embryogenesis and gametogenesis, its presence does not seem to be necessary for normal development and spermatogenesis. Knowing how parsimonious nature is with genetic information, one must be skeptical at dismissing a gene's need in the face of its tightly regulated expression. Although it seems that the study of the *RET* oncogene will have great relevance in approaching MEN 2, it is not easy to dismiss the phenomenon of tissue-specific, *c-mos*-mediated transformation in transgenic mice. As previously mentioned, the *mos* oncogene serves as a useful paradigm in the study of other oncogenes. It does so in showing us how much insight can be gained from their study and how much remains to be discovered.

See Also the Following Articles

CELL CYCLE CONTROL • C-MYC PROTOONCOGENE • FOS ONCOGENE • MYB • TRANSGENIC MICE IN CANCER RESEARCH

Bibliography

Colledge, W. H., Carlton, M. B. L., Udy, G. B., and Evans, M. J. (1994). Disruption of c-mos causes parthenogenetic development of unfertilized mouse eggs. *Nature* **370,** 65–68.

Daar, I., Nebreda, A. R., Yew, N., Sass, P., Paules, R., Santos, Wigler, M., and Vande Woude, G. F. (1991). The ras oncoprotein and M-phase activity. *Science* **253,** 74–76.

Hashimoto, N., Watanabe, N., Furuta, Y., Tamemoto, H., Sagata, N., Yokoyama, M., Okazaki, K., Nagayoshi, M., Takeda, N., Ikawa, Y., and Aizawa, S. (1994). Parthenogenetic activation of oocytes in c-mos deficient mice. *Nature* **370,** 68–71.

Masui, Y., and Markert, C. L. (1971). Cytoplasmic control of nuclear behaviour during meiotic maturation of frog oocytes. *J. Exp. Zool.* **177,** 129–146.

Mulligan, L. M., *et al.* (1993). Germ-line mutations of the RET proto-oncogene in multiple endocrine neoplasia type 2A. *Nature* **363,** 458–460.

Nurse, P. (1990). Universal control mechanism regulating onset of M-phase. *Nature* **344,** 503.

Okazaki, K., and Sagata, N. (1995). MAP kinase activation is essential for oncogenic transformation of NIH3T3 cells by Mos. *Oncogene* **10,** 1149–1157.

Oskarrson, M., McClements, W. L., Blair, D. G., Maizel, J. V., and Vande Woude, G. F. (1980). Properties of a normal mouse cell DNA sequence (sarc) homologous to the src sequence of Moloney sarcoma virus. *Science* **207,** 1222–1224.

Propst, F., and Vande Woude, G. F. (1985). C-Mos protooncogene transcripts are expressed in mouse tissues. *Nature* **315,** 516–518.

Sagata, N., Watanabe, N., Vande Woude, G. F., and Ikawa, Y. (1989). The c-Mos protooncogene product is a cytostatic factor (CSF) responsible for meiotic arrest in vertebrate eggs. *Nature* **342,** 512–518.

Schulz, N. T., *et al.* (1992). Pheochromocytomas and C-cell thyroid neoplasms in transgenic c-mos mice: A model for the human multiple endocrine neoplasia type 2 syndrome. *Cancer Res.* **52,** 450–455.

Wasserman, W. J., and Masui, Y. A. (1976). Cytoplasmic factor promoting oocyte maturation: Its extraction and preliminary characterization. *Science* **191,** 1266–1268.

Watanabe, N., Vande Woude, G. F., Ikawa, Y., and Sagata, N. (1989). Specific proteolysis of the c-mos protooncogene product by calpain upon fertilization of *Xenopus* eggs. *Nature* **342,** 505–511.

Zhou, R., Oskarrson, M., Paules, R. S., Schulz, N., and Vande Woude, G. F. (1991). The c-mos proto-oncogene product polymerizes with and phorphorylates tubulin. *Science* **251,** 671–675.

c-myc Protooncogene

Lawrence B. Gardner
Linda A. Lee
Chi V. Dang

The Johns Hopkins University School of Medicine

GLOSSARY

apoptosis An orderly, molecular process involving specific proteases that results in the commitment and execution of cell death.

contact inhibition Cell growth arrest exhibited by cells that contact other cells.

gene amplification A process that results in an abnormal increase in gene copy number through repeated replication of DNA in a specific region of the genome.

transactivation The process of increasing transcription of a gene through the action of a transcription factor.

Warburg effect Displayed by tumor cells that convert glucose primarily to lactic acid through glycoloysis rather than to water and carbon dioxide through the tricarboxylic acid cycle.

C-MYC is the prototype for oncogene activation by gene amplification and chromosomal translocation. In contrast to the tightly regulated expression of c-myc in normal cells, c-myc expression is frequently deregulated in human cancers. The c-myc gene produces an oncogenic transcription factor that affects many cellular processes including cell growth, cell proliferation, apoptosis, and cellular metabolism. Hence, c-myc acts as an integrator and accelerator of cellular metabolism and proliferation.

I. INTRODUCTION

In 1911, Peyton Rous observed that chicken sarcoma could be transmitted by means of cell-free extracts, suggesting that a virus could be the etiologic agent behind avian tumor formation. Based on the work of Bishop and Varmus, studies of a specific subgroup of avian retrovirus which induces myeloid leukemia, sarcomas, liver, kidney, and other tumors in chickens, led to the identification of the v-myc oncogene. The discovery of a homologous sequence in normal human cellular DNA, termed c-myc, supported the view that oncogenic avian retroviruses could molecularly capture and activate cellular growth regulatory genes. The finding that human cancers frequently display altered expression of c-myc initiated the search for other oncogenes and ushered in the modern age of cancer genetics.

Significant progress has been made over the last two decades in our understanding of the function of c-myc in both normal and abnormal cells. It is clear that the deregulated expression of c-myc plays a significant role in human tumorigenesis. Immunocytochemical staining for the c-Myc protein and analyses of the c-myc gene and its expression indicate that this oncogene is overexpressed in a wide variety of human cancers. Eighty percent of breast cancers, 70% of colon cancer, 90% of gynecological cancers, 50% of hepatocellular carcinomas, and a variety of hematological tumors possess abnormal myc expression. It is estimated that approximately 70,000 U.S. cancer deaths per year are associated with changes in the c-myc gene or its expression. The importance of myc in cancer is underscored not only by the prevalence of genetic alterations of myc in human cancers, but also by its clinical significance. For example, N-myc amplification is a prognostic indicator for neuroblastoma, and the sine qua non of Burkitt's lymphoma is deregulated expression of c-myc that results from chromosomal translocations.

Over the past decade, the protein c-Myc has emerged as a transcription factor, able to regulate gene expression. This article reviews the structure of c-Myc, the other cellular homologues N-Myc and L-Myc, the mechanism of Myc transactivation, and some of the genes c-Myc upregulates or represses. The function of Myc in normal cellular function, particularly in proliferation and differentiation, will be examined. Specific mechanisms for Myc overexpression in cancer and the effect of this overexpression on the cell cycle, apoptosis, differentiation, and genomic instability will be discussed.

II. MYC STRUCTURE AND FUNCTION

The human c-myc gene is located on chromosome 8q24. It consists of three exons, and transcription may be initiated at one of three promoters. The translational AUG start site is located in the second exon. The gene encodes for a major 439 amino acid, 64 kDa c-Myc protein. Alternative translational initiation start sites result in both longer and shorter forms of the protein, termed p67 Myc and MycS, respectively. The c-Myc protein is glycosylated and phosphorylated, and these modifications may have an effect on function. Analysis of the c-Myc sequence reveals several conserved N-terminal domains, which are termed Myc boxes that are found in the closely related proteins N-Myc and L-Myc. The C-terminal end is likewise conserved in the Myc family. The conservation of these sequences suggests that they are important functional domains (Fig. 1).

The C-terminal region of c-Myc contains a helix–loop–helix leucine zipper (HLH LZ), which is a dimerization motif found in several transcription factors. The HLH LZ domain mediates homotypic or heterotypic dimerization with selected other HLH LZ proteins. The c-Myc dimerization domain is necessary for cellular transformation, and in 1991 the bHLH LZ protein Max was identified as a c-Myc-binding protein. The Max RNA and protein have long half-lives (3 and >24 h, respectively) as compared to those of c-Myc (30 and 20 min, respectively) and in most systems studied, Myc appears to be the limiting, regulated component of the heterodimer. Immediately adjacent to the HLH dimerization domain is a region rich in basic amino acids that directly contacts specific DNA sequences, termed E boxes (5'-CACGTG-3' or variations thereof). In addition to Myc, Max can bind to other bHLH LZ Mad family proteins. While Mad–Max heterodimers bind the E box to antagonize c-Myc transactivation, it is likely that the sets of target genes of Mad–Max and Myc–Max complexes are not identical. Mad levels, as opposed to Myc, increase during differentiation, and decreased expression of Mad2/Mxi-1 protein has been implicated in carcinogenesis (Fig. 2).

Studies to date suggest that DNA-bound Myc–Max complexes activate transcription through the amino-terminal 143 amino acids of c-Myc. A small segment of this region is also required for Myc-mediated transcriptional repression, although the mechanism for this is not well understood. This 143 amino acid N-terminal transregulatory domain of c-Myc is required for transformation, and it is intriguing to note

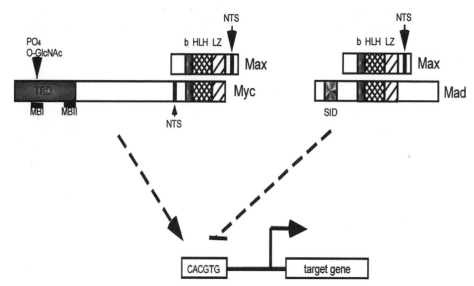

FIGURE 1 Heterodimerization of Max with either c-Myc or Mad proteins. Heterodimeric transcription factors regulate transcription of a hypothetical target gene through the E-box element, 5'-CACGTG-3'. c-Myc–Max activates transcription possibly through histone acetylation and direct interaction with the transcriptional machinery. Mad–Max complexes recruit Sin3, other corepressors, and histone deacetylases to repress transcription. The c-Myc, Mad, and Max functional domains are shown with all three proteins containing the basic helix–loop–helix leucine zipper (bHLH LZ). NTS, nuclear-targeting signal; TRD, transregulatory domain; SID, Sin3 interacting domain. MBI and MBII are Myc boxes or conserved sequences among MYC family of proteins. Phosphorylation and glycosylation sites in Myc box I are represented by PO4 and O-GlcNAc, respectively. Other phosphorylation sites of c-Myc are not shown.

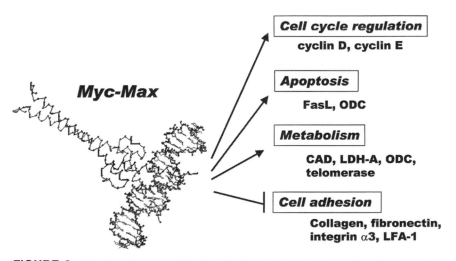

FIGURE 2 The Myc–Max basic helix–loop–helix leucine zipper heterodimer binds a target DNA site, termed E box. c-Myc regulates downstream target genes, resulting in activation cell cycle regulation, apoptosis, or inhibition of cell adhesion. Examples of c-Myc target genes associated with different cellular functions are listed.

that transformation appears to be highly dependent on Myc-mediated transrepression.

Recent progress has yielded insights into how c-Myc transactivates genes. c-Myc heterodimerizes with Max and binds the canonical 5'-CACGTG-3' E-box sequence, as well as noncanonical sites, which are variations of the consensus CANNTG sequence. The DNA-bound Myc–Max heterodimer interacts through the Myc N-terminal region with a variety of proteins involved in transcription. These include the TATA-binding protein (TBP) and another protein, TRRAP, which associates with histone acetylase. Acetylation of histones may then open up chromatin to allow access of transcription factors that belong to the general transcriptional machinery, such as TBP, to DNA. Other putative Myc-binding proteins have been implicated in regulating Myc-transactivating properties, including p107 and Miz-1. In contrast to Myc–Max complexes, Mad–Max complexes recruit histone deacetylases, which induce compact chromatin structures that limit the access of transcription factors to DNA.

III. MYC FUNCTION IN NORMAL DEVELOPMENT

Expression of c-*myc* in the normal cell is exquisitely regulated by external cues, such as growth factors and extracellular matrix contacts, as well as by internal clocks, such as the cell cycle. The resting cell normally expresses little to no c-*myc*, whereas cells stimulated by growth factors to proliferate robustly increase c-*myc* expression as an immediate early gene. The c-*myc* gene then returns to its basal quiescent state in resultant resting daughter cells. Ectopic overexpression of c-*myc* in primary cells, however, appears to activate a protective pathway through the induction of p19/p14ARF that results in a p53-dependent cell death pathway. Through this means, normal cells that overexpress c-*myc* and deviate toward neoplasia are eliminated from the host organism through apoptosis.

Regulated expression of c-*myc*, as well as other family members during embryogenesis, is required for normal development. Mice in which both alleles of c-*myc* have been deleted die in early embryonic de-

velopment, most likely as a result of the lack of primitive hematopoiesis. Through gene replacement studies, N-*myc* is able to substitute for c-*myc* during embryogenesis. The lack of a distinct phenotype in L-*myc* null animals suggests that L-*myc* is not required for embryogenesis, although it may be necessary for the proper function of specific cellular types in the adult mouse. Embryonic fibroblasts from animals lacking c-*myc* show a marked decrease in proliferation rate and viability. The fruitfly *Drosophila* with mutated *myc* alleles are viable, but are much smaller than wild-type flies, indicating that *myc* participates in the control of normal cell and organismal size.

IV. MECHANISMS OF MYC OVEREXPRESSION IN CANCER

Overexpression of Myc occurs by several mechanisms in human cancers. The normal c-*myc* gene may be activated by a chromosomal translocation, as in the case of Burkitt's lymphoma, where translocations place the c-*myc* locus adjacent to immunoglobulin genes that are highly transcriptionally active in B cells. Another common mechanism of *myc* overexpression is gene amplification. This is found most dramatically in other members of the *myc* family, where over 200 copies per cell of N-*myc* can be found in neuroblastoma, and over 50 copies per cell of c-*myc*, N-*myc*, or L-*myc* may be found in small-cell lung cancers. Alterations of c-*myc* gene transcription may account for the observed elevation of Myc in human colon carcinoma. In this case, it is currently hypothesized that catenins, which are inactivated when bound to the adenomatous polyposis coli (APC) protein, might activate *myc* expression in the absence of APC through the LEF/TCF4 transcription factor. Mutant, transcriptionally active β-catenin proteins may contribute to deregulated Myc expression in colon, liver, and other cancers.

Other mechanisms of c-*myc* overexpression have also been uncovered in the experimental setting. For example, removal of 3' UTR-destabilizing sequences causes an elevation of *myc* mRNA. Insertion of retroviruses adjacent to the *myc* locus activates its expression. Oncogenic *ras* appears to stabilize the Myc protein through an unknown mechanism. All of these modes of elevating *c-myc* expression have not, however, been established in human cancers.

V. MYC FUNCTION IN CANCER

In the 1970s, Weinberg and co-workers showed that rat embryo cells could be transformed when *c-myc* and *ras* were cotransfected. Since then a variety of models have clearly indicated that *c-myc* is oncogenic. When immortalized fibroblasts are engineered to overexpress *c-myc*, they acquire the ability to grow in soft agar, signifying loss of contact inhibition commonly found in tumor cells. Transgenic animals overexpressing *c-myc* form tumors in a variety of tissues. More recently it has been shown that the conditional induction of *c-myc* *in vivo* in keratinocytes or hematopoeitic cells can lead to proliferation and clonal expansion, a hallmark of neoplasia.

Although a link between *c-myc* and cancer is quite established both *in vivo* and *in vitro*, the mechanism of *c-myc*-mediated transformation is not fully known. Recent work has established a role for *c-myc* in cell cycle progression, metabolism, apoptosis, and genomic instability. One model proposes that *c-myc* promotes cell proliferation and genomic instability by accelerating cells through G1 and S phases of the cell cycle, abrogating cell cycle checkpoints, and increasing cell metabolism. In many settings, these alterations lead to apoptosis, or cell death. However, in the background of additional mutations that activate antiapoptotic signals, *c-myc* can lead to full-blown neoplasm.

To better understand c-Myc function and its role in neoplasia, recent efforts have concentrated on identifying genes that are induced or repressed by c-Myc. Direct targets of c-Myc are defined as those target genes whose expression is directly altered due to c-Myc binding at their promoter or intronic sequences. Indirect targets are those activated two or more steps downstream of Myc (i.e., induced by transcription factors, which have been induced by a c-Myc-mediated event).

c-Myc target genes have been identified using several techniques, generally comparing cell lines that overexpress *c-myc* with ones that do not. With the availability of cells that are null for *c-myc*, it is now possible to begin to study the role of c-Myc in normal cell homeostasis. Hence, it is important to distinguish between c-Myc targets induced in normal cell homeostasis versus those induced in pathophysiological conditions in which c-Myc is overexpressed. Myc target genes have been identified in a variety of ways, including DNA microarray analysis. While none of the Myc responsive genes by itself recapitulates the complete Myc phenotype, many have been implicated in *myc* functions, such as apoptosis, cell cycle control, and cell adhesion.

A. Cell Cycle Effects and Genomic Instability

Despite the facts that *c-myc* is an early response gene, that *c-myc* knockout fibroblasts proliferate more slowly than wild-type cells, and that *c-myc* overexpressing cells proliferate faster than wild-type cells, literature concerning the effects of *c-myc* overexpression on the cell cycle is inconsistent. Most work has focused on the effect of c-Myc on regulatory proteins of the G1–S phase transition of the cell cycle. This transition is promoted when cyclin-dependent kinases (CDKs) complex with and activate cyclins. Cyclin-dependent kinase inhibitors (CDKIs) inhibit this activation. c-Myc has been implicated in inducing cyclin D1 and D2, cyclin E, CDK4, and cdc25a, a phosphatase, which activates CDK2 and CDK4. c-Myc has also been shown to lower the amounts or inhibit the function of the CDK inhibitor, p27, potentially by increasing cyclin D levels, which can then sequester p27.

A highly regulated cell cycle permits cells to repair DNA damage before replicating, thus promoting genomic fidelity. Inappropriate cell cycle proliferation can lead to genomic instability, resulting in new mutations and abnormal chromosome number and structure. c-Myc overexpression, even transiently, can induce genomic instability that is characterized by gene amplification, aneuploidy, and polyploidy.

B. Apoptosis and Immortality

Interestingly, Burkitt's lymphoma has long been noted to have not only a high mitotic index, but also a high apoptotic rate. c-Myc-induced apoptosis was initially recognized in studies of the 32d.3 myeloid progenitor cell line. In the absence of IL-3, enforced c-myc expression drives cells into S phase and accelerates the rate of cell death. Fibroblasts that overexpress c-myc undergo apoptosis in response to several environmental stresses, including low serum, hypoxia, and low glucose. The regions of Myc that are required for apoptosis are also those that are required for transcription. Although several myc target genes, such as ornithine decarboxylase (ODC) and lactate dehydrogenase A (LDH-A), appear to be involved in myc-induced apoptosis, the mechanism of myc action in apoptosis is not clear. In the case of primary cells, p19/p14ARF is likely to be a relevant downstream effector of Myc-induced apoptosis.

Myc has been noted to activate telomerase, an enzyme that sustains telomere length and leads to immortalization of cells (i.e., an ability to be passaged indefinitely). The relevant clinical correlation is the intriguing observation that both N-myc amplification and telomerase levels are parallel predictors of poor outcome in neuroblastoma. This observation might be construed to suggest that N-myc is responsible for the elevation of telomerase in neuroblastoma; however, hard evidence for this and for the connection between Myc and telomerase in human cancers remains sparse.

C. Metabolism

It stands to reason that increased proliferation requires increased energy and availability of biosynthetic substrates and would therefore necessitate increase metabolic rates. It is well established that the major component of a eukaryotic cell is its ribosomal mass, which constitutes up to 40% of total mass and accounts for 90% of cellular RNA mass. It is also notable that as a cell traverses through the G1 phase of the cell cycle, its mass gradually increases prior to the initiation of DNA synthesis in S phase. The regulation of cell mass is linked to the cell cycle, although the molecular basis for this regulation is largely unknown. Intriguingly, mutation of the Drosophila myc gene results in small flies that resemble flies that bear mutant ribosomal protein genes. These small flies are small not because they have fewer cells, but rather their cells are smaller in size. These observations suggest that myc participates in the regulation of cell

mass, and this notion has gained support from observations in specific mammalian cells that overexpress c-Myc. Studies have suggested that c-Myc overexpression results in an elevated expression of genes encoding translational factors and ribosomal proteins, which in turn may contribute to increased cellular mass.

Both large and small tumors are often hypoxic as a result of diminished, disordered neovascularization. Survival and rapid proliferation of a tumor in a hostile environment are often accompanied by a switch of cancer cells to use glucose as an energy source without oxygen and lead to an overproduction of lactic acid. The transcription factor, HIF-1, is induced by hypoxia and transactivates many glycolytic enzymes necessary for this switch. Interestingly, HIF-1 binds to a DNA motif in the promoter of these genes that is very similar to the Myc E box. Myc is able to transactivate many of these same glycolytic genes and the glucose transporter GLUT-1. Hence, the widespread deregulation of c-myc in human cancers may contribute to enhanced tumor glycolysis, known as the Warburg effect.

As cells prepare for S phase, adequate substrates must accumulate to ensure the fidelity of DNA replication. Genes that are important in nucleotide biosynthesis and DNA metabolism are also implicated as Myc targets, such as carbamoyl phosphate synthase (CAD), ODC, dihydrofolate reductase, and thymidine kinase. Although little is known about the possible role of c-Myc in regulating cellular metabolism during the second cell cycle gap, G2, and during mitosis, a complex role for c-Myc in regulating cellular metabolism has clearly emerged from recent studies.

VI. SUMMARY

The study of c-Myc has its roots in simple observations made by Peyton Rous some 90 years ago, and the understanding of its role as an oncogenic switch has evolved through various paradigm shifts over the past two decades. It is currently regarded as a central transcriptional oncogenic switch that regulates a large variety of cellular functions through altering gene expression. The repertoire of cellular functions affected by c-Myc, including cell cycle, metabolism, and apoptosis, may be further fine-tuned in the context of specific cell types and other transcriptional regulators that also converge on Myc target genes. Although rudimentary, our understanding of the role c-Myc has already yielded promising insights that might be of therapeutic importance.

See Also the Following Articles

CELL CYCLE CONTROL • c-MOS PROTOONCOGENE • FOS ONCOGENE • MYB • TELOMERES AND TELOMERASE • TP53 TUMOR SUPPRESSOR GENE

Bibliography

Amati, B., Alevizopoulos, K., and Vlach, J. (1998). Myc and the cell cycle. *Front Biosci.* **3**, D250.

Cole, M. D., and McMahon, S. B. (1999). The Myc oncoprotein: A critical evaluation of transactivation and target gene regulation. *Oncogene* **18**, 2916.

Dang, C. V. (1999). c-Myc target genes involved in cell growth, apoptosis, and metabolism. *Mol. Cell Biol.* **19**, 1.

Elend, M., and Eilers, M. (1999). Cell growth: Downstream of Myc - to grow or to cycle? *Curr Biol.* **9**, R936.

Facchini, L. M., and Penn, L. Z. (1998). The molecular role of Myc in growth and transformation: Recent discoveries lead to new insights. *FASEB J.* **12**, 633.

Grandori, C., and Eisenman, R. N. (1997). Myc target genes. *Trends Biochem Sci.* **22**, 177.

Klein, G. (2000). Dysregulation of lymphocyte proliferation by chromosomal translocations and sequential genetic changes. *Bioessays* **22**, 414.

Luscher, B., and Larsson, L. G. (1999). The basic region/helix-loop-helix/leucine zipper domain of Myc proto-oncoproteins: Function and regulation. *Oncogene* **18**, 2955.

Nesbit, C. E., Tersak, J. M., and Prochownik, E. V. (1999). MYC oncogenes and human neoplastic disease. *Oncogene* **18**, 3004.

Obaya, A. J., Mateyak, M. K., and Sedivy, J. M. (1999). Mysterious liaisons: The relationship between c-Myc and the cell cycle. *Oncogene* **18**, 2934.

Pelengaris, S., Rudolph, B., and Littlewood, T. (2000). Action of Myc in vivo: Proliferation and apoptosis. *Curr. Opin. Genet. Dev.* **10**, 100.

Prendergast, G. C. (1999). Mechanisms of apoptosis by c-Myc. *Oncogene* **18**, 2967.

Schmidt, E. V. (1999). The role of c-myc in cellular growth control. *Oncogene* **18**, 2988.

Schreiber-Agus, N., and DePinho, R. A. (1998). Repression by the Mad(Mxi1)-Sin3 complex. *Bioessays* **20**, 808.

Thompson, E. B. (1998). The many roles of c-Myc in apoptosis. *Annu. Rev. Physiol.* **60**, 575.

ISBN 0-12-227556-X